A Special Issue of
*Cognitive Neuropsychology*

# The organisation of conceptual knowledge in the brain: Neuropsychological and neuroimaging perspectives

Edited by

Alex Martin
*National Institute of Mental Health, Bethesda, MD, USA*

and

Alfonso Caramazza
*Harvard University, Cambridge, MA, USA*

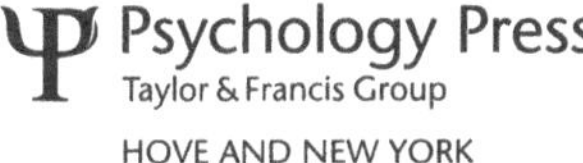


HOVE AND NEW YORK

Published in 2003 by Psychology Press Ltd
27 Church Road, Hove, East Sussex, BN3 2FA

Simultaneously published in the USA and Canada
by Taylor & Francis Inc.
711 Third Avenue, New York, NY 10017

First issued in paperback 2015

*Psychology Press is an imprint of the Taylor & Francis Group, an informa business*



*British Library Cataloguing in Publication Data*
A catalogue record for this book is available from the British Library

ISSN 0264-3294

This book is also a special issue of the journal *Cognitive Neuropsychology* and forms Issues 3, 4, 5, and 6 of Volume 20 (2003).

Cover design by Joyce Chester
Typeset in the UK by Quorum Technical Services, Cheltenham, Glos

ISBN 13: 978-1-138-87794-8 (pbk)
ISBN 13: 978-1-8416-9947-9 (hbk)

# COGNITIVE NEUROPSYCHOLOGY

Volume 20 Issue 3/4/5/6 May–September 2003

**Contents**

# COGNITIVE NEUROPSYCHOLOGY

This journal promotes the study of cognitive processes from a neuropsychological perspective. Cognition is understood very broadly, as including for example perception, attention, object recognition, planning, language, thinking, memory, and action. It covers neuropsychological work bearing on our understanding of normal cognitive processes as well as neuropsychological disorders of cognition arising at any stage of life span. All manuscript submissions should be addressed to Sophie Forster, Journals Editorial Assistant, Psychology Press Ltd, 27 Church Road, Hove, East Sussex BN3 2FA, UK. Notes for contributors are available from the publisher on request.

**Subscription information**

*Cognitive Neuropsychology* is published by Psychology Press Ltd, a member of the Taylor & Francis Group.

*New subscriptions and changes of address should be sent to:* Psychology Press, c/o Taylor & Francis Ltd, Rankine Road, Basingstoke, Hampshire, RG24 8PR, UK. Send change of address notices at least six weeks in advance, and include both old and new addresses.

Subscription rates to Volume 20, 2003 (8 issues) are as follows (prices inclusive of postage and packing):

To individuals: £176.00 (UK); $290.00 (Rest of world)

To institutions: £544.00 (UK); $897.00 (Rest of world)

*Cognitive Neuropsychology* (USPS permit number 016265) is published eight times per year in February, March, May, June, July, September, October, and December. The 2003 US Institutional subscription price is $897.00. Periodicals postage paid at Champlain, NY, by US Mail Agent IMS of New York, 100 Walnut Street, Champlain, NY. US Postmaster: Please send address changes to pCGN, PO Box 1518, Champlain, NY 12919, USA.



Information about Psychology Press journals and other publications is available from http://www.psypress.co.uk

Go to http://www.tandf.co.uk/journals/pp/02643294.html for current information about this journal, including how to access the online version or to register for the free table of contents alerting service.

*Cognitive Neuropsychology* is covered by the following abstracting, indexing, and citation services: Current Contents (ISI); ASSIA; APA PsycINFO; Sociological Abstracts; Biosciences Information Service; MLA International Bibliography; EMBASE; LLBA; Neuroscience Citation Index (ISI); Research Alerts (ISI); Social SciSearch (ISI); Social Science Citation Index (ISI); Social Services Abstracts; SciSearch (ISI); CDAB; UnCover; Linguistics Abstracts.

Printed in the United Kingdom by Henry Ling Limited, at the Dorset Press, Dorchester, DT1 1HD.

This publication has been produced with paper manufactured to strict environmental standards and with pulp derived from sustainable forests.

COGNITIVE NEUROPSYCHOLOGY, 2003, 20 (3/4/5/6), 195–212

# NEUROPSYCHOLOGICAL AND NEUROIMAGING PERSPECTIVES ON CONCEPTUAL KNOWLEDGE: AN INTRODUCTION

Alex Martin
*National Institute of Mental Health, Bethesda, USA*

Alfonso Caramazza
*Harvard University, Cambridge, USA*

The modern era of study of the representation of object concepts in the human brain began in 1983 with a report by Warrington and McCarthy of a patient with preserved knowledge for animals, foods, and flowers, relative to inanimate objects (Warrington & McCarthy, 1983). This was followed the next year by a report of four patients with the opposite pattern of preserved and impaired category knowledge (Warrington & Shallice, 1984). Specifically, these patients presented with a relatively selective impairment for knowing about living things and foods. Since publication of these seminal case studies, over 100 patients have been reported with a category-specific deficit for biological categories (living things, especially four-legged animals), relative to inanimate objects (especially tools and other artifacts), and more than 25 cases with the opposite pattern of deficit (Figure 1). Heightened appreciation of the importance of these clinical cases for understanding the organisation of conceptual knowledge, as well as for object recognition, the organisation of the lexicon, and the storage of long-term memories, has also motivated an increasing number of functional brain-imaging studies of object category representation in the normal human brain. The goal of this special issue of *Cognitive Neuropsychology* is to provide a forum for new findings and critical, theoretical analyses of existing data from patient and functional brain-imaging studies.

## THE THEORIES OF CONCEPT ORGANISATION

A number of different theoretical positions have been advanced to explain category-specific deficits. However, as described by Capitani, Laiacona, Mahon, and Caramazza (2003-this issue), much of the current debate centres on whether concepts are organised by property or by category.[1] Most investigators assume that the deficits are a direct consequence of the organisation of object properties in the brain. The best known property-based model of semantic category-specific deficits is the sensory/functional theory (S/FT), proposed by Warrington, Shallice, and McCarthy (Warrington & McCarthy, 1987; Warrington & Shallice, 1984).

[1] Note, however, that the two types of organisation need not be mutually exclusive. It is possible that concepts are organised into domains and within domains the organisation may very well be by property type or correlation (Caramazza, 1998; see also Mahon & Caramazza, 2003-this issue).

Requests for reprints should be addressed to Alex Martin, PhD, Laboratory of Brain and Cognition, National Institute of Mental Health, Building 10, Room 4C-104, 10 Center Drive MSC 1366, Bethesda, Maryland 20892-1366, USA (Email: alex@codon.nih.gov).



http://www.tandf.co.uk/journals/pp/02643294.html
DOI:10.1080/02643290342000050

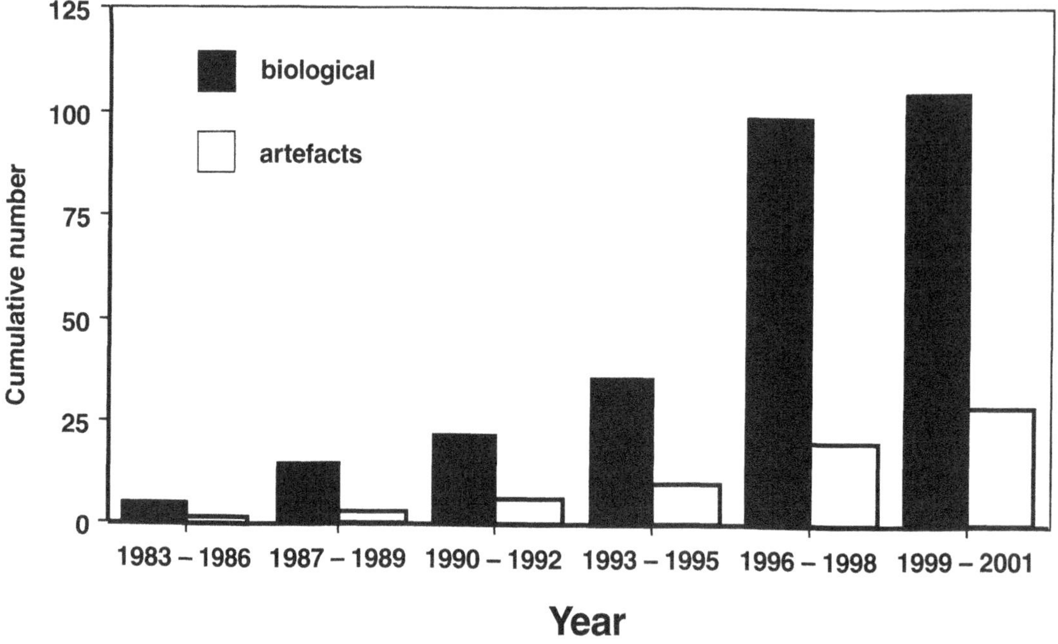


Figure 1. *Cumulative number of patients with category-specific disorders for biological objects and artefacts reported in the literature since 1983. Based on the review provided by Capitani et al. (2003-this issue).*

Although there are important differences among them, similar accounts have been proposed by a number of other investigators (e.g., Damasio, 1989; Humphreys & Forde, 2001; Martin, Ungerleider, & Haxby, 2000). The central idea behind S/FT-like theories is that conceptual knowledge about objects is organised by sensory features (e.g., form, motion, colour, smell, taste) and functional properties (the motor habits related to their use, typical location where they may be found, their social value, etc.).[2] Categories differ as to the importance or weight assigned to each of these properties. In this view, category-specific (C-S) semantic disorders occur when a lesion disrupts knowledge about a particular property or set of properties critical for defining that object category and for distinguishing among its members. Thus damage to regions where information about object form is stored will produce a C-S disorder for animals. This is because visual appearance is assumed to be a critical property for defining animals, and because the distinction between different animals is assumed to be heavily dependent on knowing about subtle differences in their visual form (e.g., distinguishing among four-legged animals). A critical component of these models is that the lesion should affect

[2] Theories differ as to what is meant by "functional" properties. In the early literature, "functional" was used together with "associative" (functional-associative) to distinguish sensory from nonsensory properties of objects (e.g., Farah & McClelland, 1991). When used in the context of S/FT it has generally been interpreted in this sense. However, in some theories the term "functional" is restricted to the sense "use" and in others to the sense "motor habit." Sensory/motor theories of the representation of objects have tended to favour the latter sense (Martin et al., 2000). However, if we were to restrict "functional" to mean "motor habit" we would only be able to use the term "function" for a very small set of objects—primarily tools. This can be easily appreciated when we consider the functions of various artefacts. Thus, although some functions are associated with fairly specific motor patterns (e.g., scissors: used for cutting with a highly specific motor pattern), others are not associated with any specific motor pattern (e.g., car: used for transportation; house: used for shelter; shoes: used to protect feet; wedding ring: used to indicate a particular social status; etc.). These examples illustrate that "function" cannot be reduced to a specific sensorimotor system.

knowledge of all object categories with these characteristics, not only animals. In a similar fashion, damage to regions where information about how an object is used should produce a C-S disorder for tools, and all other categories of objects defined by the way in which they are manipulated.

Correlated structure accounts represent a related approach. These theories propose that the organisation of conceptual knowledge is dictated by the way in which properties of objects are statistically related to one another in the world, rather than by organisation of brain systems (for prominent examples of this approach, see Caramazza, Hillis, Rapp, & Romani, 1990; Devlin, Gonnerman, Andersen, & Seidenberg, 1998; Garrard, Lambon Ralph, Hodges, & Patterson, 2001; Tyler & Moss, 1997). S/FT-like models focus on constraints dictated by brain organisation, while correlated structure approaches focus on constraints determined by properties of the objects themselves. Nevertheless, both theories are property, rather than category, based.

The alternative to these property-based theories is the domain-specific theory (Caramazza & Shelton, 1998). On this account, our evolutionary history provides the major constraint on the organisation of conceptual knowledge in the brain. Specifically, the theory proposes that selection pressures have resulted in dedicated neural machinery for solving, quickly and efficiently, computationally complex survival problems. One implication of this theory is that the types of C-S disorders should be severely constrained. Likely candidate domains offered are animals, conspecifics, and plant life (and possibly tools). This account remains silent on the organisation of conceptual knowledge within domains; it could be organised either along the lines of correlated structure or sensory-motor theories, or of some other principle (see Mahon & Caramazza, 2003-this issue).

## THE EVIDENCE FROM PATIENTS

The issue begins with an exhaustive review of the literature by Capitani and colleagues. Following a description of the theories along the lines set out above, the authors address two critical questions about C-S disorders. First, what are the categories of C-S disorders? Second, is there an association between the type of C-S deficit and type of conceptual knowledge deficit? For example, do patients with C-S deficits for animals have disproportionate difficulty retrieving sensory information? To answer these questions they offer a critical review of the "entire" published literature since Warrington and McCarthy's report in 1983. They conclude that two facts emerge from the review of the literature. One, the categories of C-S disorders are animate objects (animals), inanimate biological objects (fruits and vegetables), and artifacts. Thus, the authors argue that the categories of C-S disorders are more fine-grained than would be predicted by property-based models like S/FT, and are consistent with the predictions of the domain-specific account. Two, there is no association between type of C-S deficit and type of conceptual knowledge deficit. In fact, the authors show that knowledge of both sensory and functional information is equally impaired in the overwhelming majority of C-S cases. Thus, what the authors view as the central prediction of S/FT models, a relationship between type of C-S deficit and type of conceptual knowledge deficit, is simply untenable. These are strong claims. Yet the authors allow others to substantiate them by providing a description of the findings in each case study, including those that were deemed acceptable for their analysis, and those that were not. This description of behavioural performance, along with the information on lesion location, should prove useful for the field.

Evidence consistent and contrary to the claims of Capitani and colleagues is presented in the papers on patients with C-S disorders included in this Special Issue. Humphreys and Riddoch present a case series analysis of seven patients with C-S disorders for living things. The case-by-case analysis of individual patients on the same battery of tests provides a powerful means of testing specific hypotheses (a similar strategy is employed by Lambon Ralph, Patterson, Garrard, & Hodges, 2003-this issue; and Borgo & Shallice, 2003-this issue). One of the implications of the Capitani et al. review is that C-S disorders of a particular type, say for animate objects, are relatively homogeneous disorders. In all patients, all types of knowledge about the impaired domain should be compromised, and the impairment should not be linked obligatorily with a selective impairment for a nonbiological category of objects (e.g., musical instruments). The patients studied by Humphreys and Riddoch (2003-this issue) suggest that the disorder may be more heterogeneous than the literature suggests. Although all of their patients showed an object naming deficit for living things, further testing revealed important differences. Moreover, these differences were related to differences in lesion location. As predicted by the domain-specific account, three of the seven cases had impaired knowledge for visual and functional information limited to living things. The others, however, had disproportionate difficulty with visual versus functional information. These latter patients also had particular difficulty with musical instruments. Humphreys and Riddoch interpret these and other aspects of the behaviour of their patients as posing difficulties for both the domain-specific and the standard form of S/FT. They go on to argue that the heterogeneous set of findings they report can be accommodated by the Hierarchical Interactive Theory (HIT; Humphreys & Forde, 2001).

The paper by Lambon Ralph and colleagues (2003-this issue) also offers data that are not easily accommodated by present views. Six patients with semantic dementia were evaluated. The logic here was to compare the performance of a single patient with a C-S disorder for living things with five other patients with a similar degree of semantic deficit as the target patient, but without a C-S disorder. As predicted by S/FT-type theories, the patient with a C-S disorder for living things had a greater impairment for sensory than functional information. However, contrary to S/FT, the other patients did as well. Thus, a greater difficulty for sensory than functional information is not causally related to C-S impairment for living things. The authors discuss how their cases present problems for all of the existing theories, and suggest that individual differences in the extent and quality of premorbid category knowledge may contribute to the observed variability in performance.

One of the key predictions of S/FT-like theories is that patients with C-S disorders for living things should also show a C-S deficit for other categories that are disproportionately dependent on sensory information. Borgo and Shallice (2003-this issue) provide a theory-driven approach to this question by testing a patient with a C-S disorder for living things on a set of "sensory-quality" categories. The logic here is that if a C-S disorder for living things is due to impaired knowledge of sensory properties, then the patient should also necessarily be impaired on categories defined primarily by sensory information (i.e., colour, texture). The categories assessed were edible substances (e.g., sauces, cheeses), drinks, and materials (e.g., metals, precious stones). As in the reports of Humphreys and Riddoch, and Lambon Ralph and colleagues, a multiple case-study approach is employed. The performance of a target patient with a C-S disorder for living things, MU, was contrasted to other patients matched with MU on performance with artefacts (see Borgo & Shallice, 2001, for a previous study of this patient). MU was impaired on the sensory-quality categories, and showed a much greater impairment for sensory than for functional properties for these categories. However, knowledge of both sensory and functional information was impaired for living things, but not artefacts. Moreover, the patients' pattern of performance on a property knowledge task differed depending on whether knowledge was probed using verification or production paradigms. Like the patients described by Lambon Ralph and colleagues, a greater deficit was found for sensory than functional information for all categories. Borgo and Shallice interpret their results as being consistent with the main predictions of S/FT. It is not clear, however, how the S/FT can account for MU's equal performance on probes of sensory and functional information for the category "living things." Furthermore, the reported association of a deficit for living things and sensory-quality categories is not a necessary one since Laiacona, Capitani, and Caramazza (in press) have reported a patient (EA) very similar to MU in all respects (including aetiology) except that he shows a dissociation between poor performance for living things and spared knowledge for sensory-quality categories.

A central feature of S/FT-like models is that they predict that the deficit should generalise over categories that share a common sensory foundation, as exemplified by the patient described by Borgo and Shallice. In contrast, the domain-specific account predicts the existence of fine-grained category-specific deficits—in particular, that knowledge of fruits and vegetables can be dissociated from knowledge about animals. Although there have only been a few prior reports of such fine-grained dissociation, compelling evidence for the dissociation is presented in this issue for two new cases: one described by Crutch and Warrington (2003-this issue), the other by Samson and Pillon (2003-this issue). Both cases had a lesion of the left occipito-temporal cortex. The fact that these cases occur is problematic for the standard S/FT model, but Crutch and Warrington argue that the patient's behaviour can readily be accommodated by a multiple sensory and motor processing channel model along the lines initially proposed by Warrington and McCarthy (1987). On this view, the category fruit and vegetables can be dissociated from animals because colour and taste knowledge play a more important role for the former category than for animals. However, although knowledge of colour was not investigated in their patient, it was in the case studied by Samson and Pillon. Although this patient had impaired knowledge of many properties of fruits and vegetables, colour knowledge was intact (and see Miceli, Fouch, Capasso, Shelton, Tamaiuolo, & Caramazza, 2001, for a patient with the opposite dissociation). Clearly, the existence of these fine-grained C-S disorders is problematic for the standard form of S/FT, although perhaps less so for the multiple channel approach described by Crutch and Warrington. Nevertheless, there seems to be no principled reason why any property-based account would predict a C-S disorder for fruits and vegetables rather than any other object category. The fact that the domain-specific account does make this strong prediction needs to be addressed.

The domain-specific theory makes another strong prediction. Because domain-specific knowledge systems are innate, they should be present from birth and, if damaged, recovery of function should be minimal. Farah and Rabinowitz (2003-this issue) provide favourable evidence here for both these predictions. Their subject, Adam, sustained bilateral damage to occipitotemporal cortices at the age of 1 day. Tested at the age of 16 years, Adam showed a profound deficit for living but not for nonliving things (Adam also has a severe prosopagnosia, see Farah, Rabinowitz, Quinn, & Liu, 2000). Also consistent with the domain-specific account, retrieval of sensory and functional information were equally impaired for living, but spared for nonliving, things. Clearly, whatever was damaged at birth in this subject had profound implications for learning about certain categories of objects and not others. How best to characterise what was damaged is difficult to determine. Consistent with the domain-specific account, Farah and Rabinowitz suggest damage to a semantic category-specific component. Nevertheless, as the authors note, even in this case a property-based explanation cannot be ruled out.

All of these reports describe patients with C-S disorders for biological kinds. This bias in the frequency of C-S deficits for biological objects has been evident since the first reports by Warrington and colleagues (Figure 1). Nevertheless, a reasonably large number of patients with knowledge disorders effecting nonbiological categories have been reported. The contribution of Tranel, Kemmerer, Adolphs, Damasio, and Damasio (2003-this issue) focuses on the nonbiological category that has received the most attention; tools. The reason for this focus is self-evident. Tools are defined largely by their functional properties, which, in turn, are strongly correlated with shape. Moreover, these "functional" properties are clearly linked to sensory and motor systems involved in object manipulation and use. Thus, they are an ideal category for testing ideas about the functional neuroanatomy associated with the sensory and motor properties of objects. Tranel and colleagues tested a group of 90 subjects with unilateral lesions on two measures probing tool and action knowledge. Twenty-six subjects were identified who were impaired on one or both of the measures, and all but one patient showed intact knowledge of famous persons. Because this was the only other category assessed, the selectivity of their deficit cannot be determined. However, unlike the reports discussed above, the goal of this study was not to explore the selectivity or nature of the deficit. Rather, the goal was to identify a group of patients with poor performance on the tool knowledge tasks in order to identify the locus of lesions.

The results of an analysis of lesion overlap were quite revealing. Three regions were identified, all lateralised to the left hemisphere. One included premotor and nearby prefrontal cortex, another involved parietal cortex, and the third was in the posterior part of the middle temporal gyrus. Each of these sites has, in turn, been linked to specific sensorimotor aspects of tool use. For example, single cell recording studies in monkeys have identified regions in ventral premotor and intraparietal cortices involved in grasping and manipulating objects. Cells in these regions also fire when monkeys see objects they have previously manipulated (see Jeannerod, 2001, for review). The site in the posterior part of the middle temporal gyrus was near, if not including, cortex involved in perceiving visual motion in monkeys and humans. Moreover, as will be discussed below, functional brain-imaging studies on tool representation have identified these same regions, and have also provided evidence for the functional properties of these regions along the lines discussed above. Thus, these findings provide evidence for a property-based network of regions in the human left hemisphere critical for knowing about tools.

The contribution by Mahon and Caramazza (2003-this issue), however, poses a serious challenge to this view. First, the authors clarify that the domain-specific account does not deny the possibility that one constraint on the organisation of conceptual knowledge in the brain is modality or type of information. However, the domain-specific theory does demand that the information within a modality- or property-specific semantic subsystem must be organised by category. According to the sensory/motor account (Martin et al., 2000), knowledge is stored in the sensory and motor systems active when information was acquired (in this case, information about tools). When this system is damaged, knowledge about tools is impaired. Mahon and Caramazza reason that if the above statement were true, then it should not be possible to dissociate conceptual knowledge about an object from the ability to demonstrate and know about the use of that object. However, as they discuss, patients have been reported who indicate that these types of knowledge can be doubly dissociated. For example, patient WC (Buxbaum, Veramonti, & Schwartz, 2000), had a left parietal lesion and damage to sensorimotor representations, as evidenced by impaired knowledge of tool use, but intact knowledge of other aspects of tools (e.g., knowing that, for example, a radio and a phonograph have related functions, even though they are manipulated differently). Mahon and Caramazza argue that the existence of such cases makes the strong form of a sensory/motor property-based model untenable. Alternatively, however, one could argue from a sensory/motor perspective that patient WC's selective loss of knowledge about how objects are manipulated is because of damage to a region where this information, and only this type of information, is represented (i.e., motor sequences associated with an object's use). The best candidate regions would be left premotor and/or parietal cortices. In this way, one might be able to accommodate the dissociation of different types of conceptual knowledge about tools. However, this would entail abandoning the strong version of the theory, which holds that functional knowledge is directly represented in motor representations. Interestingly, Mahon and Caramazza also note that WC's modality-related dissociation between types of knowledge within a domain would be problematic for a domain-specific account that did not include a clear distinction between functional knowledge and the possible motor schemes for its realisation.

The patients discussed in these reports each pose challenges to the prevailing views on concept organisation in the brain. In their contribution, Simmons and Barsalou (2003-this issue) offer a new theoretical perspective. Their goal was to build on each of the three types of theories outlined above (S/FT-like, domain-specific, and correlated structure approaches), to form a theory that incorporates the most important features of each position. The proposal also incorporates much of the thinking developed by Barsalou (1999) on how conceptual knowledge can be represented by perceptual symbol systems. Their proposal also draws heavily on Damasio's theory of convergence zones (Damasio, 1989; and see Crutch & Warrington, 2003-this issue, and Tranel et al., 2003-this issue, for other discussions of the role of convergence zones in the organisation of conceptual knowledge). Central to Simmons and Barsalou's model is the "similarity-in-topography principle", which proposes a mechanism to account for both property-level and category-level representations within a hierarchically organised system of convergence zones. Much like the HIT (Humphreys & Forde, 2001), this theory assumes a large number of principles in order to account for different patterns of C-S knowledge deficits (e.g., single category, multiple categories, disproportionate loss of sensory information, equal loss of sensory and functional knowledge) and lesion locations. One danger of these types of proposals, however, is that they may be so powerful that they can account for any pattern of impairment. To their credit, Simmons and Barsalou address this concern by providing specific predictions generated by their theory for both patterns of deficit and lesion locations. They also address differences between their proposal and related accounts (e.g., HIT).

## FUNCTIONAL BRAIN-IMAGING STUDIES OF NORMAL INDIVIDUALS

To provide a context for the functional brain-imaging contributions, we first provide a brief review of findings from previous studies. For details, the interested reader can consult recent reviews by Bookheimer (2002); Josephs (2001); Martin (2001); Martin and Chao (2001); and Thompson-Schill (2002).

1. The brain regions most commonly associated with object category representation are ventral occipitotemporal, lateral temporal, posterior parietal (especially the intraparietal sulcus), and ventral premotor cortices.[3]

2. Activity within these regions is modulated by category. Objects belonging to different semantic categories produce different patterns of activity in these regions.

3. All objects tested to date show different patterns of activity in ventral occipito-temporal cortex. The most studied objects have been human faces, houses, animals, and tools. However, distinct object category-related patterns of activity have been reliably discriminated among relatively large sets of object categories (7 by Haxby, Gobbini, Furey, Ishai, Schouten, & Pietrini, 2001; 7 by Spiridon & Kanwisher, 2002; 10 by Cox & Savoy, 2002). Biological objects (faces, animals) typically show peak activity in the lateral portion of the fusiform gyrus, whereas the peak for artefacts (tools) is typically located in the medial portion of the fusiform. Ventral occipital regions (especially the inferior occipital gyrus) typically respond more strongly to biological objects (faces, animals) than to artefacts. However, activity associated with each object category is not confined to a specific location, but may cover a broad expanse of occipito-temporal cortex.

4. Each "category-specific" region in ventral temporal cortex (e.g., the fusiform face area) also responds, to a lesser extent, to other object categories. Controversy exists as to whether these smaller activations are nonspecific responses to the presence of a visual stimulus, or whether they are object category-related and thus of functional significance. At least some evidence favours the latter view (Chao, Weisberg, & Martin, 2002).

[3] The claim that the regions identified are implicated in semantic representation of objects is not beyond criticism. Some of the regions may be involved in representing the structure of objects or the motor plans associated with the use of objects. Whether or not such information should be considered part of a semantic system or part of perceptual and motor systems is not resolved (for discussion, see Mahon & Caramazza, 2003-this issue)

5. In contrast to ventral cortex, lateral temporal cortex responds to a more limited number of object categories. The most common finding has been activation of the superior temporal sulcus (STS) in response to faces and animals (typically stronger in the right than the left hemisphere), and activation of the middle temporal gyrus in response to tools (MTG, typically stronger in the left than the right hemisphere). Objects shown moving in their characteristic fashion produce enhanced, category-related activity in this region. In contrast, category-related patterns in ventral cortex are relatively the same for static and moving images (Beauchamp, Lee, Haxby, & Martin, 2002).

6. Activation of the intraparietal and ventral premotor cortices has been strongest to tools and other manipulable objects. This activity is nearly always confined to the left hemisphere.

Much remains to be determined about the processing characteristics and/or type of information represented in these regions. Nevertheless, two conclusions may be drawn from these findings. First, the regions discussed above are involved in both perceiving and representing (storing) information about different object properties such as form (ventral occipito-temporal), motion (lateral temporal, with STS particularly responsive to biological motion, and MTG particularly responsive to tool-associated motion), and object use (intraparietal and ventral premotor regions). There are considerable data from monkey neurophysiology and lesion studies, as well as from human functional brain-imaging studies to support this view (for example, that STS is critical for detecting biological motion). Second, at least some of these purported object–property regions also appear to be organised by category. This seems most clear for posterior regions of the temporal cortex. In the fusiform gyrus animate objects produce more activity in the lateral fusiform than do manipulable artefacts, while the medial fusiform shows the opposite bias. In lateral temporal cortex, STS responds more to animate objects than to artefacts, while MTG responds more to manipulable artefacts than animate things.

With these findings in mind, we now turn to the neuroimaging papers. The section begins with a detailed analysis and review of the cognitive and associated anatomical components of a domain that has yet to be considered, the representation of number concepts. In their paper, Dehaene, Piazza, Pinel, and Cohen (2003-this issue) argue that number is a good candidate for a biologically determined semantic domain: Elementary number-processing ability has been documented in nonhuman primates without training, and in children prior to language development. In addition, as reviewed in their paper, functional brain-imaging studies and neuropsychological investigations suggest the existence of a distinct neural circuit for number processing. The authors propose that this circuit is composed of three separate regions in parietal cortex, each serving a specific function in the support of arithmetic operations. For our present discussion, the most interesting region is localised in the horizontal segment of the intraparietal sulcus (HIP). Dehaene and colleagues make a strong case that this region is essential for the semantic representation of numbers as quantities. One piece of evidence for this claim is that HIP is consistently more active for numbers relative to other object categories. In particular, HIP is more active when number names are contrasted to animal names, and when comparing numbers versus objects along a non-numerical scale (e.g., the ferocity of animals). As mentioned above, naming and making semantic judgements about tools also activates the intraparietal sulcus. This raises the intriguing possibility of a neural correspondence between the regions involved in representing properties associated with manipulating objects, and those involved in number representation. Although comparisons of locations of activity across tasks and laboratories must be made with caution, it may be noteworthy that the peak of activity, reported by Dehaene et al. across several studies, places the activity on the dorsal bank of the sulcus, while the peak activity reported across several studies of tools places the activity in a different location, deep within the sulcus (e.g., Beauchamp et al., 2002; Chao & Martin, 2000; Chao et al., 2002). Thus these regions may be anatomically distinct, but perhaps functionally linked.

Next follows a group of papers on the relationship between perceptual and conceptual processing. This issue is particularly relevant for functional brain imaging because it is often difficult to distinguish activity associated with perception of stimulus features from activity associated with higher-level visual and conceptual processes. In addition, the interaction between perceptual and conceptual processing is an important component of some formulations of property-based theories (e.g., Humphreys & Forde, 2001; Humphreys & Riddoch, 2003-this issue; Martin, 1998; Simmons & Barsalou, 2003-this issue). For example, in the HIT model (Humphreys & Forde, 2001), a lesion affecting the structural description system can produce a category-specific disorder for living things because of the overlap, or similarity, between the structural descriptions of items within this category (and see Humphreys & Riddoch, 2003-this issue). Because of the interactive nature of the system, a mild problem in accessing visual knowledge could result in a naming deficit for those categories that depend heavily on visual knowledge in order to distinguish among their members. On this view, a lesion to the structural description system should not lead to a deficit for artefacts. In contrast, the domain-specific account predicts that, just like conceptual knowledge, structural descriptions will be organised by domain (see Caramazza & Shelton, 1998). However, this theory makes no claims about the interaction between perceptual and conceptual processes.

The neuropsychological literature offers some, but not overwhelming, evidence for this interaction. One piece of evidence comes from patient ELM whose ability to learn new object–name paired-associates was influenced by the semantic relationship between the names paired with the objects. Semantically-related names resulted in poorer learning than semantically unrelated names (e.g., Arguin, Bub, & Dudek, 1996; but see comments on this and other putative cases of semantic agnosia by Capitani et al., 2003-this issue). There is also some evidence for perceptual/conceptual interactions in normal subjects. For example, repetition blindness (assumed to be a purely visual phenomenon) can be influenced by semantic factors (Parasuraman & Martin, 2001), and performing an object decision task interferes more with retrieving words based on semantic (category fluency) than on spelling (letter fluency) constraints (a motor task produced the opposite pattern of interference; Martin, Wiggs, Lalonde, & Mack, 1994).

In their paper, Gauthier, James, Curby, and Tarr (2003-this issue) directly address this issue in normal individuals. Specifically, they ask whether performance on a visual task (in this case, object matching) can be influenced by conceptual knowledge. Using a procedure modelled after the studies carried out with ELM, they provide evidence that the ability to make a perceptual decision (visual matching of novel objects) is faster and more accurate when these objects were paired with semantically unrelated object names, or a dissimilar set of feature names, than when the names were from the same semantic category or when there was substantial feature overlap. One implication of these results is that they call into question our ability to firmly rule out conceptual influences on "perceptual" processes and perceptual impairments.

Neuroimaging evidence for a more intimate link between conceptual and perceptual processes is provided in the paper by Kan, Barsalou, Solomon, Minor, and Thompson-Schill (2003-this issue). Their primary goal was to obtain evidence consistent with the idea that conceptual knowledge is grounded in the perceptual system (see Barsalou, 1999). The study was motivated by previous reports of activation of a "visual area" (posterior region of the left fusiform) when generating mental images of objects (D'Esposito et al., 1997) and when answering questions about visual object properties (Thompson-Schill, Aguirre, D'Esposito, & Farah, 1999; but see comment by Caramazza, 1999). To test this idea, subjects performed a property-verification task. As predicted, activation was found in the left fusiform region, and this occurred only when the experimental design required subjects to retrieve semantic information to perform the property-verification task. The authors argue that the results provide additional evidence that conceptual knowledge is organised visually and grounded in perception.

Further evidence for the interaction of perceptual and conceptual processing comes from studies showing that animate objects (faces, animals) activate early visual processing areas (specifically, medial occipital cortex and the inferior occipital gyrus) to a greater extent than tools and other inanimate objects (e.g., houses). For example, relative to tools, enhanced occipital activity has been found for naming line drawings and photographs of animals (Chao, Haxby, & Martin, 1999; Damasio, Grabowski, Tranel, Hichwa, & Damasio, 1996; Martin, Wiggs, Ungerleider, & Haxby, 1996), naming silhouettes of animals (Martin et al., 1996), making same/different judgements with animal pictures (Perani et al., 1995, 1999), matching-to-sample, and simply viewing animal pictures (Chao et al., 1999). The paper by Tyler and colleagues (2003-this issue) adds to this growing list of reports. Positron emission tomography (PET) was used to record brain activity while subjects performed a semantic categorisation task with object pictures (animals, tools, vehicles, fruits and vegetables). The inferior occipital gyrus was found to be more active for animals than any of the other categories tested (the activity was reported to extend anteriorly into the right cerebellum; we return to this finding below). It was previously suggested (e.g., Martin et al., 1996, 2000) that greater activation of occipital cortex for naming animals than tools might reflect top-down activation of lower-level visual processing regions when detailed information is needed to distinguish between category members (e.g., to distinguish between different four-legged animals in order to name them), in much the same way that occipital cortex is activated during certain visual imagery tasks (Kosslyn et al., 1999; and see Hochstein & Ahissar, 2002, for a review of the role of top-down modulation in visual perception). Tyler and colleagues offer a similar explanation for their finding but attribute it to bottom-up visual processing of the stimuli. As they note, however, the enhanced occipital activity for semantic processing of the animal pictures was not due to visual complexity per se. Visual complexity failed to play a role in either the behavioural or imaging results in their study. Moreover, a bottom-up explanation is difficult to reconcile with findings of increased activation of inferior occipital cortex for animals relative to tools in studies that used written names, rather than pictures (Chao et al., 1999; Perani, Schnur, Tettamanti, Garno-Tempini, Cappa, & Fazio, 1999; and see Price, Noppeney, Phillips, & Devlin, 2003-this issue).

Aside from the occipital and cerebellar (but see below) findings for animals, no other category-related differences were found. However, this null finding is exactly what the authors predicted based on their conceptual structure model (Tyler & Moss, 1997, 2001). In their view, category-specific deficits emerge as a function of the content and structure of concepts within a non-differentiated distributed neural system. Within this system, category-specific deficits occur because some concepts are more protected from damage than others due to their structure. Living things have many shared properties that are highly intercorrelated (eyes, breathe), and fewer distinctive features, and these are weakly correlated with other properties of animals. In contrast, tools have the opposite arrangement of shared and distinctive properties. It is this disadvantage for distinctive relative to shared properties of living things compared to artefacts that results in the disproportionate number of patients with a deficit for living things. A direct prediction of this account is that there should be no category specificity in the normal brain (Tyler et al., 2003-this issue). Thus, support for an undifferentiated semantic system is dependent on showing that category-related differences in neural activity do not exist. This would seem to be a difficult position to defend given the neuropsychological and neuroimaging evidence reviewed thus far (and see previously cited reviews).

Tyler and colleagues (2003-this issue) do report two findings consistent with much of the functional imaging literature. First, performance on the semantic tasks was associated with activity in a widespread network including occipital, temporal, parietal, and frontal areas. Second, each of these areas responded to multiple object categories. However, in contrast to previous reports, no differences were observed between categories in any of the regions.

The authors pay particular attention to the fusiform gyrus because of prior reports that categories of living things, including human faces and animals, show enhanced activity in the more lateral portion of the fusiform, whereas tools show enhanced activity in the medial portion of the fusiform. These category-related activations are anatomically close and in fact, are overlapping (see Chao et al., 2002; Haxby et al., 2001; Haxby, Ishai, Chao, Ungerleider, & Martin, 2000; Martin & Chao, 2001; and Spiridon & Kanwisher, 2002, for evidence and discussion of these findings). Thus, one possibility for their failure to find differential activity is that PET lacks the spatial resolution to resolve distinct peaks of activation when they are generated from anatomically close sites. (For evidence that PET may fail to reveal category-related differences in the fusiform gyrus, whereas fMRI does reveal such differences, see discussion and Figure 6.4 in Martin, 2001.) This explanation, however, appears unlikely given that PET has revealed enhanced medial fusiform activity for naming tools versus naming animals (Whatmough, Chertkow, Murtha, & Hanratty, 2002), and greater activity in the lateral fusiform for animals relative to tools across a variety of semantic tasks (Price et al., 2003-this issue). Moreover, a lack of spatial resolution cannot explain a failure to find enhanced activity for tools in lateral temporal cortex, specifically the posterior region of the left middle temporal gyrus, as this has been reported multiple times using PET as well as fMRI (see above-cited reviews).

Tyler et al. (2003-this issue) used stringent criteria for the identification of category-specific regions. The area should respond more to one category versus the others combined, as well as more to that category versus each of the others separately. Nevertheless, even with these stringent criteria, activity specific for animals was found in the posterior region of the right hemisphere, extending anteriorly from the right inferior occipital cortex (as discussed above), to the right cerebellum. However, the location reported for this cerebellar activity was at 40–55–19 (standard coordinates measure in mm along three axes). This location is, in fact, essentially identical to the location Tyler and colleagues used as their target region for the lateral fusiform gyrus (39–54–17, based on Chao et al., 1999). Thus, one possibility is that the activity was not in the cerebellum (a unique finding for a region responding more to animals than other object categories), but rather was in the lateral fusiform gyrus. Greater activity in the lateral fusiform for animals relative to tools has been reported multiple times (including Price et al., 2003-this issue, at 40–54–14, which they label as the posterior region of the right lateral fusiform). In addition, this lateral portion of the fusiform is activated by faces (the so-called fusiform face area, FFA; along with the inferior occipital gyrus; see Haxby, Hoffman, & Gobini, 2000, for review). The coordinates for this face-responsive region are again nearly identical to those reported by Tyler and colleagues (40–55–19 reported as right cerebellum by Tyler et al., 2003-this issue, vs. the right FFA reported at 40–59–22 by McCarthy, Puce, Gore, & Allison, 1997; 39–59–16 by Haxby et al., 1999; 36–51–24 by Henson, Shallice, Gorno-Tempini, & Dolan, 2002; and 40–55–10 by Kanwisher, McDermott, & Chun, 1997, to cite a few locations from what is now a large and consistent literature). Thus, the activity reported by Tyler et al. may have been in the lateral portion of the right fusiform, not the cerebellum. If so, then their report may provide some of the strongest evidence for category selectivity in the lateral fusiform; in their study this area responded more strongly to animals vs. tools, animals vs. fruits, and animal vs. vehicles.

Of course, having established that a category of objects can differentially activate a region of the fusiform gyrus does not, in and of itself, tell us what the activation means. Price and colleagues (2003-this issue) directly address this critical question in this issue, and in so doing, return us to the thorny problem of the relationship between perceptual and conceptual processing. Based on previous findings by their group and others, the authors note that there may be an important distinction between activity in the posterior and anterior regions of the fusiform gyrus. Specifically, that posterior fusiform activity may be driven to a greater extent by visual features of the stimuli than by semantic variables, whereas activity in the anterior fusiform may be more sensitive to semantic than visual variables. Evidence in support of this division of labour was obtained by a combined analysis of seven experiments in which subjects performed a variety of semantic tasks on natural kinds (including animals) and man-made objects (including tools), two experiments that required retrieval of semantic information about object-associated properties (colour, size), and one experiment on detection of simple features of meaningless visual stimuli—false fonts.

Consistent with previous findings, results of these analyses demonstrated an advantage for natural kinds (animals, fruits and vegetables) over man-made objects (tools, vehicles, and furniture) in the posterior region of both the left and right lateral fusiform gyrus. Moreover, both animals and fruits and vegetables showed more activity than tools. However, these category-related differences were found only for pictures of objects, not words. In addition, these posterior fusiform regions were activated by the feature detection task. Thus, the authors argue, the posterior fusiform may be a unimodal visual processing area. As a result, category-related differences may be driven bottom-up from visual input when the task requires increased structural differentiation (as emphasised by Humphreys and colleagues; see Humphreys & Riddoch, 2003-this issue). This could not, however, be due to the visual complexity of the objects because this region was strongly activated by fruits and vegetables, which have simple visual forms (see also Tyler et al., 2003-this issue). Price and colleagues also suggest that this unimodal region of the fusiform can be driven top-down depending on task demands. This proposal was supported by appeal to studies showing category-related differences in this region of the fusiform using mental imagery tasks (e.g., Ishai, Ungerleider, & Haxby, 2000) and word-processing tasks that required subjects to make decisions on the structural details of objects (e.g., Chao et al., 1999).

In contrast to these results, a more anterior region of the fusiform was activated only by the tasks requiring retrieval of visual information from object names. This area was strongly lateralised to the left hemisphere and did not overlap with the more posterior region where category-related differences were observed. Price and colleagues argue that this more anterior fusiform region may be a polymodal association area. Moreover, they suggest that visual information can be retrieved from this region without recourse to the more posterior category-sensitive regions. It should be kept in mind, however, that the information retrieval tasks focused on specific object properties, like colour, not on object categories per se. Nevertheless, as their report stresses, within a relatively circumscribed region (i.e., the left fusiform gyrus), there may be important differences in the processing characteristics mapped along a posterior-to-anterior gradient. As Price and colleagues note, these differences are consistent with anatomical and neurophysiological studies of monkey temporal cortex, and may help to explain some differences in patterns of performance in C-S patients (see Humphrey & Riddoch, 2003-this issue).

The final contribution to this issue, by Martin and Weisberg (2003-this issue), also offers data germane to the issue of the relationship between perceptual and conceptual processes and category-related activity in the fusiform gyrus and other brain regions. In contrast to the approach taken by Price and colleagues, in which differences between regions were based on how they were modulated by category and task demands, Martin and Weisberg took a different tack. Specifically, they sought to determine whether the pattern of category-related activity previously reported for living things (animals and faces) and artefacts could be found when the same visual objects were used to represent both categories. This would eliminate the concern that the category-related activity in posterior cortex was due completely, or in part, to bottom-up processing of visual differences in the shape or colour of the stimuli used to represent these categories.

To accomplish their goal, they developed a set of animations composed of simple geometric forms in motion. The study was modelled after the now classic demonstration by Heider and Simmel (1944), that simple geometric forms in motion can be interpreted, with little effort, as depicting animate beings with specific intentions. In their study, subjects were shown animated vignettes designed to elicit concepts related to social interactions (e.g., children playing baseball, sharing ice-cream) or mechanical devices (a factory conveyor belt, a pinball machine). The results showed the same dissociation in ventral and lateral temporal cortices as seen for animate objects and artefacts. In ventral temporal cortex, vignettes interpreted as conveying social interactions elicited heightened activity in the lateral fusiform, while the mechanical vignettes led to heightened activity in the medial fusiform gyrus. In lateral temporal cortex, the social vignettes elicited bilateral activation of STS (stronger in the right than left hemisphere), as is typically seen with animate objects, whereas the mechanical vignettes showed activation in left MTG, as is typically seen for tools. The activity in the fusiform gyrus included both the posterior and anterior regions identified by Price and colleagues (2003-this issue). However, posterior and anterior sectors were not analysed separately. Nevertheless, these results can-not be due to bottom-up processing of the visual stimuli. The same geometric forms were used in both the social and mechanical animations. Thus, these category-related differences seem to reflect top-down influences.

In addition to these findings, Martin and Weisberg reported that the social vignettes activated a number of regions associated with social processing (for a recent review, see Adolphs, 2001). Specifically, stronger activity for social than mechanical vignettes was found in the anterior regions of STS, the amygdala, and in ventromedial prefrontal cortex. Activity in these areas was strongly lateralised to the right hemisphere. The sites associated with the social vignettes closely replicated and extended the findings reported by Castelli and colleagues using a different set of animations (Castelli, Happé, Frith, & Frith, 2000). By including the mechanical condition in the current study, Martin and Weisberg were able to distinguish between regions associated with processing within a specific conceptual domain (social, mechanical), from those involved in more general purpose, problem-solving aspects of the tasks. Within a property-based framework, the authors speculate that higher-order concepts such as "animacy" may be represented in a network of regions composed of areas that store knowledge of what animate objects look like (lateral fusiform gyrus), how they move (STS), coupled with areas for representing and modulating affect (amygdala and ventromedial frontal cortex).[4] It was also noted that a network dedicated to processing within the social domain is consistent with a domain-specific account. Specifically, it could be argued that selection pressures have equipped us with a dedicated neural system for quick and efficient problem solving within the social domain.

The functional imaging data seem to suggest that object concepts may be organised, in part, by property.[5] These data also seem to suggest that, within these regions, object concepts may be organised by category. This seems to be especially true of regions in posterior ventral and lateral temporal cortices. Thus one central question will be to determine how the cortex got this way. For domain-specific accounts, the answer is straightforward. An organisation by specific category types is a natural

[4] This discussion overlooks some rather difficult issues. For example, the property "animate" is stated to be represented in a distributed network that includes information of various modalities, and therefore there is no need to postulate the existence of an independent, abstract representation "animate" in addition to the possible grounding of this property in a distributed network. But this seems unlikely to be correct. Consider the stimuli used by Martin and Weisberg. Animacy was inferred by the subjects from the pattern of movements of geometric shapes. This implies that "movement pattern" is sufficient to ascribe animacy to an object. Similarly, animacy may be assigned strictly on the basis of visual form without movement (a picture of a dog, say). But this means that no individual feature is necessary for the concept animate. Instead it seems that the property "animate" is triggered if any one of a set of specific properties (e.g., being capable of experiencing emotion) is present, implying a non correspondence between any one part and the whole concept. This implies, in turn, that "animate" is an abstraction from diverse patterns of features of different sorts—social, emotional, perceptual, and motor—and is not reducible to a sensory/motor pattern.

[5] It is important to highlight "in part" to stress that the concept of "dog" or "hammer" includes much more than sensory- and motor-related properties. We know a great deal about objects beyond what they look like, how they move, how they are used, how they feel, etc. Neuroimaging studies have, to date, revealed little if anything about where this other information is represented, even though most of our semantic memory must include this type of nonsensory/motor-based knowledge.

consequence, and the primary prediction of the theory. Property-based theories must impose additional constraints to explain how these category-related regions of activity emerge as a consequence of experience. Yet potential mechanisms are beginning to be identified that could account for the development of spatially organised clusters of neurons that respond to similar object properties (e.g., Erickson, Jagadeesh, & Desimone, 2000). This, and other potential mechanisms, may account for the development of an object category-like organisation in the brain.

## FINAL COMMENTS AND FUTURE DIRECTIONS

We have discussed the papers in this Special Issue primarily in the terms used by the authors themselves. A major emphasis has been on whether the results support one or another theory of the organisation of conceptual knowledge in the brain. In this effort, we have presented the three major theories of the causes of category-specific deficits as if they constituted mutually exclusive proposals. However, a more accurate characterisation of the state of the art would be to argue that the three proposals actually represent three principles (domain, modality, property structure) about the organisation of conceptual knowledge that need not necessarily be mutually exclusive. That is, each theory can be seen as making assumptions at a different level in a hierarchy of questions about the organisation of conceptual knowledge (Caramazza & Mahon, 2003-this issue). At the broadest level is the question of whether or not domain-specific constraints play a role in the organisation of conceptual knowledge. Independently of the answer we give to this question, we would still need to answer the question of how concepts are represented and structured in the brain. The second question concerns whether conceptual representations are stored in separate modality-specific subsystems or a single amodal system. Thus, it is entirely possible that conceptual knowledge is organised by domains, and within domains by type of modality (see discussion in Mahon & Caramazza, 2003-this issue). Once again, independently of how one answers the second-level question, we would still want to know how specific properties of objects are related to each other. Here, the focus would be on questions about how the distribution of the properties that characterise an object might shape the way individual property information is represented. Of course, it could turn out that some version of the correlated structure theory could account for all the facts from neuropsychology and neuroimaging without appealing to either domain-specific principles or modality-specific organisation. This outcome seems implausible given the evidence presented in this Special Issue. Alternatively, it could turn out that a new variant of the modality-based accounts would be able to explain all the data reviewed here. This outcome, too, seems implausible. Perhaps the time has come to consider how the three principles that underlie the different explanations of category-specific deficits might be integrated into a more comprehensive proposal. The combined consideration of neuropsychological and neuroimaging research is beginning to provide answers to these questions.

We believe that the papers included in this Special Issue of *Cognitive Neuropsychology* serve to highlight what we know (or think we know) and, more importantly, what we still need to know in order to begin to understand category-specific disorders and the representation of concepts in the human brain. Here we mention a few of these goals. First, much of the debate about the patients relies on their ability to retrieve information about sensory and functional object properties. To fully understand these patterns of deficit will require a much finer-grained analysis of these properties (see for example Cree & McRae, in press). Second, studies of patients who sustained damage very early in life (see Farah & Rabinowitz, 2003-this issue), and studies of patients with developmental disorders limited to a single domain (e.g., developmental prosopagnosia; De Haan, & Campbell, 1991) should be helpful in characterizing the nature of innate mechanisms. Third, the relationship between neuroanatomy and category-specific disorders is poorly understood and the functional imaging data have done little to clarify this issue.

Some of the imaging data fit well with the lesion data; especially with regard to knowledge of tools and other manipulable objects (see Gainotti, 2000; Tranel, Damasio, & Damasio, 1997; and Tranel et al., 2003-this issue). In contrast, the relevance of the complex organisation in ventral temporal cortex to category-specific disorders is unknown. Given the complex organisation of overlapping representations in this region revealed by fMRI, it seems highly unlikely that a lesion could selectively carve out one category-responsive region from another. This suggests that some of the critical regions for producing category-specific disorders, especially for living things, reside elsewhere in the brain. Detailed neuropsychological investigations of individual patients coupled with neuroimaging should help to clarify this issue (e.g., Mummery, Patterson, Wise, Vandenberghe, Price, & Hodges, 1999).

## REFERENCES


Adolphs, R. (2001). The neurobiology of social cognition. *Current Opinion in Neurobiology*, *11*, 231–239.

Arguin, M., Bub, D., & Dudek, G. (1996). Shape integration for visual object recognition and its implication in category-specific visual agnosia. *Visual Cognition*, *3*, 221–275.

Barsalou, L. W. (1999). Perceptual symbol systems. *Behavioral and Brain Sciences*, *22*, 577–660.

Beauchamp, M. S., Lee, K. E., Haxby, J. V., & Martin, A. (2002). Parallel visual motion processing streams for manipulable objects and human movements. *Neuron*, *34*, 149–159.

Bookheimer, S. (2002). Functional MRI of language: New approaches to understanding the cortical organisation of semantic processing. *Annual Review of Neuroscience*, *25*, 151–188.

Borgo, F., & Shallice, T. (2001). When living things and other "sensory quality" categories behave in the same fashion: A novel category specificity effect. *Neurocase*, *7*, 201–220.

Borgo, F., & Shallice, T. (2003). Category-specificity and feature knowledge. evidence from new sensory-quality categories. *Cognitive Neuropsychology*, *20*, 327–353.

Buxbaum, L. J., Veramonti, T., & Schwartz, M. F. (2000). Function and manipulation tool knowledge in apraxia: Knowing "what for" but not "how." *Neurocase*, *6*, 83–97.

Capitani, E., Laiacona, M., Mahon, B., & Caramazza, A. (2003). What are the facts of semantic category-specific deficits? A critical review of the clinical evidence. *Cognitive Neuropsychology*, *20*, 213–261.

Caramazza, A. (1998). The interpretation of semantic category-specific deficits: What do they reveal about the organisation of the conceptual knowledge in the brain? *Neurocase*, *4*, 265–272

Caramazza, A. (1999). Minding the facts: A comment on Thompson-Schill et al.'s "A neural basis for category and modality specificity of semantic knowledge." *Neuropsychologia*, *38*, 944–949.

Caramazza, A., Hillis, A. E., Rapp, B. C., & Romani, C. (1990). The multiple semantics hypothesis: Multiple confusions? *Cognitive Neuropsychology*, *7*, 161–189.

Caramazza, C., & Mahon, B. Z. (2003). *The organization of conceptual knowledge: The evidence from category-specific semantic deficits.* Manuscript submitted for publication.

Caramazza, A., & Shelton, J. R. (1998). Domain-specific knowledge systems in the brain: The animate–inanimate distinction. *Journal of Cognitive Neuroscience*, *10*, 1–34.

Castelli, F., Happé, F., Frith, U., & Frith, C. (2000). Movement and mind: A functional imaging study of perception and interpretation of complex intentional movement patterns. *Neuroimage*, *12*, 314–325.

Chao, L. L., Haxby, J. V., & Martin, A. (1999). Attribute-based neural substrates in temporal cortex for perceiving and knowing about objects. *Nature Neuroscience*, *2*, 913–919.

Chao, L. L., & Martin, A. (2000). Representation of manipulable man-made objects in the dorsal stream. *NeuroImage*, *12*, 478–484.

Chao, L. L., Weisberg, J., & Martin, A. (2002). Experience-dependent modulation of category-related cortical activity. *Cerebral Cortex*, *12*, 545–551.

Cox, D., & Savoy, R. (2002). *FMRI "brain reading": A statistical pattern recognition approach to fMR imaging of visual object recognition and imagery.* Paper presented at The fMRI Experience IV, Bethesda, MD, USA.

Cree, G. S., & McRae, K. (in press). Analyzing the factors underlying the structure and computation of the meaning of chipmunk, cherry, chisel, cheese, and cello (and many other such concrete nouns). *Journal of Experimental Psychology: General.*

Crutch, S. J., & Warrington, E. K. (2003). The selective impairment of fruit and vegetable knowledge: A multiple processing channels account of fine-grain category specificity. *Cognitive Neuropsychology, 20,* 355–372.

Damasio, A. R. (1989). Time locked multiregional retroactivation: A systems level proposal for the neural substrates of recall and recognition. *Cognition, 33,* 25–62 .

Damasio, H., Grabowski, T. J., Tranel, D., Hichwa, R. D., & Damasio, A. R. (1996). A neural basis for lexical retrieval. *Nature, 380,* 499–505.

De Haan, E. H. F., & Campbell, R. (1991). A 15 year follow-up of a case of developmental prosopagnosia. *Cortex, 27,* 489–509.

Dehaene, S., Piazza, M., Pinel, P., & Cohen, L. (2003). Three parietal circuits for number processing. *Cognitive Neuropsychology, 20,* 487–506.

D'Esposito, M., Detre, J. A., Aguirre, G. K., Stallcup, D., Alsop, D. C., Tippett, L. J., & Farah, M. J. (1997). A functional MRI study of mental image generation. *Neuropsychologia, 35,* 725–730.

Devlin, J., Gonnerman, L., Anderson, E., & Seidenberg, M. (1998). Category-specific deficits in focal and widespread damage: A computational account. *Journal of Cognitive Neuroscience, 10,* 77–94.

Erickson, C. A., Jagadeesh, B., & Desimone, R. (2000). Clustering of perirhinal neurons with similar properties following visual experience in adult monkeys. *Nature Neuroscience, 3,* 1143–1148.

Farah, M. J., & McClelland, J. L. (1991). A computational model of semantic memory impairment: Modality specificity and emergent category specificity. *Psychological Review, 120,* 339–357.

Farah, M. J., & Rabinowitz, C. (2003). Genetic and environmental influences on the organisation of semantic memory in the brain: Is "living things" an innate category? *Cognitive Neuropsychology, 20,* 401–408.

Farah, M. J., Rabinowitz, C., Quinn, G. E., & Liu, G. T. (2000). Early commitment of neural substrates for face recognition. *Cognitive Neuropsychology, 17,* 117–123.

Gainotti, G. (2000). What the locus of brain lesion tells us about the nature of the cognitive defect underlying category-specific disorders: A review. *Cortex, 36,* 539–559.

Garrard, P., Lambon Ralph, M. A., Hodges, J. R., & Patterson, K. (2001). Prototypicality, distinctiveness and intercorrelation: Analyses of semantic attributes of living and nonliving concepts. *Cognitive Neuropsychology, 18,* 125–174.

Gauthier, I., James, T. V., Curby, K. M., & Tarr, M. J. (2002). The influence of conceptual knowledge on visual discrimination. *Cognitive Neuropsychology, 20,* 507–523.

Haxby, J. V., Gobbini, M. I., Furey, M. L., Ishai, A., Schouten, J. L., & Pietrini, P. (2001). Distributed and overlapping representations of faces and objects in ventral temporal cortex. *Science, 293,* 2425–2430.

Haxby, J. V., Hoffman, E. A., & Gobbini, M. I. (2000). The distributed neural system for face perception. *Trends in Cognitive Neuroscience, 4,* 223–233.

Haxby, J. V., Ishai, A., Chao, L. L., Ungerleider, L. G., & Martin, A. (2000). Object form topology in the ventral temporal lobe. *Trends in Cognitive Neuroscience, 4,* 3–4.

Haxby, J. V., Ungerleider L. G., Clark, V. P., Shouten, J. L., Hoffman, E. A., & Martin, A. (1999). The effect of face inversion on activity in human neural systems for face and object perception. *Neuron, 22,* 189–199.

Heider, F., & Simmel, M. (1944). An experimental study of apparent behavior. *American Journal of Psychology, 57,* 243–249.

Henson, R. N. A., Shallice, T., Gorno-Tempini, M. L., & Dolan, R. J. (2002). Face repetition effects in implicit and explicit memory tests as measured by fMRI. *Cerebral Cortex, 12,* 178–186.

Hochstein, S., & Ahissar, M. (2002). View for the top: Hierarchies and reverse hierarchies in the visual system. *Neuron, 36,* 791–804.

Humphreys, G. W., & Forde, E. M. E. (2001). Hierarchies, similarity, and interactivity in object recognition: "Category-specific" neuropsychological deficits. *Behavioral and Brain Sciences, 24,* 453–509.

Humphreys, G. W., & Riddoch, M. J. (2003). A case series analysis of "category-specific" deficits of living things: The HIT account. *Cognitive Neuropsychology, 20,* 263–306.

Ishai, A., Ungerleider, L. G., & Haxby, J. V. (2000). Distributed neural systems for the generation of visual images. *Neuron, 26,* 979–990.

Jeannerod, M. (2001). Neural simulation of action: A unifying mechanism for motor cognition. *Neuroimage, 14,* S103–S109.

Josephs, J. E. (2001). Functional neuroimaging studies of category specificity in object recognition: A critical review and meta-analysis. *Cognitive, Affective, and Behavioral Neuroscience, 1,* 119–136.

Kan, I. P., Barsalou, L. W., Solomon, K. O., Minor, J. K., & Thompson-Schill, S. L. (2003). Role of mental imagery in a property verification task: fMRI evidence for perceptual representations of conceptual knowledge. *Cognitive Neuropsychology, 20*, 525–540.

Kanwisher, N., McDermott, J., & Chun, M. M. (1997). The fusiform face area: A module in human extrastriate cortex specialised for the perception of faces. *Journal of Neuroscience, 17*, 4302–4311.

Kosslyn, S. M., Pascual-Leone, A., Felician, O., Camposano, S., Keenan, J. P., Thompson, W. L., Ganis, G., Sukel, K. E., & Alpert, N. M. (1999). The role of Area 17 in visual imagery: Convergent evidence from PET and rTMS. *Science, 284*, 167–170.

Laiacona, M., Capitani, E., & Caramazza, A. (in press). Category-specific semantic deficits do not reflect the sensory/functional organisation of the brain: A test of the "sensory quality" hypothesis. *Neurocase*.

Lambon Ralph, M. A., Patterson, K., Garrard, P., & Hodges, J. R. (2003). Semantic dementia with category specificity: A comparative case-series study. *Cognitive Neuropsychology, 20*, 307–326.

Mahon, B. Z., & Caramazza, A. (2003). Constraining questions about the organisation and representation of conceptual knowledge. *Cognitive Neuropsychology, 20*, 433–450.

Martin, A. (1998). The organisation of semantic knowledge and the origin of words in the brain. In N. G. Jablonski & L. C. Aiello (Eds.), *The origins and diversification of language* (pp. 69–88). San Francisco: California Academy of Sciences.

Martin, A. (2001). Functional neuroimaging of semantic memory. In R. Cabeza & A. Kingstone (Eds.), *Handbook of functional neuroimaging of cognition* (pp. 153–186). Cambridge, MA: MIT Press.

Martin, A., & Chao, L. L. (2001). Semantic memory and the brain: Structure and processes. *Current Opinion in Neurobiology, 11*, 194–201.

Martin, A., Ungerleider, L. G., & Haxby, J. V. (2000). Category-specificity and the brain: The sensory-motor model of semantic representations of objects. In M. S. Gazzaniga (Ed.), *The cognitive neurosciences* (2nd edition). Cambridge, MA: MIT Press.

Martin, A., & Weisberg, J. (2003). Neural foundations for understanding social and mechanical concepts. *Cognitive Neuropsychology, 20*, 575–587.

Martin, A., Wiggs, C. L., Lalonde, F. L., & Mack, C. (1994). Word retrieval to letter and semantic cues: A double dissociation in normal subjects using interference tasks. *Neuropsychologia, 32*, 1487–1494.

Martin, A., Wiggs , C. L., Ungerleider, L. G., & Haxby, J. V. (1996). Neural correlates of category-specific knowledge. *Nature, 379*, 649–652.

McCarthy, G., Puce, A., Gore, J. C., & Allison, T. (1997). Face-specific processing in the human fusiform gyrus. *Journal of Cognitive Neuroscience, 9*, 605–610.

Miceli, G., Fouch, E., Capasso, R., Shelton, J. R., Tamaiuolo, F., & Caramazza, A. (2001). The dissociation of color from form and function knowledge. *Nature Neuroscience, 4*, 662–667

Mummery, C. J., Patterson, K., Wise, R. J. S., Vandenberghe, R., Price, C. J., & Hodges, J. R. (1999). Disrupted temporal lobe connections in semantic dementia. *Brain, 122*, 61–73.

Parasuraman, R., & Martin, A. (2001). Interaction of semantic and perceptual processes in repetition blindness. *Visual Cognition, 8*, 103–118.

Perani, D., Cappa, S. F., Bettinardi, V., Bressi, S., Gorno-Tempini, M., Matarrese, M., & Fazio, F. (1995). Different neural systems for the recognition of animals and man-made tools. *NeuroReport, 6*, 1637–1641.

Perani, D., Schnur, T., Tettamanti, M., Gorno-Tempini, M., Cappa, S. F., & Fazio, F. (1999). Word and picture matching: A PET study of semantic category effects. *Neuropsychologia, 37*, 293–306.

Price, C. J., Noppeney, U., Phillips, J., & Devlin, J. T. (2003). How is the fusiform gyrus related to category-specificity? *Cognitive Neuropsychology, 20*, 561–574.

Samson, D., & Pillon, A. (2003). A case of impaired knowledge for fruit and vegetables. *Cognitive Neuropsychology, 20*, 373–400.

Simmons, W. K., & Barsalou, L. W. (2003). The similarity-in-topography principle: Reconciling theories of conceptual deficits. *Cognitive Neuropsychology, 20*, 451–486.

Spiridon, M., & Kanwisher, N. (2002). How distributed is visual category information in human occipito-temporal cortex? An fMRI study. *Neuron, 35*, 1157–1165.

Thompson-Schill, S. L. (2002). Neuroimaging studies of semantic memory: Inferring "how" from "where". *Neuropsychologia, 41*, 280–292.

Thompson-Schill, S. L., Aguirre, G. K., D'Esposito, M., & Farah, M. (1999). A neural basis for category and modality specificity of semantic knowledge. *Neuropsychologia, 37*, 671–676.

Tranel, D., Damasio, H., & Damasio, A. R. (1997). A neural basis for the retrieval of conceptual knowledge. *Neuropsychologia, 35*, 1319–1327.

Tranel, D., Kemmerer, D., Adolphs, R., Damasio, H., & Damasio, A. R. (2003). Neural correlates of conceptual knowledge for actions. *Cognitive Neuropsychology*, *20*, 409–432.

Tyler, L. K., Bright, P., Dick, E., Tavares, P., Pilgrim, L., Fletcher, P., Greer, M., & Moss, H. (2003). Do semantic categories activate distinct cortical regions? Evidence for a distributed neural semantic system. *Cognitive Neuropsychology*, *20*, 541–559.

Tyler, L. K., & Moss, H. E. (1997). Functional properties of concepts: Studies of normal and brain-damaged patients. *Cognitive Neuropsychology*, *14*, 511–545.

Tyler, L. K., & Moss, H. E. (2001). Towards a distributed account of conceptual knowledge. *Trends in Cognitive Sciences*, *5*(6), 244–252.

Warrington, E. K., & McCarthy, R. (1983). Category specific access dysphasia. *Brain*, *106*, 859–878.

Warrington, E. K., & McCarthy, R. A. (1987). Categories of knowledge. Further fractionations and an attempted integration. *Brain*, *110*, 1273–1296.

Warrington, E. K., & Shallice, T. (1984). Category specific semantic impairments. *Brain*, *107*, 829–854.

Whatmough, C., Chertkow, H., Murtha, S., & Hanratty, K. (2002). Dissociable brain regions process object meaning and object structure during picture naming. *Neuropsychologia*, *40*, 174–186.

COGNITIVE NEUROPSYCHOLOGY, 2003, 20 (3/4/5/6), 213–261

# WHAT ARE THE FACTS OF SEMANTIC CATEGORY-SPECIFIC DEFICITS? A CRITICAL REVIEW OF THE CLINICAL EVIDENCE

E. Capitani
*Milan University, Italy*

M. Laiacona
*S. Maugeri Foundation, Italy.*

B. Mahon
*Harvard University, Cambridge, USA*

A. Caramazza
*Harvard University, Cambridge, USA and Cognitive Neuroscience Sector, SISSA, Trieste, Italy*

In this study we provide a critical review of the clinical evidence available to date in the field of semantic category-specific deficits. The motivation for undertaking this review is that not all the data reported in the literature are useful for adjudicating among extant theories. This project is an attempt to answer two basic questions: (1) what are the categories of category-specific deficits, and (2) is there an interaction between impairment for a type of knowledge (e.g., visual, functional, etc.) and impairment for a given category of objects (e.g., biological, artefacts, etc.). Of the 79 case studies in which the reported data are sufficiently informative with respect to the aims of our study, 61 presented a disproportionate impairment for biological categories and 18 presented a disproportionate impairment for artefacts. Less than half of the reported cases provide statistically and theoretically interpretable data. Each case is commented upon individually. The facts that emerge from our critical review are that (1) the categories of category-specific semantic deficits are animate objects, inanimate biological objects, and artefacts (the domain of biological objects fractionates into two independent semantic categories: animals, and fruit/vegetables); (2) the types of category-specific deficits are not associated with specific types of conceptual knowledge deficits. Other conclusions that emerge from our review are that the evidence in favour of the existence of cases of reliable category-specific agnosia or anomia is not very strong, and that the visual structural description system functions relatively autonomously from conceptual knowledge about object form.

Requests for reprints should be addressed to Erminio Capitani, Milan University, Clinic for Nervous Diseases, S. Paolo Hospital, via Di Rudinì 8, 20142 Milan, Italy (Email: erminio.capitani@unimi.it).

We are grateful to Riccardo Barbarotto and Anna Basso for their permission to report data unpublished in the original papers describing some patients. Glyn Humphreys and Raffaella Rumiati kindly discussed some data regarding patient SRB. We are also grateful to Rosemary Allpress for her linguistic revision of a section of the text.

This project was supported in part by NIH grant DC 04245 to Alfonso Caramazza, by a MURST grant to Erminio Capitani, and by MURST "Cofin" Grant MM06571713-05.





http://www.tandf.co.uk/journals/pp/02643294.html DOI:10.1080/02643290244000266

## INTRODUCTION

A central issue in the cognitive brain sciences is the organisation of conceptual knowledge in the human brain. The neuropsychological phenomenon of category-specific semantic deficits, in which the ability to identify specific categories of objects can be selectively impaired while performance with other categories remains relatively intact, provides an empirical basis for theories directed at the organisation of conceptual knowledge in the brain. Such theories can be divided into two groups, according to their underlying basic principle: the *correlated structure principle*, which assumes that the organisation of conceptual knowledge in the brain is a reflection of the statistical co-occurrence of the properties of objects, and the *neural structure principle*, which assumes that the organisation of conceptual knowledge is governed by representational constraints imposed by the brain itself.

The central assumption shared by theories based on the *correlated structure principle* is that any structure in the organisation of conceptual knowledge in the brain reflects the way in which properties of objects are statistically related to one another in the world. One proposal based on the correlated structure principle is the Organised Unitary Content Hypothesis (OUCH) (Caramazza, Hillis, Rapp, & Romani, 1990). In this account, conceptual space is lumpy, in that objects that share many properties tend to be represented together. For instance, the semantic representations of things that are made of a certain kind of stuff, have similar shapes, or are capable of self-generated movement might cluster together. If it is assumed that brain damage can selectively affect lumpy areas of conceptual space, either because these conceptual clusters are neurally contiguous and thus susceptible to selective damage, or because damage to a given property will propagate to highly correlated properties, then it is possible for specific categories of objects to be damaged (relatively) independently of one another. Other OUCH type models contrast the "distinctiveness" of object properties with the "correlation" of object properties (Garrard, Lambon Ralph, Hodges, & Patterson, 2001; Tyler & Moss, 1997). For instance, in one account, the highly correlated properties of items from biological categories would reinforce each other, thus making the category of living things less susceptible to impairment under conditions of moderate brain damage (Devlin, Gonnerman, Andersen, & Seidenberg, 1998). Contrastively, other authors have argued that the representations of artefacts should be less susceptible to moderate brain damage due to the high correlation between the distinctive form of an artefact and its function (Moss, Tyler, Durrant-Peatfield, & Bunn, 1998).

The crucial aspect to all OUCH-type theories is that the organising principle of conceptual knowledge in the brain is not semantic (e.g., animate vs. inanimate), but the degree to which properties of objects tend to co-occur in the world. Because of this, theories of category-specific deficits based on the correlated structure principle make two predictions: (1) any category that is sufficiently compact in conceptual space (either because its members map onto conceptual clusters or because of links among their highly correlated properties) is a candidate for selective damage/sparing; (2) selective damage to a semantic category will equally affect all types of knowledge of that category.

Two types of theories based on the *neural structure principle* have been proposed. Common to these theories is the assumption that the organisation of conceptual knowledge is determined by representational constraints internal to the brain. However, the first class of theories and, until recently, the received view, assumes that category-specific impairments arise from a noncategorically organised semantic system. Instead, this class of theories holds that conceptual knowledge is distributed across functionally and neuroanatomically distinct modality-specific semantic subsystems, each dedicated to storing and processing a specific type of information: e.g., visual, motor, auditory, etc. It is also assumed by this class of theories that the ability to identify different categories of objects depends differentially on the integrity of processes internal to distinct modality-specific subsystems. In the original account (Farah & McClelland, 1991; Warrington & McCarthy, 1983, 1987; Warrington & Shallice, 1984), the ability to identify living things depends differentially upon processes internal to the visual semantic subsystem, while the ability to identify nonliving things depends differentially upon processes internal to the functional/associative semantic subsystem: the sensory/functional theory (SFT). Throughout this paper we will use the terms "functional/associative" and "perceptual" to refer to different aspects of conceptual knowledge because these terms are widely employed in the literature; however, it should be made clear that their contrast is not based on a corroborated theory of how knowledge is acquired or represented. In particular, it is not clear if the contrast between functional/associative and perceptual semantic information (and, according to some authors, between correspondingly distinct semantic subsystems) depends on how (i.e., along which channel) the information is acquired, or on the format according to which the information is encoded or stored (for discussion, see Shelton & Caramazza, 2001). In the practice of most authors, the operational meaning of "functional/ associative" knowledge has a rather wide scope, encompassing many different aspects of conceptual knowledge, which may or may not coincide for items from different categories: e.g., what an object is used for, how it is used, where it is usually found, whether it moves and how it moves, etc. The term "perceptual" knowledge is sometimes used in reference to information about the visual appearance (i.e., the shape and texture of an object), but it is sometimes also used to refer to information that can be directly perceived in the presence of the object through perceptual channels different from the visual modality.

In recent years, several variants of the SFT have emerged, each modifying the details of how different categories of objects depend differentially on different modality-specific systems. For instance, Humphreys and Forde (2001; see also Humphreys, Riddoch, & Quinlan, 1988) assume that living things are more visually similar, with the result that there will be more perceptual crowding among the structural descriptions of living things compared to those of nonliving things. Thus, damage to the (visual) structural description system will tend to affect the category living things disproportionately compared to the category nonliving things. Also recently, Borgo and Shallice (2001) have assumed that the identification of living things, as well as several other "sensory quality categories" such as nonedible materials, liquids, and edible substances, depends differentially on colour and texture information. On this account, these "sensory quality categories" (i.e., living things, nonedible materials, liquids, edible substances) should never dissociate from one another under conditions of brain damage. Finally, Martin, Ungerleider, and Haxby (2000) have proposed a third variant of the SFT: the sensory/motor theory (SMT). The SMT makes the same assumption regarding living things as the original SFT, but assumes that for manipulable artefacts, the ability to identify such objects depends upon intact knowledge of how to use them.

The common assumption shared by modality-specific theories is that category-specific impairments are not truly categorical impairments, but are rather impairments to a modality of knowledge (e.g., visual, functional, etc.) upon which the ability to identify exemplars from certain domains of objects differentially depends. Thus, *all modality-specific theories are committed to the prediction that there will be an association between an impairment to a type of knowledge (e.g., visual, functional, etc.) and an impairment to a category of objects (e.g., biological objects, artefacts, etc.)*. Specifically, three predictions are made: (1) An impairment to the visual modality implies an impairment for the category of biological objects, while an impairment to the functional modality implies an impairment for the category of artefacts; (2) an impairment for biological objects implies a deficit for visual knowledge, while an impairment for artefacts implies a deficit for functional/ associative knowledge; and (3) the grain of category-specific deficits must necessarily be coarse, reflecting the relative importance of different modalities of conceptual knowledge for identifying different semantic categories. The latter prediction follows from the assumption that if a type of modality-specific knowledge is damaged it will necessarily result in impairment of *all* the categories for which this type of knowledge is central. For example, damage to visual conceptual knowledge should result in impairment for at least the categories animals, musical instruments, and fruits and vegetables. Stated differently, we should not observe category-specific deficits restricted to the category of animals or the category of fruits and vegetables.

The second class of theories based on the neural structure principle is the domain-specific account (Caramazza & Shelton, 1998; see also Santos & Caramazza, 2002; Shelton & Caramazza, 2001). In this account, the broadest dimension for the organisation of conceptual knowledge in the brain is determined by the role that objects have played in our evolutionary history. Specifically, it is assumed that selection pressures have resulted in *domain-specific neural circuits* dedicated to solving, quickly and efficiently, computationally complex survival problems (for example, avoiding predators and finding food). Obvious candidate domains are animals, conspecifics, and plant life (and possibly tools; see Hauser, 1997, for discussion of this possibility). The domain-specific account makes two predictions: (1) brain damage can result in category-specific semantic deficits only for evolutionarily defined domains; (2) selective damage to a semantic category will equally affect all types of knowledge about that category.

The literature on category-specific deficits is currently quite large (see recent reviews in Caramazza, 1998; Forde & Humphreys, 1999; Gainotti, 2000; Humphreys & Forde, 2001). About three quarters of reported cases present a greater impairment for biological categories, and about one quarter present the opposite pattern. For most of the reported cases, category-specific naming deficits have been interpreted as reflecting an impairment to semantic knowledge; however, some cases have been interpreted as reflecting damage to pre-semantic, object recognition systems (e.g., damage to the structural description system: agnosic patients), while some cases have been interpreted as reflecting damage to post-semantic, that is, lexical representations. The term "agnosia" classically refers to those deficits of object identification restricted to a given input channel, in the absence of elementary sensory impairments affecting the same channel. With respect to visual agnosia, the historical distinction between apperceptive agnosia (referring to damage to very preliminary stages of perception) and associative agnosia (referring to the missed "association" between what is actually perceived and the stored "generalised' shape of an object) is certainly a simplification. It is commonly assumed that information about the "generalized" or "canonical" shape of a given object is stored separately from semantic information, and is represented in a "structural description system" that only contains information about the visual properties but not other types of information about the stimulus. Furthermore, the semantic system itself certainly contains information about the visual/perceptual properties of objects. However, we neither have a corroborated theory about the relationship between the representations stored in the structural description system and those stored in the semantic system(s), nor do we know exactly how these representations dynamically interact while a subject performs a cognitive task.

Not all of the data reported in the category-specific literature is useful for adjudicating among the extant theories of category-specific deficits, for several reasons. First, many of the early reports did not control for various "nuisance" variables known to affect performance. For example, early studies did not always control for stimulus familiarity or visual complexity. However, it is now clear that the phenomenon of category-specific deficit cannot be dismissed as the result of uncontrolled stimulus factors, as many cases have since been reported in which the relevant concomitant variables have been controlled. Second, many authors did not collect the kind of data required to distinguish between the various theories that have been proposed to explain category-specific deficits. And third, the reported results are at times not sufficiently clear to permit unambiguous interpretation. Thus, it is crucial to critically review and evaluate the literature on category-specific deficits in order to separate those cases that are useful in distinguishing among theories from those that are not. As such a project, this article is driven by an attempt to answer two questions that will allow for an evaluation of the alternative theoretical accounts that have been advanced to account for category-specific semantic deficits. The core issues addressed in this review are as follows. First: What are the categories of category-specific deficits? This is an important theoretical question, as different theories make different predictions as to the type and distribution of category effects that may be observed. Second: Is there an interaction between impairment for a type of knowledge (e.g., visual, functional, etc.) and impairment for a given category (e.g., biological, artefacts, etc.)? The status of the modality-specific theories turns on the answer to this question, as all such theories require that there be an association between a type of knowledge impairment and a specific pattern of category-specific deficit. The predictions made by the principal theories are summarised in Table 1.

We wish to emphasise that the scope of the analyses reported here is limited to consideration of the issues discussed above. It is not our intention to evaluate individual, specific theories of the causes of semantic category-specific deficits or specific theories of the organisation of conceptual knowledge. Instead, our objective is to establish as clearly as possible the *facts* that emerge from neuropsychological investigations of semantic category-specific deficits, insofar as they concern (1) the grain of the categories affected and (2) the type (modality) of conceptual knowledge that is affected in the various types of category-specific deficits.

The paper is organised as follows. We begin with a description of the database on which our critical review is based. This is followed by the results of several analyses, the details of which are reported in appendices so as not to clutter the presentation of the results. First, we report the analysis of the attested types of category-specific deficits, focusing on the patterns of relationship between category-specific deficits and impairments of types of knowledge about objects. Specifically, we consider whether patients with category-specific deficits for biological categories are also disproportionately impaired for knowledge of the visual properties of objects. That is, we attempt to answer the question: What is the nature of the deficit in patients with category-specific deficits? Second, we report an analysis of the grain of the observed deficits. Here we consider both the issue of whether the category of biological concepts fractionates into finer-grained category-specific deficits as well as whether there are specific patterns of associations as predicted by the SFT. That is, we answer the question: What are the categories of category-specific deficits? We conclude with a brief assessment of what we consider to be the core facts that emerge from our analysis of the literature (at least with respect to the grain of category-specific deficits and the relationship between modality of knowledge and category effects).

## ANALYSIS OF THE DATABASE

### The database for a critical review

Beginning with the first informative study in the literature (Warrington & Shallice, 1984), we have evaluated all the published papers on semantic category-specific deficits through the year 2001. This survey focuses on the dissociation (in either direc-

**Table 1.** *Schematic representation of the basic predictions entailed by the main types of explanations of category-specific deficits*

| | *Categories selectively or disproportionately impaired* | *Type of knowledge defective in the (most) impaired categories* | *Type of knowledge defective in the (relatively) spared categories* |
|---|---|---|---|
| | *Theories based on the correlated structure principle* | | |
| OUCH-type | Any category sufficiently compact in conceptual space | All types of knowledge | No specific impairment |
| | *Theories based on the neural structure principle* | | |
| SFT-types | All categories for which the crucial modality-specific subsystem is damaged (e.g., biological categories) | Semantic information crucial for the impaired category (e.g., visual) | Semantic information crucial for the impaired category (e.g., visual) |
| D-S account | Only evolutionarily salient categories (e.g., animals, fruit and vegetables, conspecifics (tools?)) | All types of knowledge | No specific impairment |

tion) between biological and artifact categories. We found 79 case studies in which the reported data are sufficiently informative with respect to the aims of our study. We did not consider those cases in which the data are not clearly reported or were not submitted to a statistical analysis, even if such data could be potentially relevant (e.g., Damasio, 1990, cases AN and PSD; Goldenberg, 1992; Laurent et al., 1990, Case 9). We also excluded cases of developmental category-specific deficit (e.g., Temple, 1986). Appendix A lists all the cases included in this database: Section 1 lists single cases presenting a disproportionate impairment for living categories ($n$ = 61); Section 2 lists cases presenting a disproportionate impairment for nonliving categories ($n$ = 18).

For each case listed in Appendix A1 and A2, demographic data, aetiology, and lesion site are reported. Moreover, we report all available data that bears on the disproportionately impaired categories, emphasising which level of representation was determined by the authors to be the locus of the deficit, and indicating if other categories were affected outside the classical realms of living and nonliving.

From group studies or multiple single case studies 76 patients were found who presented with a disproportionate category-specific impairment: 42 were more impaired for biological categories, and 34 for artefacts. Appendix B summarises the relevant information reported in the reference papers. These studies, however, were too limited, or only summary accounts were presented; therefore, these patients were not considered for further evaluation.

## What is the nature of the deficit in putative cases of semantic category-specific deficit?

In this section we address several issues. We begin by identifying those patients for whom we have sufficient data to address the core question: "What is the nature of the deficit in patients with semantic category-specific deficits?" These patients are then classified according to whether they have a conceptual level deficit for a particular semantic category, and whether the deficit is uniform across perceptual and functional knowledge about category members. This classification will then serve as the basis for drawing empirical generalisations about the nature of category-specific deficits and for a general evaluation of the major theories of the organisation of conceptual knowledge in the brain.

### Authors' classification of cases of category-specific deficit

Table 2 reports the authors' claims regarding the level and type of deficit for the cases listed in Appendix A. These are all the cases for which a first-pass analysis suggests that the reported data may be sufficient to permit conclusions regarding three specific questions: (1) the type of semantic knowledge (perceptual or functional) that is impaired in each patient; (2) whether this impairment applies to all categories or only those for which the patient's performance is disproportionately impaired; and (3) whether the (visual) structural description system is impaired, and if so, whether this pre-semantic impairment is itself category-specific. The table is partitioned into sections, reporting separately those cases presenting a disproportionate impairment for biological categories (Table 2a), and those presenting the opposite dissociation (Table 2b). In the table are also reported patients with category dissociations interpreted by the authors as reflecting purely agnosic or lexical deficits.

### Classification of cases of category-specific deficits following reanalysis of the reported results

The cases reported in Table 2 were submitted to a critical analysis. Bibliographic and other information about the cases are listed in Appendix A. The results of the critical review are reported separately for each case in Appendix E. Comments on the case reports are listed in alphabetical order according to the patients' initials; patients are separated into those presenting a disproportionate impairment for natural categories, and those presenting the opposite dissociation. In Appendix E we comment on whether or not the claims made by the respective authors are empirically well founded.

**Table 2(a).** *Author's classification of the nature of the cognitive impairment: Cases with category-specific impairment involving the biological categories*

| *Level of impaired knowledge* | *Structural description system* | *Cases* |
|---|---|---|
| *Semantic deficit* | Spared. | No cases. |
| Perceptual attributes worse than | Defective for biological categories. | SRB[a]. |
| functional/associative attributes for all categories. | Defective overall. | DM94, EC. |
| *Semantic deficit* | Spared. | KR. |
| Perceptual attributes worse than functional/ associative attributes only for biological categories. | Defective for biological categories. | FELICIA, GIULIETTA, HELGA, LH, MICHELANGELO. |
| | Not tested or inconclusive. | LA. |
| *Semantic deficit* | Spared. | EA (2nd 3rd exam), FM, JENNIFER, LF, SB. |
| Perceptual and functional/associative attributes evenly impaired for biological categories. | Defective for biological categories. | CA, DB[a], EA (1st exam), EMMA[a], EW, GR, JBR[a], MF. |
| | Defective overall. | MU. |
| | Not tested or inconclusive. | RC. |
| *Semantic deficit* | Spared. | BD, SE (contradictory data). |
| Data insufficient for determining which | Defective for biological categories. | DM97[a]. |
| type of knowledge is more impaired. | Not tested or inconclusive. | C(CW97), FA, FB, FI, GP97, ING, JH, JMC, JV, KB, KG, MB, MC, NV, PR, PS, RM, SBY, TOB, TS, VG. |
| *Deficit level not determined* | Defective for biological categories. | IL. |
| | Not tested. | GC, NR. |
| *Deficit classified as agnosic* | Spared. | MR. W. |
| | Spared on object reality decision, but impaired on heads test. | JB. |
| | Defective for animals. | ELM. |
| | Defective. | NA[a]. |
| | Defective with outline drawings, spared with silhouette. | HJA. |
| | Not tested. | FS, MS. |
| *Deficit classified as lexical* | Borderline. | DANTE. |
| | Not tested. | MD, TU, 5 cases by H. Damasio et al., 1996. |

Deficits are classified in terms of the type of category and the type of knowledge (perceptual vs. functional/associative) that are hypothesized to be impaired. The status of patients' structural description system is also reported.
[a]Artefacts not reliably tested.

We also provide our interpretation of the locus of impairment with respect to three levels of representation: semantic, lexical, or pre-semantic (agnosia). The criteria for including cases of dissociation between biological categories and artefacts, and between sensory and functional properties, were (1) a detailed quantitative report of differences in performance, (2) a comparison with control data obtained using the same materials, and (3) a statistical significance assessment, unless the pattern of data was self-evident. In general, the reported cases presented a disproportionate impairment of one category or of one type of knowledge. Less frequently, the impairment was restricted to a given category, while performance on other categories was within normal limits: remarks on this latter type of case profile can be found for the relevant cases in Appendix E. For those cases in which the reported data analyses did not permit a definitive classification, we have attempted to supplement the analyses provided by the authors with new analyses based on the available published data. The type of analysis we have performed is based on the study of 2 × 2 × 2 contin-

**Table 2(b).** *Author's classification of the nature of the cognitive impairment: Cases with category-specific impairment involving artefacts*

| *Level of impaired knowledge* | *Structural description system* | *Cases* |
|---|---|---|
| *Semantic deficit*<br>Perceptual attributes worse than functional/ associative attributes for all categories. | Spared.<br>Defective. | IW.<br>SM. |
| *Semantic deficit*<br>Perceptual attributes worse (or better) than functional/associative attributes only for artefacts. | | No cases. |
| *Semantic deficit*<br>Perceptual and functional/associative attributes evenly impaired for artefacts. | Spared.<br>Not tested or inconclusive. | PL.<br>CN98, ES. |
| *Semantic deficit*<br>Data insufficient for determining which type of knowledge is more impaired. | Not tested or inconclusive. | CN94, CW92, JJ, KE, M.LUCIEN, NB, PJ, VER, VP, YOT. |
| *Deficit classified as agnosic* | Spared. | DRS. |
| *Deficit classified as lexical* | Not tested. | CG, GP98, 7 cases by H. Damasio et al., 1996. |

Deficits are classified in terms of the type of category and the type of knowledge (perceptual vs. functional/associative) that are hypothesized to be impaired. The status of patients' structural description system is also reported.

gency tables. These report the frequency of (1) correct and incorrect responses of (2) patients and controls, according to (3) the impairment/ sparing of perceptual and functional/associative knowledge of biological categories. As a minimal approach, the reanalysis considered the percentage correct performance of the patient and the controls for perceptual and functional/associative knowledge of biological category items. The crucial analysis concerns the interaction between the patient/control classification and the type of impaired knowledge, i.e., whether the difference between perceptual and functional/associative knowledge is greater for the given patient than for the control group. Details of these analyses are extensively reported for the relevant cases in Appendix E. These data can be analysed with either a log-linear or a logit-linear model. We are aware that this approach offers only an approximate answer to the lack of a proper experimental design. That is, because this analysis requires that all controls be collapsed into a single cell, it cannot take into account any variation within the normal controls. It is thus possible that a single patient's performance falls within the central 95% of the controls' distribution, while at the same time it is significantly different from the controls' performance when the latter is collapsed into a single data point. Notwithstanding this caveat, we consider significant findings as a suggestive piece of evidence whose reliability can be evaluated within a wider theoretical context. A further comment is necessary regarding the general risk of type II errors: In principle, it is possible that we have at times accepted the null hypothesis (no difference in performance between perceptual and functional/associative knowledge) in some cases where a greater number of stimuli and thus a greater statistical power could have revealed a significant difference. However, the complexity of the statistical design (based on the study of generalised linear models) and the need to consider the significance of interactions makes it impossible to calculate the risk of type II error for this type of analysis.

The result of this critical analysis is a new classification of the reported cases, which may or may not be consistent with that proposed by the authors of the original reports. This new classification and the data in support of it will be considered the core set of facts for interpreting the phenomenon of category-specific deficits.

Table 3 reports the revised classification of those patients presenting a *semantic* deficit. This table will serve as the basis for evaluating different pro-

**Table 3(a).** *Revised classification of the relationship between the type of category and type of knowledge that is damaged in each patient: Cases with biological categories semantic impairment*

| *Level of impaired knowledge* | *Structural description system* | *Cases* | *Lesion site* |
|---|---|---|---|
| *Semantic deficit*<br>Perceptual attributes worse than functional/associative attributes for all categories | | No cases | |
| *Semantic deficit*<br>Perceptual attributes worse than functional/associative attributes only for biological categories | Defective for biological categories | GIULIETTA<br>MICHELANGELO | MRI: Bilateral T<br>CT: Bilateral T, anterior |
| *Semantic deficit*<br>Perceptual and functional/associative attributes evenly impaired for biological categories | Spared | EA (2nd 3rd exam)<br>FM<br>JENNIFER<br><br>SB | MRI: Left T<br>CT: Left F-T<br>CT: Atrophy of posterior left hemisphere<br>CT: Left T (oedema) |
| | Defective for biological categories | CA<br>DB<br><br>EA (1st exam)<br>EMMA[a]<br><br>EW<br>GR<br>JBR[a]<br>MF | CT: Left sylvian atrophy<br>MRI: Diffuse bilateral and mesial T atrophy<br>MRI: Left T<br>MRI: Bilateral T, right more than left<br>CT: Left posterior F and P<br>CT: Left F-T<br>CT: T-bilateral<br>MRI: Right T severe. Left T mildly involved later |
| | Defective overall | MU | MRI: Bilateral F T; right O |
| | Not tested | RC | MRI: Bilateral T, left more severe |

The classification is based on a critical evaluation of the evidence reported by the authors and, where possible, the results of new analysis of data reported by the authors. The cases are also classified in relation to the integrity of their structural description system. Patients' lesion sites, indicating if the imaging data were derived from CT-scan or from MRI, are also reported.
[a]Artefacts not reliably tested.

posals of the causes of category-specific semantic deficits, and the organisation of conceptual knowledge in the brain.

Table 3 reveals that patients with a disproportionate impairment for biological categories are of three types: (1) patients with a prevailing deficit for perceptual knowledge and impairment in object reality decision for biological category items (Michelangelo and Giulietta); (2) patients with balanced deficits for perceptual and functional/associative knowledge but no impairment in object reality decision (e.g., cases Jennifer and EA, 2nd examination); (3) patients with balanced deficits for perceptual and functional/associative knowledge and impaired object reality decision for biological category items (e.g., cases EW and GR).

As discussed in the Introduction, competing accounts of category-specific semantic deficits make different predictions regarding (1) the types of conceptual knowledge (perceptual vs. functional/associative) that should be impaired given a certain pattern of category-specific deficit, and (2) the semantic categories that should be disproportionately impaired given a certain pattern of impairment of perceptual vs. functional/associative knowledge. Table 3 clarifies the relationship between impaired semantic categories and types of conceptual knowledge. The strongest conclusion is

**Table 3(b).** *Revised classification of the relationship between the type of category and type of knowledge that is damaged in each patient: Cases with semantic impairment for the domain of artefacts*

| *Level of impaired knowledge* | *Structural description system* | *Cases* | *Lesion site* |
|---|---|---|---|
| *Semantic deficit*<br>Functional/associative attributes worse than perceptual attributes for all categories | | No cases | |
| *Semantic deficit*<br>Functional/associative attributes worse than perceptual attributes only for artefacts | | No cases | |
| *Semantic deficit*<br>Perceptual attribute worse than functional/associative attributes for all categories | Spared | IW | MRI: atrophy of the left T lobe (reduction of the inferior T gyrus) |
| *Semantic deficit*<br>Functional/associative and perceptual attributes evenly impaired for artefacts; both spared or evenly impaired for biological categories | Spared | PL | MRI: Left F-T atrophy |
| | Defective for artefacts | No cases | |
| | Defective overall | No cases | |
| | Not tested or inconclusive | CN98 | MRI: Left anterior and inferior mesial T. |
| | | ES | MRI: Bilateral atrophy of inferior T lobes, more extensive on the right. |

The classification is based on a critical evaluation of the evidence reported by the authors and, where possible, the results of new analysis of data reported by the authors. The cases are also classified in relation to the integrity of their structural description system. Patients' lesion sites, indicating if the imaging data were derived from CT-scan or from MRI, are also reported.

that impairment of specific semantic categories is *not* associated with damage to a particular type of conceptual knowledge (perceptual vs. functional/associative). Our reanalysis shows that a disproportionate deficit for perceptual knowledge restricted to biological categories is only found in two cases, Giulietta and Michelangelo,[1] while in 11 cases perceptual and associative knowledge are impaired to equivalent degrees. Furthermore, the only case of global impairment for visual-perceptual knowledge (case IW) presented a relative impairment for artefacts (although the effect was not impressive). This pattern of results is clearly inconsistent with the classical SFT account of the causes of semantic category-specific deficits.

For those cases presenting a prevailing semantic deficit for biological categories, object reality decision was impaired in 11 cases and was spared in 4. Therefore, damage to pre-semantic visual knowledge is *not* required for disproportionate impairment of the biological categories. This finding is inconsistent with models which assume that a disproportionate deficit for living things arises because the structural descriptions of their category members are more similar to each other than those of nonliving things, and thus more susceptible to error when the structural description or the semantic system is damaged (e.g., Humphreys & Forde, 2001). Furthermore, Table 3 clearly demonstrates that an impairment for object reality decision is not necessarily associated with an impairment for semantic perceptual knowledge compared to functional/associative knowledge. Only in cases Giulietta and Michelangelo was a disproportionate impairment for perceptual knowledge observed; however, in nine cases the

[1] These two patients were examined in the same laboratory, and presumably with the same materials. It should also be noted that in our statistical reanalysis of the published data, we have decided to ignore certain weaknesses inherent in the experimental design. Therefore, this pattern is in strong need of confirmation with fresh data.

impairments for perceptual and associative knowledge were equivalent.

Although the great majority of cases presenting reliable category-specific dissociations can be interpreted as deficits arising at the semantic level (as indicated, for example, by the fact that they are impaired in verifying property statements), for some cases the respective authors have suggested a pre-semantic or post-semantic level of impairment. Here we briefly consider these cases (but see Appendix E for details).

*Are there cases of category-specific agnosia?* Some authors have suggested that category-specific impairments can originate at early ("apperceptive") stages of visual perception. Funnell (2000) hypothesised that case NA suffered from apperceptive category-specific agnosia. However, the category effect in naming was not strong and the pictorial stimuli from biological and artefact categories were not strictly matched for their visual characteristics. For cases FS, MS, and MrW experimental data are insufficient to support clear interpretation, and the reader is referred to Appendix E for discussion of those cases.

HJA was classified as a case of "integrative agnosia". The evidence in favour of an agnosic deficit is not direct but is based on the observation of a category-specific impairment in picture naming (and drawing from memory) combined with relatively intact semantic knowledge. The authors considered the "contour overlap" of the pictures (supposedly greater for biological items) as the critical variable responsible for the observed category effects. However, our reanalysis of the reported data is not in line with this claim. We have also reconsidered the purported role of contour overlap in other cases (JB, SRB) with a similarly negative conclusion (see also case NA, Appendix E).

The case study of ELM focused on fine-grained aspects of a purported visual perception deficit for biological stimuli. On the whole, an agnosic component of the category-specific deficit is probable, but a semantic deficit for the same categories cannot be excluded. This case has some similarity to the cases Michelangelo and Giulietta, for whom the respective authors have indicated the structural description system to be the locus of the observed category-specific effects. We do not have an articulated theory of the relationship between the "structural description system" (generally considered to be a pre-semantic, modality-specific cognitive stage) and stored perceptual knowledge, which can be directly accessed through the verbal system. Therefore, it is not clear whether these cases present agnosic or semantic deficits.

With respect to cases presenting a possible agnosia for artefacts, DRS was classified as having associative agnosia for objects, but this conclusion is weakened by the fact that "nuisance" factors were not strictly controlled for the different categories.

Summing up, claims about the existence of category effects at an early perceptual level are not given clear support by our critical review. Category discrepancies in naming by patients affected by visual agnosia do not exclude the possibility that a semantic deficit coexists with their visual disorder.

*Are there cases of category-specific anomia?* Evidence supporting the existence of category-specific anomia will necessarily be weak, since it mainly rests on negative findings about possible pre-semantic or semantic impairments. We cannot exclude the possibility that in such cases a subtle semantic deficit was not detected due to the relatively low difficulty of comprehension tasks (relative to production tasks). This conclusion applies to cases Dante and TU, who presented impairments for biological categories, and to case GP98, who presented the opposite dissociation. For cases MD and CG see comments in Appendix E. Thus, although category-specific anomias are certainly theoretically possible (perhaps reflecting disconnection from semantics to the lexical system or systems) evidence for their existence is not particularly strong.

## What are the categories of category-specific deficits?

In this section we discuss which categories are impaired in category-specific semantic deficits. This general point includes a number of distinct issues, which will be discussed under separate headings. We begin by considering the "grain" of category-specific deficits. We address the issue of whether there is convincing evidence for further fractionations within the categories of living and nonliving things. We also consider the status of the categories "food," "musical instruments," and "body parts." This seemingly arbitrary selection of categories for special consideration has empirical and theoretical motivations. On the empirical side, it has been observed that these categories appear to violate the living/nonliving dichotomy. For example, it has been claimed that musical instruments tend to be impaired in patients with damage to the category living things. On the theoretical side, it has been claimed that deficits that appear to be category-specific in nature are really deficits to noncategorical, modality-based conceptual knowledge subsystems that disproportionately affect all categories that are differentially dependent on those subsystems. Therefore, the putative association of, for example, musical instruments and living things is of great theoretical significance.

### *Is there evidence for further fractionations within the biological and artefact domains?*

The study of category-specific deficits has focused mainly on the contrast between biological and artefact categories. However, the stimuli from these categories are not always comparable from one study to another (see Appendix A). With respect to biological categories, nearly all authors have included animal stimuli; some authors indicate as animals only the subset of "four-legged animals," and separately consider insects, birds, and fish. Less consistently, plant life has been included in the category living things, generally comprised of fruit and vegetables, and more rarely flowers. With respect to artefacts, the stimuli employed most often include tools, vehicles, and furniture, and less consistently, kitchen utensils and clothing.

Generally, authors have not explicitly addressed the issue of homogeneity within the domains of biological and artefact categories. Because of this, the number of stimuli employed from each sub-category have seldom allowed for fine-grained comparison within the broad domains of biological and artefact categories. However, there are now a number of cases that seem to show fine-grained dissociations. Table 4 reports those cases presenting with dissociations within the biological category, sorted on the basis of the degree of evidence. Two points are relevant. First, there is a double dissociation between an impairment for animals and an impairment for plant life. Second, a severe deficit for fruit and vegetables has been reported only for male patients (eight males, i.e., MD, EA, JJ, ELM, GR, JV, SRB, TU); for the category animals no clear gender effect emerges (two females, i.e., EW, LA; two males, i.e., LH, KE). We will return to this point below.

Within the domain of nonliving categories, YOT shows a trend toward a more severe impairment for small manipulable "indoor" objects compared to large outdoor objects. However, this case is extremely complicated and presents with different category patterns across different tasks.

**Table 4.** *Evidence for further fractionation within the biological domain*

| | *Strong evidence* | *Possible evidence or trend* |
|---|---|---|
| Animals more impaired than fruit and vegetables. | EW selective impairment of animals. | LA<br>LH<br>KE relative preservation of fruit and vegetables. |
| Fruit and vegetables more impaired than animals. | MD selective impairment of fruit and vegetables.<br>EA substantial impairment of fruit and vegetables.<br>JJ substantial advantage for animals. | ELM<br>GR<br>JV<br>SRB<br>TU |

*The status of the categories "food," "body parts," and "musical instruments"*

The category "food" includes both naturally occurring items as well as manufactured food. It is thus of theoretical interest whether the category food behaves like other "natural" categories. Interest in this issue is also motivated by the observation, especially in the early studies of category-specific deficits, that an impairment for the category "food" is often associated with an impairment for living things (see Appendix C). In order to deconfound the category "food" from other natural categories, for instance, fruit and vegetables, we will limit our discussion to those studies in which the category "food" did not include fruit and vegetable stimuli in the form that they naturally appear. A reliable impairment for the category "food" was observed in Felicia, JBR, and SB, all of whom also presented with a general impairment for biological categories. Furthermore, in case JJ, who presented a selective sparing of animals, performance on the category "food" was similar to performance on fruit and vegetables—both categories were impaired. These findings would suggest that the category "food" has a deep similarity to fruits and vegetables. However, in both case MD, who presented a reliable impairment for fruit and vegetables, and case PS, who was impaired for animals and vegetables, food was spared. Thus, it would seem that impairment for the category of food dissociates from impairment for biological categories such as animals and fruit and vegetables. The question concerning the nature of the broader category "food" remains open.

The a priori classification of body parts and musical instruments seems to be unequivocal: Strictly speaking, body parts are natural items and musical instruments are artefacts. However, authors who have studied these stimuli in semantically impaired patients have often been puzzled by the observation that performance for these two categories of objects can dissociate from performance on biological and artefact categories, respectively. Somewhat paradoxically, it has been suggested that musical instruments are similar to living category items, since the ability to identify musical instruments, it is argued, depends upon their visual attributes (Dixon, Piskopos, & Schweizer, 2000). It has also been suggested, paradoxically, that body parts are more similar to artefacts, since, it has been argued, both body parts and artefacts depend upon functional/associative information for their identification (Warrington & McCarthy, 1987).

The suggestion of a close relationship between musical instruments and biological categories on the one hand, and body parts and artefacts, on the other, is primarily based on cases presenting a prevailing deficit for biological categories, with less impaired or even normal performance on body part stimuli. In Appendix D we report data for only those patients who presented with a deficit for body parts as well as a dissociation between living and nonliving things. It should be emphasised that the statements reported in this appendix are based on inspection of the reported data; the labels "spared/impaired" do not necessarily endorse the conclusion that a real effect is actually present or would survive covariance for the relevant "nuisance" variables.

If there actually is an association between body parts and artefacts, then those cases presenting a prevailing impairment for artefacts should also present a greater impairment for body parts compared to biological categories. An inspection of the literature does not offer convincing evidence that body parts are systematically more impaired than biological categories in these patients: cases GC, GP98, and PL presented a disproportionate impairment for artefacts, but were not correspondingly impaired for body parts.

The relationship between musical instruments and biological categories is even less uniform: there are cases of impairment for biological categories where performance on musical instruments is at, or near, the normal level (BD, CW, EW, Felicia, and SE), and cases where performance falls near the level for biological categories, or even at a lower level (see Appendix D). With respect to the opposite dissociation, in which performance for biological categories is better than for artefacts, there are cases that present with poor performance on musical instruments (CG, CW92, PL, SM, YOT). Only for case GP98 was the naming impairment for musical instruments intermediate between that for artefacts and that for biological categories.

On the whole, if any definite point emerges for the categories of body parts and musical instruments from the literature on semantic memory patients, it is that body parts tend to be spared and musical instruments tend to be impaired beyond the biological categories/artefacts dissociation. As a consequence, other factors that might influence the pattern of patients' performance should be taken into account in order to allow a clearer interpretation of the status of these two categories. The relationship between the categories "musical instruments" and "body parts" and the domains "living things" and "nonliving things" has recently been investigated by Barbarotto, Capitani, and Laiacona (2001), by means of a latent variables analysis carried out on a sample of semantically impaired patients. In line with the impression drawn from the literature, the raw mean performance of the patients in this study indicate that body parts are the most preserved category while musical instruments are the least preserved category. However, after covariance, this profile was no longer observed; the result can be explained at the group level as arising from the influence of unmatched "nuisance" variables, such as age of acquisition and lexical frequency. This does not of course exclude the possibility that, in single cases, there may be selective impairment or sparing of body parts (see Shelton, Fouch, & Caramazza, 1998, for discussion). However, the outcome of the latent variables analysis indicated that body parts were related only to artefacts, and that musical instruments showed a significant relationship to artefacts but only a marginal relationship to biological categories. For more in-depth discussion of these findings, the readers are referred to the original paper.

An association between impairment for biological categories and impairment for other categories has been suggested (e.g., with precious stones for case JBR) but is not supported by sufficient experimental evidence. More recently, Borgo and Shallice (2001) reported case MU, who was impaired for biological categories as well as for the "sensory quality" categories (liquids, edible substances, materials). However, this pattern of association, too, is not a necessary one since sensory quality categories dissociate from biological kind objects in at least one patient, EA (Laiacona, Capitani, & Caramazza, in press).

## DISCUSSION

Neuropsychological investigations provide one of the richest sources of data for constraining theories of normal cognition and its possible neural basis. Practice and analysis have shown that the methodology of single-patient investigation generates the most reliable observations for this purpose. Nonetheless, as for any method, there are intrinsic limitations that must be considered when interpreting data from single-patient reports. These limitations are well known (Caramazza, 1986). Because patients are experiments of nature, we do not have control over the exact transformations to the cognitive system introduced by brain damage. This means that replication is pragmatically of limited utility in this type of research: patients present with varying degrees of severity, clinical profiles may evolve rapidly, and the configuration of noncritical cognitive deficits and associated brain lesions vary considerably across patients. This last feature is crucial, since it ends up constraining the tasks that can be administered to any given patient, thus making it impossible to "replicate" tasks used with other, similar patients. The end result is that the cases relevant to a theoretical issue consist of many "partial" experiments, since there are always questions that remain open given alternative theoretical perspectives. And, yet, we have no choice but to consider the set of partial experiments as they are given to us. For the reasons listed above, there is no simple way to "complete" the experiments. Nonetheless, within the set of potentially useful case studies we can distinguish those that are theoretically useful from those whose status is more problematic. This is what we have tried to do in this critical review. We have pulled out from the large set of patients with semantic category-specific deficits those studies which present data that are statistically reliable on tasks that tap the integrity of perceptual and functional/associative knowledge. In the end, the most useful way to determine the theoretical value of a single case study is not the mere, faithful "replication" of the case (which would clearly be important but, as pointed out, may be pragmatically nearly impossible) but an assessment of the pattern of results obtained across theoretically relevant cases. That is, convergence of results rather than straight replication is the more realistic tool available to researchers working with neurological cases.

The picture that emerges from our critical review of the published cases has the following general contour—we say "contour" because, as we will argue below, the internal details of the picture remain unclear. The most reliable form of semantic category-specific deficit is found for the domain of biological objects.[2] However, this domain fractionates into two independent semantic categories: the categories of animals (animate objects) and fruits and vegetables (inanimate biological objects) can be damaged/spared independently of each other. Furthermore, although impairment of the biological domain is often associated with impairment to the categories of manufactured foods and musical instruments, these associations are *not* necessary. The category of body parts clearly dissociates from animals and fruits and vegetables, and is most often impaired together with artefacts. However, there are case reports (see Appendix D) confirming the dissociation of this category from the domain of artefacts (see also Shelton et al., 1998, for such a case and review of other relevant cases). No reliable fractionations have been reported for the domain of artefacts (see critical review of YOT in Appendix E). Therefore, in answer to the question "What are the categories of category-specific semantic deficits?" the most cautious answer would seem to be "the categories of animate objects, inanimate biological objects, and artefacts."

The other major question addressed in this review concerns the relationship between type of category-specific deficit and type of conceptual knowledge deficit. More specifically, the question concerns whether there is a necessary association between impairment to the domain of biological objects and impairment to knowledge of the visual properties of objects, and between impairment to the domain of artefacts and impairment to knowledge of the functional/associative properties of objects. The results of our review are clear on one aspect of this question: Types of category-specific deficits are *not* associated with specific types of conceptual knowledge deficit. In fact, the vast majority of patients with category-specific deficit for biological objects are equally impaired for visual and functional/associative properties of objects.

The facts that have emerged from our critical review of the cases of category-specific deficits have clear, if limited, implications for theories of the causes of these deficits. First, the categories of category-specific deficits are far more fine-grained than predicted by SFT accounts. That is, there is convincing evidence that the domain of living things fractionates into two distinct domains: animate objects and the domain of fruit and vegetables. Second, category-specific deficits are generally associated with uniform damage to conceptual knowledge independently of whether such knowledge concerns form, function, or other conceptual properties of objects. These results are clearly inconsistent with core expectations derived from SFT accounts; they are somewhat problematic for OUCH-type theories; but they are fully consistent with evolutionarily based domain-specific accounts.

As noted in the Introduction, SFT-type accounts predict that the categories of category-specific deficits are determined by the type of conceptual knowledge that is damaged in a given patient. Of particular relevance here is the claim that damage to "visual semantic" representations will necessarily result in disproportionate difficulty for living things, as well as other categories such as musical instruments that presumably also depend crucially on this type of conceptual knowledge for distinguishing among the members of the category. Thus, the SFT predicts the necessary co-occurrence of damage to animals, fruit/vegetables, musical instruments, and sensory quality categories (liquids and substances) (e.g., Borgo & Shallice,

[2] This type of dissociation is more frequent among males than females. Considering cases affected by prevailing biological categories deficit and by a disease whose incidence is not related to gender such as herpetic encephalitis, males were 21/28, and this proportion is significantly different from chance ($p = .006$).

2001). The fact that the categories animals and fruit/vegetables can be damaged independently of each other is highly problematic for SFT accounts. Also highly problematic for these theories is the fact that selective impairment for living things is not associated with disproportionate impairment for visual relative to other types of object knowledge.

The pattern of results that have emerged from our review are not entirely consistent with OUCH-type accounts. To be sure, these accounts correctly predict that category-specific deficits should not necessarily result in greater damage for one type of conceptual knowledge (i.e., visual vs. functional) than another. However, they fail to predict the disproportionate occurrence of category-specific deficits for the biological categories. By contrast, the latter two results are exactly as predicted by the Domain-specific theories. The latter class of theories assume that the domains of biological kinds have a special status in virtue of their fundamental evolutionary value. Although the picture of the empirical facts about category-specific deficits that we have painted is clear in its outlines, the details remain indistinct and uncertain. For example, the relationship between impairment to manufactured and natural foods remains unresolved, although there are indications that the two may dissociate. Also problematic for interpretation is the fact that all the reported cases presenting greater difficulty for fruit/vegetables than for animals were males, and it has been observed that relative to women, men are less familiar with fruit and vegetables than they are with animals. For a broader discussion of gender effects, see Barbarotto, Laiacona, Macchi, and Capitani (2002). More importantly, the relationship between impaired category and impaired type of knowledge is rather complicated. The complication comes from the fact that three distinct patterns of relationship between knowledge of object form and type of impaired category have been reliably documented. These patterns are schematically represented in Figure 1. The first pattern corresponds to selective deficits in object decision and in conceptual knowledge about the perceptual properties of living things. The second pattern corresponds to uniform damage to conceptual knowledge pertaining to the properties of biological kind objects, but spared ability to make object decisions for all objects. The third and most common pattern consists of selective damage to the category biological objects in object decision tasks and impairment for all types of conceptual knowledge about those objects.

Difficulties in object decision tasks have typically been interpreted as reflecting damage to the structural description system—a system that represents the visual form of objects for recognition. Available data indicate that the structural description system is organised into separate domains of knowledge such that they can be damaged independently of each other (see Table 3). This view entails the existence of pure category-specific agnosias, but our review has failed to find such cases (that are statistically reliable). Moreover, the different patterns of deficits in the object decision and conceptual knowledge tasks suggest that the structural description system functions relatively autonomously from conceptual knowledge about object form. This conclusion is motivated by the fact that there is no necessary association between difficulties in object decision and conceptual knowledge tasks, whether the latter tap knowledge about object form or their function: In particular, the same pattern (balanced semantic impairment of perceptual and functional/associative knowledge) can coexist with the sparing and with the impairment of the structural description system. However, two cases in which the structural description system was damaged in a categorical fashion (Michelangelo and Giulietta) were apparently affected by selective damage to perceptual semantic knowledge of biological categories in association with damage to the structural descriptions of the same categories. Some authors (Sartori & Job, 1988) have interpreted the latter pattern as indicating that the integrity of the structural descriptions of biological objects is necessary for the integrity of the semantic knowledge of the perceptual attributes of those objects.

This hypothesis has interesting implications. If the pattern of performance characterised by category-specific object decision impairment and modality-independent conceptual knowledge impairment (e.g., cases EW, GR, etc.) were to

A. Perceptual attributes worse than associative attributes only for natural categories: Structural description impaired only for natural categories (Giulietta and Michelangelo)

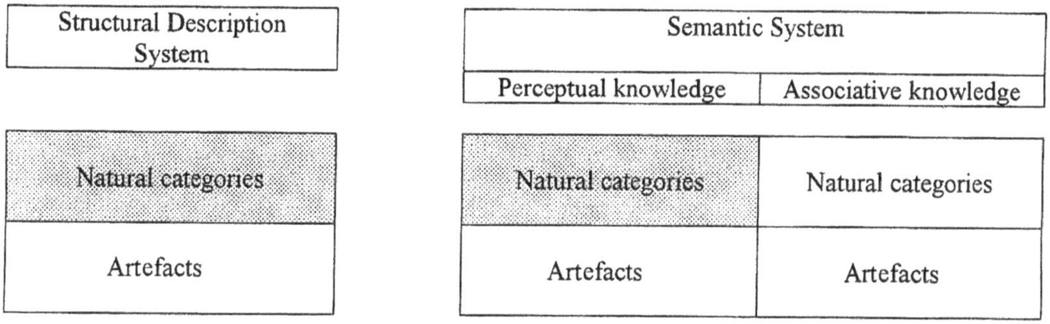

Structural Description System

Natural categories

Artefacts

Semantic System

| Perceptual knowledge | Associative knowledge |
|---|---|
| Natural categories | Natural categories |
| Artefacts | Artefacts |

B. Balanced deficit for perceptual and associative attributes of natural categories: Structural description spared (EA 2nd–3rd, FM, Jennifer, SB)

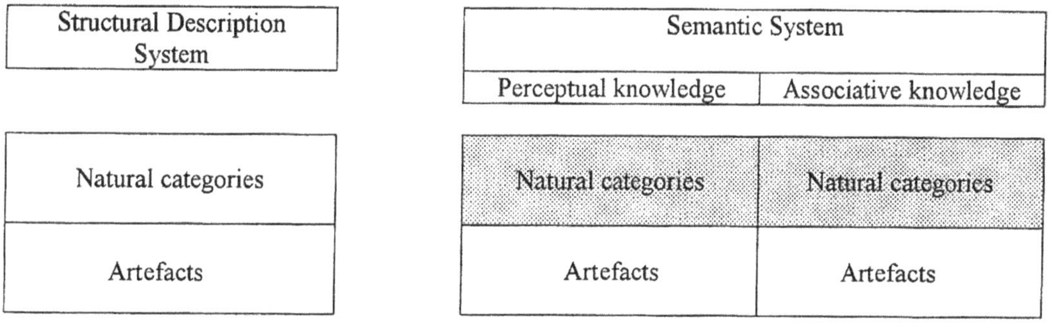

Structural Description System

Natural categories

Artefacts

Semantic System

| Perceptual knowledge | Associative knowledge |
|---|---|
| Natural categories | Natural categories |
| Artefacts | Artefacts |

C. Balance between the deficit for perceptual and associative attributes of natural categories: Structural description impaired for natural categories (CA, DB, EA 1st, Emma*, EW, GR, JBR*, MF, MU; * = artefacts were not reliably tested in the object reality decision)

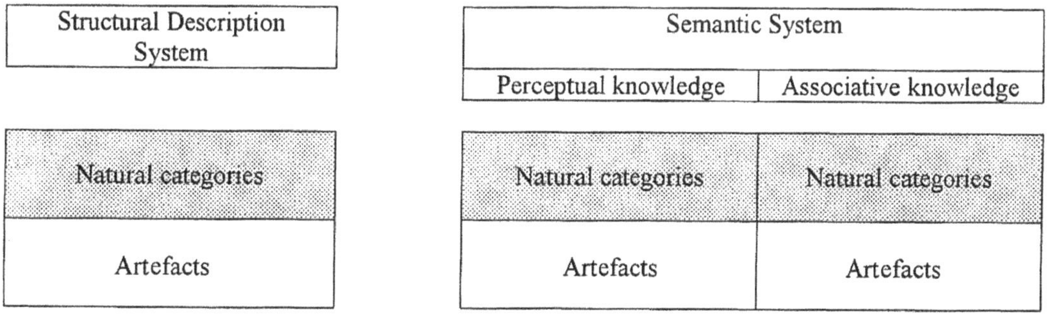

Structural Description System

Natural categories

Artefacts

Semantic System

| Perceptual knowledge | Associative knowledge |
|---|---|
| Natural categories | Natural categories |
| Artefacts | Artefacts |

**Figure 1.** *Deficits of perceptual and associative attributes.*

result from damage to both a categorically organised structural description system and a categorically organised homogeneous semantic system, it would be reasonable to expect that (1) these patients would in general be affected by a semantic deficit that is more severe for perceptual than functional/associative semantic knowledge, and (2) that they would tend to show more severe deficits in naming objects than patients with damage to only the conceptual system (e.g., patients FM, Jennifer, etc.). The analysis of the type of semantic impairment and of the severity of naming impairment across subgroups of patients (see Appendix F) failed to show this pattern of results: After angular transformation, the mean severity of the group with no damage to the structural description system (38. 6% correct) was not milder than the mean severity of the group with damage to the structural description system (44. 12% correct). This difference was not significant, $t(10) < 1$, n.s.

In conclusion, there are two clear facts that have emerged from this investigation of semantic category-specific deficits. First, the domain of biological kinds can be damaged independently of all other semantic categories tested and, furthermore, this domain of knowledge further fractionates into animate and inanimate domains. Second, the vast majority of category-specific semantic deficits typically involve to equal degrees all types of object properties (perceptual and functional/associative) in the affected categories. Theories of the organisation of conceptual knowledge that cannot account for these facts must be considered with suspicion.

## REFERENCES

(The cases described in each paper are shown in parentheses.)

Arguin, M., Bub, D., & Dudek, G. (1996). Shape integration for visual object recognition and its implication in category-specific visual agnosia. *Visual Cognition*, *3*, 221–275. (ELM)

Barbarotto, R., Capitani, E., & Laiacona, M. (1996). Naming deficit in herpes simplex encephalitis. *Acta Neurologica Scandinavica*, *93*, 272–280. (LF, EA, FA, FI)

Barbarotto, R., Capitani, E., & Laiacona, M. (2001). Living musical instruments and inanimate body parts? *Neuropsychologia*, *39*, 406–414.

Barbarotto, R., Capitani, E., Spinnler, H., & Trivelli, C. (1995). Slowly progressive semantic impairment with category specificity. *Neurocase*, *1*, 107–119. (MF)

Barbarotto, R., Laiacona, M., Macchi, V., & Capitani, E. (2002). Picture reality decision, semantic categories and gender. A new set of pictures, with norms and an experimental study. *Neuropsychologia*, *40*, 1637–1653.

Basso, A., Capitani, E., & Laiacona, M. (1988). Progressive language impairment without dementia: A case with isolated category specific semantic defect. *Journal of Neurology, Neurosurgery and Psychiatry*, *5*, 1201–1207. (NV)

Borgo, F., & Shallice, T. (2001). When living things and other "sensory-quality" categories behave in the same fashion: A novel category-specific effect. *Neurocase*, *7*, 201–220. (MU)

Breedin, S. D., Martin, N., & Saffran, E. M. (1994a). Category specific semantic impairments: An infrequent occurrence? *Brain and Language*, *47*, 383–386. (VP, CN94, PJ, DM94)

Breedin S. D., Saffran E. M., & Coslett, B. H. (1994b). Reversal of the concreteness effect in a patient with semantic dementia. *Cognitive Neuropsychology*, *11*, 617–660. (DM94)

Bunn, E. M., Tyler, L. K., & Moss, E. (1997). Patient JBR: The role of familiarity and property type in a selective deficit for living things. *Brain and Language*, *60*, 10–12. (JBR)

Capitani, E., & Laiacona, M. (2000). Classification and modelling in neuropsychology: From groups to single cases. In F. Boller & J. Grafman (Eds.), *Handbook of neuropsychology*, *Vol. 1* (2nd ed., pp. 53–76). Amsterdam: Elsevier.

Capitani, E., Laiacona, M., & Barbarotto, R. (1993). Dissociazioni semantiche intercategoriali. Parte II: procedura automatica di analisi di una batteria standardizzata. *Archivio di Psicologia, Neurologia e Psichiatria*, *54*, 457–476. (CA)

Cappa, S. F., Frugoni, M., Pasquali, P., Perani, D., & Zorat, F. (1998). Category-specific naming impairment for artefacts: A new case. *Neurocase*, *4*, 391–397. (GP98)

Caramazza, A. (1986). On drawing inferences about the structure of normal cognitive systems from the analysis of patterns of impaired performance: The case for single-patient studies. *Brain and Cognition*, *5*, 41–66.

Caramazza, A. (1998). The interpretation of semantic category-specific deficits: What do they reveal about the organisation of the conceptual knowledge in the brain? *Neurocase, 4*, 265–272

Caramazza, A., Hillis, A. E., Rapp, B., & Romani, C. (1990). The multiple semantics hypothesis: Multiple confusion? *Cognitive Neuropsychology, 7*, 161–189.

Caramazza, A., & Shelton, J. R. (1998). Domain-specific knowledge systems in the brain: The animate-inanimate distinction. *Journal of Cognitive Neuroscience, 10*, 1–34. (EW)

Carbonnel, S., Charnallet, A., David, D., & Pellat, J. (1997). One or several semantic systems? Maybe none: Evidence from a case study of modality and category-specific "semantic" impairment. *Cortex, 33*, 391–417. (EC)

Cardebat, D., Demonet, J.-F., Celsis, P., & Puel, M. (1996). Living/nonliving dissociation in a case of semantic dementia: a SPECT activation study. *Neuropsychologia, 34,* 1175–1179. (GC)

Damasio, A. R. (1990). Category-related recognition defects as a clue to the neural substrates of knowledge. *Trends in Neuroscience, 13*, 95–98.

Damasio, H., Grabowski, T. J., Tranel, D., Hichwa, R. B., & Damasio, A. R. (1996). A neural basis for lexical retrieval. *Nature, 380*, 499–505.

De Haan, E. H. F., Young, A. W., & Newcombe, F. (1992). Neuropsychological impairment of face recognition units. *Quarterly Journal of Experimental Psychology, 44A*, 141–175. (NR)

De Renzi, E., & Lucchelli, F. (1994). Are semantic systems separately represented in the brain? The case of living category impairment. *Cortex, 30*, 3–25. (Felicia)

Devlin, J. T., Gonnerman, L. M., Andersen, E. S., & Seidenberg, M. S. (1998). Category-specific semantic deficit in focal and widespread brain damage: A computational account. *Journal of Cognitive Neuroscience, 10*, 77–94.

Dixon, M. J. (1999). Tool and bird identification in a patient with category-specific agnosia. *Brain and Cognition, 40*, 97–100. (ELM)

Dixon, M. J., & Arguin, M. (1999). Shape-set dimensionality vs. structural distance effects in a patient with category-specific visual agnosia. *Brain and Cognition, 40*, 101–104. (ELM)

Dixon, M. J., Bub, D. N., & Arguin, M. (1997). The interaction of object form and object meaning in the identification performance of a patient with category-specific visual agnosia. *Cognitive Neuropsychology, 14*, 1085–1130. (ELM)

Dixon, M. J., Piskopos, K., & Schweizer, T. A. (2000). Musical instrument naming impairments: the crucial exception to the living/nonliving dichotomy in category-specific agnosia. *Brain and Cognition, 43*, 158–164. (FS)

Etcoff, N. L., Freeman, R., & Cave, K. R. (1991). Can we lose memories of faces? Content specificity and awareness in a prosopagnosic. *Journal of Cognitive Neuroscience, 3*, 25–41. (LH)

Farah, M. J. (1997). Distinguishing perceptual and semantic impairments affecting visual object recognition. *Visual Cognition, 4*, 199–206. (Mr.W)

Farah, M. J., Hammond, K. M., Mehta, Z., & Ratcliff, G. (1989). Category-specificity and modality-specificity in semantic memory. *Neuropsychologia, 27*, 193–200. (LH)

Farah, M. J., & McClelland, J. L. (1991). A computational model of semantic memory impairment: Modality specific and emergent category specificity. *Journal of Experimental Psychology General, 120*, 339–357.

Farah, M. J., McMullen, P. A., & Meyer, M. M. (1991). Can recognition of living things be selectively impaired? *Neuropsychologia, 29*, 185–193. (LH, MB)

Farah, M. J., Meyer, M. M., & McMullen, P. A. (1996). The living/nonliving dissociation is not an artifact: giving an a priori implausible hypothesis a strong test. *Cognitive Neuropsychology, 13*, 137–154. (LH, MB)

Farah, M. J., & Wallace, M. A. (1992). Semantically-bounded anomia: Implications for the neural implementation of naming. *Neuropsychologia, 30*, 609–621. (TU)

Forde, E. M. E., Francis, D., Riddoch, M. J., Rumiati, R. I., & Humphreys, G. W. (1997). On the links between visual knowledge and naming: A single case study of a patient with a category-specific impairment for living things. *Cognitive Neuropsychology, 14,* 403–458. (SRB)

Forde, E. M. E., & Humphreys, G. W. (1999). Category-specific recognition impairments: A review of important case studies and influential theories. *Aphasiology, 13*, 169–193.

Funnell, E. (2000). Apperceptive agnosia and the visual recognition of the object categories in dementia of the Alzheimer type. *Neurocase, 6*, 451–463. (NA)

Funnell, E., & De Mornay Davies, P. (1996). JBR: A reassessment of concept familiarity and a category-specific disorder for living things. *Neurocase, 2*, 461–474. (JBR)

Gaillard, M. J., Auzou, P., Miret, M., Ozsancak, C., & Hannequin, D. (1998). Trouble de la dénomination pour les objets manufacturés dans un cas d'encéphalite herpétique. *Révue Neurologique, 154*, 683–689. (CN98)

Gainotti, G. (2000). What the locus of brain lesion tell us about the nature of the cognitive defect underlying category-specific disorders: A review. *Cortex, 36*, 539–559.

Gainotti, G., & Silveri, M. C. (1996). Cognitive and anatomical locus of lesion in a patient with a category-specific semantic impairment for living beings. *Cognitive Neuropsychology, 13*, 357–389. (LA)

Garrard, P., Lambon Ralph, M. A., Hodges, J. R., & Patterson, K. (2001). Prototypicality, distinctiveness and intercorrelation: Analyses of semantic attributes of living and nonliving concepts. *Cognitive Neuropsychology, 18*, 125–174.

Garrard, P., Patterson, K., Watson, P., & Hodges, J. R. (1998). Category-specific semantic loss in dementia of Alzheimer's type. Functional-anatomical correlations from cross-sectional analyses. *Brain, 121*, 633–646. (Case identity unspecified)

Gentileschi, V., Sperber, S., & Spinnler, H. (2001). Cross-modal agnosia for familiar people as a consequence of right infero-polar temporal atrophy. *Cognitive Neuropsychology, 18*, 439–463. (Emma)

Goldenberg, G. (1992). Loss of visual imagery and loss of visual knowledge: A case study. *Neuropsychologia, 30*, 1081–1099.

Gonnerman, L. M., Andersen, E. S., Devlin, J. T., Kempler, D., & Seidenberg, M. S. (1997). Double dissociation of semantic categories in Alzheimer disease. *Brain and Language, 57*, 254–279. (NB, GP97)

Hanley, J. R., Young, A. W., & Pearson, N. A. (1989). Defective recognition of familiar people. *Cognitive Neuropsychology, 6*, 179–210. (BD)

Hart, J., Berndt, R. S., & Caramazza, A. (1985). Category-specific naming deficit following cerebral infarction. *Nature, 316*, 439–440. (MD)

Hart, J., & Gordon, B. (1992). Neural subsystems for object knowledge. *Nature, 359*, 60–64. (KR)

Hauser, M. D. (1997). Artifactual kinds and functional design features: What a primate understands without language. *Cognition, 64*, 285–308.

Hécaen, H., & De Ajuriaguerra, J. (1956). Agnosie visuelle pour les objets inanimées par lésion unilatérale gauche. *Révue Neurologique, 94*, 222–233. (M. Lucien)

Hillis, A. E., & Caramazza, A. (1991). Category-specific naming and comprehension impairment: A double dissociation. *Brain, 114*, 2081–2094. (JJ, PS)

Hillis, A. E., Rapp, B., Romani, C., & Caramazza, A. (1990). Selective impairment of semantics in lexical processing. *Cognitive Neuropsychology, 7*, 191–243. (KE)

Humphreys, G. W., & Forde, E. M. E. (2001). Hierarchies, similarity, and interactivity in object recognition: "Category-specific" neuropsychological deficits. *Behavioural and Brain Sciences, 24*, 453–509.

Humphreys, G. W., Riddoch, M. J., & Price, C. J. (1997). Top-down processes in object identification: Evidence from experimental psychology, neuropsychology and functional anatomy. *Philosophical Transactions of the Royal Society (B), 352*, 1275–1282. (SRB, DM97)

Humphreys, G. W., Riddoch, M. J., & Quinlan, P. T. (1988). Cascade processes in picture identification. *Cognitive Neuropsychology, 5*, 67–103. (JB)

Laiacona, M., Barbarotto, R., & Capitani, E. (1993). Perceptual and associative knowledge in category specific impairment of semantic memory: A study of two cases. *Cortex, 29*, 727–740. (FM, GR)

Laiacona, M., Barbarotto, R., & Capitani, E. (1998). Semantic category dissociation in naming: Is there a gender effect in Alzheimer disease? *Neuropsychologia, 36*, 407–419. (no. 1, 2, 3, 4, 5, 6, 7, 8 / no. 24, 25, 26)

Laiacona, M., & Capitani, E. (2001). A case of prevailing deficit of nonliving categories or a case of prevailing sparing of living categories? *Cognitive Neuropsychology, 18*, 39–70. (PL)

Laiacona, M., Capitani, E., & Barbarotto, R. (1997). Semantic category dissociation: A longitudinal study of two cases. *Cortex, 33*, 441–461. (LF, EA)

Laiacona, M., Capitani, E., & Caramazza, A. (in press). Category-specific semantic deficits do not reflect the sensory- functional organisation of the brain: A test of the "sensory- quality" hypothesis. *Neurocase.*

Lambon Ralph, M. A., Howard, D., Nightingale, G., & Ellis, A. W. (1998). Are living and nonliving category-specific deficits causally linked to impaired perceptual or associative knowledge? Evidence from a category-specific double dissociation. *Neurocase, 4*, 311–338. (DB, IW)

Laurent, B., Allegri, R. F., Michel, D., Trillet, M., Naegele-Faure, B., Foyatier, N., & Pellat, J. (1990). Encéphalites herpétiques à prédominance unilatérale. Etude neuropsychologique au long cours de 9 cas. *Revue Neurologique, 146*, 671–681.

Laws, K. R. (1998). Leopards never change their spots: A reply to Moss, Tyler, and Jennings. *Cognitive Neuropsychology, 15*, 467–479. (SE)

Laws, K. R., Evans, J. J., Hodges, J. R., & McCarthy, R. A. (1995). Naming without knowing and appearance without associations: Evidence for constructive processes in semantic memory? In R. A. McCarthy (Ed.), *Semantic knowledge and semantic representations* (pp. 409–433). Hove, UK: Lawrence Erlbaum Associates Ltd. (SE)

Lecours, S., Arguin, M., Bub, D., Caille, S., & Fontaine, S. (1999). Semantic proximity and shape feature integration effects in visual agnosia for biological kinds. *Brain and Cognition*, *40*, 171–173. (IL)

Magnié, M. N., Ferreira, C. T., Giusiano, B., & Poncet, M. (1999). Category specificity in object agnosia: Preservation of sensorimotor experiences related to objects. *Neuropsychologia*, *37*, 67–74. (JMC)

Martin, A., Ungerleider, L. G., & Haxby, J. V. (2000). Category specificity and the brain: The sensory/motor model of semantic representations of objects. In M. S. Gazzaniga (Ed.), *The new cognitive neurosciences* (pp. 1023–1036). Cambridge, MA: MIT Press.

Mauri, A., Daum, I., Sartori, G., Riesch, G., & Birbaumer, N. (1994). Category-specific semantic impairment in Alzheimer's disease and temporal lobe dysfunction: A comparative study. *Journal of Clinical and Experimental Neuropsychology*, *16*, 689–701. (Helga, Michelangelo)

McCarthy, R. A., & Warrington, E. K. (1988). Evidence for modality-specific meaning systems in the brain. *Nature*, *334*, 428–430. (TOB)

McCarthy, R. A., & Warrington, E. K. (1990). The dissolution of semantics. *Nature*, *343*, 599. (TOB)

Mehta, Z., Newcombe, F., & De Haan, E. (1992). Selective loss of imagery in a case of visual agnosia. *Neuropsychologia*, *30*, 645–655. (MS)

Moss, H. E., & Tyler, L. K. (1997). A category-specific semantic deficit for nonliving things in a case of progressive aphasia. *Brain and Language*, *60*, 55–58. (ES)

Moss, H. E., & Tyler, L. K. (2000). A progressive category-specific semantic deficit for nonliving things. *Neuropsychologia*, *38*, 60–82. (ES)

Moss, H. E., Tyler, L. K., Durrant-Peatfield, M., & Bunn, E. M. (1998). "Two eyes of a see-through": Impaired and intact semantic knowledge in a case of selective deficit for living things. *Neurocase*, *4*, 291–310. (RC)

Moss, H. E., Tyler, L. K., & Jennings, F. (1997). When leopards lose their spots: Knowledge of visual properties in category-specific deficits for living things. *Cognitive Neuropsychology*, *14*, 901–950. (SE)

Parkin, A. J. (1993). Progressive aphasia without dementia: A clinical and cognitive neuropsychological analysis. *Brain and Language*, *44*, 201–220. (TOB)

Pietrini, V., Nertempi, P., Vaglia, A., Revello, M. G., Pinna, V., & Ferro-Milone, F. (1988). Recovery from herpes simplex encephalitis: Selective impairment of specific semantic categories with neuroradiological correlation. *Journal of Neurology, Neurosurgery and Psychiatry*, *51*, 1284–1293. (RM, JV)

Riddoch, M. J., & Humphreys, G. W. (1987a). A case of integrative visual agnosia. *Brain*, *110*, 1431–1462. (HJA)

Riddoch, M. J., & Humphreys, G. W. (1987b). Visual object processing in optic aphasia: A case of semantic access agnosia. *Cognitive Neuropsychology*, *4*, 131–185. (JB)

Riddoch, M. J., Humphreys, G. W., Gannon, T., Blott, W., & Jones, V. (1999). Memories are made of this: The effects of time on stored visual knowledge in a case of visual agnosia. *Brain*, *122*, 537–559. (HJA)

Rumiati, R. I., & Humphreys, G. W. (1997). Visual object agnosia without alexia or prosopoagnosia: Arguments for separate knowledge stores. *Visual Cognition*, *4*, 207–217. (MrW)

Rumiati, R. I., Humphreys, G. W., Riddoch, M. J., & Bateman, A. (1994). Visual object agnosia without prosopoagnosia or alexia: Evidence for hierarchical theories of visual recognition. *Visual Cognition*, *1*, 181–225. (MrW)

Sacchett, C., & Humphreys, G. W. (1992). Calling a squirrel a squirrel but a canoe a wigwam: A category-specific deficit for artifactual objects and body parts. *Cognitive Neuropsychology*, *9*, 73–86. (CW92)

Samson, D., Pillon, A., & De Wilde, V. (1998). Impaired knowledge of visual and nonvisual attributes in a patient with a semantic impairment for living entities: A case of a true category-specific deficit. *Neurocase*, *4*, 273–290. (Jennifer)

Santos, L. R., & Caramazza, A. (2002). The domain specific hypothesis: A developmental and comparative perspective on category-specific deficits. In E. M. E. Forde & G. W. Humphreys (Eds.), *Category-specificity in brain and mind* (pp. 1–23). Hove, UK: Psychology Press.

Sartori, G., Coltheart, M., Miozzo, M., & Job, R. (1994a). Category specificity and informational specificity in neuropsychological impairment of semantic memory. In C. A. Umiltà & M. Moscovitch (Eds.), *Attention and performance XV* (pp. 537–550). Cambridge, MA: MIT Press. (Michelangelo)

Sartori, G., & Job, R. (1988). The oyster with four legs: A neuropsychological study on the interaction between vision and semantic information. *Cognitive Neuropsychology, 5*, 105–132. (Michelangelo)

Sartori, G., Job, R., & Coltheart, M. (1993a). The organisation of object knowledge: Evidence from neuropsychology. In D. E. Meyer & S. Kornblum (Eds.), *Attention and performance XIV* (pp. 451–465). Cambridge, MA: MIT Press. (Michelangelo, Dante)

Sartori, G., Job, R., Miozzo, M., Zago, S., & Marchiori, G. (1993b). Category-specific form-knowledge deficit in a patient with herpes simplex virus encephalitis. *Journal of Clinical and Experimental Neuropsychology, 15*, 280–299. (Giulietta)

Sartori, G., Miozzo, M., & Job, R. (1993c). Category-specific naming impairments? Yes. *Quarterly Journal of Experimental Psychology, 46(A)*, 489–504. (Michelangelo)

Sartori, G., Miozzo, M., & Job, R. (1994). Rehabilitation of semantic memory impairments. In M. J. Riddoch & G. W. Humphreys (Eds.), *Cognitive neuropsychology and cognitive rehabilitation* (pp. 103–124). Hove, UK: Lawrence Erlbaum Associates Ltd. (Giulietta, Michelangelo)

Shelton, J. R., & Caramazza, A. (2001). The organisation of semantic memory. In B. Rapp (Ed.), *The handbook of cognitive neuropsychology* (pp. 423–443). Hove, UK: Psychology Press.

Shelton, J. R., Fouch, E., & Caramazza, A. (1998). The selective sparing of body part knowledge: A case study. *Neurocase, 4*, 339–351.

Sheridan, J., & Humphreys, G. W. (1993). A verbal-semantic, category-specific recognition impairment. *Cognitive Neuropsychology, 10*, 143–184. (SB)

Silveri, M. C., & Gainotti, G. (1988). Interaction between vision and language in category-specific semantic impairment, *Cognitive Neuropsychology, 5*, 677–709. (LA)

Silveri, M. C., Gainotti, G., Perani, D., Cappelletti, J. Y., Carbone, G., & Fazio, F. (1997). Naming deficit for non-living items: Neuropsychological and PET study. *Neuropsychologia, 35*, 359–367. (CG)

Silveri, M. C., Perri, R., & Cappa, A. (2000). *I deficit selettivi per il nome e per il verbo hanno origine a livello semantico?* Paper presented at the Autumn Meeting of the Italian Neuropsychological Society, Bologna, November 17–18. (CG)

Sirigu, A., Duhamel, J.-R., & Poncet, M. (1991). The role of sensorimotor experience in object recognition. *Brain, 114*, 2555–2573. (FB)

Swales, M., & Johnson, R. (1992). Patients with semantic memory loss: Can they relearn lost concepts? *Neuropsychological Rehabilitation, 2*, 295–305. (JH)

Takarae, Y., & Levin, D. T. (2001). Animals and artifacts may not be treated equally: Differentiating strong and weak fonts of category-specific visual agnosia. *Brain and Cognition, 45*, 249–264. (ELM, LH, MB)

Teixeira Ferreira, C., Giusiano, B., & Poncet, M. (1997). Category-specific anomia: Implication of different neural networks in naming. *Neuroreport, 8*, 1595–1602. (MC, PR, VG)

Temple, M. C. (1986). Anomia for animals in a child. *Brain, 109*, 1225–1242.

Tippett, L. J., Glosser, G., & Farah, M. J. (1996). A category-specific naming impairment after temporal lobectomy. *Neuropsychologia, 34*, 139–146. (Case identity not specified)

Turnbull, O. H., & Laws, K. R. (2000). Loss of stored knowledge of object structure: Implication for "Category-specific" deficits. *Cognitive Neuropsychology, 17*, 365–389. (SM)

Tyler, L. K., & Moss, H. E. (1997). Functional properties of concepts: Studies of normal and brain damaged patients. *Cognitive Neuropsychology, 14*, 511–545. (RC)

Warrington, E. K., & McCarthy, R. A. (1983). Category specific access in dysphasia. *Brain, 106*, 859–878. (VER)

Warrington, E. K., & McCarthy, R. A. (1987). Categories of knowledge. Further fractionation and an attempted integration. *Brain, 110*, 1273–1296. (YOT)

Warrington, E. K., & McCarthy, R. A. (1994). Multiple meaning systems in the brain: A case for visual semantics. *Neuropsychologia, 32*, 1465–1473. (DRS)

Warrington, E. K., & Shallice, T. (1984). Category specific semantic impairments. *Brain, 107*, 829–854. (KB, JBR, SBY, ING)

Wilson, B. A. (1997). Semantic memory impairments following nonprogressive brain injury: A study of four cases. *Brain Injury, 11*, 259–269. (KG, TS, JBR, CW97)

Wilson, B. A., Baddeley, A. D., & Kapur, N. (1995). Dense amnesia in a professional musician following herpes simplex virus encephalitis. *Journal of Clinical and Experimental Neuropsychology, 17*, 668–681. (C)

Young, A. W., Newcombe, F., Hellawell, D., & De Haan, E. (1989). Implicit access to semantic information. *Brain and Cognition, 11*, 186–209. (MS)

# APPENDIX A

## Cases presenting a category dissociation

We report all the cases to our knowledge that showed a category dissociation in picture naming or in any other task. We did not consider cases whose data were not clearly reported or submitted to a statistical analysis even if they could potentially be relevant (e.g., Laurent et al., 1990, Case 9; Goldenberg, 1992; Damasio, 1990). In section 1 are grouped the single cases showing a prevailing natural categories impairment and in section 2 cases presenting a prevailing artefacts impairment. For the complete reference see Appendix E. Cases of finer-grained dissociations within biological categories are italicised (strong evidence) or underlined (possible evidence; see also Table 4).

### *1. Primary biological categories impairment*

| *Case/Authors* | *Age, gender* | *Disproportionately impaired categories* | *Aetiology* | *Lesion site* |
|---|---|---|---|---|
| BD<br>Hanley et al., 1989 | 55, M | Animals, fruit and vegetables | HSE | Right T (posterior part of superior T gyrus) |
| C (CW97)<br>Wilson, 1997;<br>Wilson et al., 1995 | 46, M | Animals (other biological categories not examined) | HSE | Bilateral: T poles, hippocampus, amygdala, Mam-b; Left: inferior, middle and superior T gyri, insula, medial F, striatum; Right: inferior T gyrus, insula. |
| CA<br>Capitani et al., 1993 | 68, M | Biological categories (animals, fruit and vegetables not analysed separately) | Progressive aphasia | Left sylvian atrophy |
| DANTE<br>Sartori et al., 1993a | 22, M | Animate (not further specified) | Encephalitis | Not reported |
| DB<br>Lambon Ralph et al., 1998 | 86, F | Animals (fruit and vegetables not tested in most tasks) | DAT | Bilateral general and mesial T atrophy |
| DM94<br>Breedin et al., 1994a, 1994b | 56, M | Animals, insects (fruit and vegetables not tested) + musical instruments | Focal degenerative | MRI = normal<br>SPECT = inferior T-O (more severe to left) |
| DM97<br>Humphreys et al., 1997 | 44, F | Animate stimuli (not further specified) | Brain abscess | Left medial and inferior T-O |
| EA<br>Barbarotto et al., 1996;<br>Laiacona et al., 1997 | 47, M | Biological categories (animals, fruit and vegetables not analysed separately) and musical instruments. After 9 years animals and musical instruments were still defective, but less impaired than fruit and vegetables | HSE | Left T: middle, inferior, fusiform and lingual; parahippocampal gyrus was spared, partial involvement of hippocampus |
| EC<br>Carbonnel et al., 1997 | 55, M | Animals (plants slightly impaired) | Anoxia | No lesion on MRI |
| ELM<br>Arguin et al., 1996;<br>Dixon, 1999; Dixon & Arguin, 1999; Dixon et al., 1997;<br>Takarae & Levin, 2001 | 68, M | Fruit and vegetables; animals less severe | Stroke | Bilateral inferior T |
| EMMA<br>Gentileschi et al., 2001 | 60, F | Biological (not further specified) | Focal degeneration | Bilateral infero-polar T, right more severe than left |

| Case/Authors | Age, gender | Disproportionately impaired categories | Aetiology | Lesion site |
|---|---|---|---|---|
| EW<br>Caramazza & Shelton, 1998 | 72, F | Animals (sparing fruit and vegetables and all the other categories) | Stroke | Left posterior F and P |
| FA<br>Barbarotto et al., 1996 | 56, M | Biological categories (animals, fruit and vegetables not analysed separately) | HSE | Left T lateral, mainly middle and inferior; Right F, rectus and cingulate gyri |
| FB<br>Sirigu et al., 1991 | 19, M | Animals and food | HSE | Bilateral T: pole and inferior neocortex, hippocampus, amygdala |
| FELICIA<br>De Renzi & Lucchelli, 1994 | 49, F | Biological categories (animals, fruit, vegetables and flowers) + food | HSE | Left F-T and insula; right T-insula |
| FI<br>Barbarotto et al., 1996 | 68, M | Biological categories (animals, fruit and vegetables were not analysed separately) | HSE | Left T (hippocampus, parahippocampus and basal), insula and F basal; right deep peri-ventricular white matter |
| FM<br>Laiacona et al., 1993 | 20, M | Biological categories (animals, fruit and vegetables not analysed separately) and musical instruments | Head injury | Left F-T |
| FS<br>Dixon et al., 2000 | 50, M | Animals and musical instruments (four items each) (other LC categories not tested) | HSE | Not reported |
| GC<br>Cardebat et al., 1996 | 72, F | Animals (fruit and vegetables not tested) | Progressive aphasia | Left T atrophy, mesial and posterior |
| GIULIETTA<br>Sartori et al., 1993b | 55, F | Animals (fruit and vegetables in a preliminary test) | HSE | Bilateral T and hippocampus |
| GP97<br>Gonnerman et al., 1997 | 61, M | Biological (fruit and vegetables) more impaired than artefacts (furniture, vehicles, clothing, weapons). Animals not included | DAT | Mild cerebral atrophy consistent with the subject's age |
| GR<br>Laiacona et al., 1993 | 22, M | Biological categories (animals, fruit and vegetables not analysed separately, *but possible greater impairment of fruit and vegetables*). Musical instruments impaired | Head injury | Left F-T |
| HELGA<br>Mauri et al., 1994 | 60, F | Animals and vegetables (not analysed separately) | DAT | No atrophy on CT-scan |
| HJA<br>Riddoch & Humphreys, 1987a;<br>Riddoch et al., 1999 | 61, M | Animals, fruit and vegetables (and body parts, see comments) | Stroke | Bilateral inferior T, OT, fusiform, lingual |
| IL<br>Lecours et al., 1999 | 75, M | Biological items | HSE | Not reported |
| ING<br>Warrington & Shallice, 1984 | 44, F | Animals, food | HSE | T-bilateral |
| JB<br>Riddoch & Humphreys, 1987b;<br>Humphreys et al., 1988 | 45, M | Animals, fruit and vegetables. Their impairment on picture naming was balanced. Body parts were relatively spared. | Head injury | Left PO |

| *Case/Authors* | *Age, gender* | *Disproportionately impaired categories* | *Aetiology* | *Lesion site* |
|---|---|---|---|---|
| JBR<br>Warrington & Shallice, 1984; Bunn et al., 1997; Funnell & De Mornay Davies, 1996; Wilson, 1997 | 23, M | Biological categories and foods. Musical instruments impaired and body parts spared in a word definition task | HSE | T-bilateral |
| JENNIFER<br>Samson et al., 1998 | 22, F | Animals, fruit, vegetables (not significantly different) | Head injury | Atrophy of posterior L hemisphere |
| JH<br>Swales & Johnson, 1992 | 53, M | Animals, fruit and vegetables | HSE | Left T |
| JMC<br>Magniè et al., 1999 | 58, M | Animals, fruit, vegetables, musical instruments | Post-anoxic | CT-scan: no lesion |
| JV<br>Pietrini et al., 1988 | 47, M | *Plants (more severe than animals)* | HSE | Left: anterior and middle T, F basal, insula; Right: insula |
| KB<br>Warrington & Shallice, 1984 | 60, F | Animals, food | HSE | T-bilateral, left more severe |
| KG<br>Wilson, 1997 | 27, F | Animals (other natural categories not examined) and musical instruments | Head injury | Left T antero-lateral, P inferior |
| KR<br>Hart & Gordon, 1992 | 70, F | Animals (see Appendix E) | Para-neoplastic | Diffuse, especially T lobes bilaterally |
| LA<br>Silveri & Gainotti, 1988; Gainotti & Silveri, 1996 | 54, F | *Animals possibly more severe than flowers. Fruit and vegetables.* Food intermediate (1st exam), more severe at 2nd exam. Musical instruments (2nd exam) impaired | HSE | Bilateral inferior T (L more severe). On the left: hippocampus and amygdala. |
| LF<br>Barbarotto et al.,1996; Laiacona et al., 1997 | 43, M | Biological categories (animals, fruit and vegetables), not analysed separately | HSE | Left whole T, part of F, hippocampus, and parahippocampal gyrus. Right: T basal, fusiform and parahippocampal gyrus |
| LH<br>Farah et al., 1989, 1991, 1996; Etcoff et al., 1991; Takarae et al., 2001 | 36, M | Biological categories: *more severe with animals*, probably intermediate with fruit and vegetables (Etcoff et al.). Musical instruments intermediate and body parts just mildly impaired | Head injury | Right: very severe T and F; Left: subcortical O-T; bilateral P-O |
| MB<br>Farah et al., 1991, 1996; Takarae et al., 2001 | 30, F | Biological categories (not further distinguished). Musical instruments intermediate and body parts spared | Head injury | Left T swelling, without focal damage |
| MC<br>Teixeira Ferreira et al., 1997 | 59, M | Animals (other natural categories not tested) | Stroke | Left medial-inferior T; right inferior T |
| MD<br>Hart et al., 1985 | 34, M | Fruit and vegetables (other categories spared, including animals and food) | Stroke | Left F and basal ganglia |
| MF<br>Barbarotto et al., 1995 | 60, M | Biological categories (animals, fruit and vegetables not analysed separately). Musical instruments were intermediate | Progressive focal degeneration | Right T severe atrophy, involving hippocampus and parahippocampal gyrus. Left T mildly involved later |

| *Case/Authors* | *Age, gender* | *Disproportionately impaired categories* | *Aetiology* | *Lesion site* |
|---|---|---|---|---|
| MICHELANGELO<br>Sartori & Job, 1988; Sartori et al., 1993a, 1993b, 1994a, 1994b; Mauri et al., 1994 | 38, M | Animals and vegetables | HSE | T anterior, bilateral |
| MS<br>Young et al., 1989;<br>Mehta et al., 1992 | 41-43, M | Biological categories | HSE | Bilateral T-O |
| MU<br>Borgo & Shallice, 2001 | 30, M | Biological categories, liquids, edible substances, nonedible materials | HSE | Bilateral T lobes and F lobes (medial portions); right O lobe (medial portion) |
| NA<br>Funnell, 2000 | 70, F | Possible greater impairment of biological categories (especially insects) | DAT | Bilateral T-P atrophy (more marked on the right) |
| NR<br>De Haan et al., 1992 | 29, M | Biological categories | Head injury | Right P and left T-P |
| NV<br>Basso et al., 1988 | 73, M | Biological categories and musical instruments | Progressive aphasia | Left T atrophy |
| PR<br>Teixeira Ferreira et al., 1997 | 69, M | Animals (other biological categories not tested) | HSE | Left medial-inferior T; right inferior T |
| PS<br>Hillis & Caramazza, 1991 | 45, M | Animals and vegetables (fruit intermediate, foods spared) | Head injury | Bilateral T subdural haematoma; left F haematoma; right F epidural haematoma |
| RC<br>Tyler & Moss, 1997;<br>Moss et al., 1998 | 37, M | Animals, fruit and vegetables (balanced impairment) | HSE | Bilateral T, left more severe |
| RM<br>Pietrini et al., 1988 | 23, M | Animals and plants | HSE | Left T and F basal |
| SB<br>Sheridan & Humphreys, 1993 | 19, F | Animals, food (including fruit and vegetables) | HSE | Left T oedema |
| SBY<br>Warrington & Shallice, 1984 | 48, M | Biological categories and food | HSE | Bilateral T |
| SE<br>Laws et al., 1995;<br>Laws, 1998;<br>Moss et al., 1997 | 60, M (left-handed) | Biological categories (main focus on animals) | HSE | Left nearly normal (slight signal alteration on uncus and amygdala); right: inferior and lateral T, uncus, hippocampus, parahippocampal gyrus, insula |
| SRB<br>Forde et al., 1997;<br>Humphreys et al., 1997 | 38, M | Biological categories (*fruit and vegetables probably more impaired than animals*) | AVM haemorrhage | Left: T (inferior medial), O; right: Thalamic infarction |
| TOB<br>McCarthy & Warrington, 1988, 1990; Parkin et al., 1993 | 63, M | Biological categories (not further split) were disproportionately impaired only in a spoken names definition task | Progressive aphasia | Left T (at PET scan) |

| Case/Authors | Age, gender | Disproportionately impaired categories | Aetiology | Lesion site |
|---|---|---|---|---|
| TS<br>Wilson, 1997 | 31, M | Animals (other biological categories not examined) | Head injury | Generalised atrophy, especially left superior T |
| TU<br>Farah & Wallace, 1992 | 51, M | *Fruit and vegetables (animals probably intermediate)* | AVM haemorrhage | Left O |
| VG<br>Teixeira Ferreira et al., 1997 | 48, F | Animals (other biological categories not tested) | HSE | Left medial-inferior T |
| MR. W<br>Rumiati et al., 1994; Rumiati & Humphreys, 1997; Farah, 1997 | 88, M | Biological categories ("structurally similar categories") inconsistently worse | ? | Cerebral and cerebellar atrophia |

## 2. *Primary artefacts impairment*

| Case/Authors | Age, gender | Disproportionately impaired categories | Aetiology | Lesion site |
|---|---|---|---|---|
| CG<br>Silveri et al., 1997, 2000 | 66, M | Artefacts more impaired than biological items or animals. Artefacts were not explicitly contrasted. Musical instruments were very close to artefacts | Progressive atrophy | Left T |
| CN94<br>Breedin et al., 1994a | Not reported | Tools more impaired than animals | Stroke | Left FP |
| CN98<br>Gaillard et al., 1998 | 25, F | Impaired artefacts (on naming: not further distinguished; on the questionnaire: tools). Spared biological items (on naming: not further distinguished; on the questionnaire: fruit and vegetables) | HSE | Left anterior and infero-mesial T |
| CW92<br>Sacchett & Humphreys, 1992 | 39, M | Artefacts (not analysed at a finer level of fractionation) and musical instruments more impaired than animals | Stroke | Left FP |
| DRS<br>Warrington & McCarthy, 1994 | 59, M | Common objects more impaired than animals, vehicles, and flowers | Stroke | Right P and left OT |
| ES<br>Moss & Tyler, 1997, 2000 | 67, F[a] | Artefacts more impaired than biological categories, without further distinction | Progressive aphasia | Cerebral atrophy, inf T lobes bilaterally more extensive on the right |
| GP98<br>Cappa et al., 1998 | 27, M | Tools, furniture, more impaired than vehicles, musical instruments, vegetables and animals; Fruit and body parts probably spared on naming | Bleeding of AVM plus polectomy | Left anterior T |
| IW<br>Lambon Ralph et al., 1998 | 53, F[b] | Artefacts more impaired than biological categories (no further distinguished) | Progressive degeneration | Atrophy of the left T lobe |
| JJ<br>Hillis & Caramazza, 1991 | 67, M | The categories different from animals, i.e., vegetables, fruit, food, body parts, clothing, furniture; transportation was intermediate | Stroke | Left T and basal ganglia |

| *Case/Authors* | *Age, gender* | *Disproportionately impaired categories* | *Aetiology* | *Lesion site* |
|---|---|---|---|---|
| KE<br>Hillis et al., 1990 | 52, M | Taking into account the mean percentage of errors over 6 tasks, body parts, furniture and clothing were the most impaired, whereas food, *vegetables and fruit the least, water animals, transport, other animals and birds intermediate* | Stroke | Left F-P |
| M. LUCIEN<br>Hécaen & De Ajuriaguerra, 1956 | 64, M | Artefacts | Neoplasia | Left mesial O, extending to P and slightly to T lobe |
| NB<br>Gonnerman et al., 1997 | 80, F | Artefacts (furniture, vehicles, clothing, weapons) more impaired than biological items (fruits and vegetables), without distinction within artefacts and biological items. | DAT | Mild cerebral atrophy |
| PJ<br>Breedin et al., 1994a | Not reported | Tools more impaired than animals | Stroke | Left FP |
| PL<br>Laiacona & Capitani, 2001 | 76, F | Artefacts (tools, furniture, and vehicles not analysed separately) more impaired than biological categories (animals, fruit and vegetables not analysed separately). Musical instruments were the worst category | Progressive aphasia | Left: FT atrophy |
| SM<br>Turnbull & Laws, 2000 | 84, M | According to the authors, on naming artefacts are more impaired than biological items. Nonliving and biological categories data are further fractionated, but data are not analysed; musical instruments were the worst category | Infarction | Right: posterior and inferior OT region, thalamus and internal capsule |
| VER<br>Warrington & McCarthy, 1983 | 68, F | Objects more impaired than food, flowers and animals; no further distinction between subtypes of objects | Stroke | Left: FP |
| VP<br>Breedin et al., 1994a | Not reported | Tools more impaired than animals | Stroke | Left FP |
| YOT<br>Warrington & McCarthy, 1987 | 50, F | *Small manipulable objects* and furniture, body parts more impaired than large man-made objects and animals, occupation, vegetables, fabrics. Musical instruments were also impaired | Stroke | Left TP |

[a]Left-handed. [b]Ambidextrous?

# APPENDIX B

## Other cases from group studies not included in the database

### *1. Primary biological categories impairment*[a]

| *Cases/Authors* | *Disproportionately impaired and spared categories* | *Etiology* | *Comments* |
|---|---|---|---|
| No. 1, 2, 3, 4, 5, 6, 7, 8 Laiacona et al., 1998 | Biological categories (animals, fruit and vegetables, not separately analysed) more impaired than artefacts (tools, vehicles, and furniture not separately analysed) | DAT | Seven patients out of 8 were males. Only picture naming was analysed. Concomitant variables were strictly controlled in the statistical comparison carried out separately for each patient |
| 18 cases out of 58 Garrard et al., 1998 | Animals more impaired than objects and vehicles, which are not distinguished | DAT | Semantic probes and objects decision were not investigated |
| Exp. 1[b]: 1 case Gonnerman et al., 1997<br><br>Exp. 2: 10 cases | Exp. 1: vehicles, furniture, clothing, and weapons less impaired than than fruit and vegetables.<br>Exp. 2: as above but tools replaced weapons, and animals were added | DAT | The authors claim that 10 patients out of 15 (Experiment 2), and some other cases from Experiment 1 (which included 15 different patients) showed a prevailing impairment of biological categories. The authors suggest that the relative impairment of biological categories is observed among the more severe patients. However, no statistical comparison supports the category effect within each subject |
| 5 cases H. Damasio et al., 1996 | Animals only | Not detailed | Anterior sector of left inferior T region. The authors claim that the defect was restricted to lexical retrieval, but this conclusion seems unwarranted (for a thorough comment see Caramazza & Shelton, 1998) |

## 2. *Primary artefacts impairment*[a]

| *Cases/Authors* | *Disproportionately impaired and spared categories* | *Etiology* | *Comments* |
|---|---|---|---|
| No. 24, 25, 26<br>Laiacona et al., 1998 | Artefacts (tools, vehicles, and furniture not separately analysed) more impaired than biological categories (animals, fruit and vegetables, not separately analysed) | DAT | All three patients were females. Only picture naming was analysed. Concomitant variables were strictly controlled in the statistical comparison carried out separately for each patient. |
| 3 cases out of 58<br>Garrard et al., 1998 | Vehicles and objects more impaired than animals | DAT | Semantic probes and object decision were not investigated |
| Exp. 1: 1 Case[c]<br>Gonnerman et al., 1997<br><br>Exp. 2: 3 cases | Exp. 1: vehicles, furniture, clothing, and weapons more impaired than fruit and vegetables.<br>Exp. 2: as above but tools replaced weapons, and animals were added | DAT | The authors claim that 3 patients out of 15 (Exp. 2), and some other cases from Exp. 1 (which included 15 different patients) showed a prevailing impairment of nonliving categories. They suggest that the relative impairment of artefacts is associated with a mild severity. However, no statistical comparison supports the category effect within each subject |
| 17 cases out of 31<br>Tippett et al., 1966 | Speeded picture naming<br>14 right T: no deficits<br>17 left T: impaired, more severely on artefacts than biological categories | T lobectomy for intractable epilepsy | This study concerns the mean of the performances of the left T lobectomy patients. These data are uninformative with respect to semantic knowledge or the structural description system. They are not in line with the role suggested by Damasio for the left T pole |
| 7 cases<br>H. Damasio et al., 1996 | Tools only | Not detailed | Posterior sector of left inferior-T and the most anterior part of the lateral O region. The authors claim that the defect was restricted to lexical retrieval, but this conclusion seems unwarranted (for a thorough comment see Caramazza & Shelton, 1998) |

[a]Due to their limited or summary study, these patients will not be considered for further classification.
[b]One patient had a clear advantage for artefacts (100% vs. 67%).
[c]One patient had a clear advantage for biological categories (92% vs. 54%).

# APPENDIX C

## Details about the status of "food" in patients presenting category dissociations

*1. Patients with biological categories impairment*

| *Name* | *Age, gender* | *Impaired categories* | *Meaning and extension of the label "food"* |
|---|---|---|---|
| FB | 19, M | Animals and food. | No details given (a category of plant life is not separately considered). |
| FELICIA | 49, F | Biological items (animals, fruit, vegetables and flowers) food. | Food is listed among NLC, and separately from fruit and vegetables. |
| ING | 44, F | Animals, food. | 15 items (Exp. 8; items not reported in Appendix). |
| JBR | 23, M | Biological categories and food. | Food is considered separately from fruit and vegetables (Bunn et al., 1997), but is mixed with fruit and vegetables in Warrington and Shallice's (1984) Exp. 4. |
| KB | 60, F | Animals, food. | 5 items only (Exp. 8; items not reported in Appendix). |
| LA | 54, F | Animals possibly more severe than flowers. Fruit and vegetables. Food intermediate (1st exam), more severe at 2nd exam. | Food distinguished from fruit and vegetables. |
| MD | 34, M | Fruit and vegetables (animals and food spared). | Food distinguished from fruit and vegetables. |
| MU | 30, M | Biological categories; liquids, substances, edible materials. | Edible liquids (e.g., olive oil) and solid edible substances (e.g., nutella cream). No separate data for edible/non-edible liquids. |
| PS | 45, M | Animals and vegetables (fruit intermediate, food spared). | Food distinguished from fruit and vegetables. |
| RS | 63, M | Disproportionate impairment of fruit and vegetables and food. | Manufactured food. |
| SB | 19, F | Animals, food (including fruit and vegetables). | Food includes fruit and vegetables in naming (Exp. 1). In Exp. 2. real food naming is distinguished into different subtypes: SB was 1/21 correct for fruit and vegetables, and 3/41 correct for the remainder. |
| SBY | 48, M | Natural categories and food. | Food composition (Exp. 5, stimuli taken from Snodgrass and Vanderwart set) is not detailed. |

*2. Patients with artefacts impairment*

| *Name* | *Age, gender* | *Impaired categories* | *Meaning and extension of the label "food"* |
|---|---|---|---|
| JJ | 67, M | Impairment of the categories different from animals, i.e., vegetables, fruit, food, body parts, clothing, furniture. | Food distinguished from fruit and vegetables. |
| KE | 52, M | Taking into account the mean percentage of errors over six tasks, body parts, furniture and clothing were the most impaired, whereas food, vegetables and fruit were the least; water animals, transportation, other animals and birds intermediate. | Food distinguished from fruit and vegetables. |
| VER | 68, F | Objects more impaired than food, flowers, and animals; no further distinction between subtypes of objects. | Food stimuli were photographs cut out of recipe books: part of food consisted of fruit and vegetables, part of prepared dishes (e.g., soup and steak). |

## APPENDIX D

### Status of musical instruments and body parts in patients presenting the opposite types of LC/NLC category dissociation[a]

| *Case* | *Balance between biological categories and artefacts* | *Status of body parts* | *Musical instruments* |
|---|---|---|---|
| BD | Biological categories impairment | Unexplored | Spared |
| C(CW97) | Animals impairment | Unexplored | Spared (the patient was a musician) |
| CA | Biological categories impairment | Spared | Intermediate |
| DM | Animals impairment | Slightly impaired | Severely impaired |
| EA | Biological categories impairment | Spared | Impaired (animals and musical instruments recovered more than fruit and vegetables) |
| EW | Animals impairment | Spared | Nearly spared |
| FELICIA | Biological categories impairment | Spared | Spared |
| FM | Biological categories impairment | Spared | Impaired |
| FS | Animals impairment | Unexplored | Impaired (four items only) |
| GR | Biological categories impairment | Spared | Impaired |
| HJA | Biological categories impairment | Impaired | Unexplored |
| JB | Biological categories impairment | Relatively spared | Unexplored |
| JBR | Biological categories impairment | Spared | Impaired |
| JH | Biological categories impairment | Spared | Unexplored |
| JMC | Biological categories impairment | Unexplored | Impaired |
| KG | Animals impaired | Unexplored | Impaired |
| LA | Biological categories impairment | Spared | Impaired |
| LF | Biological categories impairment | Spared | Impaired |
| LH | Biological categories impairment | Mildly impaired | Intermediate |
| MB | Biological categories impairment | Spared | Intermediate |
| MD | Fruit and vegetables (animals spared) | Spared | Unexplored |
| MF | Biological categories impairment | Spared | Intermediate |
| MU | Biological categories impairment | Spared | Intermediate |
| NV | Biological categories impairment | Spared | Impaired |
| PS | Biological categories impairment | Spared | Unexplored |
| RC | Biological categories impairment | Spared | Unexplored |
| SE | Biological categories impairment | Spared | Minimally impaired or spared |
| CG | Artefacts impairment | Spared | Impaired |
| CW92 | Artefacts impairment | Only two stimuli, both failed | Impaired |
| GP98 | Artefacts impairment | Spared | Moderately impaired |
| JJ | Categories other than animals | Impaired | Unexplored |
| KE | Furniture and clothing most impaired | Impaired | Unexplored |
| PL | Artefacts impairment | Relatively spared | Severely impaired |
| SM | Artefacts impairment | Impaired | Severely impaired |
| YOT | Small manipulable objects | Impaired | Impaired |

[a]Data generally refer to picture naming or picture identification; different tasks are indicated.

# APPENDIX E

## Critical comments on the data base

In this appendix we critically review the cases listed in Appendix A, arguing whether or not the claims made by the respective authors are well founded. When the original data analyses were not exhaustive, we have tried to supplement these analyses with our own on the basis of the published data. We have used generalised linear model analyses to study the logistic regression of correct/incorrect responses; the resulting linear model includes several relevant variables. In some instances we could study reported frequencies with multi-dimensional contingency tables, considering as main factors (1) correct vs. incorrect responses, (2) patients vs. controls, and (3) answers to probes concerning perceptual vs. associative knowledge. This analysis was often only possible for living categories. Such data can be analysed equivalently with either a log-linear or a logit-linear model (Capitani & Laiacona, 2000). We are aware that this approach offers only approximate answers: collapsing control subjects into a single cell does not take into account variation within normals, thus treating them as a whole. In this situation it is possible that a single patient's performance could still be within the central 95% of the controls' distribution, while at the same time being significantly different from the collapsed controls. Notwithstanding this caveat, we will consider significant findings as a suggestive piece of evidence.

### *1. Cases presenting a disproportionate impairment for natural categories*

BD (Hanley, Young, & Pearson, 1989)
This case was studied primarily for his difficulties in identifying people. He was impaired at identifying pictures of fruit, flowers, and vegetables. The patient was also impaired in naming animals and fruit from spoken definition. The concomitant nuisance variables were not strictly controlled. Musical instruments were not noticeably impaired. Perceptual and associative knowledge were not investigated. Object reality decision was within normal limits.

C(CW97) (Wilson, Baddeley, & Kapur, 1995; Wilson, 1997)
This case is reported with different initials in two studies (C and CW). The patient presented a semantic deficit for animals but was not examined for other biological categories. Musical instruments were substantially spared on different tasks (picture naming and picture recognition); it should be noted that the patient was a professional musician. Perceptual and associative knowledge were not investigated.

CA (Capitani, Laiacona, & Barbarotto, 1993)
Separate data for perceptual and associative probes were not reported in the original paper. However, for perceptual knowledge, CA was 45% correct (27/60 ) for biological categories and 78% correct (47/60) for artefacts. For associative knowledge, CA was 53% correct (32/60) for biological categories, and 68% correct (41/60) for artefacts. The interaction between type of knowledge and category was not significant after adjusting for the level of difficulty of the questions. This case, affected by a progressive cerebral atrophy, was only examined with CT-scan. Left sylvian atrophy was evident, but we are not sure that the atrophy was confined to the lateral aspects of the left hemisphere, as details of inferior and mesial temporal structures are not evident on axial CT-scan slices.

DANTE (Sartori, Job, & Coltheart, 1993a)
This patient had a disproportionate impairment for naming pictures of biological items; the impairment disappeared after phonological cue. Biological categories were not further distinguished. Semantic knowledge of perceptual properties was assessed by means of a sentence verification task, and Dante performed within the normal range for both animals and objects. Perceptual knowledge was also investigated with visual tasks. Associative knowledge was not investigated. The authors claim that the naming impairment for biological stimuli was purely lexical, due to retrieval difficulties from the phonological output lexicon. This conclusion does not seem entirely warranted: Successful naming improvement after phonemic cue may also reflect the disambiguation of uncertain identification of the stimulus within a group of semantically similar alternatives.

The patient scored within the normal range for both biological stimuli and artefacts on object reality decision. However, on visual part–whole matching, only investigated for animals, performance was not normal (13/16 correct, which corresponds to a $z$-score of -3.14 with respect to the control group, which was nearly at ceiling). This seems to be at odds with the conclusion of a purely anomic deficit.

DB (Lambon Ralph, Howard, Nightingale, & Ellis, 1998)
This patient, examined on several different picture naming tasks, presented a consistent advantage for artefacts that was more significant for low-familiarity items. Subsets of biological stimuli were not distinguished.

Semantic knowledge was examined with three tasks. Using well-controlled materials, neither a difference due to type of question, nor an interaction between category and stimulus type was detected. Performance on object reality decision tasks, examined with BORB as well as another battery, indicated a deficit for animals.

DM94 (Breedin, Saffran, & Coslett, 1994b)
This report focuses on a reversed concreteness effect. Category effects were observed with a task in which the patient had to pick the odd one out of a triplet of names. The patient was at chance with animals and musical instruments; on a restricted subset of matched stimuli DM was worse with animals than with tools.

The patient was also examined on semantic probes, but the data is not completely reported. For the semantic probes, a category effect was no longer evident (biological categories were slightly better, although not significantly), and on a subset of the questions DM was better with associative than perceptual attributes. However, the results are not divided into all combinations of semantic categories and knowledge types. Object reality decision was below normal range, but a controlled comparison between animals and other stimuli was not carried out.

Due to the inconsistency of the category effects and the limits of the experimental design, this case provides no information as to the relationship between semantic categories and perceptual and associative knowledge.

DM97 (Humphreys, Riddoch, & Price, 1997)
This patient was disproportionately impaired for naming biological items: 46% correct (35/76) for biological items, vs. 75% (57/76) for artefacts. The patient was also examined on naming from definitions based on perceptual or functional information: the patient performed poorly on perceptual definitions, both for animate stimuli 34% (13/38) and artefacts 50% (19/38). For the same perceptual definitions, controls were 81% correct (31/38) for animate stimuli and 66% correct (25/38) for artefacts. The data for naming from functional definitions are not reported separately for each object category: 89% (68/76) for DM(97) and 93% (71/76) for controls. A reanalysis of this patient's data is not possible because the number of controls is not indicated. By inspection, however, the difference between DM(97) and the controls' average is clear for animate stimuli (34% vs. 81%) but is much smaller for artefacts (50% vs. 66%). We should point out that the controls' performance reported in this paper is different from the controls' data reported in Forde et al. (1997: patient SRB) in which the patient was presumably administered the same test.

Object reality decision was impaired; however, the materials used do not permit a comparison between categories.

EA (Barbarotto, Capitani, & Laiacona, 1996; Laiacona, Capitani, & Barbarotto, 1997)
This patient presented a clear semantic deficit for biological categories, with no difference between perceptual and associative information as examined with verbal semantic probes. The deficit was detected on three successive examinations separated by long time intervals. At the outset, EA also presented an impairment for musical instruments, while body parts were nearly spared. On an object reality decision task, EA was slightly impaired for biological categories on the first administration (80% correct, normal ≥87%), but was 100% correct at the second administration.

A re-examination of the patient 9 years later (unpublished data) revealed that the patient was still impaired for biological categories, although picture naming was also still defective for artefacts. On this re-examination, the patient had a greater impairment for fruit and vegetables on word–picture matching as well as on a verbal questionnaire. A slight discrepancy between animals and plant life was evident at the first assessment, and animals recovered to a greater extent. On the last assessment, animal stimuli were 100% correct on word–picture matching, compared to 60% for plant life. On semantic probes, EA was 75% correct with animals, and 52% correct with plant life. The recovery of musical instruments was similar to that of animals. Also on the re-examination, the integrity of the structural description system was further confirmed by the normal performance of EA on an object decision test carried out with new and strictly controlled materials.

EC (Carbonnel, Charnallet, David, & Pellat, 1997)
This patient is reported to have an impairment for perceptual knowledge across object categories; however, the impairment for associative knowledge was limited to animals. In addition, EC was impaired for all categories on a number of pre-semantic visual tests.

The study of perceptual and associative knowledge was limited to the analysis of the correct elements given by the patient in a word definition task, thus providing only weak evidence. If supported by stronger data, a possible interpretation of this pattern could be an association between visual agnosia and a semantic deficit limited to animals.

ELM (Arguin, Bub, & Dudek, 1996; Dixon, Bub, & Arguin, 1997; Dixon & Arguin, 1999; Dixon, 1999; Takarae & Levin, 2001)
The authors label the patient as having a category-specific visual agnosia, and the investigations focused on fine-grained analyses of basic visual processes. On picture naming ELM was 39% correct for stimuli belonging to biological categories, and 88% correct for artefact stimuli. However, ELM was also impaired on a sentence verification task tapping visual semantic properties of animals (55% correct, chance = 50%); on questions tapping associative knowledge, the patient was 85% correct, which is slightly below normal range. However, neither the number of stimuli nor control data are provided for the sentence verification task, and we are not sure if the difficulty of the task is comparable for perceptual and associative questions. Semantic properties of artefacts were not explored.

The lack of a controlled and exhaustive comparison between perceptual and associative knowledge pertaining to different object categories makes it problematic to interpret the pattern of semantic knowledge impairment. A deficit on an object reality decision task is reported for animals (59% correct) but not for artefacts (93% correct); however, the number of stimuli is again not reported, and control data are not provided.

The merits of this study are its concentration on fine-grained aspects of the deficit for visual perception of biological stimuli. On the whole, an agnosic component to the category-specific deficit is probable, but a degree of a semantic deficit for the same categories cannot be excluded. In this case impaired object reality decision for biological categories is associated with the possible loss of stored visual-perceptual knowledge for the same categories: this is reminiscent of cases Michelangelo and Giulietta.

The original data have recently been reanalysed by Takarae and Levin (2001) with an extended set of form-related variables, and the category dissociation was confirmed.

EMMA (Gentileschi, Sperber, & Spinnler,2001)
This patient presented a deficit for knowledge pertaining to people, not limited to prosopagnosia, but also involving the retrieval

of relevant biographical knowledge from a given name. As a marginal finding, the authors report a disproportionate impairment for semantic information concerning biological categories, with a balanced deficit for perceptual and associative knowledge. This category-specific effect was assessed with only a semantic memory questionnaire. On a visual object reality decision, the patient scored below normal range, but the materials employed for this task (BORB) do not permit a reliable comparison between categories.

EW (Caramazza & Shelton, 1998)
This case presented a semantic deficit restricted to animals, with sparing of fruit and vegetables as well as other categories, including body parts and musical instruments. EW's category-specific deficit for animals was not modality-specific (for visual knowledge). In various attribute-processing tasks she consistently performed equally poorly for visual and functional/associative statements for animals and, in contrast, within normal limits for all attributes pertaining to inanimate objects. Object reality decision was impaired for only animals.

FA (Barbarotto, Capitani, & Laiacona, 1996)
The published report indicates a picture naming deficit for items from biological categories. On a revisitation of the clinical record, we found that the same pattern was evident in word–picture matching, which suggests that FA's impairment was probably located at the semantic level. Further tasks could not be given because the patient was uncooperative. Therefore, more detailed information about the pattern of semantic knowledge impairment is not available.

FB (Sirigu, Duhamel, & Poncet, 1991)
This patient probably had a greater naming impairment for animals and food than for artefacts. The study focused on fine-grained aspects of tools knowledge. Animals and food were severely impaired on naming, but on matching to sample animals were better than food; however, it is possible that the materials were not matched for the relevant nuisance variables. Perceptual and associative knowledge of animals and food was impaired in a classification task (e.g., "does it live in France?"). The patient was also examined on a naming to description task that contrasted perceptual and functional descriptions, but apparently the experimental design did not include biological category items. Drawing of biological category items was impaired.

FELICIA (De Renzi & Lucchelli, 1994)
This patient presented a reliable categorical dissociation in naming, for which biological categories were disproportionately impaired. By inspection, it would seem that animals were more severely affected than fruit and vegetables; however, the conclusion of a finer-grained dissociation between biological categories is not warranted, as the difficulty of the materials has not been controlled, and because flower naming was even more impaired than animal naming. The patient was also impaired at naming food as well as professions: The interpretation of the latter deficit is not clear, as this category seems to not be comparable with concrete items (i.e., biological categories or artefacts). Interestingly, neither musical instruments nor body parts were considerably impaired.

This study presents some problems. Stimuli belonging to different categories were not matched for all of the relevant concomitant variables. It is not specified whether each item was investigated with both perceptual and associative questions, or whether different stimuli were used for different types of questions. For associative questions, control data are not reported and were not considered in the statistical comparison; also, it could be that the associative questions were easier. We will ignore whether the difference in performance between different types of knowledge is greater for the patient than for controls. For biological categories, some aspects of associative knowledge were also impaired, as in questions such as (1) "does the animal live in Italy?" and (2) the categorisation of animals according to the way they move. The number of perceptual and functional/associative questions is not specified. On the whole, a selective or disproportionate impairment for perceptual knowledge of biological categories is possible, but is not definitively demonstrated; it is evident that some functional/associative information was not available to the patient.

Object reality decision was impaired for only animal stimuli.

Felicia was observed twice, with more than 2 years separating the two assessments. The bulk of reported data is from the second examination. The authors hypothesise that perceptual knowledge was initially impaired for all categories, and that the recovery of perceptual knowledge was limited to artefacts. However, perceptual knowledge of artefacts was not evaluated at the first examination.

FI (Barbarotto, Capitani, & Laiacona, 1996)
This patient presented a disproportionate naming impairment for biological categories. Data concerning the balance between perceptual and associative knowledge of different categories is not available.

FM (Laiacona, Barbarotto, & Capitani, 1993)
A semantic deficit for biological categories was evident in naming, word–picture matching, and semantic probes. Perceptual and associative knowledge of items from biological categories were impaired to comparable levels.

Data for object reality decision was not reported in the original paper. However, data recovered from the clinical record shows that object reality decision was within the normal range for biological categories: 87% correct (26/30); normal range 87% and above, as well as for nonliving categories: 97% (29/30); normal range: 83% and above.

Animals, fruit and vegetables were impaired to an equivalent degree. Musical instruments were impaired on all semantic tasks while body parts were spared.

FS (Dixon, Piskopos, & Schweizer, 2000)
Although the authors classified this case as a category-specific agnosia, only picture naming was evaluated. The integrity of

associative and perceptual knowledge and of the structural description system were not assessed. The evidence in favour of a category-specific impairment is based on the patient's performance on four items from each of the categories artefacts, musical instruments, and animals, although the items were repeated five times. The stimuli were matched for frequency, familiarity, and visual complexity, but apparently were not matched for name agreement, image agreement, and prototypicality. The small number of stimuli from each category does not permit strong general conclusions.

GC (Cardebat, Demonet, Celsis, & Puel, 1997)
The paper describes a case affected by left temporal lobe degeneration, who presented a deficit for semantic knowledge of animals (other biological categories were not tested). The study is focused on SPECT data and does not provide relevant information regarding either the type of knowledge impairment or the sparing/impairment of the structural description system.

GIULIETTA (Sartori, Miozzo, & Job, 1994b; Sartori, Job, Miozzo, Zago, & Marchiori, 1993b)
This patient presented an impairment for naming pictures of biological items; there did not seem to be a substantial difference between animals and plants (30% vs. 41% correct respectively). On semantic probe questions about animals the patient was 93% correct (54/58) for associative questions, and 62.5% correct (50/80) for perceptual questions; the control average for perceptual questions was 86.6% correct (69.3/80); however, associative questions were not administered to controls. The patient made errors on rather easy associative probe questions about animals ("The elephant is typical of Christmas day" and "The leopard lives in our region"). On an object reality decision task, Giulietta was impaired for only animals (she correctly judged all the real elements but rejected nonexistent ones at chance). The evolution of this case is reported by Sartori, Miozzo, and Job (1994b): The patient did not recover after 8 months of cognitive rehabilitation.

A disproportionate impairment for perceptual knowledge of animals is possible, but a strong conclusion cannot be drawn on the basis of the published analysis due to inadequacies in the experimental design: (1) the semantic probes tapping visual and associative knowledge of animals were not administered for the same stimuli; (2) no control data is provided for associative probes; thus, it could be that these probes were easier than the perceptual probes; (3) the task was slightly different for associative and perceptual probes, since in the former the patient was given a list of names and asked to indicate which item was (e.g.) ferocious, whereas the perceptual probe questions were administered one at a time. No direct comparison is made between associative and perceptual knowledge of biological categories.

A reanalysis of the available data might yield further information; however, no control data have been given for associative probes. Let us then consider only natural categories, in order to check whether or not the patient is in fact more impaired on probes tapping visual properties compared to probes tapping associative properties. It is reasonable to presume that, on associative probes of biological stimuli, controls would perform at a level between the score of Giulietta and ceiling (i.e., 100% correct). Let us first assume that the 10 controls were at the level of Giulietta, i.e., 54/58 correct. Their correct answers would be 540/580. For the visual probes, Giulietta was correct on 50/80 probes, and controls were 693/800 correct. Analysing the above frequency by means of a log-linear model, the overall difference between Giulietta and the control group is significant, $\chi^2(1) = 19.118$, $p < .0001$, and the difference between visual and nonvisual probes is significant, $\chi^2(1) = 28.042$, $p < .0001$. The interaction between the above factors is also significant, $\chi^2(1) = 6.168$, $p = .013$. This indicates that Giulietta had a disproportionate deficit for perceptual probes pertaining to natural categories. An even more significant outcome is observed if the performance of controls is assumed to be at ceiling, $\chi^2 = 9.928$, $p = .002$.

One limit to our approach comes from the possibility that the associative probes were so easy that a deficit could not be detected in the patient; however, at the same time, performance on associative probes has often been impaired in similar cases (see, e.g., Felicia, who was defective in judging if an animal lives in Italy). Thus, we think that this case provides some evidence in favour of a disproportionate deficit for the visual knowledge of animals.

GP97 (Gonnerman, Andersen, Devlin, Kempler, & Seidenberg, 1997)
This patient was examined on three tasks: picture naming, word–picture matching, and superordinate comprehension (e.g., pointing to a "gun" as the examiner gives the word "weapon"). The artefact categories examined were furniture, vehicles, weapons, and clothing; the biological categories examined were fruit and vegetables. Items from different categories were matched only for prototypicality. Performance for biological categories was more impaired than performance for artefacts, with this pattern being consistent across all time slices (four examinations). Different aspects of semantic knowledge were not examined.

GR (Laiacona, Barbarotto, & Capitani, 1993)
This patient had a possible sparing of animals compared to fruit and vegetables (in picture–word matching animals were 95% correct while fruit and vegetables were 65% correct; on semantic probes animals were 63% correct while fruit and vegetables were 50% correct). However, a controlled comparison of performance for the different categories was not carried out. Musical instruments were severely impaired in naming (20% correct), but only slightly impaired in word–picture matching (85% correct) as well as on semantic probes (83% correct). Body parts were spared.

For this patient, object reality decision was not reported in the original paper. Data recovered from the clinical record reveal that object reality decision was impaired for living categories (53% correct, 16/30; normal range: 87% and above) but was normal for nonliving categories (93% correct, 28/30; normal range: 83% and above).

**HELGA** (Mauri, Daum, Sartori, Riesch, & Birbaumer, 1994)
This patient was impaired on naming items from biological categories (animals and vegetables were not distinguished). For the remainder of the study only animals were considered. The items used to investigate perceptual and associative knowledge of animals were probably not the same, and the authors did not directly compare these types of knowledge. For animals, perceptual probes were 24/30 correct while nonperceptual probes were 40/44 correct, $\chi^2(1) = 1.816$, n.s.. No control data is provided for associative questions. The evidence provided by this case is inconclusive with respect to the contrast between associative and perceptual semantic knowledge. Object reality decision and part-whole matching were impaired for animals.

**HJA** (Riddoch & Humphreys, 1987a; Riddoch, Humphreys, Gannon, Blott, & Jones, 1999)
This case, classified as "integrative visual agnosia," was first reported in 1987 and then re-examined 10 years later. We will comment only on the data concerning the category-specific impairment as well as the performance of the patient on semantic probe questions. Data reported in 1987 show that HJA named fewer "structurally similar" items (animals, birds, insects, fruit and vegetables) than structurally distinct items (body parts, furniture, household items, tools, vehicles). In the Appendix all the stimuli are reported together with their name frequency as well the naming success. The authors claim that only structural similarity can account for the observed outcome, because name frequency had no effect on HJA's naming; they also maintain that the animate/inanimate distinction was not the right explanation because, for instance, "body parts" are animate but are structurally distinct. However, this is problematic because the literature suggests that body parts should not be collapsed with other categories (for a review, see Barbarotto, Capitani, & Laiacona, 2001).

We have reanalysed HJA's naming data excluding body parts stimuli, as well as one unique musical instrument (piano) and one item with no reported word frequency (lettuce). One might claim that the elimination of body parts disrupts the balance between the remaining living and nonliving categories, or between the remaining structurally distinct and structurally similar categories; however, excluding body parts cannot influence whether or not there is an effect of contour overlap on naming success for the remaining stimuli. On the other hand, HJA successfully named only three body parts out of nine, and this militates against the general rule, suggested by the authors, that in this patient distinct categories are the least impaired. In the logistic regression analysis the dependent variable was the response (correct or incorrect) while the model variables were word frequency and category. Frequency did not have an influence on naming, $\chi^2 < 1$; nor did frequency influence performance after logarithmic transformation, $\chi^2(1) = 1.202$, n.s. In contrast, stimulus category did account for the observed outcome, yielding a $\chi^2(1) = 7.860, p = .005$, and $\chi^2(1) = 7.623, p = .006$ when the frequency effect was partialled out.

At this point the question becomes: What does "category" really mean? The authors claim that the relevant distinction is that between structurally similar and structurally distinct exemplars; however, after eliminating body parts, the dichotomy between biological items and artefacts works just as well. In their subsequent paper (1999) the authors clarify what is meant by structural similarity ("overall contour overlap and listed number of parts in common"); quantitative measures are provided in other papers (Riddoch & Humphreys, 1987a; Humphreys et al., 1988). Therefore, it was possible to compute directly the effect of contour overlap for the majority of the items belonging to biological categories (32/35) and artefacts (22/30) in the 1987 study. In the logistic regression analysis performed on this subset of 54 stimuli, the model included word frequency (logarithmic), category, and contour overlap. Again, in this subset of stimuli, frequency was not influential, $\chi^2 < 1$, whereas category was highly significant, both when considered alone, $\chi^2(1) = 6.664, p = .01$, as well as within a model that included all three predictors, $\chi^2(1) = 6.682, p = .01$. On the contrary, contour overlap never yielded a significant chi-square (< 1 both when considered alone as well as within the model including all three variables). Furthermore, an examination of the interaction between category and contour overlap revealed that the effect of the latter variable was not different for artefacts and biological categories, $\chi^2(1) = 2.303, p = .129$, n.s. It is also interesting to check if contour overlap was influential within only biological items ("structurally similar" categories); thus, we investigated its role separately for natural entities and artefacts. For biological categories, the effect of contour overlap fell far short of significance, $\chi^2 < 1$, whereas for artefacts there was a trend, $\chi^2(1) = 3.023, p = .08$. For biological items, the contour overlap of items that were correctly and incorrectly named was almost identical; for artefacts, stimuli that were named correctly tended to have (paradoxically) greater amounts of contour overlap (although this did not reach significance, see above). Summing up, it seems better justified to denote these two groups of stimuli as biological items and artefacts, than to distinguish them on the basis of their structural similarity.

On probe questions, which concerned only biological items, HJA performed well when the stimuli were presented auditorily but poorly with pictorial presentation of the same items, suggesting that semantic knowledge was preserved. Visual knowledge was still unimpaired more than 10 years later on forced-choice tasks ("is A larger than B?").

With respect to the structural description system, HJA performed poorly on an object decision task with line drawings (69/120), but showed a significant improvement with silhouettes (63/88), approaching normal range (65–85). The authors therefore suggest that HJA is impaired in integrating local part information with information about global shape. This pattern of impairment was confirmed in 1997. However, deterioration of drawing from memory was observed and the authors suggest that ongoing reinforcement of the input is important to preserve visual properties in long-term memory. A general decrease in HJA's semantic knowledge was not observed; nevertheless, on definition tasks, the production of visual attributes decreased for structurally similar (biological) items.

The authors interpreted HJA's deficit as a case of integrative visual agnosia (a form of apperceptive agnosia). Data is not provided by category for object decision, so we do not know if there was a category-specific effect in this task. However, if there was a category-specific impairment for picture naming, as well as for drawing from memory, and if stored semantic knowledge was spared at the first examination, then it is possible that HJA originally suffered from a categorical impairment at a pre-semantic stage.

**IL** (Lecours, Arguin, Bub, Caille, & Fontaine, 1999)
This patient presented a reliable category-specific impairment for biological categories in picture naming. Object reality decision was more impaired for pictures representing animals, fruit and vegetables, compared to pictures of artefacts. Perceptual and associative semantic knowledge were not investigated.

**ING** (Warrington & Shallice, 1984)
This patient was only examined on word–picture matching. Neither attribute knowledge nor object reality decision were directly examined. Processing difficulty of the materials was not controlled. The impairment for food (85% correct) was intermediate between animals (80% correct) and inanimate objects (97%).

**JB** (Riddoch & Humphreys, 1987b; Humphreys, Riddoch, & Quinlan, 1988)
This patient was classified by the authors as a case of semantic access agnosia and optic aphasia. JB had a severe naming deficit, but was not impaired on an object reality decision task, suggesting that his stored perceptual knowledge was spared at the pre-semantic level of the structural description system. (However, performance on the "Heads" test, drawing completion, and drawing from memory was impaired.)

The patient was more impaired at naming pictures for stimuli belonging to "structurally similar" compared to "structurally distinct" categories. This distinction largely overlaps with the contrast between, respectively, biological categories and artefacts, with the exception of body parts, which are natural but are also, according to the authors, a structurally distinct category. Based on the patient's good naming performance for body parts, the authors suggest that the natural–artefact contrast cannot account for the pattern of naming impairment. However, many cases have now demonstrated that body parts cannot be collapsed with animals and plant life in the study and discussion of category effects (for a review, see Barbarotto et al., 2001). The authors further suggest that the crucial variable here is the degree of contour overlap, which differentiates biological categories (high overlap) from artefacts (low overlap). However, the degree of contour overlap did not correlate with the naming success within each category, and on this basis the authors have suggested a more complex and general interpretation of the role of this variable in the process of naming.

To disentangle the relevance of the category classification from that of contour overlap, we have reanalysed the data reported in Appendix D (Riddoch & Humphreys, 1987b) eliminating the 10 body parts stimuli and the unique musical instrument (bell). For the four stimuli whose name frequency is not indicated in the paper, we have introduced the value of zero: presumably, their low number should not alter the general outcome of the analysis. In the remaining set of 77 stimuli, the names of items from natural categories were of lower frequency and their contour overlap was higher (16.67) than that of artefacts (10.76). In the logistic regression analysis the dependent variable was the response (correct or incorrect); the model variables were word frequency (logarithmic), contour overlap, and category. Frequency and category were highly significant, both when considered one at a time and within a model including all three predictors: in the latter cases, $\chi^2(1) = 14.984$ for category and 11.257 for frequency effects. On the contrary, contour overlap never yielded a significant chi-square (3.568 when considered alone and 1.606 within the three-variables model). Moreover, the interaction between category and contour overlap was not significant, $\chi^2(1) = 0.003$, n.s., showing that the effect of the latter variable was not different between artefact items and *natural* category items.

A further relevant point for the interpretation of this case is the status of semantic knowledge; it was examined with probes tapping functional-associative properties of natural categories, using pictorial and spoken-name presentation of the stimulus. The patient performed worse with pictorial presentation and was more impaired with specific than with general questions. Interestingly, specific questions with spoken name presentation were 76% correct, a relatively poor performance considering that the patient responded by choosing among two or a few presented alternatives. This raises the question of whether associative verbal knowledge of animals was spared or impaired, as it would be problematic for the interpretation of this case provided by the authors if associative verbal knowledge was impaired. Unfortunately, no control data is provided, and the authors simply concluded that: "JB's relatively poor performance on the specific questions… in the spoken name version of the cued definition tasks may reflect his general intellectual level." The patient was also given questions regarding stored knowledge of visual attributes, but only colour knowledge was investigated; also, as was the case for functional-associative knowledge, the patient performed worse when the stimuli were presented pictorially compared to presentation of the spoken name. However, performance on spoken name presentation was only 48% correct. The deficit for animals, fruit and vegetables was balanced (about 15% correct). Performance on body parts was relatively spared (80%). Musical instruments were not included.

In conclusion, this is a complex case, but the available data and their reanalysis do not exclude the likelihood of (at least) some degree of general semantic impairment affecting biological categories. The hypothesis that category effects are apparent and should be traced back to a crucial role of contour overlap is supported by neither the data nor our own reanalysis of the data.

JBR (Warrington & Shallice, 1984; Bunn, Tyler, & Moss, 1997; Funnell & De Mornay Davies, 1996; Wilson, 1997)
This patient has been reported in several different papers. In the original study by Warrington and Shallice (1984) the patient was more severely impaired for biological stimuli and foods than for inanimate objects in naming and verbal definition tasks. In Experiment 7, the authors examined the ability of the patient to give a definition to 12 stimulus words from each of 26 different categories. Animals were not significantly worse than was expected on the basis of their lexical frequency; whereas, according to the same criterion, other inanimate categories such as precious stones and diseases, were impaired. As a general pattern, the results of Experiment 7 confirm that the set of 26 categories cannot be considered as a whole: Most artefacts were included among the categories showing better performance, and with the biological categories mostly showing worse performances. However, this experiment does not permit conclusions to be drawn at the level of each of the 26 categories. The expected value for each category was calculated solely on the basis of a categorised frequency effect with a different set of names, and other variables were not considered; moreover, only one control subject was examined, and chi-square significance levels were not adjusted for repeated testing. Anyway, JBR was proficient with body parts, and impaired with musical instruments.

An informative study of semantic knowledge was performed by Funnell and De Mornay Davies (1996) by means of a property verification task. In the same study, the patient performed within the pathology range on object reality decision using BORB stimuli, which include mostly animals. Thus we will ignore whether or not the performance of the patient on object reality decision for artefacts was spared or impaired. With respect to the comparison between perceptual and associative knowledge, the authors intentionally included, within both categories, stimuli that had been named or defined correctly (50% of the items) and named or defined incorrectly (the other 50%). Consequently, the category effect is not discernible in this analysis.

JENNIFER (Samson, Pillon, & De Wilde, 1998)
This patient was impaired for natural categories on a number of different naming tasks. By inspection, performance for animals was more severely impaired than for fruit and vegetables (on average, naming was 22% correct for animals, 51% correct for fruit and vegetables, and 73% correct for artefacts) but the contrast between different natural categories was not significant after covariance for a number of concomitant variables. The results are somewhat inconsistent regarding the status of associative knowledge of natural categories. This type of knowledge was impaired in an attribute verification task, but was spared in a categorisation task (sorting animal names on the basis of the country in which they live). However, the categorisation task was presumably easier; thus, the conclusion that visual and nonvisual attributes of natural categories were not differently impaired seems justified. Object reality decision was examined with the BORB as well as with an original task. Whereas with the BORB the results were "slightly below the published norms", on the other task Jennifer performed "quite well," i.e., within the normal range (she was correct on 65 instances out of 72, i.e., 90%); the authors conclude that she "did not appear to be impaired in retrieving the stored structural description of the objects depicted in pictures".

JH (Swales & Johnson, 1992)
This patient presented a deficit for pictures of animals, fruit and vegetables. After rehabilitation, biological category items improved, but after 6 weeks only performance on fruit and vegetables confirmed the recovery, whereas the patient showed a decline for animals. The contrast between animals and fruit and vegetables was not the aim of this study; the difficulty of the questions was not controlled, and the small number of items from each of these subcategories (five animals and five fruits and vegetables) does not permit a sound conclusion to be drawn on the basis of this result.
Perceptual and associative information were not investigated separately.

JMC (Magnié, Ferreira, Giusiano, & Poncet, 1999)
Although the materials used to study this patient were probably not strictly controlled, the category effect in object recognition seems striking (0% for natural items vs. 60% or more for artefacts). Perceptual and associative knowledge pertaining to the different categories was not examined.

JV (Pietrini, Nertempi, Vaglia, Revello, Pinna, & Ferro-Milone, 1988)
This patient presented a deficit for natural categories (animals and plants) on picture naming, word–picture matching, word definition, and naming from description. Also, the patient was impaired in naming man-made objects. The authors claim that plants were "selectively impaired." The impairment was possibly more severe for this category, but the performance of the patient on animals was also below normal range in many instances; furthermore, stimuli corresponding to the categories of animals and plants were not matched for frequency, familiarity, etc. However, while the impairment definitely affected the semantic system, perceptual and associative information were not tested separately.

KB (Warrington & Shallice, 1984)
This patient was examined on only word–picture matching. Factors affecting the difficulty of processing of the materials were not controlled. An impairment for food (55% correct) was intermediate between an impairment for animals (45% correct) and one for inanimate objects (85%). Neither attribute knowledge nor object reality decision were directly tested.

KG (Wilson, 1997)
This patient presented a slight semantic deficit for animals (other biological categories were not examined). Also, performance on musical instruments was impaired. However, some of the reported data seem inconsistent, and perceptual and associative knowledge were not investigated.

KR (Hart & Gordon, 1992)
The interpretation of this case presents some problems. Property verification for the spared categories and associative knowledge of animals were nearly always 100% correct. The patient was much worse than chance on perceptual property judgement of animals with pictorial stimuli, and was consistent on incorrect responses. When given the choice between a previously given incorrect response and the correct response, she almost always chose the wrong response, as if she had consistently false beliefs or as if, in some way, she had decided to give a meditated wrong response. As the task had only two alternatives, it is not possible to disentangle the two possible interpretations envisaged above.

LA (Silveri & Gainotti, 1988; Gainotti & Silveri, 1996)
This patient was examined twice, with an interval of about 8 years. In the first examination, LA presented a balanced deficit for naming coloured pictures of animals, fruit, and vegetables, while performance for food was intermediate. Semantic knowledge of animals was examined with a naming to definition task: The patient made more errors on perceptually based definitions than on definitions based on associative features. However, in this task the set of animals defined on the basis of perceptual features was not the same as the set defined on the basis of functional/encyclopaedic features.

On the second assessment, considering the full set of stimuli, animals were 10% correct, plant life 37% correct, food 15% correct, musical instruments 20% correct, other artefacts 69% correct, and body parts were 90% correct. Animals were named significantly worse than vegetables; however, if only high frequency items are taken into account, the difference is not significant. Semantic knowledge of animals and objects was examined by means of a new naming to definition task, as well as by a sentence verification task. In the former, perceptual and associative definitions were given for the same stimulus. Animals were still disproportionately impaired on naming after perceptual definition, but this condition was also more difficult for control subjects. A data reanalysis indicates that LA was worse than controls, $\chi^2(1) = 53.187$, $p < .0001$, and that perceptual definitions were more difficult, $\chi^2(1) = 7.962$, $p = .005$, but the interaction between these effects was not significant, $\chi^2(1) = 0.748$, n.s. On the sentence verification task, the patient performed poorly on probes concerning perceptual attributes of animals and vegetables (respectively, 13% and 33% correct, with a chance level of 25%). Probes tapping functional properties of animals and vegetables yielded a higher proportion of correct judgments (56%, 9/16, and 67%, 4/6 respectively). In this task, however, controls were at ceiling and latency data could not be analysed; on this basis, as acknowledged by the authors, one cannot exclude the possibility that the living/perceptual condition was more difficult. A disproportionate impairment for perceptual knowledge of natural items is possible, but cannot be considered to be a definite finding.

Data from picture reality decision are not reported.

LF (Barbarotto, Capitani, & Laiacona, 1996; Laiacona, Capitani, & Barbarotto, 1997)
This patient presented with a clear category-specific naming impairment that mildly affected semantic knowledge of items from biological categories. Animals, fruit and vegetables were impaired at a similar level. On picture naming, musical instruments were the most impaired category while body parts were spared. LF was examined twice and was largely recovered at the time of the second examination. The performance on the semantic probes was impaired but too mild for investigating the balance between perceptual and associative knowledge. Notwithstanding the large lesion, which included the left hippocampus and parahippocampal gyrus, the cognitive deficit of the patient was mild, and he showed a remarkable recovery.

LH (Farah, Hammond, Mehta, & Ratcliff, 1989; Farah, Meyer, & McMullen, 1996; Etcoff, Freeman, & Cave, 1991; Takarae & Levin, 2001)
Farah and her coworkers (1989) conclude that LH presented a selective deficit for perceptual knowledge pertaining to natural categories (this was also the most difficult task for controls). The statistical analysis used to support this claim is questionable. The authors compared the performance of LH with that of 12 controls: They first divided the observed scores of the patient by the standard deviation of the controls, and then compared this ratio with the $t$-distribution. For the visual properties of natural items the control distribution is highly skewed; thus, this does not permit the use of the normal or the $t$-distribution for determining the position of a single subject. With such distributions, only nonparametric techniques can determine whether or not a single subject's score is within the normal range. Even for unidirectional tolerance limits, the size of the normal sample should be at least 60 subjects. A probability point yielded by the t-distribution tables is not informative. Thus, in this case we have no real statistical basis for judging whether or not a single score is within the normal range, nor can we judge whether or not the performance on two tests was significantly different for a single subject. This analysis does not really contribute to the comparison between perceptual and associative knowledge impairments.

However, in their 1989 paper, Farah et al. report the data necessary for a more well-founded comparison of the performance of LH on tasks tapping visual and nonvisual knowledge of items from biological and artefact categories. Let us consider biological category stimuli. If the hypothesis of Farah et al. is correct, the difference between visual and nonvisual knowledge of LH should be significantly greater than that of the control group. The sum of correct responses given by controls for visual and nonvisual questions can be reconstructed as follows. For biological categories, correct visual responses were 80.4% × 95 (number of questions) × 12 (number of controls) = 916; correct nonvisual responses were 88.5% × 93 × 12 = 988.

The above frequencies can be entered into a log-linear or into a logit-linear model and compared to the performance of LH. LH performed correctly on 60/95 for visual responses and 79/93 for nonvisual responses; for controls, performance was 916/1140 correct for visual responses and 988/1116 correct for nonvisual responses. The statistical analysis with a log-linear model yields $\chi^2(1)$ = 12.310 for the difference between LH and controls and = 38.417 for the difference between visual and nonvisual questions (both highly significant); and $\chi^2$ = 2.229 for the interaction ($p$ = .135, n.s. This means that the greater difficulty LH had with visual than nonvisual questions was not significantly different from that of the control group.

The severe prosopagnosia of this patient was examined by Etcoff et al. (1991). In this study LH was 51% correct with animals and 75% with some fruit and vegetables, but we do not know if the stimuli were of comparable difficulty. These authors also gave LH an object reality decision task, on which the patient was 49% correct with animals and 85% correct with artefacts. No separate data are given for subgroups of the biological categories, possibly because only animals were examined.

On the naming of Snodgrass and Vanderwart pictures, reported in the 1996 paper, the patient was 63.6% correct for musical instruments and 72.3% correct for body parts (the reported percentages correct for natural categories and artefacts were 52% and 84.1%, respectively).

The original data have recently been reanalysed by Takarae and Levin (2001) with an extended set of form-related variables, and the category dissociation was confirmed.

MB (Farah, Meyer, & Mc Mullen, 1996; Takarae & Levin, 2001)

On picture naming with the Snodgrass and Vanderwart set, performance on items from living categories was 33.4% correct, and 76.7% correct for nonliving categories. The data reported in the 1996 paper allow a separate evaluation of musical instruments (49.8% correct) and body parts (83.3% correct). Perceptual and associative knowledge were not examined.

The original data have recently been reanalysed by Takarae and Levin (2001) with an extended set of form-related variables: the category effect was not confirmed on the covariance analysis.

MC (Teixeira Ferreira, Giusiano, & Poncet, 1997)

Naming was examined for only animals and tools. Perceptual and associative knowledge were examined, but separate data are not reported.

MD (Hart, Berndt, & Caramazza, 1985)

The authors report that when asked judgements about category, size, colour, texture, and shape, the patient gave correct responses for all properties, although the responses were hesitant for fruit and vegetables. However, the probes were not controlled and the data are not explicitly given. On categorisation tasks with pictures, the patient's errors consisted entirely of confusions involving the categories fruit and vegetables. Therefore, the deficit does not seem restricted to a problem in accessing lexical representations.

MD named body parts correctly as well as food products outside the categories of fruit and vegetables.

MF (Barbarotto, Capitani, Spinnler, & Trivelli, 1995)

This patient was affected by a severe progressive semantic deficit for biological categories, and by prosopagnosia. In addition he was severely impaired for his knowledge of architecture, a field that had been the patient's profession and the subject of his university teaching; this last deficit involved both pictorial and encyclopaedic knowledge. For a long time MF was still competent in the forensic and managing aspects of his job. For a great part of the progression of the semantic impairment, artefacts were spared and biological categories were severely impaired. Perceptual and associative knowledge of biological categories were not differently impaired. Data regarding musical instruments and body parts were not reported in the original paper, but were available from the original record. Body parts were 100% correct in the December 1989 examination. At the same time, musical instruments were 30% correct in picture naming, 90% correct in word–picture matching, and 75% correct on a verbal semantic questionnaire. Biological categories were 37% correct in naming, 75% correct in word–picture matching, and 63% correct in the questionnaire, whereas artefacts were 87%, 97%, and 97% correct, respectively. Musical instruments were somewhat intermediate between living and nonliving categories on word–picture matching as well as on the semantic questionnaire, even if for naming the patient was severely impaired. Object reality decision was impaired for natural categories.

MICHELANGELO (Sartori, Job, & Coltheart, 1993a; Sartori, Miozzo, & Job, 1993c; Sartori, Coltheart, Miozzo, & Job, 1994a; Sartori, Miozzo, & Job, 1994b; Sartori & Job, 1988; Mauri, Daum, Sartori, Riesch, & Birbaumer, 1994)

This patient is reported in several papers appearing from 1988 to 1994; not all tasks were administered in each of the different examinations. In the original study, the patient was impaired at naming animals and vegetables to an approximately equivalent degree (in a different examination vegetables seemed less impaired than animals, but the former category was collapsed with food). In the 1993 paper, the authors report a disproportionate impairment on a perceptual attributes decision task for animate stimuli compared to inanimate stimuli; in the 1994 paper a substantial sparing of knowledge of nonvisual properties of animals is reported. It is reasonable to assume that the patient did not improve between the two examinations, given that a long time had elapsed since the occurrence of acute encephalitis. It is also worth noting that the patient did not benefit from cognitive rehabilitation (Sartori et al., 1994b).

A disproportionate impairment for perceptual knowledge of biological categories cannot be considered a definite finding on the basis of the published analyses. On perceptual questions concerning biological categories, Michelangelo scored 60% correct (48/80); controls scored 86.9% (69.5/80). On perceptual questions concerning artefacts Michelangelo scored 88.7% correct (71/80); controls scored 90.7% (72.6/80). On associative questions about biological stimuli Michelangelo scored 87.5% correct (35/40). No control data are given, but, as argued for

Giulietta, it is reasonable to suppose that controls were at least at the same level of the patient.

A reanalysis of the available data might yield an approximated evaluation. Let us consider natural categories, in order to see if there was in fact a disproportionate deficit for visual properties compared to associative properties. It is reasonable to presume that the level of control performance on associative probes of biological stimuli was between that of Michelangelo and ceiling (i.e., 100% correct). Let us first assume that the 10 controls were performing at the level of Michelangelo, who was 35/40 correct. Their collapsed correct answers would be 350/400. On visual probes, Michelangelo was 48/80 correct, and controls were 695/800 correct. Analysing the above data with a log-linear model, the overall difference between Michelangelo and the control group is significant, $\chi^2(1) = 23.140$, but the difference between visual and nonvisual probes is not significant, $\chi^2(1) = 2.270$. The interaction between the above factors is significant, $\chi^2(1) = 0.213$, $p = .004$. That is, Michelangelo's deficit is disproportionately severe for visual probes pertaining to biological categories. An even more significant outcome is observed if the missing values of controls are replaced by ceiling performance, $\chi^2(1) = 11.680$, $p = .0006$.

The results of this analysis would support the reality of a greater impairment for perceptual knowledge of biological categories, but should be viewed with caution. In particular, perceptual and associative knowledge were probably assessed in different periods, and the different types of questions were not based on the same stimuli.

On object reality decision, Michelangelo was impaired for animal stimuli but not for artefacts.

MS (Mehta, Newcombe, & De Haan, 1992; Young, Newcombe, Hellawell, & De Haan, 1989)

This patient (reported by the authors as suffering from severe object agnosia) was examined with RT experiments in which a category membership judgment was made for a given noun; the results indicate a deficit for biological categories. No data are reported in support of the presence of a category-specific agnosia (in the strict sense). In a third experiment, the patient showed a priming effect in a lexical decision task for the category names of words belonging to biological and artefact categories. Perceptual and associative knowledge were not investigated. The purported semantic impairment for natural categories is inferred on the basis of the patient's poorer performance on a fluency task as well as on identification from definitions.

The visual imagery ability of this patient was investigated in a distinct study. The patient was impaired at imaging living items, whereas he performed at control level for nonliving items. He showed a definite deficit for both perceptual and factual information about living material given the item's name ("which two of three items were similar" in terms of some visual or nonvisual property).

Summing up, this case presented a disproportionate deficit for living categories across a wide set of tasks, some of which were purely verbal and involved nonperceptual knowledge. Furthermore, the imagery task for living category items had a verbal input. No data demonstrate that the reported object agnosia is reliably category-specific.

MU (Borgo & Shallice, 2001)

This patient presented a disproportionate semantic deficit for biological categories. This deficit was evident in several naming tasks (different visual confrontation naming tasks as well as naming from description), in matching tasks and on semantic probe questions. Perceptual and functional/associative knowledge were equivalently impaired for biological categories: MU's naming of biological items was much poorer than naming of man-made artefacts from both functional/associative and perceptual descriptions; moreover, on a verbal questionnaire MU presented a comparable deficit for perceptual and functional knowledge attributes. With respect to visual-perceptual tasks, MU was slightly impaired on colour naming and identification. With semantic probes, MU showed sparing of body parts (97%) and an intermediate performance for musical instruments (78%). The patient was impaired on object decision tasks (BORB) as well as with silhouettes and progressive silhouettes in the VOSP test: In this latter task no difference was detected between biological categories and artefacts.

The authors have examined the status of the patient's knowledge of other categories, which have seldom been investigated in semantic memory patients: i.e., liquids, edible substances, and materials; the authors argue for a deep similarity between the latter set and biological categories.

NA (Funnell, 2000)

This patient was affected by a progressive cerebral degeneration: She presented a form of apperceptive visual agnosia which caused, according to the author, a disproportionate picture naming impairment for biological categories. Semantic and lexical knowledge were spared: NA correctly responded to 26/28 questions about biological category items, and to 27/28 for artefacts; her few errors occurred in response to functional questions. NA presented a clear visual perceptual disturbance, but the evidence that the category-specific deficit for naming arose at the perceptual level is only indirect. The pictures representing items from biological categories were more visually complex; however, the naming errors made by the patient were not influenced by the visual complexity of the stimuli: This independence seems to not be in agreement with the diagnosis of apperceptive visual agnosia. According to the author, the patient was sensitive to a number of other perceptual characteristics of the stimuli, (such as "joints" between separable parts, etc.); it would have been interesting to check if the stimuli corresponding to biological categories and artefacts were balanced for all these perceptual aspects.

At the first examination body part naming was 69% correct (9/13) and musical instrument naming was 100% correct (5/5).

NA certainly presented an apperceptive visual disturbance, but its categorical specificity can only be inferred from the moderate category effect in picture naming, where the patient performed worse for biological category items on only one out of three tasks. As such, the claim for a categorical organisation of apperceptive stages of visual processing is not supported by strong evidence.

NR (De Haan, Young, & Newcombe, 1992)
This patient was affected by prosopagnosia and amnesia and was impaired on visuospatial perception tests and on name retrieval. A category effect on naming is marginally reported, but object category effects were not further investigated.

NV (Basso, Capitani, & Laiacona, 1988)
This study has been revisited after taking into account the structure of the semantic memory questionnaire, which was not reported in the original paper. On the basis of this revision, we conclude that the comparison between perceptual and associative knowledge is not reliable, as controls were not examined, and all of the stimuli were not investigated with balanced associative and perceptual questions. In particular, perceptual probes concerned only animal stimuli. Therefore, the conclusion of the authors that the patient's impairment disproportionately affected perceptual knowledge is not warranted, as perceptual knowledge was confounded with animal knowledge. Musical instruments were impaired and body parts were spared.

PR (Teixeira Ferreira, Giusiano, & Poncet, 1997)
Naming was only examined for animals and tools. Perceptual and associative knowledge were examined, but separate data are not reported.

PS (Hillis & Caramazza, 1991)
On a picture naming task, the patient was impaired for animals and vegetables; in contrast, fruit was less impaired (although worse than any artefact category). Food and body parts were spared. This association of impaired categories was confirmed in a follow-up examination.

The patient was administered a word definition task, but responses were not analysed in terms of the perceptual and associative information produced by the patient.

RC (Moss, Tyler, Durrant-Peatfield, & Bunn, 1998; Tyler & Moss, 1997)
This case was first reported in 1997 and more extensively described and commented upon in 1998. As the results reported in each account are not in full agreement, we will refer to the latter study. On naming Snodgrass and Vanderwart pictures RC showed an equivalent impairment for animals, fruit and vegetables (9% correct); artefacts were 50% correct while body parts were relatively spared (92%). Similar percentages were observed using a new set of coloured pictures. The patient was examined on a naming from spoken description task (descriptions were based on either functional or visual properties). There were 15 perceptual definitions and 15 functional descriptions for biological items, and the same for artefacts; however, different stimuli were used for perceptual and functional descriptions. Regardless, there was no difference in the patient's ability to identify targets from descriptions based on either functional or perceptual properties for either category (for biological categories, hits were 0 for both perceptual and associative descriptions; for artefacts, hits were 47% and 53%, respectively). With respect to the null performance on associative definitions of living things, there is good evidence for an equivalent impairment to both visual and functional knowledge of natural categories, notwithstanding the lack of strict controls on the materials. Object reality decision data are not reported.

RM (Pietrini, Nertempi, Vaglia, Revello, Pinna, & Ferro-Milone, 1998)
This patient was examined twice. At the first examination, RM was impaired for biological categories on naming, word–picture matching (plants), and word definitions (animals). An equivalent deficit for animals and plants was observed on three tasks, but on word definitions animals were significantly more impaired. However, this latter finding should be viewed with caution due to the possible influence of nuisance variables, the low significance level, and the inflation of type I error risk due to repeated testing. After 18 months, only naming tasks were impaired for both biological categories. Even at the last examination, a subtle semantic deficit cannot be excluded. The criteria for judging if the word definitions were correct are not given. A comparison between perceptual and associative knowledge is not possible.

SB (Sheridan & Humphreys, 1993)
This patient was equally impaired at naming animals and food, the latter of which included many items from the categories of fruit and vegetables. The patient presented an equivalent impairment for stored visual and nonvisual knowledge of biological categories, assessed with an attribute judgment task. Object reality decision and the "Heads" test were within normal range. SB was impaired on drawing from memory.

SBY (Warrington & Shallice, 1984)
This patient was impaired at naming and identifying animals and food, but relatively spared for artefacts. The patient was not administered a separate examination for perceptual and associative knowledge.

SE (Laws, 1998; Laws, Evans, Hodges, & McCarthy, 1995; Moss, Tyler, & Jennings, 1997)
This case was described with contrasting conclusions by Laws et al. (1995) and by Moss et al. (1997), with a further reply by Laws (1998). Laws et al. claimed that the patient, examined 5 years after acute encephalitis, suffered from a very mild naming deficit for biological categories, but the remainder of the study concentrated only on animals. Although the authors report relatively intact naming performance for both animals and objects on a restricted set of stimuli, for the whole Snodgrass and Vanderwart set SE correctly named only 69% (54/78) of animals, fruit, and vegetables. Body parts were 100% correct and musical instruments were 58% correct. On an object decision task, SE scored within the normal range. In the authors' opinion, SE was affected by a disproportionate or selective impairment for associative knowledge of biological categories.

Moss and her colleagues independently re-examined SE and reported that he was 86% correct with artefacts (body parts were 100% and musical instruments were 90% correct), 63% correct with animals (including also birds and insects), and 60% correct for fruit and vegetables. With respect to type of knowledge impairment, Moss and colleagues came to the opposite conclusion to that of the original report, i.e., that the patient had a selective impairment for the visual properties of biological categories. The arguments of Moss and her colleagues can be found in their original paper. The main impairment was found with distinctive visual properties of biological categories, but this deficit was mild (accuracy of SE was .84, whereas the worst control scored .89). A similar conclusion was suggested by other tasks, i.e., definition generation and priming effects.

In his final reply, Laws (1998) argued that the set of stimuli used by Moss and colleagues in their rebuttal study were not appropriate, and further commented on theoretically relevant points. On the basis of these contrasting findings, however, it seems conservative to not classify SE with respect to the degree of impairment for visual and associative semantic knowledge of natural entities.

**SRB** (Forde, Francis, Riddoch, Rumiati, & Humphreys, 1997; Humphreys, Riddoch, & Price, 1997)

This patient has been reported in two papers. The patient presented a deficit for natural categories that was more severe for fruit and vegetables (58% correct in picture naming) than for animals (81% correct). This difference was consistent across different tasks. SRB also had reading problems (letter-by-letter reading).

In the main study (Forde et al., 1997) the authors investigated picture naming latencies, analysing whether the contour overlap of the stimuli was a better predictor of the performance than the living/nonliving distinction within a model that also included familiarity, frequency, visual complexity, and prototypicality. They concluded that contour overlap was a better predictor than category classification. However, this analysis is not convincing. The set of stimuli used for this analysis included more animals than fruit and vegetables: The full set reported by Humphreys et al. (1988) included 26 animals and 12 fruit and vegetables. Moreover, within this set, only those stimuli named correctly could be considered, thus (probably) further reducing the number of items from the categories of fruit and vegetables.

Relevant data for assessing the balance between perceptual and associative knowledge are reported in both studies, with a naming to definition task contrasting visual-perceptual definitions and functional-associative definitions. However, a comparison of the data reported by Forde et al. (1997) with that reported by Humphreys et al. (1997) reveals several discrepancies (see Table E1). It can be seen that:

(a) The data for perceptual definitions of biological categories and artefacts are crossed in the two papers.

(b) SRB's correct naming performance for the associative condition is (overall) 73/76 in Forde et al. and 70/76 in Humphreys et al.

(c) Control data are not consistent at several points.

Table E1

| | *Visual-perceptual definitions* | | *Functional-associative definitions* | |
|---|---|---|---|---|
| *Reference* | *Biological* | *Artefacts* | *Biological* | *Artefacts* |
| *Forde et al. (1997)* | | | | |
| SRB | 23/38 | 16/38 | 35/38 | 38/38 |
| Controls | 32.25/38 | 32.50/38 | 37.00 | 37.50 |
| Range | (30–34) | (21–38) | (36–38) | (37–38) |
| *Humphreys et al. (1997)* | | | | |
| SRB | 16/38 | 23/38 | – | – |
| Controls | 31/38 | 25/38 | – | – |
| Overall | | | | |
| SRB | 39/76 | | 70/76 | |
| Controls (*SD*) | 56/76 (4.0) | | 71/76 (2.1) | |

SRB was marginally impaired on object reality decision (BORB) (27/32 correct vs. a control mean of 29.8/32), but this battery includes an overwhelming majority of living category items. In drawing from memory, drawings of natural category items (animals, fruit and vegetables) were worse than those of man-made objects.

Due to the limits of this experiment, this patient does not appear to be informative for the contrast between perceptual and associative knowledge in category-specific dissociations.

**TOB** (McCarthy & Warrington, 1988, 1990; Parkin, 1993)

This patient was affected by surface dyslexia and dysgraphia. When asked to define pictures and spoken words, the patient was clearly impaired in defining spoken names of biological things, but not in defining pictorially presented stimuli. On this basis McCarthy and Warrington argue for the existence of distinct modality and category-specific cerebral meaning systems. In a later study (Parkin, 1993) the patient did not present a category effect in picture naming when materials were controlled. The impairment for giving specific definitions to spoken names was confirmed for animals but was not present for vegetable names.

The study of TOB does not contribute information regarding the contrast between perceptual and associative knowledge.

**TS** (Wilson, 1997)

This patient presented a possible semantic deficit for animals (other biological categories were not examined).

**TU** (Farah & Wallace, 1992)

According to the authors, TU presented a selective naming deficit for fruit and vegetables, with spared semantic knowledge of the same categories. The selectivity of the impairment to fruit and vegetables was inferred from an investigation of naming latencies: In a linear regression model, the classification "fruit and vegetables vs. all other categories" resulted in the most significant factor; however, it was included in the model together with the classification "living vs. nonliving." This statistical design is not optimal; it would have been preferable to include the living vs. nonliving classification and the contrast (fruit + vegetables) vs. animals (excluding nonliving stimuli from the latter analysis). Table 1 of the paper suggests that animals were probably intermediate between fruit/vegetables and artefacts (Furthermore, the use of logistic regression does not seem appropriate, and other linear models are better suited for an analysis of naming latencies.)

Regarding semantic knowledge, the authors report that "TU had adequate knowledge about fruits and vegetables," but the analysis of the semantic knowledge is rudimentary and details are not given.

The authors claim that the patient was impaired at the lexical level, because phonemic cueing influenced naming success. However, the influence of a phonemic cue may also arise from the disambiguation of poor identification of the stimulus within a group of semantically similar alternatives.

VG (Teixeira Ferreira, Giusiano, & Poncet, 1997)
Naming was only examined for animals and tools. Perceptual and associative knowledge were examined, but separate data are not reported.

MR.W (Rumiati, Humphreys, Riddoch, & Bateman, 1994; Rumiati & Humphreys, 1997; Farah, 1997)
According to the authors, MrW presented with object agnosia without alexia or prosopoagnosia (a claim that has been criticised by Farah, 1997, and further maintained by Rumiati & Humphreys, 1997). The patient was impaired on a "heads and tail" test, but object decision was within the normal range. On a subset of the materials, the patient had a prevailing naming deficit for structurally similar categories, but this was not confirmed on the whole set of stimuli when data were submitted to simultaneous regression analyses with name agreement and other concomitant variables included in the model. The patient probably has a semantic impairment, but the authors do not specify how semantic knowledge of nonliving categories has been examined. The reported data is not exhaustive and is not detailed with respect to individual categories.

## *2. Cases presenting a disproportionate impairment for artefacts*

CG (Silveri, Gainotti, Perani, Cappelletti, Carbone, & Fazio, 1997; Silveri, Perri, & Cappa, 2000)
The authors claim that this patient was affected by a progressive picture naming impairment, with disproportionate severity for artefacts. In their opinion, this deficit was purely lexical in nature; however, a word of caution is suggested as a subtle semantic deficit may have escaped detection. In fact, close scrutiny and reanalysis of the data suggest that the conclusion of a category-specific lexical impairment may not be warranted. The authors administered three different naming tasks; for all three tasks, the category discrepancy appeared only as the disease progressed. On a reanalysis of the contingency tables reported in the first assessment, the category effect was never significant, $\chi^2(1) =$ 1.184 for test 1; 1.002 for test 2; and 2.464 for test 3. Presumably at the same time, word–picture matching and a semantic verbal questionnaire were at ceiling, but these tests were not repeated on subsequent examinations when a category effect was evident. (Even at subsequent examinations, a clear-cut category effect was evident only with naming test 3, whereas differences were marginal or not significant with tests 1 and 2.) Therefore, it is possible that a semantic deficit was present at the later examinations. Interestingly, and consistent with this last possibility, verbal comprehension was impaired on later examinations of this patient (Silveri, Perri, & Cappa, 2000); this suggests a diagnosis of semantic dementia. At first assessment we can presume that the structural description system was spared, as the patient's performance on a word–picture matching task was flawless. Different artefact categories were not explicitly contrasted. Available data indicate that naming of musical instruments was 60% correct, a level closer to that of artefacts (56.7%) than biological items (70%). Performance on body parts was flawless.

CN94 (Breedin, Martin, & Saffran, 1994a)
This patient was given an oddity task on triplets of names (pick the odd one out). Several categories were considered, but only animals and tool stimuli were of comparable mean frequency. The statistical comparison is not clear: a contingency table analysis might indicate more errors on tool stimuli than on animal stimuli. However, it is not clear that the difficulty of the task was balanced across categories, as control performance was at ceiling for both categories. On this basis the evidence in favour of a dissociation is insufficient. Furthermore, the type of knowledge tapped by the triplets is not specified, and could differ between different categories.

CN98 (Gaillard, Auzou, Miret, Ozsancak, & Hannequin, 1998)
The patient presented a relative deficit for artefacts over three assessments on a naming task. The comparison between perceptual and associative knowledge was made with only tools and fruit/vegetables. We have reanalysed the reported data by means of a Fisher exact test: Perceptual and associative information were not differentially affected for biological categories, nor for tools, and the same outcome was observed collapsing these categories together. However, no controls were examined. Given the small number of probes included in this experiment, the statistical comparison between perceptual and functional/associative knowledge would have had sufficient power only if underlying differences were of considerable size.

CW92 (Sacchett & Humphreys, 1992)
The patient was administered picture naming tests, as well as word–picture and picture-word matching. In only one of the picture naming tasks were the stimuli corresponding to artefacts and animals matched for frequency; here, an advantage for animals was evident. (Within the set of artefacts the authors also included five musical instruments and two body parts: However, even eliminating the latter stimuli, the category effect would probably be preserved.) Animal naming was 19/20 correct,

artefacts 6/13 correct, musical instruments 1/5 correct, and body parts were 0/2 correct. In this experiment perceptual and associative knowledge was not distinguished, and an object decision task was not administered. The data are not relevant for a direct verification of any hypothesis about the origin of the category effect. Concerning a possible fragmentation within artefacts, the small number of stimuli used in picture naming for each category prevents a finer grained analysis (the highest number of stimuli was five for clothing and musical instruments, and the smallest was one for vehicles; the number of body parts stimuli was two). For the other tests detailed data are not reported.

DRS (Warrington & Mc Carthy, 1994)
This patient was impaired in the identification of common objects (no other categories were considered in the first part of the study). The authors conclude that DRS presented a category-specific visual associative agnosia affecting artefacts ("... the locus of the deficit appears to lie within those components...that assign meaning to a structured percept, or in access to them"). A study of category-specific effects was then carried out with visual-visual matching of drawings (common objects vs. animals or vehicles) and word–picture matching (common objects vs. animals and flowers or vs. animals and vehicles). According to the authors, the recognition of common objects was disproportionately impaired. However, no control data are given, and stimuli from different categories were not clearly matched for the relevant concomitant variables. The structural description system is reported to be spared on the basis of an object reality decision task (although this conclusion is based on the performance of the patient on VOSP silhouettes, and it is not granted that the patient would have been normal with full-detail drawings). Perceptual and associative knowledge were not tested verbally. The fact that nuisance variables were not controlled makes it problematic to accept the conclusion that artefacts were disproportionately impaired.

ES (Moss & Tyler, 1997, 2000)
This patient, affected by a progressive degenerative disease, was examined from 1994 to 1996. The authors report that she was more impaired for artefacts, and that the category effect became more evident as the disease progressed. They claim that there was a crossover of the category effect in naming from the first to the last examination (with a greater impairment for biological categories at the outset, and for artefacts at the later stage). The initial impairment for biological categories was evident with the whole set of Snodgrass and Vanderwart pictures, but not with a subset in which the stimuli were matched for familiarity (Moss & Tyler, 1997). A reanalysis of the published data concerning the property verification task (Moss & Tyler, 2000) does not confirm a significant advantage for artefacts at the early stage of testing. Visual and associative properties were not differently affected with respect to the stimulus category.

The authors discuss the distinction between shared and distinctive properties for biological and artefact items. We reanalysed the data of the last assessment published in Moss and Tyler (2000) with a logit-linear model that included as factors category type, the shared/distinctive classification, and the type of knowledge (visual or associative) investigated. Here, only the factor of stimulus category significantly influenced the probability of success, whereas neither property type (shared vs. distinctive) nor the visual/associative classification were significant. None of the first order interactions were significant.

No data were given concerning the structural description system.

GP98 (Cappa, Frugoni, Pasquali, Perani, & Zorat, 1998)
This patient presented a disproportionate naming impairment for artefacts, even when musical instruments and body parts were not considered. At the same time, the performance of the patient on a word–picture matching task and on a semantic questionnaire were, respectively, normal and mildly impaired. The stimuli used in the naming task were probably not matched for all of the relevant concomitant variables: The authors divided the items into low and high familiarity groups, and the category effect was confirmed in both subsets. However, this does not rule out the possibility that in both subsets nonliving stimuli were less familiar, or that living and nonliving stimuli were not balanced for other lexical or pictorial variables. Moreover, with respect to the stimuli considered in the main analysis, it would seem that the latter analysis has been carried out on different sets of artefacts ($n$ = 111 vs. 64) and biological items ($n$ = 69 vs. 94). The interpretation that the categorical deficit was confined to the lexical level does not seem entirely warranted for two reasons: First, the patient's performance on the semantic questionnaire was mildly impaired despite the fact that it was very easy (the three controls scored 100% correct, and the format of the test was a fixed-choice task with only two alternatives). As the authors acknowledge, the possibility of a subtle semantic *impairment* cannot be ruled out. Second, in a word–picture verification test, the patient made 9 errors out of 88 trials (10.2%): all of the errors except 1 were on stimuli that the patient also failed to name.

The impairment for artefacts does not seem homogeneous, as vehicles were relatively spared with respect to tools and furniture. Naming of musical instruments was just moderately impaired.

IW (Lambon Ralph, Howard, Nightingale, & Ellis, 1998)
This patient presented a greater impairment for artefacts than for biological items on several different naming tasks, although the effect was not impressive (raw data were 33% vs. 42% correct); the effect became significant only after covariance for familiarity and other psycholinguistic factors. Interestingly, this patient presented a relative loss of perceptual over associative knowledge for all categories, and her structural description system, examined with a number of different tests, was preserved. This case militates against the necessity of explaining the deficit for biological categories in terms of a loss of perceptual knowledge.

The reported data do not provide details useful to distinguish within animate categories and within artefacts.

JJ (Hillis & Caramazza, 1991)
This patient presented a substantial advantage for animals on oral and written naming and auditory word–picture verification. All other categories examined were severely impaired, the only exception being the category of transportation, which was intermediate. A word definition task was administered at a later stage, but the results were not subjected to a quantitative evaluation in order to investigate different components of semantic knowledge. The structural description system was not investigated.

KE (Hillis, Rapp, Romani, & Caramazza, 1990)
This patient was examined with a set of six tasks tapping comprehension and production of words belonging to 10 semantic categories; the rank of errors observed in each category was consistent across different tasks. Averaging across the six tasks, body parts, furniture, and clothing were the most impaired categories, while fruit, vegetables, and food were the least impaired. However, items were not matched for the relevant concomitant variables. On a sorting task, superordinate knowledge was preserved, as were some aspects of perceptual knowledge of animals (size and colour). Neither different types of knowledge, nor the integrity of the structural description system, were assessed.

M.LUCIEN (Hécaen & De Ajuriaguerra, 1956)
This patient was probably affected by visual agnosia, the type of which is not well defined. The examination focused on visual naming; artefacts seemed more impaired than animals. However, the results were not given a quantitative evaluation, and the other crucial cognitive aspects were not examined.

NB (Gonnerman, Andersen, Devlin, Kempler, & Seidenberg, 1997)
This patient was examined with three tasks: picture naming, word–picture matching, and superordinate comprehension (e.g., pointing to a gun when the examiner gave the word weapon). The artefact categories examined were furniture, vehicles, weapons, and clothing; biological categories included only fruit and vegetables. No distinction was made within either artefacts or biological stimuli. The items from different categories were matched for only prototypicality. The patient was examined four times in 4 years: In the first assessment no discrepancy was evident, but starting from the second examination the patient showed a greater impairment for artefacts (most evident at the third examination and less evident at the final one). Different aspects of semantic knowledge were not examined.

PJ (Breedin, Martin, & Saffran, 1994a)
This patient was given an oddity task on triplets of names (pick the odd one out). Several categories were considered, but only animals and tool stimuli were of comparable mean frequency. The statistical comparison is not clear: A contingency table analysis might indicate more errors on tool stimuli than on animal stimuli. However, it is not clear that the difficulty of the task was balanced across categories, as control performance was at ceiling for both categories. On this basis the evidence in favour of a dissociation is insufficient. Furthermore, the type of knowledge tapped by the triplets is not specified, and could be discrepant between different categories.

PL (Laiacona & Capitani, 2001)
This patient presented a disproportionate impairment for artefacts in naming and word–picture matching, as well as on a verbal semantic questionnaire. In the statistical analyses the comparisons were carried out taking into account a wide set of nuisance variables and some difficulty indices. The authors found neither differences between perceptual and associative knowledge, nor an interaction between knowledge type and category. The patient performed within normal range on an object decision task for all categories. In a follow-up examination, the pattern of category impairment was confirmed, notwithstanding the worsening of the overall cognitive level. No statistical comparison was attempted within the domains of biological categories and artefacts. However, some evidence points toward a possible fractionation of artefacts categories. At picture naming (first examination) biological categories were 37% correct, artefacts 13% correct, body parts 60% correct, and musical instruments 20% correct. Data from the other tasks and follow-up data suggest that, on the whole, body parts were the most preserved category, and musical instrument the least preserved.

SM (Turnbull & Laws, 2000)
The evidence in favour of a disproportionate naming impairment for artefacts is not strong for this case. A category effect was present only among low familiarity stimuli, and a main effect of category was significant for neither high- nor middle-familiarity stimuli, nor for the overall set. Moreover, the naming errors of this patient mirror the performance of controls, as even the latter group presented a disproportionate difficulty with low familiarity artefacts. (The controls' performance, entered alone as a model variable in a data reanalysis with logistic regression, explains 84% of the variability.)

Regarding the verbal semantic probes used to investigate visual and associative knowledge, visual knowledge was slightly more impaired than associative knowledge, but no category dissociation was evident. Concerning object reality decision, SM performed poorly on the VOSP battery; on the BORB battery, SM scored below normal range, but the category effect could not be evaluated due to the low number of artefacts included.

On naming the Snodgrass and Vanderwart picture set, body parts were 42% correct (5/12), and musical instruments were 13% correct (1/8, i.e., the worst performance).

VER (Warrington & McCarthy, 1983)
This patient presented a global aphasia with sparing of object recognition as judged by performance on a picture-object matching task. The category-specificity of her deficit was investigated by comparing spoken word–picture matching of objects and food (Exp. 10) as well as objects, animals, and flowers (Exp. 11). Subtypes of objects were not investigated separately. In both experiments, objects fared worse. The type of semantic knowledge that was spared/impaired was not investigated.

VP (Breedin, Martin, & Saffran, 1994a)
This patient was administered an oddity task on triplets of names (pick the odd one out). Several categories were considered, but only animal and tool stimuli were equated for mean frequency. The statistical comparison is not clear: A contingency table analysis might indicate that more errors were made on tools than on animals. However, the difficulty of the task may not have been equated across categories, as the performance of controls was at ceiling for both categories. On this basis the evidence in favour of a dissociation is insufficient. Also, subtypes of biological and artefact categories cannot be reliably compared. The type of knowledge tapped by the triplets is not specified, and could differ between different categories.

YOT (Warrington & McCarthy, 1987)
This patient presented a global aphasia and phonological dyslexia with impaired comprehension of visual stimuli as judged from a visual–visual matching task. The category-specificity of her deficit was investigated by comparing spoken word–picture matching and spoken word–written word matching. In the former task, indoor objects fared worse than food, flowers, and animals, and in a further analysis small manipulable objects were more impaired than food and large outdoor man-made objects. In tasks of the second type (spoken word written word matching), the most preserved categories were animals, occupations, vegetables, and fabrics, whereas the most severely impaired categories were body parts and furniture. The type of semantic knowledge that was spared/impaired was not investigated. Evidence in favour of a fractionation within the category of artefacts is provided by the spoken word–picture matching task, in which indoor objects were 58% correct compared to 78% for outdoor objects. The former subset mainly included tools, implements and kitchen utensils, whereas the latter mainly included vehicles and buildings. Chance performance in this task is indicated as 20%. In a further spoken word–picture matching experiment, it was found that musical instruments were impaired (33% correct). However, stimuli were not controlled for the relevant concomitant variables.

## APPENDIX F

### Picture naming severity for those patients presenting a disproportionate semantic impairment for biological categories and for which perceptual and functional/associative knowledge could be reliably compared

*1. Perceptual attributes worse than associative attributes only for biological categories: Structural description impaired only for biological categories*

| *Case* | *Biological categories* | *Artefacts* | Δ | *Mean* |
|---|---|---|---|---|
| GIULIETTA | 56.25% | 87.50% | 31.25 | 71.87% |
| MICHELANGELO | 32.90% | 74.90% | 42.00 | 53.90% |
| Mean | 44.57% | 81.20% | 36.63 | 62.88% |

*2. Balanced deficit for perceptual and functional/associative attributes of biological categories: Structural description spared*

| *Case* | *Biological categories* | *Artefacts* | Δ | *Mean* |
|---|---|---|---|---|
| EA (2nd exam) | 3.00% | 43.00% | 40.00 | 23.00% |
| FM | 20.00% | 70.00% | 50.00 | 45.00% |
| JENNIFER | 36.1% | 77.80% | 41.70 | 56.95% |
| SB | 9.50% | 35.00% | 25.50 | 22.25% |
| Mean | 17.15% | 56.45% | 39.30 | 36.80% |

*3. Balanced deficit for perceptual and functional/associative attributes of biological categories: Structural description impaired for biological categories*

| *Case* | *Biological categories* | *Artefacts* | Δ | *Mean* |
|---|---|---|---|---|
| CA | 3.30% | 20.00% | 16.07 | 11.65% |
| DB | 58.00% | 81.00% | 23.00 | 69.50% |
| EA (1st exam) | 0.00% | 17.00% | 17.00 | 8.50% |
| EW[a] | 34.00% | 90.40% | 56.40 | 62.20% |
| GR | 13.00% | 73.00% | 60.00 | 43.00% |
| JBR[b] | 26.00% | 58.00% | 32.00 | 42.00% |
| MF | 37.00% | 87.00% | 50.00 | 62.00% |
| MU | 33.30% | 75.00% | 41.70 | 54.15% |
| Mean | 25.57% | 62.67% | 37.10 | 44.12% |

[a]For case EW the reported figures refer to animals vs. tools, furniture, and vehicles.
[b]The reported data for case JBR are drawn from Bunn, Tyler, and Moss (1997).

COGNITIVE NEUROPSYCHOLOGY, 2003, 20 (3/4/5/6), 263–306

# A CASE SERIES ANALYSIS OF "CATEGORY-SPECIFIC" DEFICITS OF LIVING THINGS: THE HIT ACCOUNT

Glyn W. Humphreys and M. Jane Riddoch
*University of Birmingham, UK*

We report a case series analysis of a group of seven patients with apparent "category-specific" disorders affecting living things. On standard diagnostic tests, a range of deficits were apparent, with some cases appearing to have impaired visual access to stored knowledge, some with impaired semantic knowledge (across modalities), and some with an impairment primarily at a name retrieval stage. Patients with a semantic deficit were impaired for both visual and associative/functional knowledge about living things, whilst patients with a modality-specific access deficit showed worse performance when stored visual knowledge was probed. In addition, patients with impaired access to visual knowledge were affected when perceptual input was degraded by masking, and all patients showed an interaction between perceptual similarity and category when matching pictures to names or defining statements. We discuss the results in terms of the Hierarchical Interactive Theory (HIT) of object recognition and naming (Humphreys & Forde, 2001). We also discuss evidence on lesion sites in relation to research from functional brain imaging on category differences in object identification in normal observers.

## INTRODUCTION

Since Warrington and Shallice's (1984) first experimental paper on the topic, there have been numerous reports of patients with problems in recognising and naming objects belonging to particular categories of object. Most commonly patients have been reported with impaired recognition and naming of living things, but the opposite impairment, for nonliving things, has also been noted on several occasions (see Caramazza, 1998; Forde & Humphreys, 1999; Humphreys & Forde, 2001; Tyler & Moss, 2001, for recent reviews). These neuropsychological reports have been bolstered by converging evidence from normal observers studies, including: (1) studies using functional imaging to demonstrate differences in the neural substrates of recognition and naming for living and nonliving things (e.g., Chao, Haxby, & Martin, 1999; Devlin et al., 2003; Martin, Wiggs, Ungerleider, & Haxby, 1996; Perani, Schnur, Tettamanti, Gorno-Tempini, Cappa, & Fazio, 1999; Spitzer et al., 1999; though see Devlin et al., 2002), (2) differences in event-related potential signals to stimuli from the different categories (Kiefer, 2001), and (3) differences in the efficiency of processing living and nonliving things (Humphreys, Riddoch, & Quinlan, 1988; Lloyd-Jones & Humphreys, 1997). There have been claims that these differences may reflect artifactual variations in familiarity and image complexity (Funnell & Sheridan, 1992; Stewart, Parkin, & Hunkin, 1992). However, the fact that

Requests for reprints should be addressed to Glyn W. Humphreys, Behavioural Brain Sciences Centre, School of Psychology, University of Birmingham, Birmingham, B15 2TT, UK.

This work was supported by a grant from the Medical Research Council (UK). We thank all the patients for kindly taking part, Dr V. Chavda for help in transcribing the MRI scans, Adam Cooper for his help in constructing the associates for Experiment 4, and Toby Lloyd-Jones for the stimuli used in Experiment 5.





http://www.tandf.co.uk/journals/pp/02643294.html

DOI:10.1080/02643290342000023

double dissociations can occur (see Hillis & Caramazza, 1991), and that category effects remain even with covarying factors either controlled or factored out (Farah, Meyer, & McMullen, 1996; Sartori, Miozzo, & Job, 1993), suggests that they are a real consequence of the different ways in which stimuli from contrasting categories are processed and neurally represented in the brain.

Several different accounts have been offered to explain category-specific recognition and naming disorders. We discuss four.

## Domain-specific semantic knowledge

In some respects, the most straightforward argument is that the deficits represent the categorical organisation of semantic knowledge in the brain (e.g., Caramazza & Shelton, 1998). On this view, our concepts of the world are organised according to specific domains created by evolutionary pressures—for representing knowledge about animals, about plant-life (e.g., fruits and vegetables), and about other objects (possibly with some subdivision for the phylogenetically more recent category of tools; see Santos & Caramazza, 2002). Disorders affecting either living or nonliving things can then arise because of selective damage to the domain-specific representations for knowledge about each stimulus class. This can explain why deficits can arise for fruits and vegetables but not necessarily for animals (Farah & Wallace, 1992; Hart, Berndt, & Caramazza, 1985), or for animals but not for fruits and vegetables (Caramazza & Shelton, 1998). Such dissociations are difficult to explain if performance was affected by some single underlying factor (e.g., the perceptual similarity between items within each category; see below), but they would follow if semantic knowledge was represented separately for these classes of object.

## The sensory-functional account

A somewhat different view is that the impairments do not reflect the modular representation of knowledge about different categories, but rather differences in the particular types of information that living and nonliving things depend on for recognition and naming. The sensory-functional (S-F) account of category-specific disorders was first proposed by Warrington and Shallice (1984). They suggested that living things are differentiated from one another primarily on the basis of their sensory/perceptual properties. In contrast, nonliving things are individuated by their functional properties. Accordingly, damage to stored knowledge about the sensory-perceptual properties of objects may disrupt the recognition and naming of living things, whilst damage to knowledge about the functional properties of objects will impair nonliving things. According to this account, stored knowledge is not categorically organised but rather organised in terms of properties associated with, and that differentiate between, particular objects (see also Allport, 1985; Warrington & McCarthy, 1987). Neurological lesions can affect some categories of object more than others because of the varying importance of the different properties for object identification.

Warrington and Shallice (1984) reported data from two patients with problems in identifying living things, following herpes simplex encephalitis infection. One reason they proposed the S-F account was that the problems spread to some categories of nonliving thing, including musical instruments, cloths, and gems. Warrington and Shallice suggested that these nonliving things, like living things, were identified primarily on the basis of their sensory/perceptual properties; consequently damage to sensory/perceptual knowledge would affect these nonliving categories as well as living things. This last point, however, is controversial. Borgo and Shallice (2001) recently confirmed the presence of deficits with nonliving foodstuffs and other material defined by sensory properties, in a patient with an impairment for living things. In contrast, Laiacona, Capitani, and Caramazza (in press) report data on a patient with a deficit for living things with good verbal knowledge about nonliving items defined by their sensory properties. A computer simulation of the basic double dissociation between deficits for living and nonliving things, based on the assumption that these stimuli differ in terms of the number of sensory/perceptual and functional attributes they are defined by, was reported by Farah and McClelland (1991).

However, for the S-F view it is unclear why different patterns of impairments may sometimes emerge with animals, on the one hand, and fruits and vegetables on the other. In addition, for this account, a deficit for living things should be linked to poor retrieval of perceptual rather than functional knowledge about stimuli. Yet some patients with problems for living things are as impaired at answering questions about the functional properties of the affected stimuli as they are at answering questions about their perceptual properties (Borgo & Shallice, 2001; Caramazza & Shelton, 1998; Laiacona, Barbarotto, & Capitani, 1993a; Samson, Pillon & De Wilde, 1998; Sheridan & Humphreys, 1993). These findings are somewhat problematic.

## Distributed semantics

More recently, studies have shown that living and nonliving things are distinguished more by the correlations between their perceptual and functional features, rather than by the number of associated perceptual or sensory features (e.g., McRae & Cree, 2002; McRae, De Sa, & Seidenberg, 1997; Moss, Tyler, & Devlin, 2002). Most notably, living things typically have intercorrelated perceptual features, shared across members of a category, which are associated with common biological functions (breathing, eating, reproducing). Distinctive perceptual features are not associated with the object's function (e.g., the stripes of a tiger). In contrast, nonliving things have distinctive perceptual features that correlate with their function (McRae & Cree, 2002; Moss et al., 2002). Moss, Tyler, and colleagues propose that these different relations between sensory/perceptual and functional properties of objects can give rise to the observed patterns of category deficits (Durrant-Peatfield, Tyler, Moss, & Levy, 1997; Moss, Tyler, & Jennings, 1997; Moss, Tyler, Durrant-Peatfield, & Bunn, 1998; Tyler & Moss, 1997, 2001). Rather than suggesting that semantic knowledge is organised on the basis of domain-specific categories or sensory vs. functional knowledge, these investigators argue for a distributed semantic system without differentiation in terms of category or feature property. Correlated features may be more robust than distinctive features to the effects of brain damage, since degradation of part of a representation may be recovered from the interlinked features. For living things the correlated features may enable shared properties concerning (e.g.) biological function to be recovered (see Moss et al., 1997; Tyler & Moss, 1997), but identification of the specific object may be impaired since the distinctive sensory/perceptual features are not linked to functional features within the semantic system. In contrast, nonliving things may still be identified because the distinctive sensory/perceptual features are supported by functional features. A simulation of this basic result within a system with randomly distributed semantic representations was reported by Durrant-Peatfield et al. (1997; see also Tyler & Moss, 2001). Interestingly, when high levels of lesion were simulated, a small advantage emerged for living things over nonliving things. The authors attributed this to those remaining correlated features for sensory/perceptual knowledge and biological function being able to support identification of a core set of objects (there being more intercorrelated features for living things, leaving a residual core even after heavy damage). Consequently, we may expect the direction of category effects to vary as a function of the degree of deficit in a given patient (see Moss et al., 2002).

Patterns of intercorrelation between features, and whether the features are shared or distinctive, are likely to be influential factors in object recognition and naming. However, somewhat different predictions can follow from apparently small changes in models. For example, Devlin, Gonnerman, Anderson, and Seidenberg (1998) simulated the effects of lesioning to a network with interconnected semantic units that was trained to represent the perceptual and functional features of objects. Performance was less affected for living things when lesions were relatively small, whilst an advantage for nonliving things emerged as damage increased. At present it is unclear which approach to modelling is most appropriate. In addition, there are mixed data on the relations between category-specificity and the degree of deficit in patients (compare Gonnerman, Anderson, Devlin, Kempler, & Seidenberg, 1997, who found that living things were initially preserved in Alzheimer's Disease but were later impaired, with Silveri, Danieli, Giustolisi, & Gainotti, 1991, who reported the opposite—see also Garrard, Patterson, Watson, & Hodges, 1998). Furthermore, the widespread cortical changes associated with Alzheimer's disease often fail to produce clear patterns of category-specific deficit (see Garrard, Lambon Ralph, & Hodges, 2002), though on a distributed memory account, such cortical changes ought to generate category-specific losses.

It is also unclear how the distributed memory account put forward by Moss, Tyler, and colleagues fits with evidence on functional brain imaging in normal participants. Though there are disparities across those studies too, there is evidence for greater activation of the left posterior middle temporal and inferior frontal cortices when tools are named (Grabowski, Damasio, & Damasio, 1998; Martin et al., 1996; see Price & Friston, 2002). In contrast, living things have been shown to generate increased activation in regions of extra-striate and ventral occipito-temporal cortex associated with processing the visual and structural properties of objects (Martin et al., 1996; Moore & Price, 1999; Perani et al., 1995) and also in the anterior temporal lobes (Devlin et al., 2003). These data suggest that there may be some regional specialisation in object processing that underscores the category-specific deficits that arise in patients.

## The Hierarchical Interactive Theory (HIT)

The three accounts we have considered so far have been proposed in order to explain category-specific impairments in neurological patients. Yet differences in processing objects from different categories have also been reported with normal observers. For example, Humphreys et al. (1988) reported that naming times varied as a function of the "structural similarity" between category exemplars. Stimuli within high structural similarity within their category were named more slowly than those with lower structural similarity. Lloyd-Jones and Humphreys (1997) reported similar results using an object decision task in which real objects had to be distinguished from nonobjects created by combining two parts of objects from within the same category. Humphreys et al. (1988) defined structural similarity in terms of the number of common parts across category members, as listed by independent participants, and in terms of the mean overlap in the outline contours of stimuli within the same category.[1] Generally, structurally similar items come from categories of living thing (animals, fruits, vegetables), with the exception of the category body part, where the exemplars tend to have lower structural similarity. Humphreys et al. proposed that structural similarity would determine the time required to differentiate a target from competitors within the same neighbourhood in a visual recognition system (they termed this a structural description system). It was further proposed that this would have 'knock on' effects on other processes, if partial activation was transmitted in cascade, through a hierarchy of processing stages—from the structural description system through to semantic representations coding additional properties of objects (e.g., their functional attributes) or to names. In particular, the overlap in perceptual descriptions amongst items from structurally similar categories may give rise to relatively efficient access to superordinate semantic information shared across category members, but it would slow access to information about individual objects (Riddoch & Humphreys, 1987a). In addition, due to the need for greater visual differentiation within some categories, greater weight may also be placed on stored visual knowledge to "drive" the identification process. In contrast, and as suggested by the S-F account, the importance of functional differences for the identification of some nonliving things should lead to functional knowledge being weighted strongly (Humphreys, Riddoch, & Forde, 2002). Humphreys and Forde (2001) recently extended this argument to suggest that, in order to derive specific responses to individual exemplars within a structurally similar set, additional visual information may need to be recruited through re-entrant activation of visual/perceptual

[1] Using the standardised set of pictures from Snodgrass and Vanderwart (1980).

knowledge. In their Hierarchical Interactive Theory (HIT), similarity effects are transmitted through a hierarchical series of processing stages, with additional forms of information being recruited interactively to differentiate between competitors.

In addition to being distinguished by its account of normal object identification, HIT also differs from the other accounts because it holds that category effects can arise at several levels of processing. For example, a deficit in coding input into the structural description system could exacerbate the normal advantage for exemplars from structurally dissimilar rather than structurally similar categories, so that a patient would generally find living things harder to identify than nonliving things (e.g., see Riddoch & Humphreys, 1987b, for evidence). A lesion to the structural description system itself could also lead to problems with structurally similar items, since this could increase overlap within a visually defined neighbourhood. It could also generate problems for objects where visual/perceptual properties are diagnostic. In both cases, the deficit may be more serious on object naming than on other tasks, since object naming in particular requires individuation of a response to a single item. Indeed, a mild problem in accessing visual knowledge about a stimuli may masquerade as a problem in name retrieval for living things (Forde, Francis, Riddoch, Rumiati, & Humphreys, 1997; Humphreys, Riddoch, & Price, 1997).

In contrast to patients with deficits in accessing structural knowledge, a deficit at a semantic level could affect nonliving things, dependent on functional features for their identification. It is even possible for information at a semantic level to be organised categorically, so that damage could affect domains specific to (say) animals rather fruits and vegetables (see Caramazza & Shelton, 1998). Patients with semantic deficits, however, can be distinguished from those with impairments to earlier processes because the deficits affect retrieval of the functional as well as the visual/perceptual properties of stimuli (e.g., that, in addition to having horns, a cow is also used to produce milk). Semantic problems may also occur cross-modally, provided that the same semantic knowledge is accessed from different modalities (see Riddoch, Humphreys, Coltheart, & Funnell, 1988), whereas patients with a pre-semantic deficit may have intact knowledge about at least the functional properties of stimuli (Riddoch & Humphreys, 1987b). Importantly, and irrespective of the functional site of a lesion, patients with problems with living things may be sensitive to manipulations that increase the visual overlap between stimuli, since the lesion may restrict any ability to recruit visual knowledge in a top-down manner, to help differentiate between competitors.

## The present paper

In the present paper, we draw together evidence on a case series of seven patients, all of whom were selected because they had problems in identifying living things. In doing this, we generate a more powerful test than hitherto of the factors that lead to the category-specific deficits in such cases, since previous reports have typically focused on one or at most two such patients. In addition, we overcome one previous weakness in the literature, due to contrasting tests being used with different patients. The use of different tests makes it hard to compare across reports. For example, some authors have argued that functional knowledge is intact in patients with problems with living things (Forde et al., 1997), whilst others have noted deficits (Caramazza & Shelton, 1998); however, the questions used to probe functional knowledge have differed (see Humphreys & Forde, 2001, for a more detailed consideration of this issue). Here we used the same tests across all of the patients, and in so doing we are able to highlight similarities and, in addition, qualitative and quantitative differences in performance.

The data are organised into three sections. In Section 1 we present data from standardised tests of picture naming and access to semantics. These results separate the patients into three groups, according to whether they seem to have (1) a modality-specific impairment in accessing semantic knowledge from vision (patients HJA and DW), (2) an amodal deficit in semantic knowledge (patients KS, GA, and SP), or (3) a problem in name retrieval (patients DM and SRB). In Section 2 we present experiments that examine in more detail the performance of the patients with contrasting categories of object, assessing name retrieval and access to semantic, functional, and stored perceptual knowledge. In Section 3 we evaluated (1) the effects of presenting the stimuli under taxing visual conditions (with visual masks), and (2) the relative effects of category and perceptual similarity between stimuli. In the study of masking we assess whether a disruption to visual processing can affect performance in patients with deficits apparent at different levels of object naming. In the final study we present data demonstrating an interaction between structural similarity and category, so that the ability of patients to discriminate between structurally similar living things is particularly poor (compared with either structurally similar nonliving things or structurally dissimilar, but semantically similar, living things). We argue that the contrasting patterns of performance across the patients can be understood in terms of damage to different stages of object processing, covarying with the site(s) and extent of lesion. Nevertheless, at each stage of processing, performance is sensitive to perceptual overlap between stimuli. This can affect living things in particular because of a confluence of relatively high structural and semantic similarity between exemplars.

## CASE REPORTS

Data on some of the present patients have been presented before (patients HJA, SRB, DM, and DW). Here we extend those prior results with new data, whilst presenting any earlier results in the context of identical tests being performed on other patients. Transcriptions of the MRI scans for all the patients are presented in Figure 1.

In this section, we organise the patients in terms of their lesion site, beginning with those with bilateral posterior damage (HJA and DW), followed by two patients with unilateral, medial, occipito-temporal lesions (DM and SRB), and three patients with medial and anterior temporal lobe damage (unilateral in the case of patient KS, and bilateral for patients GA and SP).[2]

### HJA (dob 30.6.20; male)

HJA's case has been documented in a detailed series of papers (Chainay & Humphreys, 2001; Giersch, Humphreys, Boucart, & Kovacs, 2000; Humphreys & Riddoch, 1987; Riddoch & Humphreys, 1987b; Riddoch, Humphreys, Gannon, Blott, & Jones, 1999). He was formerly an executive working for an international company. He suffered a stroke peri-operatively in 1981, which resulted in bilateral lesions affecting inferior occipito-temporal regions of cortex (including fusiform and lingual gyri). Subsequently he had a superior altitudinal field defect. There was a range of neuropsychological deficits including: visual object agnosia, prosopagnosia, alexia without agraphia, cerebral achromatopsia, and topographical agnosia. There are grounds for arguing that HJA has a basic deficit in visual perceptual organisation, since he has problems in dealing with occlusion relations and with overlapping figures (Giersch et al., 2000; Riddoch & Humphreys, 1987b). With the "unusual views" match tests from BORB (Riddoch & Humphreys, 1993), HJA scored 16 on both the minimal-feature and foreshortened view matches, which is over 2 *SD*s lower than the control mean. Riddoch and Humphreys (1987b) noted that HJA's deficit tended to be worse with objects from structurally similar categories relative to objects from categories with structurally more dissimilar members; this is replicated here, where we report data recorded between 1999 and 2002. In follow-up tests conducted in 1997, Riddoch et al. (1999) found that HJA's basic object recognition skills had remained stable since 1981, though there was some deterioration in his stored memory for visual properties of objects when he was

[2] DW, GA, and SP also suffered some degree of frontal lobe damage. However, we suggest that this did not impinge particularly on their category-specific disorder. In screening tests with another 20 patients with damage confined to the frontal lobes, and overlapping the frontal lobe damage in DW, GA, and SP, we have failed to find evidence of category-specific deficits for living things.

required to draw or define them from memory. However, under the more constrained tests tapping visual memory here (e.g., answering visual definitions), HJA performed relatively well.

## DW (dob 10.5.39, male)

DW was a former electronic engineer and electrical tester. He had suffered long-term epilepsy before sustaining a head injury in 1985 when he fell from a ladder. The fall resulted in internal bilateral damage to the occipital lobes and unilateral damage to the right frontal lobe. He subsequently underwent a right frontal craniotomy and right frontal lobectomy. He had a left homonymous hemianopia and also a restriction to the upper right field. He was able to read both regular and irregular words relatively well (26 and 27/30 on regular and irregular words from PALPA test 35; Kay, Lesser, & Coltheart, 1992), but was surface dysgraphic. He had problems in identifying objects from vision, which was more marked for living than for nonliving things. There was evidence of some impairments in low-level visual processing. He scored 18/25 on the minimal-feature and foreshortened view match tasks from BORB, which is below the control limit for minimal-feature views. He also had difficulties with overlapping figures. Data on DW's object processing are presented in Thomas, Forde, Humphreys, and Graham (2002). The data presented here were recorded between 1987 and 1989.

## KS (dob 28.1.33, female)

KS was a former ordnance worker and housewife. She contracted herpes simplex encephalitis in 1999. This led to unilateral damage to middle and anterior regions of her left temporal lobe. Subsequently she was somewhat impaired at verbal memory (scoring 32/50 on the Warrington Recognition Memory Test with words but 39/50 with faces; Warrington, 1984); she had surface dyslexia and dysgraphia and impaired object identification which was most pronounced for living things. Early visual perception was preserved. She made no errors on the unusual view matching tasks from BORB (25/25 for both minimal-feature and foreshortened views) and had a ratio of 1:1.05 for her times to name nonoverlapping and overlapping letters. The present data were collected between 2000 and 2002.

## GA (dob 23.5.54, male)

GA was a former professional musician who suffered herpes simplex encephalitis infection in 1990. He suffered bilateral damage to the middle and anterior temporal lobe regions, which extended forward into the frontal lobes (particularly on the left). He was severely amnesic, scoring 27 and 29/50 on the Warrington Recognition Memory test with faces and words (Warrington, 1984). There was some evidence of dysexecutive syndrome. For example, he correctly sorted only two categories on the Wisconsin Card Sort Task, scoring 48 correct out of 93 trials administered (Heaton, Chelune, Talley, Kay, & Curtiss, 1993). He had a converted score of 20 (impaired) on the Hayling test of frontal lobe function (Burgess & Shallice, 1997). His performance on Stroop colour naming was poor, reporting only 11/41 colours correctly when the word was an incongruent colour name, naming instead the incongruent word. Performance on the Brixton test of frontal lobe function was somewhat better, however, where he had a scaled score of 6 (average; Burgess & Shallice, 1997). In addition to these problems, there was evidence of surface dyslexia and dysgraphia and a deficit in object identification, which was most pronounced for living things. This last deficit was the main subject of the current investigations. Data were collected between 2000 and 2002. There was no evidence of a low-level perceptual deficit. GA scored 25 and 23/25 on the minimal-feature and foreshortened-view matching tasks from BORB (Riddoch & Humphreys, 1993), which is within control levels (minimal-feature mean = 23.3, *SD* = 2; foreshortened-view mean = 21.6, *SD* = 2.6). The ratio of his naming times for nonoverlapping and overlapping letters was 1.12, again within control limits (Riddoch & Humphreys, 1993).

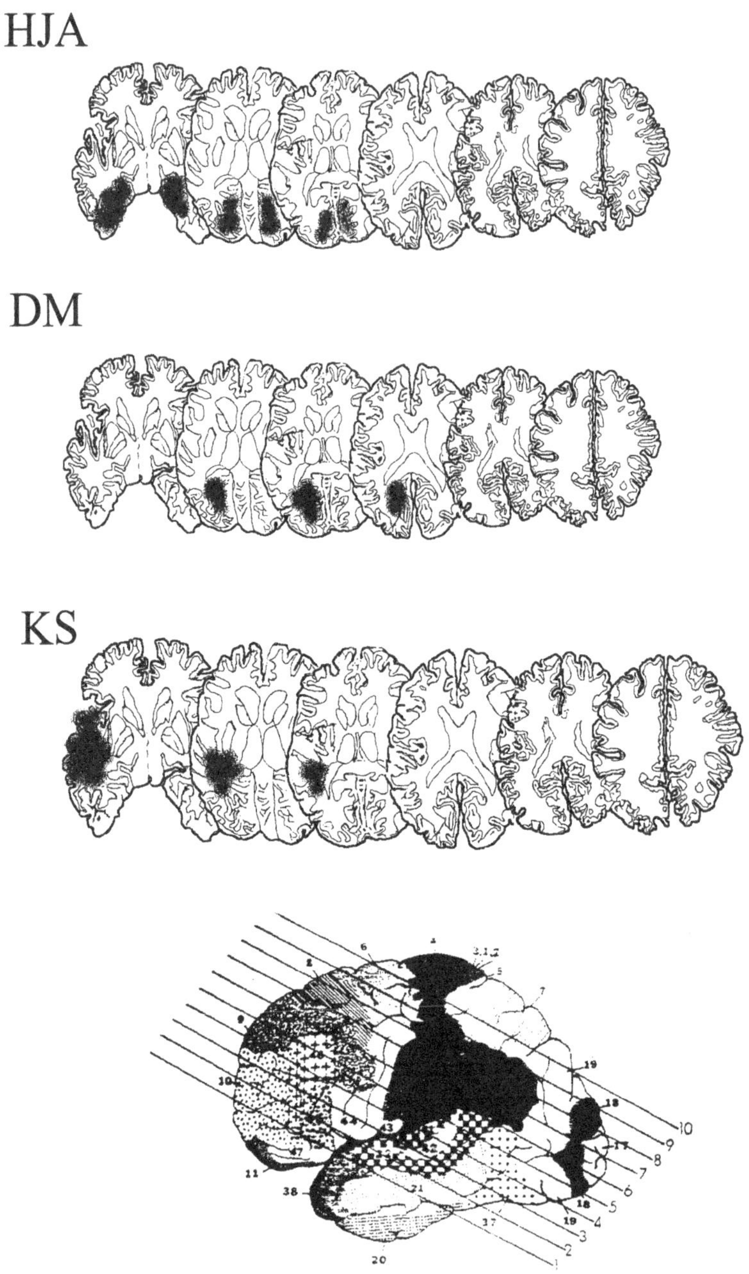


**Figure 1.** *Lesion reconstructions in the patients, from MRI scans. Lesions have been drawn onto standard slices from Gado, Hanaway, and Frank (1979). Slices 3–8 are depicted here.*

DW

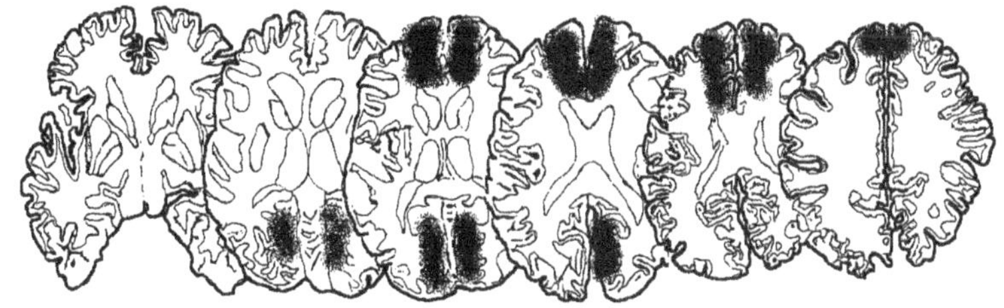

SRB

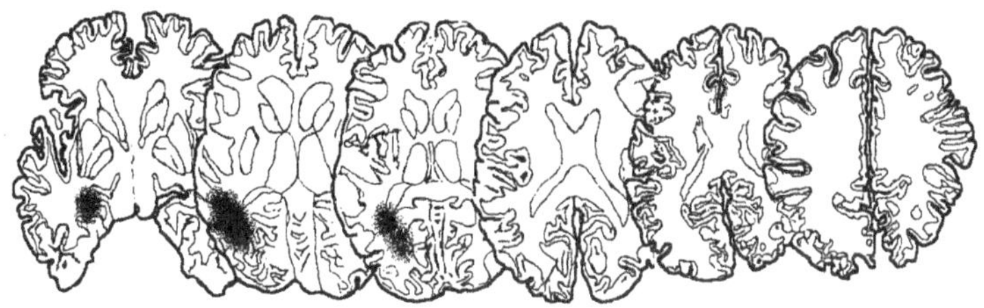

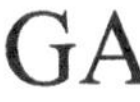


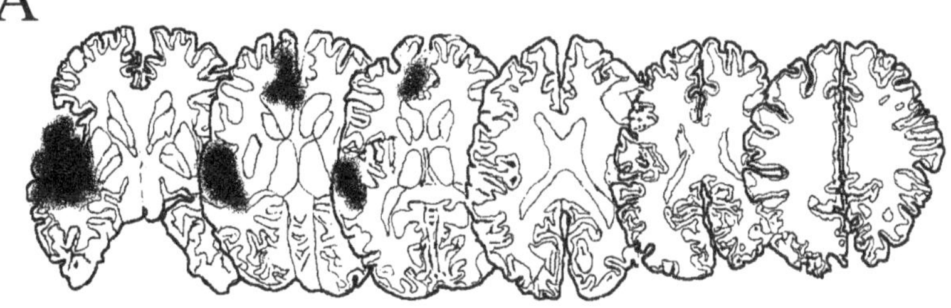

SP

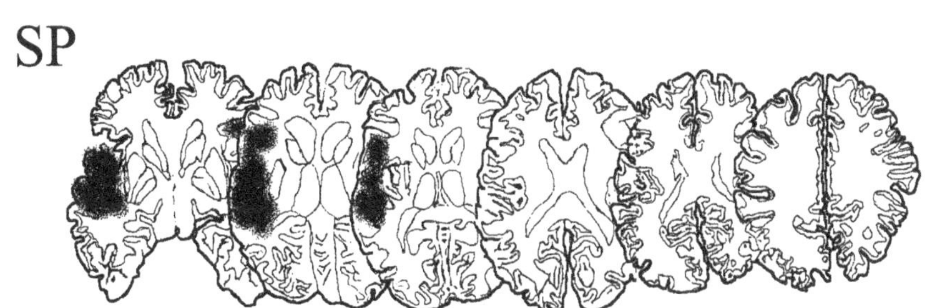

### SP (dob 16.4.53, male)

SP was a former bank manager who suffered herpes simplex encephalitis infection in 1998. This resulted in bilateral damage to middle and anterior temporal regions, which extended into the frontal lobes. He had marked anterograde and retrograde amnesia, scoring 33 and 31/50 on faces and words on the Warrington Recognition Memory Test (Warrington, 1984). As with GA, there was some evidence of dysexecutive syndrome. He had a scaled score of 2 (impaired) on the Brixton test of frontal lobe function (Burgess & Shallice, 1997) (though he named 93/94 colours correctly in an word-incongruent Stroop condition, and he sorted 7 categories correctly on the Wisconsin Card Sort Test; Heaton et al., 1993). There was also surface dyslexia and dysgraphia and a problem in object identification that was most severe for living things. Early visual processing appeared relatively preserved. He performed flawlessly on the minimal-feature and foreshortened-view matches (25/25) and he had a 1:1.03 ratio for naming nonoverlapping to overlapping letters (from BORB, Riddoch & Humphreys, 1993). The present data on SP's problems with living things was collected between 2000 and 2002.

### DM (dob 14.12.52, female)

DM was formerly a teacher. She had a brain abscess evacuated in 1994 when multiple arteriovenous malformations (AVMs) in her lungs tracked to her brain. This resulted in damage to the left medial and inferior occipito-temporal region. Subsequently DM suffered from a right hemianopia, alexia without agraphia (Osswald, Humphreys, & Olson, 2002), and problems in naming colours and living things. Low-level visual perception was relatively intact and she scored 25/25 on both the minimal-feature and foreshortened-view matches from BORB (Riddoch & Humphreys, 1993). Data on her category-specific deficit for living things were presented in Humphreys et al. (1997). In the present paper we draw on early data on picture naming and object decision from BORB. Additional data were collected between 2000 and 2002. DM's performance had remained stable during the intervening period.

### SRB (dob 9.6.56, male)

SRB, a plumber, suffered a spontaneous intracerebral haemorrhage from an underlying AVM in 1993. This produced damage in the left inferior medial occipito-temporal region. There was also evidence of a small infarct in the right thalamic region. Following the lesion, SRB had a right homonymous hemianopia and several neuropsychological deficits. He had both anterograde and retrograde amnesia, particularly for verbal material (scoring 42 and 31/50 for faces and words in the Warrington Recognition Memory test; Warrington, 1984), alexia without agraphia, and problems in identifying living things. SRB's low-level perceptual abilities appeared relatively intact. He scored 25/25 on both minimal-feature and foreshortened-view matches from BORB (Riddoch & Humphreys, 1993). Data on SRB's category-specific deficits were reported in Forde et al. (1997) and Humphreys et al. (1997). Here we draw on results with the set of 76 line drawings from BORB (Riddoch & Humphreys, 1993), and on object decisions from BORB that were reported in the original papers. The other data were recorded between 1999 and 2002. SRB's performance on retesting was very similar to that observed in our earlier sessions.

## SECTION 1: PERFORMANCE ON STANDARDISED TESTS OF OBJECT PROCESSING

### Experiment 1: Naming pictures of structurally similar and dissimilar items from BORB

In Experiment 1 we present data on the ability of the patients to identify objects used originally by Humphreys et al. (1988) to assess the effects of structural similarity on object naming. The items were drawn from categories with structurally similar (SS) exemplars (animals, fruits, vegetables) and from categories with structurally dissimilar (SD) members (body parts, clothing, furniture, kitchen utensils, vehicles). Items were assigned to the SS or SD sets according to the number of parts listed in common across category members (3.48 and 0.71 for the SS and SD items respectively), and according to the average percentage contour overlap when the pictures were overlaid (the mean overlap for SS and SD exemplars was 17.28 and 12.44% respectively; Humphreys et al., 1988). Note that the SS and SD sets employed overlap with but do not correspond exactly to the distinction between living and nonliving things, since the category "body parts" may be classed as living (see Laiacona et al., 1993a; Laiacona, Barbarotto, Trivelli, & Capitani, 1993b) but it was assigned here to the SD class based on the measures of number of common parts and outline contour overlap.

### *Method*

Each patient was tested on two separate occasions, always on different days. They were presented with line drawings of the stimuli (from the BORB manual), and asked to name one object at a time. Stimuli were presented in a random order, and presentation times were unlimited. The SS and SD items were matched for name frequency but divided into equal sets with high- and low-frequency names (above or below 10 occurrences per million in the Kuçera & Francis, 1967, norms). The stimuli within each set varied along a number of dimensions, including complexity, familiarity, and prototypicality. SD items tended to be less complex, more familiar, and less prototypical than the SS stimuli (see Humphreys et al., 1988). To ensure that any differences between the sets were not due to these other factors, the data were evaluated using analysis of covariance with complexity, familiarity, image agreement, name agreement (Snodgrass & Vanderwart, 1980), and prototypicality (Humphreys et al., 1988) entered as covariates. We also included as a further factor the reaction times (RTs) for young, normal participants to name the objects (taking RTs from Snodgrass & Yuditsky, 1996, who provide a large-scale study of naming the Snodgrass & Vanderwart, 1980, pictures). In doing this we asked whether the effects found on naming accuracy in patients could be accounted for in terms of the factors that produce latency differences between the stimuli in control participants, or whether the effects found in patients occurred over and above this. We also carried out a stepwise regression analysis with a measure of structural similarity (the percentage contour overlap between category members), along with the other factors, best predicting overall naming accuracy. In a parallel study with seven control subjects age-matched to the present patients, naming accuracy was at ceiling.

### *Results*

*Analysis of covariance.* The accuracy for each picture (scores out of 2) was used as the dependent variable, with two between-item factors (category and frequency) and with patient entered as a within-items factor. Name agreement, image agreement, familiarity, and complexity (from Snodgrass & Vanderwart, 1980), along with rated prototypicality (from Humphreys et al., 1988), and naming RTs for young, normal participants were entered as covariates. The percentage correct identification responses made to the SS and SD objects, as a function of their (Kuçera & Francis, 1967) name frequencies, are given in Figure 2. The main effect of patient failed to reach significance, $F(6, 396) = 1.17, p > .05$, but there was a reliable effect of category, $F(1, 66) = 25.8, p = .000$, even with the other variables covaried out. The effect of name frequency was not reliable, $F(1, 66) = 2.61, p > .05$. There was one borderline interaction, between patient and frequency, $F(6, 396) = 2.15, p = .05$. Most of the patients were more accurate at naming objects with high name frequencies; HJA, however, showed the opposite trend (see Figure 2). We suggest that this was because some SS items with low name frequencies had relatively distinctive shapes (e.g., giraffe, kangaroo, elephant), and HJA tended to succeed on these items. The effects of category (SS vs. SD items) were reliable for each patient (Table 1).

*Error analysis.* The naming errors made by the patients were classified using a modification of the scoring criteria proposed by Hodges, Salmon, and

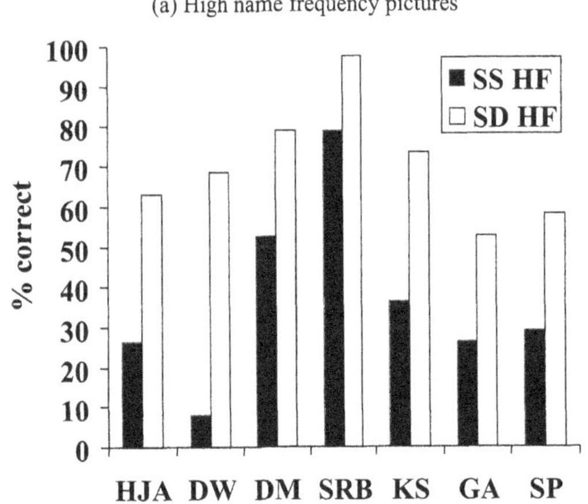


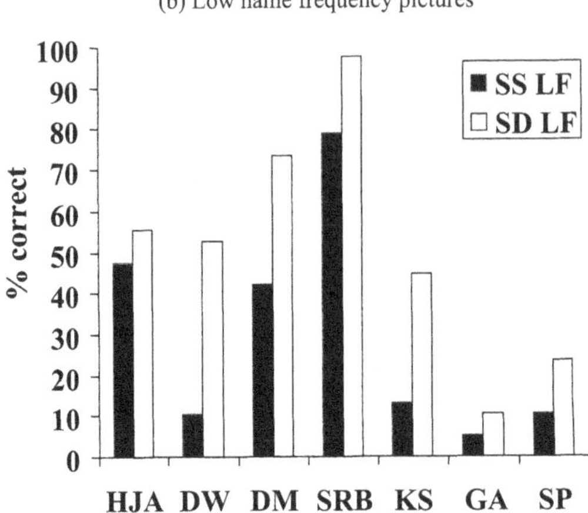


**Figure 2.** *The percentage correct identifications of pictures varying in structural similarity and name frequency, for each patient: (a) high name frequency pictures; (b) low name frequency pictures (Experiment 1).*

**Table 1.** *The effects of structural similarity and name frequency for each patient, in Experiment 1. The data were analysed using log-linear analyses with structural similarity, name frequency, and correct–error as factors. Interactions with the correct–error factor are reported, indicating proportionately more correct to error responses in the different conditions.* $\chi^2$ *values are given (1 df)*

| | *Factors* | | |
|---|---|---|---|
| *Patient* | *Structural similarity* | *Name frequency* | *Structural similarity × Name frequency* |
| HJA | 7.72** | 0.04 | 3.45 |
| DW | 47.89** | 0.73 | 1.13 |
| DM | 16.28** | 0.51 | 0.01 |
| SRB | 13.86** | 0.0 | 0.0 |
| KS | 18.67** | 10.94** | 0.02 |
| GA | 5.32* | 22.47** | 0.14 |
| SP | 8.50** | 14.50** | 0.15 |

$^*p < .01$; $^{**}p < .01$.

Butters (1991). Responses were assigned to one of the following categories: *nonresponse* (including "don't knows"), *visual errors* (mushroom → table), *visual/semantic errors* (e.g., donkey → horse), *semantic* (coordinates that were visually unrelated to targets, celery → onion; or superordinate responses, kangaroo → animal); *phonemic* (e.g., kangaroo → kanbarjew); *perseverations* (repeat of a response from the last five trials where the response seemed unrelated to the target); *unrelated* (no clear relation between target and response). In addition, and unlike Hodges et al. (1991), we separately categorised *semantic circumlocutions* (lemon → you use it on pancakes). The percentages of each type of error for each patient are shown in Table 2. It is clear from these data that different patterns of errors occurred across the patients. HJA made proportionately more visual errors than the other patients; GA and SP made proportionately more visual/semantic and semantic errors; DM, SRB, and KS made proportionately more semantic circumlocutions (though some visual errors still occurred). There were few phonological or perseverative errors.

*Stepwise regression.* The effects of category (SS vs. SD) did not interact with the factor of patient; hence, at least as far as concerns relative to deficits in naming objects from SS and SD sets, the patients may be considered a homogeneous set (even if, as we argue below, the loci of the deficits differ across patients). A stepwise regression on the data averaged across patients was conducted with the predictive factors being name agreement, image agreement, familiarity, complexity, prototypicality, and percentage contour overlap. This generated a best-fitting model with significant independent effects of familiarity and contour overlap, $t(75)$ = 5.13 and −2.67, $p$ = .00 and .01, respectively. Items high in familiarity were likely to be named correctly, whilst objects with a high percentage

Table 2. *The percentages of different error types made by the patients in Experiment 1*

| *Patients* | *No resp* | *Vis* | *Vis/sem* | *Sem* | *Phon* | *Pers* | *Unrel* | *Circum* |
|---|---|---|---|---|---|---|---|---|
| HJA | | 43 | 41 | 16 | | | | |
| DW | 36 | 14 | 12 | 38 | | | | |
| DM | | 7 | 22 | 37 | | | | 34 |
| SRB | | 10 | 25 | 30 | 5 | | | 30 |
| KS | 20 | 10 | 20 | 35 | | | | 15 |
| GA | 20 | 15 | 31 | 34 | | | | |
| SP | 8 | 10 | 36 | 33 | | | 11 | 2 |

No resp = no response; Vis = visual error; Vis/sem = visual or semantic error; Sem = semantic error; Phon = phonological error; Pers = perseveration; Unrel = unrelated error; Circum= semantic circumlocution.

contour overlap measure were likely to be misidentified. None of the other factors made an independent contribution.

### *Discussion*

The results confirm that these patients all had more difficulty in identifying objects from categories with structurally similar exemplars relative to objects from categories with structurally dissimilar exemplars. This could reflect an effect of structural similarity per se, or it could be due to the biological category that the stimuli belonged to, since the SS items were living and the majority of SD items were nonliving. Interestingly, a regression analysis carried out on the data summed across patients revealed a reliable effect of contour overlap, a measure of visual similarity between category members (Humphreys et al., 1988), in addition to an effect of familiarity. Stimuli high in structural similarity within their category, and low in familiarity, were particularly problematic. This suggests that similarity amongst category members does at least partly determine object identification when these patients are considered as a group.

At a finer-grained level, however, the error analysis indicated some differences between the patients. The two patients with bilateral occipito-temporal damage, HJA and DW, made many errors that were visually related to target pictures. The two patients with bilateral medial and anterior temporal lobe damage, GA and SP, made some visual errors along with many in which they generated rather general category labels for stimuli (bee → an animal; pear → food). In contrast to this, the patients with unilateral left-hemisphere damage, DM, SRB, and KS, all made semantic circumlocution errors in which they described where an object was used or where it might be found, but failed to come up with the object's name. To assess whether there were differences in access to semantic knowledge about objects in the different patients, Experiment 2 evaluated (a) visual recognition of objects using an object decision task (Riddoch & Humphreys, 1987c), and (b) access to semantic (associative and categorical) knowledge (using standard tests of semantic access: the associative matching test from BORB, Riddoch & Humphreys, 1993, the Pyramids and Palm Trees task, Howard & Patterson, 1992, plus a test requiring them to discriminate between fruit and vegetables).

## Experiment 2: Access to stored structural and semantic knowledge, assessed in standard tests

### *Method*

We administered one standard test of recognition of the familiar shape of an object—the "object decision task" (Riddoch & Humphreys, 1987c). The stimuli were taken from OD A Easy, from BORB (Riddoch & Humphreys, 1993). There were 16 line drawings of real objects and 16 drawings of "perceptually good" nonobjects, formed by interchanging the parts of real objects. The patients received one item at a time and had to judge whether it was a real or a meaningless object. There were no time limits. This object decision task probably requires access to stored visual knowledge about an object (Riddoch & Humphreys, 1987c). Rumiati and

Humphreys (1987) reported that 30 controls aged 65–80 had a mean of 29.8/32 (*SD* = 1.2) on this task. Three tests of access to semantic knowledge were also given: the associative matching task from BORB, the Pyramids and Palm Trees task, and a task requiring the patients to sort cards into piles separating fruits from vegetables. The associative matching test from BORB is comprised of 30 trials. On each trial a target line drawing is shown at the top of the page (e.g., hammer) along with two drawings at the bottom (e.g., nail and screw). The task is to decide which of the two items at the foot of the page is related to or used in conjunction with the target. Riddoch and Humphreys (1993) reported that controls from an age range of 57–91 scored a mean of 27.5 (*SD* 2.4). For controls age matched to the present patients, the mean level of performance was 28.9/30 (*SD1.2*). In addition to giving the associative matching test in its standard pictorial form, we also presented it in verbal form, substituting words for the pictures. The Pyramids and Palm Trees test takes a similar form. In the pictorial version, a target picture has to be matched to one of two other pictures (matching a target pyramid to either a deciduous tree or a palm tree). There are 52 trials. Howard and Patterson (1992) report that controls score above 49/52. We presented this test in both the pictorial and the verbal form (using three words instead of these pictures). In the third task, patients were presented either with 20 pictures or 20 words on cards, 10 of fruit and 10 of vegetables (the same items as used in Experiment 2). The task was to sort the cards into one pile for fruits and one for vegetables. The mean of the age-matched controls was 19.3/20 (*SD* 0.7). These tests were carried out on separate occasions with each patient. Performance was not time limited.

### *Results*

*Object decision.* The patients scored from 20/32 (HJA) and 22/32 (DW and GA) to 27/32 (KS, SP, DM, and SRB). Although these latter patients appeared less impaired at this test, all of the scores are in fact more than 2 *SD*s from the mean of controls (see Table 3; control data from Rumiati & Humphreys, 1997).

**Table 3.** *Scores of the patients and controls on the easy object decision task, version A, from BORB (Riddoch & Humphreys, 1993) (scores out of 32); control data are taken from Rumiati and Humphreys (1997)*

| *Patient* | *Score* |
|---|---|
| HJA | 20 |
| DW | 22 |
| DM | 27 |
| SRB | 27 |
| KS | 27 |
| GA | 22 |
| SP | 27 |
| Controls | 29.8 (*SD* 1.2) |

*Association match.* The percentage of correct matches made by the patients are shown in Figure 3a. DM, SRB, and KS all performed at control level, with both visual and verbal forms of the task. GA and SP fell below the control level for both modalities (> 2 *SD*s). DW and HJA scored below the control level with visual presentations but not with verbal presentations.

*Pyramids and Palm Trees.* The results for the patients are given in Figure 3b. DM and KS scored just below the control level with visual but not verbal presentation, whilst SRB was not impaired. DW and HJA were clearly impaired with visual presentations, but not with the verbal form of the task (DW was just below the control level with verbal presentations). GA and SP performed outside the level expected with controls, irrespective of the input modality.

*Categorising fruits and vegetables.* Again DM, SRB, and KS performed at the control level. DW and HJA were at the control level when the stimuli were presented verbally but they were impaired with visual presentations. GA and SP performed below the control level with both visual and verbal presentations.

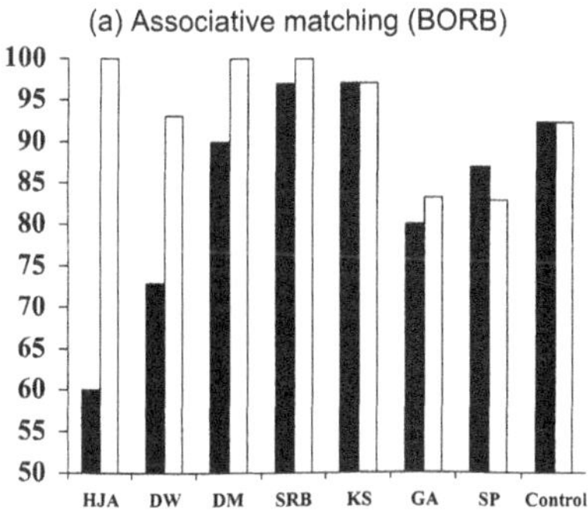


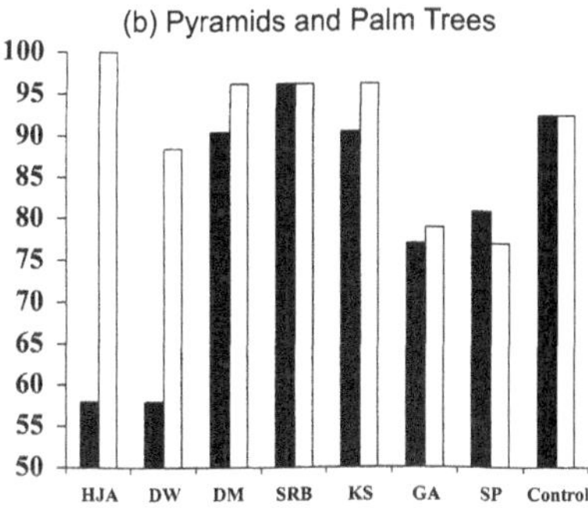


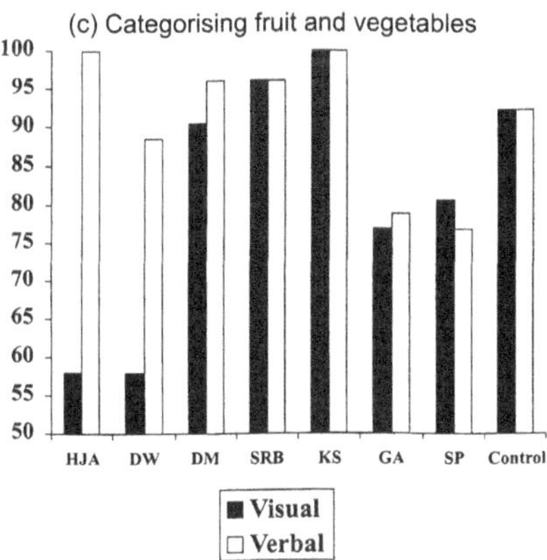


Figure 3. *The percentage correct performance on three sets of tests designed to assess access to semantic knowledge: (a) associative matching, (b) Pyramids and Palm Trees, and (c) categorising fruits and vegetables. The tests were performed either on pictures (visual) or written words (verbal). Chance is 50% in each case (Experiment 2).*

### *Discussion*

Although the patients all showed a deficit in naming pictures belonging to SS relative to SD sets (Experiment 1), contrasting impairments are revealed by the tests in Experiment 2, which assessed access to stored visual and semantic knowledge. All of the patients were impaired to some degree at object decision. In patients HJA and DW (with bilateral occipito-temporal damage), this was accompanied by a modality-specific deficit in retrieving semantic knowledge (there was an impairment with pictures but not with words as stimuli). In contrast, GA and SP (bilateral medial and anterior temporal lobe damage) had a deficit in semantic knowledge whether tested with pictures or words. The three patients with unilateral left-hemisphere damage, however, generally performed at control levels on the semantic tests, irrespective of whether the stimuli were presented as pictures or words (KS, DM, and SRB).

An account of these results can be presented along anatomical grounds. Patients with unilateral left-hemisphere damage remain able to access semantic knowledge within their right hemisphere (Coslett & Saffran, 1992), and so perform at control levels on tasks assessing semantic retrieval (KS, DM, and SRB). The patients with more posterior bilateral damage (DW and HJA) have an impairment in visual access to semantic knowledge within both hemispheres, generating a modality-specific deficit for the semantic categorisation and association matching tasks. Semantic knowledge itself, though, is not disturbed, and so the patients performed better when tested verbally (Figure 3). The patients with bilateral medial and anterior temporal lobe damage (GA and SP) have an impairment of semantic knowledge itself, within both hemispheres, and so show a deficit whether tested with pictures or words. One problem for this account, though, is that left-hemisphere damage can lead to problems in object recognition (e.g., Hillis & Caramazza, 1995; McCarthy & Warrington, 1986; Riddoch & Humphreys, 1987c). The presence of an intact right hemisphere does not guarantee intact object recognition. It can also be argued that the standard tests of semantic access do not challenge the object recognition system sufficiently to reveal a significant deficit in the patients. The Association and Pyramids and Palm Trees tasks, for instance, are not designed to contrast performance on living and nonliving things, and living things appear as targets on only a minority of trials. The fruit vs. vegetables categorisation task also assesses access to superordinate semantic knowledge, but not to precise semantic information associated with individual exemplars (see Forde et al., 1997, for discussion of this point). It is possible that a mild deficit would not be apparent on this task. This last proposal fits with the data from the object decision test, where all the patients showed some degree of deficit. Below we will present evidence indicating that KS, despite having unilateral left-hemisphere damage, does have a (mild) semantic deficit, contra to the hemisphere-specific account. This will distinguish this patient from DM and SRB, who both have more posterior lesions than KS.

## SECTION 2: EFFECTS OF BIOLOGICAL CATEGORY

Having demonstrated that these patients had reliable deficits in naming SS (living) relatively to SD (primarily nonliving) things, and that the patients appeared to differ in terms of the functional locus of their lesion (e.g., pre-semantic in HJA and DW, semantic in the case of GA and SP), we proceeded in Section 2 to evaluate in more detail whether biological category was crucial to the deficits in these patients. We report three experiments. In Experiment 3 the patients named the stimuli selected from the Snodgrass and Vanderwart (1980) norms by Laiacona et al. (1993b; see also Laiacona & Capitani, 2001). These stimuli comprise 80 items, 10 in each of four living and four nonliving categories (animals, fruits, vegetables, and body parts on the one hand, and furniture, tools, vehicles, and musical instruments on the other). Each patient was tested on two separate occasions with these stimuli presented in random order. In Experiment 4 we assessed whether there was good access to semantic knowledge about the objects used in Experiment 3, requiring patients to make associative matches to target pictures, from either other pictures or words. In Experiments 5 and 6 we evaluated whether there were deficits in accessing stored perceptual knowledge, as well as deficits in accessing more functional, semantic knowledge, for living and nonliving things. In Experiment 5 patients made object decisions to stimuli from living and nonliving categories. In Experiment 6 they answered verbal definitions stressing either perceptual or functional/semantic properties of stimuli. Are there consistent deficits for living relative to nonliving things, and do these deficits arise at a particular level of representation?

### Experiment 3: Naming pictures from Laiacona et al. (1993b)

*Method*

Each picture was given on a separate card, in a random order. Presentation times were unlimited and patients were simply asked to name each item. The pictures were also named by seven controls age-matched to the patients. Naming accuracy for the controls was at ceiling.

*Results*

The percentage correct naming responses given by each patient, for each category, are given in Figure 4.

As in Experiment 1, we conducted an analysis of covariance on the accuracy data across items, treating category as a between-items variable with eight levels and patients as a within-items factor. The covariates were name frequency, within-category prototypicality, image agreement, gender-specific familiarity, and complexity (see Laiacona & Capitani, 2001),[3] plus also latencies to name the pictures, for young control participants (again taken from Snodgrass & Yuditsky, 1996). There was no main effect of patient, $F(6, 396) = 1.27, p >$ 05, but there was a main effect of category, $F(7, 66) = 13.54, p = .000$. There was also an interaction between patient and category, $F(42, 396) = 2.13, p = .000$. This interaction arose primarily because HJA was relatively impaired at the category body part, whilst all the other patients were relatively good at naming pictures of body parts.

[3] Measures of gender specific familiarity were not available for the categories musical instrument and body part, so for these categories the familiarity ratings provided by Snodgrass and Vanderwart (1980) were used.

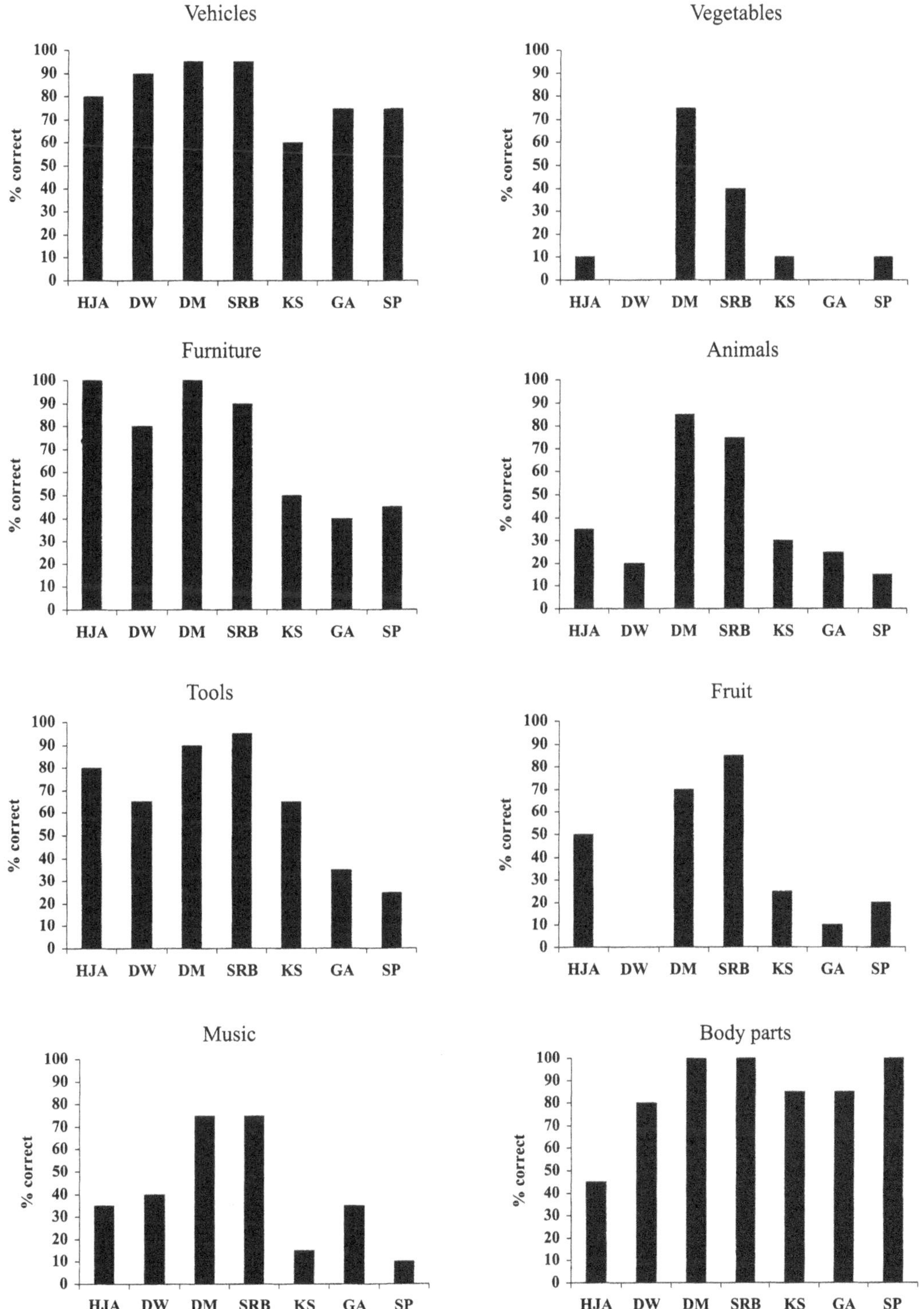


Figure 4. *The percentage of correct identifications of pictures from different categories, for each patient (Experiment 3).*

The data were also analysed taking all the subcategories together within the living and nonliving domains, respectively, to contrast living against nonliving things. There was a reliable advantage for nonliving over living things with complexity, name frequency, familiarity prototypicality, image agreement, and control naming RTs co-varied out, $F(1,71) = 22.98$, $p = .000$; the interaction of category and patient was again reliable, $F(6, 426) = 3.87$, $p = .000$.

Individual comparisons revealed that performance clustered into two broad sets that cut-across the living/nonliving distinction. Performance was relatively good on vehicles, furniture, tools, and body parts; it was poorer on animals, fruits, vegetables, and musical instruments. Taking the worst of the "good" categories, tools, performance remained better than on vegetables, $t(18) = 4.52$, $p = .000$, and on animals, $t(18) = 2.32$, $p = .03$; there was also a marginal advantage for tools over fruit, $t(18) = 1.85$, $p = .08$. However, body parts tended to be better than tools ($t < 1.0$) whilst musical instruments were identified as poorly as animals and fruits (both $t < 1.0$).

*Error analysis.* As in Experiment 1, we again analysed the errors made by the patients. The percentage of the different error types for each patient are listed in Table 4. As before, DM, SRB, and KS made a significant number of semantic circumlocutions, in which they described what the object did or where it might be found. GA and SP made a substantial number of superordinate responses along with some visual errors. HJA made errors in opposite proportions to those made by GA and SP (with visual errors predominating).

*Discussion*

Although there was some variation across the patients (particularly for the category body parts[4]), overall performance was best for the categories of vehicle, furniture, tools, and body parts, and worst for the categories of fruit, vegetables, animals, and musical instruments. In some studies of category specificity, identification has been compared across the categories of vehicle, furniture, and tools, on the one hand, and fruit, vegetables, and animals, on the other (e.g., Laiacona et al., 1993a; Laiacona & Capitani, 2001). If we take only these categories, then all the patients would present with a clear deficit for living things relative to nonliving things.

However, when all eight categories are taken into consideration, then there were also violations of the living/nonliving distinction. Body parts fell at the level found with nonliving stimuli, whilst musical instruments fell at a level found with living things. Deficits on musical instruments as well as on living things have been noted previously in the literature on category-specific deficits (Gainotti et al., 1995), though not in all cases (Barbarotto, Capitani, & Laiacona, 2001). For an account in terms of domain-specific semantics, the co-occurrence of deficits with living things and musical instruments may be a matter of association, perhaps due to the anatomical proximity of neural areas supporting semantic knowledge for living things and

**Table 4.** *The percentages of different error types made by the patients in Experiment 3*

| *Patient* | *No resp* | *Vis* | *Vis/sem* | *Sem* | *Phon* | *Pers* | *Unrel* | *Circum* |
|---|---|---|---|---|---|---|---|---|
| HJA | | 27 | 33 | 40 | | | | |
| DW | 11 | 17 | 36 | 36 | | | | |
| DM | | 9 | 41 | 32 | | | | 18 |
| SRB | | 6 | 35 | 26 | | | | 33 |
| KS | 28 | 8 | 18 | 20 | | | | 26 |
| GA | 4 | 9 | 51 | 36 | | | | |
| SP | 3 | 12 | 33 | 36 | | | 16 | |

For abbreviations see Table 2.

[4] HJA had difficulty identifying pictures of body parts that are depicted in a minimalist style in the Snodgrass and Vanderwart (1980) set.

semantic knowledge for musical instruments, and to patients having relatively large lesions (see Laiacona et al., in press). An alternative is that musical instruments may be problematic because they are relatively unfamiliar. This seems unlikely here, however. GA was formerly a professional musician and would be expected to be very familiar with the instruments tested. DM's children were also learning musical instruments and she took a keen interest in this. Nevertheless, both patients were impaired on these items compared with, say, vehicles and body parts. We suggest that other accounts need to be considered. One is the S-F account of category disorders. On this view, musical instruments may be impaired along with living things because all these items are defined primarily by their visual/perceptual properties (Warrington & Shallice, 1984). Damage to the neural systems involved in representing stored perceptual knowledge will selectively impair these stimuli. A further proposal is that musical instruments are problematic for these patients because there is substantial perceptual overlap between the members of this category. Some support for this comes from a recent simulation study by Gale, Done, and Frank (2001). They trained a Kohonen network to classify at a base-level photographic images of animals, musical instruments, clothing, and furniture. They found that animals and musical instruments tended to form local clusters within the map representation, with units within the clusters all being activated to some moderate degree by a member of the same category. Animals and musical instruments then tended to fare worse when lesions were modelled by randomly removing connections between units. Since this model was only representing stimuli based on similarity relations between their pixels, it provides objective evidence that even a low-level measure indicates relatively high similarity amongst musical instruments. On the other hand, other similarity indices do not capture this. For example, musical instruments as a category have an average contour overlap of 9.67 on the measure of Humphreys et al. (1988). This places them close to body parts (9.01) and relatively distant from fruit (20.96), vegetables (16.61), and animals (15.49). The contour overlap measure provides an index of the similarity of the outline shape of stimuli; indices of pixel overlap are sensitive to the presence of surface details and shading too. At this juncture, it is not clear which of these measures provides a better account of human performance.

We also need to take into account that body parts were generally identified at a high level. Shelton, Fouch, and Caramazza (1998) have proposed that body parts may form yet another domain-specific part of semantic memory, and this could account for either their relative sparing in some patients (Shelton et al., 1998) or their selective impairment (Suzuki, Yamadori, & Fujii, 1997). However, this is at the expense of losing some of the parsimony of this account, as it pushes the account towards positing that there is a modular representation within semantic memory for each biological category. A more parsimonious account is in terms of the S-F distinction, since body parts may be characterised by their function rather than by their visual/perceptual properties. Accordingly, body parts would be spared if damage affected visual/perceptual but not functional knowledge. Also, at least in terms of the contour overlap measure of Humphreys et al. (1988), body parts have relatively distinctive perceptual structures (see above), making them less susceptible to impairment when visual/perceptual representations are damaged. Whichever the case, the present data emphasise that body parts should not be considered as being represented along with other living things in semantic memory.

## Experiment 4: Associative matching for living and nonliving things

In Experiment 4, we examined access to semantic knowledge for a subset of the stimuli from Experiment 2. On each trial, five stimuli from a given category were presented along with another probe item that had to be matched to one of the five on the basis of an associative and/or functional relationship (being used along with one of the other stimuli). The stimuli were presented both in pictorial form and as words.

*Method*

There were 48 trials, 6 for each category (vehicles, furniture, musical instruments, tools, fruits, vegetables, animals, and body parts). The stimuli used for the matches are listed in Appendix A and two example trials (with pictures and with words) are depicted in Figure 5.[5] In addition to the patients, the tasks were carried out with six control subjects age-matched to the six patients tested (DW was not available for this study). Subjects were instructed to point to which one of the five stimuli that was related to the probe. Both the pictorial and the verbal versions of the tasks were carried out on different test occasions for both the controls and the

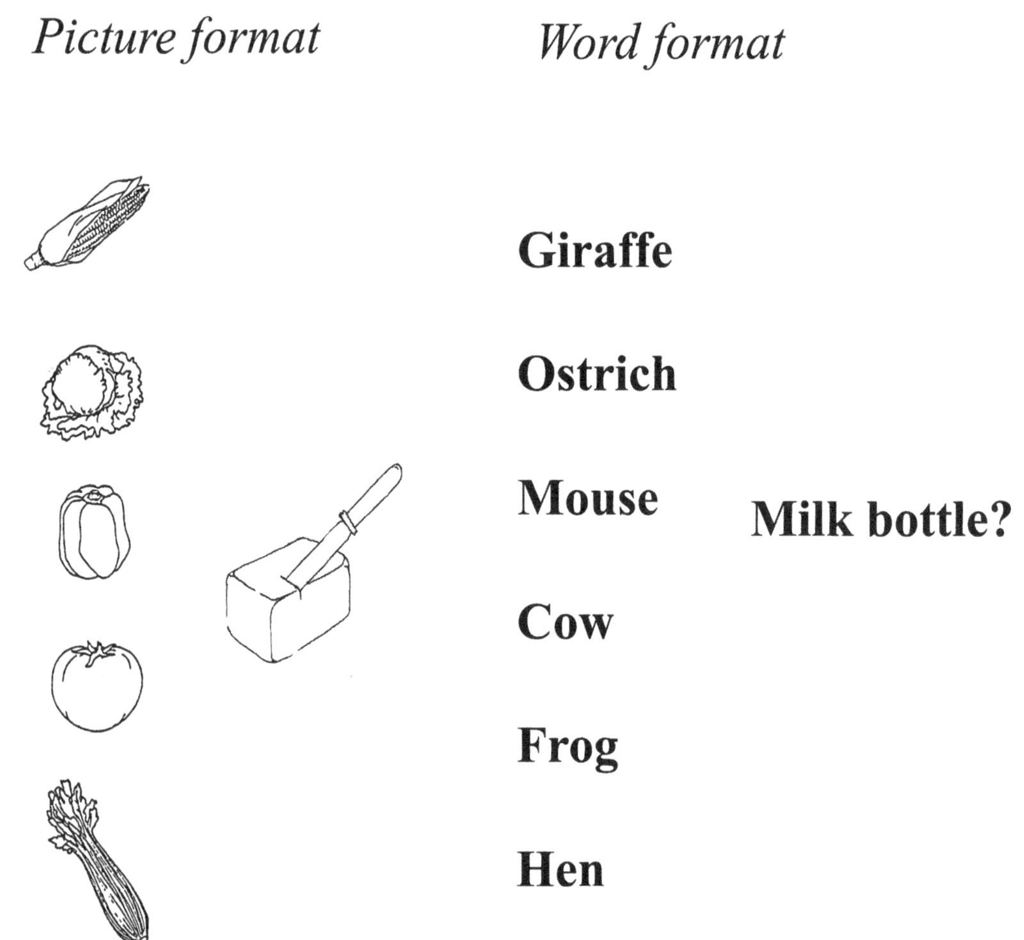


**Figure 5.** *Example stimuli used in the associative matching task for stimuli drawn from different living and nonliving categories (Experiment 4).*

[5] An anonymous referee pointed out that, for the probe TABLE, the item "lamp" might be related as well as the (target) item "chair". However, none of our controls matched TABLE to "lamp" rather than "chair." Although there is some ambiguity, we suggest that the target was by some margin the most related item in the set. With the probe SCREWDRIVER, target "screw" also shared some information in the word form, which could have facilitated matching. However, the pattern of performance remained the same with this item omitted.

patients. The patients were each tested twice on each version of the task; the controls were tested once on each version.

*Results*

The percentage correct matches made by the patients, for each category, are given in Figures 6 and 7 (with pictorial and written presentations, respectively). The means for the controls were: vehicles 94% (*SD* 0.8), furniture 92% (*SD* 1.3), musical instruments 92% (*SD* 1.1), tools 89% (*SD* 1.2), animals 92% (*SD* 1.4), fruit 94% (*SD* 0.9), vegetables 92% (*SD* 0.9), body parts 97% (*SD* 0.4). No control made more than one error for any category (83% correct). Any individual patient performing at a lower level than this also fell more than 2 *SD*s from the control mean. This was then taken as the cut-off separating normal from impaired performance.

The data for the patients overall were analysed in a mixed design analysis of variance across the items, with stimulus type (pictures vs. words) and patient as repeated measures factors (summing together the data for each patient on each item, across the two test sessions with each format), and category as a between-items factor (the eight categories, listed separately). Name frequency, prototypicality, image agreement, familiarity, complexity, and control naming RTs were entered as covariates. There was a reliable effect of category, $F(7, 33) = 4.41, p = .002$, but no overall effect of patient ($F < 1.0$) or of stimulus type ($F < 1.0$). There were no interactions. The effects of category tended to match those present in picture naming of the same stimuli (Experiment 3). Performance was better with vehicles, furniture, tools, and body parts than with fruits, vegetables, animals, and musical instruments. For example, not taking into account musical instruments and body parts, responses to vehicles tended to be lower than to the other nonliving things summed across patients, but they still tended to be better than with the two best categories of living things, animals and fruit, $t(10) = 1.86$ and 2.68 respectively, $p = .09$ and .02 respectively, analysed across items.

However, there were also some differences between the patients, especially when performance is considered relative to the controls. DM and SRB showed no differences relative to the controls (at worst scoring at the bottom of the control range), with both pictorial and written presentations. The other patients all showed some deficit. HJA's impairments were confined to pictorial presentations, whereas he performed well when the stimuli were presented verbally. For HJA there was an overall advantage for verbal over pictorial presentations, $t(47) = -4.34, p = .000$. The same also held for KS, $t(47) = -2.62, p < .025$, though, like GA and SP, she had impairments with verbal as well as with pictorial presentations (Figure 5). For KS, the deficits occurred only with the categories musical instruments, vegetables, animals, and fruit. GA and SP were also impaired on these categories, but they had further problems with vehicles and tools.

The general pattern here matched that in Experiment 2, when we tested access to superordinate knowledge for fruits and vegetables: DM and SRB have no major deficit in semantic access, HJA has a problem in visual access to semantics, and GA and SP have impaired semantic knowledge irrespective of the input modality. The main difference, though, is that KS did show impairments in this study, whereas she performed normally in Experiment 2. In the earlier experiment we assessed access to superordinate information for affected categories; in contrast, here we evaluated item-specific associative and functional knowledge. These more specific tests reveal a mild impairment in this patient.

The data from KS are interesting in two particular aspects. One is that the mild deficit arises even though KS has unilateral left-hemisphere damage. This suggests that the extent and site of damage is more critical than whether the lesion is unilateral or bilateral. KS, like GA and SP, has damage to anterior and middle regions of the temporal lobe, and this seems linked to a deficit in semantic access; however, KS's damage is less extensive (being unilateral rather than bilateral), and so the magnitude of the problem is reduced. These general conclusions, about there being a semantic impairment for KS, are confirmed in Experiment 6 below. The second interesting point is that, although KS had problems with both verbal and pictorial presenta-

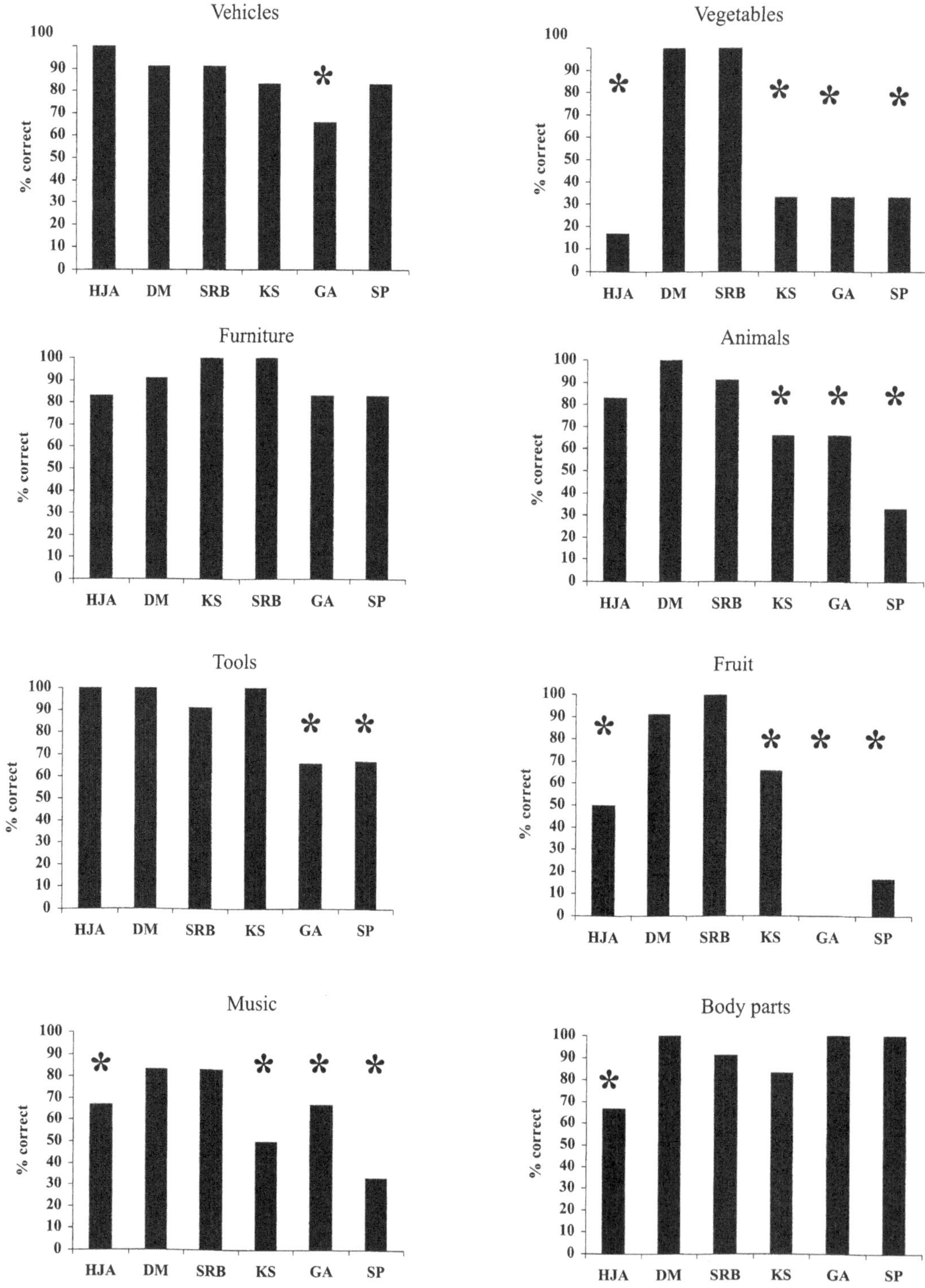


**Figure 6.** *Percentage correct associative matches with pictorial stimuli in Experiment 4. The data are separated for each category, for each patient. An asterisk (*) indicates that performance was impaired relative to controls.*

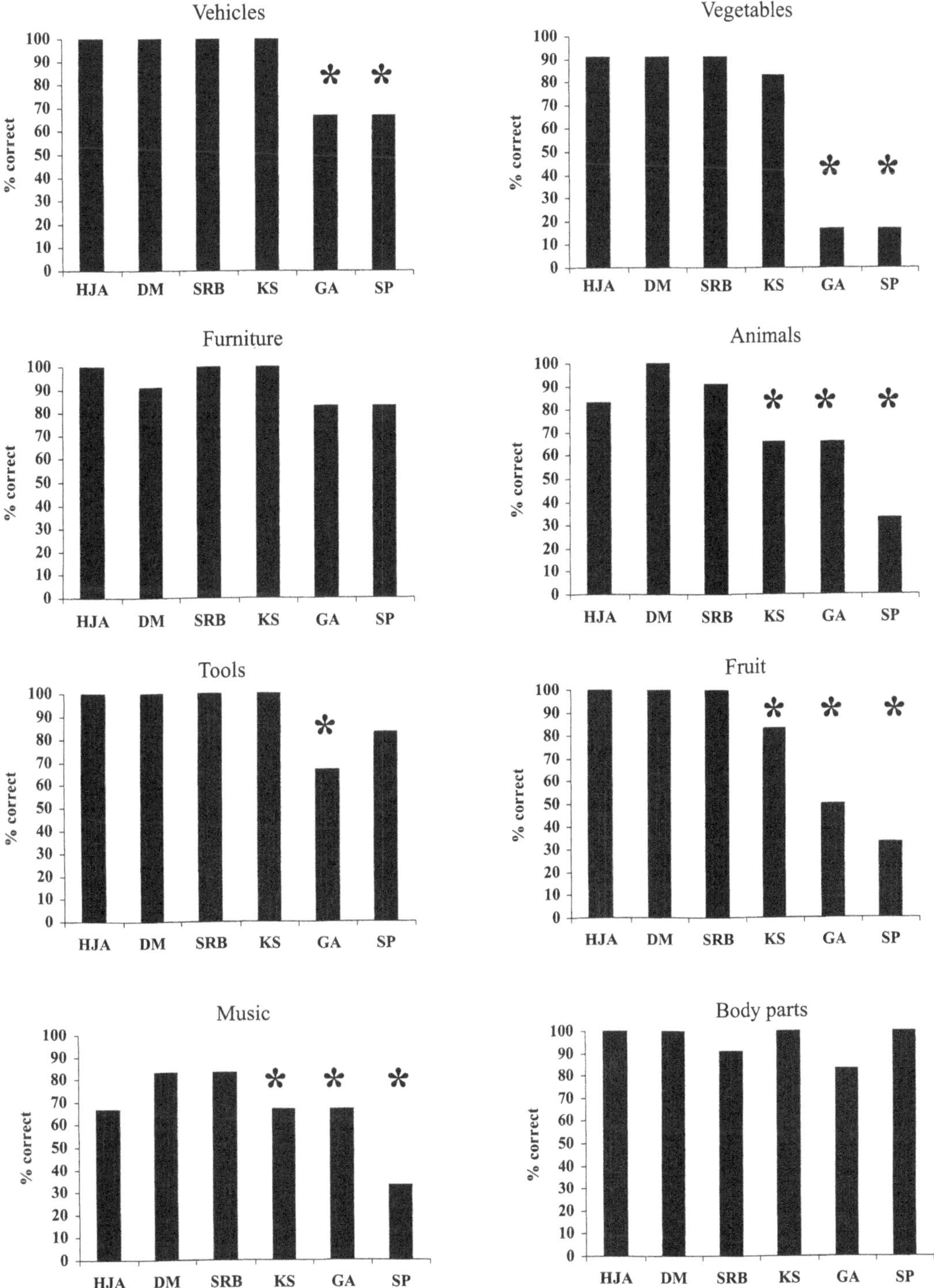


**Figure 7.** *Percentage correct associative matches with written stimuli in Experiment 4. The data are separated for each category, for each patient. An asterisk (*) indicates that performance was impaired relative to controls.*

tions (Figures 6 and 7), performance was worse with pictorial stimuli. This is consistent with the perceptual overlap between items in the impaired categories exacerbating any general difficulty in accessing associative and functional knowledge for these stimuli.

## Experiment 5: Object decision with living and nonliving things

Experiment 4 generally confirmed the data reported in the standardised tests of semantic access reported in Experiment 2 (with the exception of KS, see above). HJA has a modality-specific (visual) deficit in accessing semantic knowledge (likewise DW, in Experiment 2); GA and SP (and KS) have a deficit in semantic knowledge; DM and SRB do not appear to have a semantic deficit, even for the categories of object they find difficult to name. If there are deficits at different levels across these patients, we might also expect contrasting patterns to emerge on object decision tasks designed to evaluate perceptual knowledge about the impaired and better-preserved categories. In particular, DM and SRB ought to perform well, reflecting intact object recognition. This was tested in Experiment 5, where object decisions were carried out with stimuli from the living categories animals, fruits, vegetables, and birds, and the nonliving categories clothing, furniture, and kitchen utensils. Nonobjects were drawn from the same categories as the real objects, with the nonobjects being formed by combining parts from two different real objects. The items making up the majority of trials for four categories (fruits, vegetables, clothing, and furniture) were taken from Lloyd-Jones and Humphreys (1997).

### *Method*

There were 232 line drawings, 116 of or derived from living things (38 animals, 38 fruits and vegetables, and 40 birds), and 116 of or derived from nonliving things (38 items of clothing, 38 items of furniture, and 40 kitchen utensils). Within each category half the items were real and half were nonobjects created by joining together the parts of two different objects from that category. Example nonobjects are depicted in Figure 8. The stimuli were blocked by category (presenting all fruits and vegetables within a single block), and presented in different random orders across patients in a single session. In a subsequent session, the tests were repeated for each patient, but in an opposite order. Patients were shown one item at a time and asked to decide if it was real or meaningless. Within the fruit/vegetables set, there were 9 pictures of real fruits and 10 of real vegetables. DW was unavailable for this test. The stimuli were also presented to 10 age-matched controls.

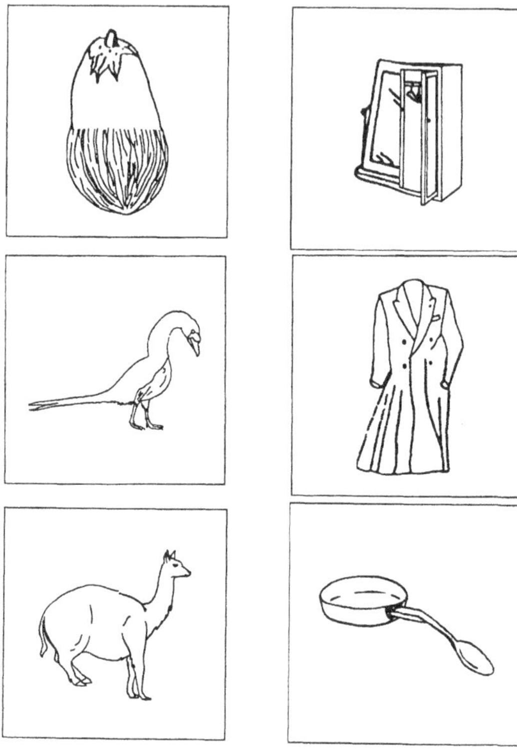

Figure 8. *Example nonobjects from the object decision task used in Experiment 5.*

### *Results*

The control means (and *SD*s) were: animals 96% (2.4), fruit/vegetables 94.7 (2.0), birds 94.5% (2.6), clothes 95.3% (2.2), furniture 95.7% (2.5) and kitchen utensils 97.5% (1.8). There were no differences across the categories ($F < 1.0$ for the effect of category).

The results for the patients are given in Figure 9. The data were analysed taking items as a random factor, with patient as a within-subjects factor and category (the six category blocks) and object type (real object vs. nonobject) as between-subjects factors (adding together the data for each patient across the test sessions). There was a main effect of category, $F(5, 220) = 18.47, p = .000$, and of patient, $F(5, 1100) = 14.08, p = .000$, but no effect of object type, $F(1, 220) = 1.18, p > .05$. There were no reliable interactions. Overall the best category of living thing for the patients was fruit/vegetables; however, performance with even this category was worse than with the worst category of nonliving thing—kitchen utensils; $F(1, 73) = 19.08, p = .000$. HJA and GA performed somewhat worse than the other patients, though all fell more than 2 *SD*s from the mean of the controls for the living items.

Although the age-matched controls all performed near ceiling in terms of accuracy, this

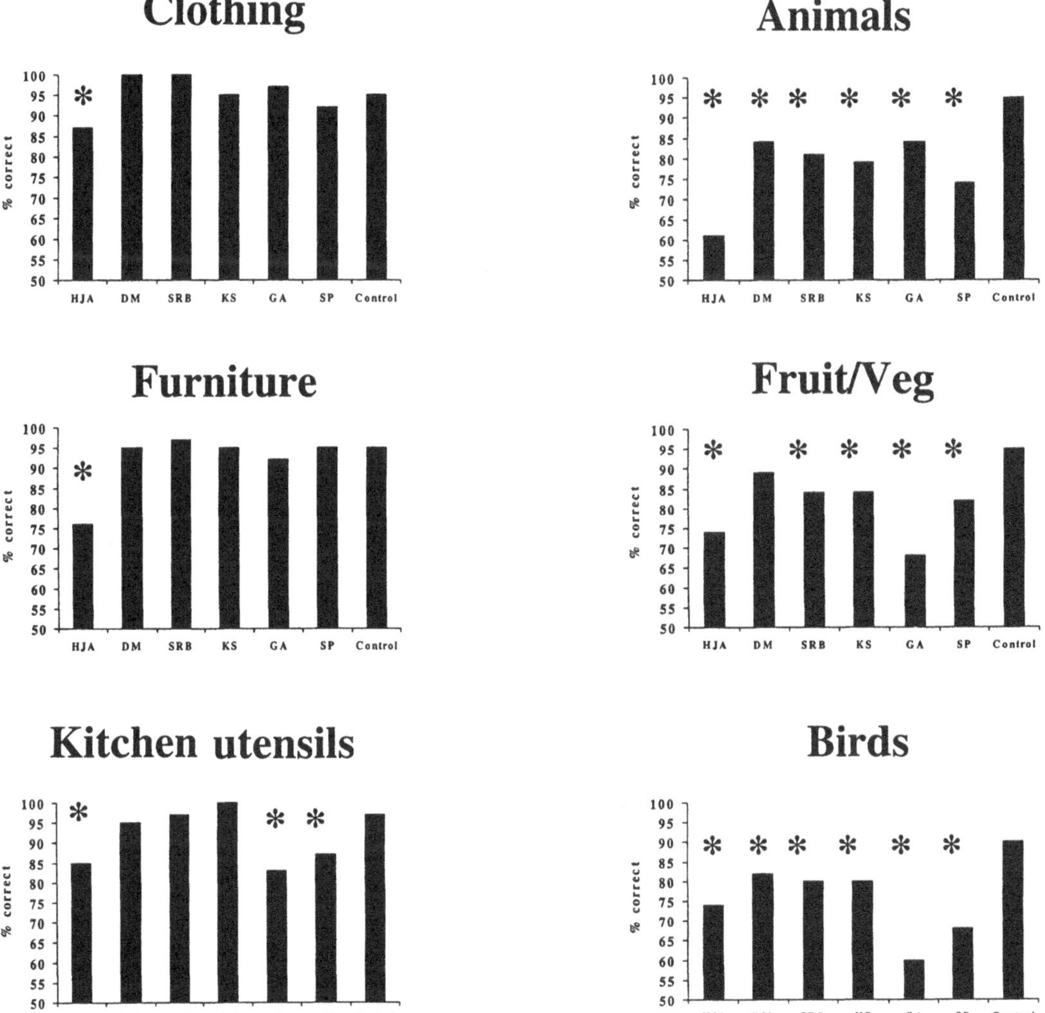


Figure 9. *Percentage correct object decisions made to each category of stimulus by each patient, in Experiment 5. An asterisk (*) indicates impaired performance relative to controls.*

measure may fail to reflect differences in task difficulty across the various categories. Lloyd-Jones and Humphreys (1997), for example, reported that young controls were slower to make object decisions to fruits and vegetables than to clothing and furniture. To assess if the effects with the patients could be accounted for in terms of the RT differences found with controls, we reanalysed the data for just the categories of fruits/vegetables, clothing, and furniture, covarying for the control RTs per item found by Lloyd-Jones and Humphreys.[6] There remained a reliable effect of category, $F(2, 50) = 6.23$, $p = .004$, but this time no effect of patient, $F(1, 50) = 1.60, p > .05$, and no interaction between patient and category, $F < 1.0$. There was no difference between furniture and clothing, $F < 1.0$, but across the patients accuracy was higher with furniture and with clothing than with fruits and vegetables, even when RT differences in controls were covaried, $F(1, 33) = 6.31, p < .025$ and, $F(1, 33) = 10.73, p < .01$, respectively, for furniture and clothing vs. fruits and vegetables.

*Discussion*

In Experiment 2 we found that all the patients fell below control levels at object decision, even though at least some of the patients (e.g., DM and SRB) performed well on semantic matching tasks. Experiment 4 replicated the good semantic matching performance for DM and SRB, even with categories of living and nonliving things. Experiment 5, however, confirmed that all the patients (including DM and SRB) had some difficulty in object decision. The patients were particularly poor at making object decisions to living things, and this deficit was apparent even when the data were covaried for differences in task difficulty across normal participants. This suggests that, despite the good semantic matching performance in some patients (DMM and SRB), there was a deficit in accessing stored visual knowledge about objects (assessed via object decision; cf. Riddoch & Humphreys, 1987c). The errors made by the patients were also not simply due to setting too lax a criterion of acceptance for living things. About half the errors across the patients were due to incorrect rejections of real objects, which occurred in addition to the false alarms to nonobjects. Consequently, there was no overall difference in accuracy on objects and nonobjects.

Forde et al. (1997) and Humphreys et al. (1997) have previously discussed similar results in DM and SRB, but where the stimuli in the object decision and semantic matching tasks were not separated by category. They suggested that this result could arise if there was a mild impairment in accessing stored perceptual knowledge about objects. This impairment would be apparent in object decision tasks, which stress fine-grained perceptual discriminations between stimuli. However, in semantic matching tasks, where choices are offered between forced-choice alternatives, this mild recognition impairment may be hidden; the information the patient can derive is sufficient to match stimuli and to reject unrelated distractors. On this view, all of the present patients have some deficit in accessing stored perceptual knowledge, though this problem is more severe for some patients than others. In each case, living things may be more vulnerable than nonliving things if living things have more overlap in their perceptual structures. Patients with a mild deficit in accessing perceptual knowledge may appear as category-specific anomics because name retrieval is more dependent on accessing fine-grained perceptual knowledge than semantic access (tested under forced-choice conditions).

## Experiment 6: Answering visual and verbal questions

In Experiment 5 we further explored stored knowledge in these patients, but now using only verbal questions. The question of whether patients showing category-specific deficits for living things have impairments to only visual/perceptual or also to functional knowledge about stimuli has been important to theories of how the deficits arise. For example, some patients have been reported as

[6] This analysis was conducted only on the real objects, since Lloyd-Jones and Humphreys (1997) only recorded RTs for these items.

having deficits not only in retrieving stored visual/perceptual knowledge about living things, but also in retrieving stored functional knowledge (e.g., Borgo & Shallice, 2001; Caramazza & Shelton, 1998; Laiacona et al., 1993a; Samson et al., 1998; Sheridan & Humphreys, 1993). This has been used to support the argument that there is damage to domain-specific semantic knowledge (affecting all knowledge about living things). In contrast, in some cases patients have been reported to be worse at retrieving visual/perceptual knowledge relative to functional knowledge, including previous reports with two of the present patients (DM and SRB; Forde et al., 1997; Humphreys et al., 1997). This last pattern of results is consistent with there being damage to stored visual/perceptual knowledge (cf. Humphreys & Forde, 2001; Warrington & Shallice, 1984). However, as we have noted, comparisons across patients are made difficult by the use of different stimuli. In Experiment 6 we sought to remedy this by probing stored visual/perceptual and verbal/functional knowledge with the same set of questions for all the present patients. Patients answered true and false questions that stressed either visual/perceptual or verbal/functional attributes of artefacts and animals (the questions were taken from Sheridan & Humphreys, 1993).

### *Method*

There were 19 questions relating to the visual/perceptual attributes of artefacts (e.g., does a bicycle have a windshield?) and 19 relating to the equivalent attributes of animals (e.g., does an elephant have a long neck?). There were 9 positive responses and 10 negative. There were also 20 questions relating to verbal/functional attributes of artefacts (e.g., do you use a hammer to bang in nails?) and a similar 20 questions for animals (e.g., do we get wool from cows?). In each set there were 10 expected positive answers (see Sheridan & Humphreys, 1993). Seven normal controls, age-matched to individual patients, made a mean of 0.07 and 0.04 errors on the visual/perceptual questions for artefacts and animals (*SD* 0.05 and 0.02). For the verbal/functional questions the control error rates were 0.01 and 0.

### *Results*

The data for the patients were subjected to a repeated measures ANOVA with the factors being type of question (visual/perceptual vs. verbal/functional) and category (artefacts vs. animals), with patients as a random factor. There was a reliable effect of question type, $F(1, 6) = 8.72, p = .026$; the effect of category and the question type × category interaction were not significant, $F(1, 6) = 3.34$ and 0.08, respectively, both $p > .05$. The patients answered the visual/perceptual questions worse than the verbal/functional questions. The results are presented in Figure 10.

Although taken as a group the patients were impaired on visual/perceptual questions, there were clear individual differences. The three patients with medial and anterior temporal lobe damage, KS, GA, and SP, all showed reliable effects of animacy. The data for each patient were subject to a log-linear analysis with the factors being question type, category, and number of correct and error responses. For each patient there was a significant interaction of category and number of correct/error responses: for KS $\chi^2(1) = 4.73$, for GA $\chi^2(1) = 21.05$, for SP $\chi^2(1) = 11.65$, all $p < .03$. There were fewer correct relative to error responses for animals than for artefacts. For SP only there was also a reliable interaction between question type and number of correct/error responses, $\chi^2(1) = 6.07$, $p < .025$; proportionately more errors occurred on visual questions. The other patients were all affected by question type rather than category. For DM, SRB, and HJA there was an overall effect of question type (Fisher exact probability, $p = .04$, .01, and .05 respectively), and no effect of category. For DW there was an effect of question type, but for animals only (Fisher exact probability, $p = .00$).

### *Discussion*

Across the group, the patients were impaired at answering visual/perceptual relative to verbal/functional questions about stimuli. However, at the level of individual patients we can distinguish two results: an effect of question type in patients DM, SRB, HJA, and DW; and an effect of animacy for KS, GA, and SP. The reliable effects of animacy for KS, GA, and SP match at least some prior results

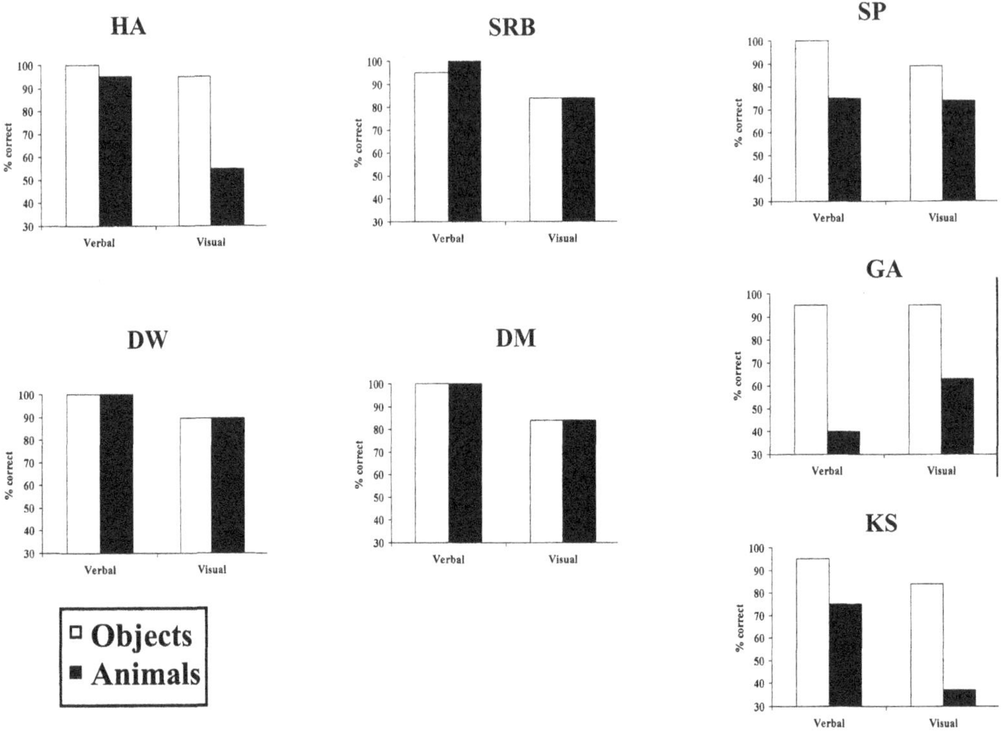


Figure 10. *Percentage correct forced-choice responses to questions stressing either the visual/perceptual or verbal/functional properties of objects, for animals and artefacts (Experiment 6).*

from patients in the literature, where difficulties with verbal/functional as well as visual/perceptual questions about living things have been demonstrated (Borgo & Shallice, 2001; Caramazza & Shelton, 1998; Laiacona et al., 1993a; Samson et al., 1998; Sheridan & Humphreys, 1993). Taken in isolation, this is consistent with an account in terms of domain-specific semantics (Caramazza & Shelton, 1998), since a deficit in domain specific semantic knowledge for living things should impair retrieval of functional as well as perceptual attributes of stimuli. On the other hand, the deficits on visual/perceptual questions, for the other patients, are consistent with there being a disturbance specifically to perceptual knowledge. This may affect living things in particular because they have overlapping perceptual structures and so are more difficult to discriminate when perceptual knowledge is damaged (Humphreys et al., 1997), or because perceptual knowledge is strongly weighted in the representation of living things (Warrington & Shallice, 1984).

## Summary of Section 2

Taken together, the data reported in Section 2 demonstrate both commonalities and differences across the patients. All the patients were impaired at naming particular categories of object (animals, fruits, vegetables, and musical instruments), they were all impaired at making object decisions to pictures of living things, and they all had difficulty in answering forced-choice definitions stressing perceptual properties of stimuli. Three of the patients, KS, GA, and SP, showed some degree of semantic impairment whether they were tested with words or pictures, and they were also impaired for questions stressing the functional properties of objects. The other patients did not have difficulty in making semantic matches with words and they did not have problems with functional questions. There is no evidence for a generalised disturbance in semantic/functional knowledge in these last patients. In two of these patients (HJA and DW), there was evidence of poor access to semantic knowledge from vision. The two remaining patients (DM and SRB) performed relatively well at semantic matching but still showed a deficit when access to stored perceptual knowledge was stressed (in object decision, and in answering perceptual questions). Interestingly, the patients with a generalised semantic deficit (across modalities and in answering all questions about living things) had more anterior lesions than those patients with deficits in accessing stored perceptual knowledge (KS, GA, and SP vs. HJA, DW, DM, and SRB). We return to this point in the General Discussion.

## SECTION 3: TESTS OF THE HIT APPROACH

The HIT approach, outlined in the Introduction, emphasises that (a) patients with damage at different stages of object processing can present with apparent category-specific deficits, but nevertheless (b) all may be prey to effects of perceptual overlap between items, which can influence several levels of processing (including name retrieval) and which can have a greater impact on living than on nonliving things (Humphreys & Forde, 2001). The data in Sections 1 and 2 here indicate that the present patients differ in the functional locus of their impairments—in some the deficit seems to be visual/perceptual in nature (HJA, DW, DM, and SRB), whilst in others the deficit seems to be explicitly semantic (and found with words as well as pictures; patients KS, GA, and SP). In Section 3 we explore the effects of perceptual overlap on the patients. Are there abnormal effects of overlap across all the patients?

### Experiment 7: Effects of masking

Experiment 5 provided evidence for some impairment in visual access to stored visual/perceptual knowledge in all the patients. In Experiment 7 we tested whether this deficit would be exacerbated under conditions of visual noise, when visual stimuli are presented with an overlapping mask. In a prior study with DM, we (Humphreys, Price, & Riddoch, 1999) reported that she was detrimentally affected when a set of pictures was presented with an overlapping mask. The result is of some interest because aspects of DM's performance suggest a problem in name retrieval rather than in semantic access (and see Experiments 2 and 4 here). The decrease in naming for "noisy" stimuli, then, suggests that the efficiency of visual access to stored knowledge can directly constrain name retrieval. For example, partial activation of stored visual knowledge may be fed through to activate both semantic and name representations for both the target and for related competitors. Any noise in visual access may lead to increased activation of competing semantic and name representations, disrupting the naming process. Experiment 7 examined whether the effects of visual noise held generally across the present patients, despite the apparent differences in any loci of damage.

#### *Method*

The stimuli were the 76 black-and-white line drawings from Experiment 1, but each was covered by a set of blue circles (radius 5 mm; see Figure 11). The circles degraded the pictures, but did not present any difficulties for 10 control participants, who identified all of the items. Patients were presented with one item at a time and asked to name it.

#### *Results*

The percentage correct naming responses for the individual patients are given in Figure 12, with the data for masked stimuli shown along with those for unmasked stimuli, from Experiment 1. The percentage correct data were analysed in a two-factor repeated measures ANOVA with patients as a random factor (with the data summed across name frequencies). There were reliable effects of the mask, $F(1, 6) = 11.06, p < .025$, and of structural similarity, $F(1, 6) = 59.79, p = .000$. The interaction was not reliable, $F < 1.0$.

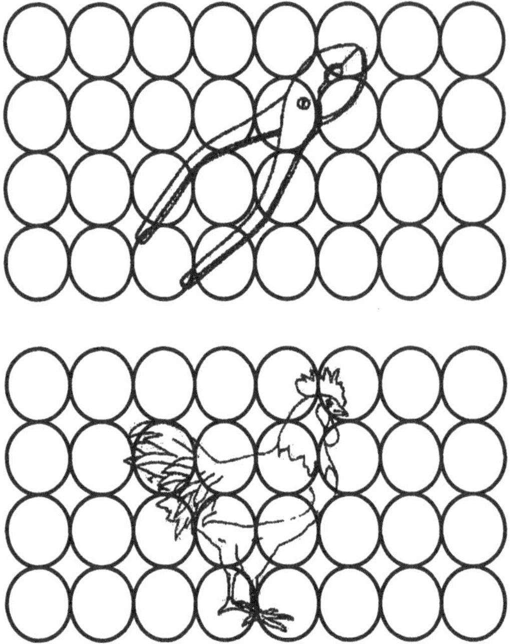

Figure 11. *Examples of masked stimuli in Experiment 7.*

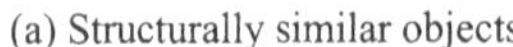


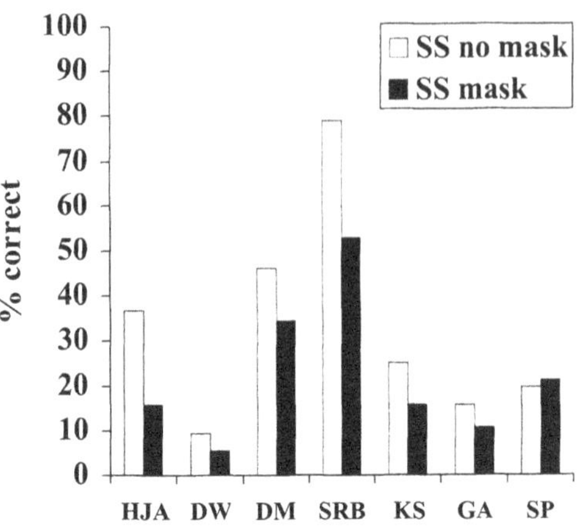


(b) Structurally dissimilar objects

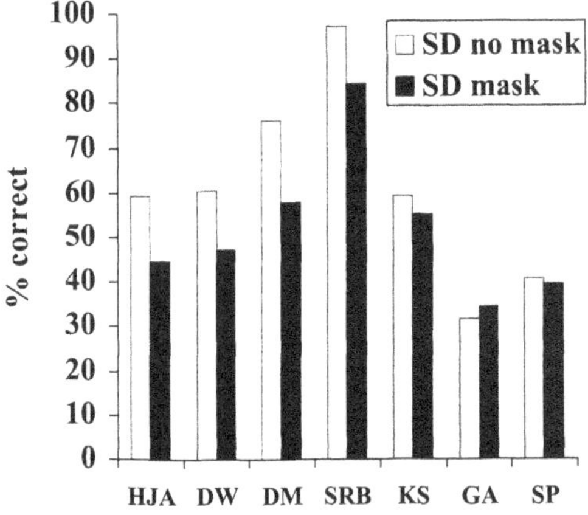


Figure 12. *The percentage correct identification responses to masked and unmasked pictures of structurally similar and dissimilar stimuli (Experiment 7): (a) structurally similar objects; (b) structurally dissimilar objects.*

Although the effects of masking were reliable when analysed across all the patients, the effects tended to be larger for the patients with more posterior lesions (HJA, DW, DM, and SRB) than for those with more anterior lesions (KS, GA, and SP). Taking just the posterior patients, the effects of both masking and structural similarity remained reliable, $F(1, 3) = 39.56$ and $35.28$, respectively, $p < .01$ (effect sizes = 31% difference in accuracy between structurally similar and dissimilar items, and a 15% difference in accuracy with masked and unmasked pictures). For the patients with more anterior lesions, KS, GA, and SP, there was no effect of masking, $F(1, 2) = 1.72, p > .05$ (an effect size of just 3%), though structural similarity remained significant, $F(1, 2) = 20.0, p < .05$ (an effect size of 26%).

The percentages of the different types of errors in naming masked stimuli are given in Table 5. The errors generally followed a similar pattern to those observed in Experiment 1. There were some increases in visual errors (cf. Table 1) and in circumlocution responses by DM and SRB.

### *Discussion*

There was a reliable effect of the masking stimulus on naming accuracy for the patients, even though the mask was not sufficient to disrupt normal naming accuracy. The disruptive effect of the mask is consistent with the patients having a deficit in visual access to stored knowledge, which is exacerbated under visually noisy conditions. With patients like HJA and DW, who have some

**Table 5.** *The percentages of different error types made by the patients in Experiment 7*

| *Patient* | *No resp* | *Vis* | *Vis/sem* | *Sem* | *Phon* | *Pers* | *Unrel* | *Circum* |
|---|---|---|---|---|---|---|---|---|
| HJA | | 56 | 32 | 12 | | | | |
| DW | 28 | 14 | 15 | 43 | | | | |
| DM | | 12 | 18 | 29 | | | | 51 |
| SRB | | 12 | 20 | 25 | | | | 53 |
| KS | 30 | 14 | 22 | 30 | | | | 4 |
| GA | 25 | 15 | 25 | 35 | | | | |
| SP | 12 | 12 | 40 | 25 | | | 11 | |

For abbreviations see Table 2.

disturbance to early perceptual processes (Riddoch & Humphreys, 1987b; Thomas et al., 2002), the effect of the mask is perhaps not surprising. The mask may increase the problems in perceptual organisation for these patients. The detrimental masking effect is more surprising with patients DM and SRB, both of whom appear to have a deficit affecting name retrieval more than semantic access. For example, DM scored 35/76 (46%) correct with masked stimuli vs. 93/152 (61%) correct with unmasked pictures. SRB named 52/76 (68% correct) of the masked pictures relative to 134/152 (88%) of the unmasked items. The effect of masking was reliable for each patient, $\chi^2(1) = 4.12$ and $11.85$, $p < .05$ and $p < .01$, respectively). To account for the result, we suggest the following. Patients HJA, DW, DM, and SRB all had some deficit in accessing stored visual/perceptual representations of objects, which was more serious than their deficit in semantic knowledge (cf. Experiment 5 with Experiments 2 and 4). Under conditions of noisy access, when the mask was present, this deficit should be exacerbated, and additional competitor representations may be activated along with the representations of the target picture. The consequence is that subsequent problems in semantic access and name retrieval are increased.

Although masking had a detrimental effect on patients with relatively posterior lesions, it did not have a reliable effect on the patients with more anterior lesions (KS, GA, and SP). For these patients, the main constraint on their object naming seems to be their poor recruitment of semantic knowledge, which limits naming even with unmasked stimuli. The results are again consistent with the functional locus of any impairment differing across patients.

The HIT account stresses that one factor that can contribute to apparent category effects in patients is perceptual overlap between exemplars, which tends to affect living things more than nonliving things. On this view, we might have expected masking to affect name retrieval for living things (making up the SS category, in Experiment 7) more than for nonliving things (making up most of the SD items), if "natural" differences in perceptual overlap are exacerbated by masking. However, we did not find this; masking was additive with the difference between SS and SD stimuli, even for those patients showing masking effects. Why might this result have occurred? One possibility is that masking obscured some of the critical local features that are used in the identification of nonliving (SD) objects, whilst leaving global shape information available, which may be more helpful for the identification of living (SS) objects (see Gerlach, 2001, for evidence with normal participants). This could have equated performance for the two sets of items, if living (SS) objects suffered more from increased competition at the structural and semantic levels from increased visual noise.

A perhaps more direct way to assess the relations between perceptual overlap and category effects is to manipulate overlap and category orthogonally. For example, although living and nonliving things tend to differ in their average perceptual overlap within their categories, at the level of individual exemplars there are clearly living things with very different perceptual structures and nonliving things with similar perceptual structures. In Experiment 8 we had patients discriminate between pairs of living and nonliving exemplars chosen so as to be either perceptually similar or perceptual dissimilar. The items comprising the dissimilar pairs were also chosen so as to be semantically closer than the items comprising the similar pairs, within each category. If category alone is important, then the patients should find it difficult to discriminate between living things irrespective of their perceptual similarity. In contrast, if perceptual similarity alone is crucial, then this factor, not category, should be crucial. A third possibility is that perceptual overlap and category interact. Living things with similar perceptual structures will tend to have some semantic overlap, and this confluence of perceptual and semantic similarity may make discrimination more difficult than when either perceptual or semantic similarity alone is manipulated (e.g., with nonliving things; see Arguin, Bub, & Dudek, 1996).

## Experiment 8: Manipulating category and perceptual overlap

### *Method*

We assembled 40 living and 40 nonliving things, which were paired together in two ways to create 20 pairs of perceptually similar and 20 pairs of perceptually dissimilar items within each category. The perceptually similar items were chosen to be semantically relatively distinct (e.g., tennis racket and frying pan, baseball bat and rolling pin, potato and orange, runner bean and banana), whilst the perceptually dissimilar items were chosen to be semantically closer than the items used in the perceptually similar conditions (tennis racket and baseball bat, frying pan and rolling pin, potato and runner bean, orange and banana). A full list of the items is given in Appendix B. The majority of stimuli were taken from Snodgrass and Vanderwart (1980), with some being redrawn to emphasise the visual similarity with the other member of their pair (in the visually similar condition). The stimuli were rated by a group of six independent observers who were asked to use a scale between 1 (low) and 7 (high) to rank the perceptual similarity and semantic similarity of each pair (participants were asked to judge semantic similarity on the basis of whether the items were "the same kind of object, were associated or used together"). The mean perceptual and semantic similarity ratings are given in Table 6. For the perceptual similarity ratings, the perceptually similar pairs were rated as being more similar than the dissimilar pairs, $F(1, 5) = 196.12, p = .000$; there was no effect of category and no interaction (both $F < 1.0$). For the semantic similarity ratings, the perceptually dissimilar pairs were ranked as being more semantically similar than the perceptually similar pairs, $F(1, 5) = 535.0$, $p = .000$, and living things were rated as more semantically similar than nonliving things, $F(1, 5) = 10.76, p < .025$. There was also an interaction between category and perceptual similarity, $F(1, 5) = 12.0$, $p < .025$. Perceptually similar living things were rated as more semantically similar than perceptually similar nonliving things, $t(5) = 4.94, p < .01$, but there was no effect of category for the perceptually dissimilar items ($t < 1.0$).

The experiment was run in two forms. In each case patients were presented with pictures of the two objects in each pair. In one trial block they were given the name and in the other they were given a semantic description of one of the objects in a pair,

**Table 6.** *Mean ratings[a] of perceptual and semantic similarity for the living and nonliving pairs of items, for Experiment 8*

| | *Category* | | | |
|---|---|---|---|---|
| | *Living things* | | *Nonliving things* | |
| *Perceptual similarity* | *Similar* | *Dissimilar* | *Similar* | *Dissimilar* |
| Perceptual similarity rating | 5.35 | 3.20 | 5.28 | 3.30 |
| Semantic similarity rating | 3.80 | 5.18 | 2.97 | 5.15 |

[a]1 = low similarity, 7 = high similarity.

and the task was to point to the member of the pair that was named/described. The pairs were repeated once within each trial block, when the other item was then named/described. Three patients had the name-match trials first, the others the description-match trials first. Each block was separated by an intervening activity. DW was not available for this study.

*Results*

The data on the name- and description-match trials were very similar and so they were summed together for each patient for the analysis. Figure 13 gives the mean percentage of correct matches for each patient for each of the four categories of stimulus: living, perceptually similar; living, perceptually dissimilar; nonliving, perceptually similar; nonliving, perceptually dissimilar. The data were analysed over items with patient and perceptual-similarity as repeated measures factors and category (living vs. nonliving) as a between-items factor. There were reliable main effects of patient, $F(5, 190) = 4.59, p = .001$, perceptual similarity, $F(1, 190) = 31.32, p = .000$, and category, $F(1, 38) = 38.68, p = .000$. HJA was worse than the other patients; matching was easier for the perceptually dissimilar pairs, and it was easier for nonliving things. In addition, there was a significant interaction between perceptual similarity and category, $F(1, 190) = 10.50, p < .01$, which was not qualified by any further interaction with patient. For both the perceptually similar pairs and the perceptually dissimilar pairs, performance was better with nonliving than with living things, $F(1, 39) = 29.67$ and $13.66$, both $p < .001$, but the interaction arose because the effect of category was larger with perceptually similar pairs.

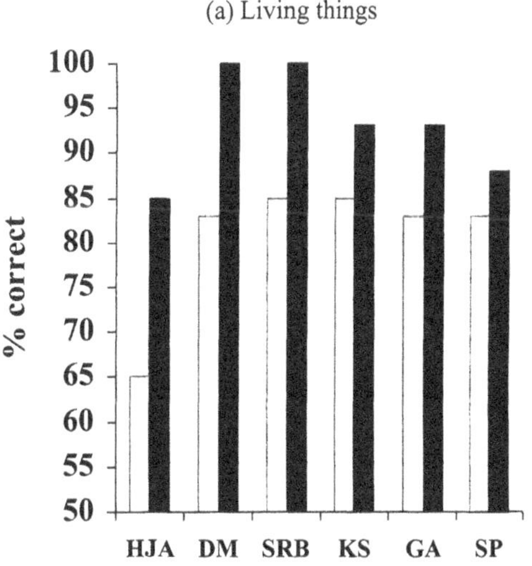


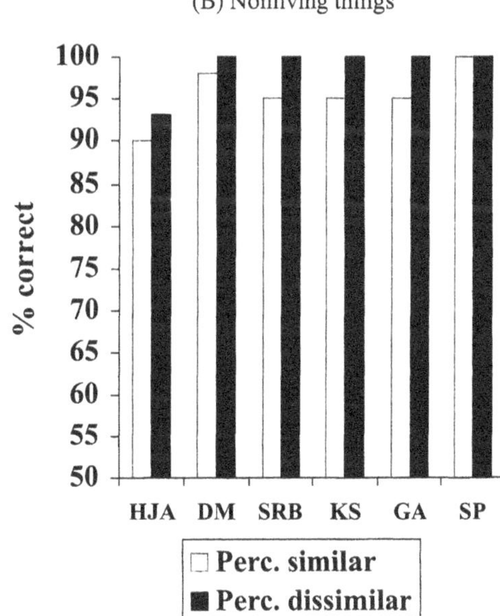


**Figure 13.** *The percentage of correct name/definition to picture matching made in Experiment 8: (a) living things; (b) non-living things.*

*Discussion*

Although all the patients found the tasks relatively easy, performance at name- and description-matching between pairs of items was affected by both perceptual similarity and category, and these two factors also interacted: The differences between the living and the nonliving items were particularly large when patients were presented with perceptually similar pairs. This greater difficulty, with perceptually similar living things, was not due to semantic similarity alone. The perceptually similar pairs were judged to be less semantically close than the perceptually dissimilar pairs, yet perceptually similar living things were the most difficult. Nevertheless, the semantic similarity between the perceptually similar living things could have been a contributory factor, since these items were more semantically similar than the perceptually similar nonliving things[7], although the living and nonliving things were matched for perceptual similarity. For example, it may be that perceptually similar living things were difficult to discriminate because there was a combination of both perceptual and semantic overlap between these items. It is also interesting that all patients showed the same tendency (Figure 13), so the combined effects of perceptual and semantic similarity had an impact on performance irrespective of whether patients seemed to have a deficit in perceptual processing or accessing perceptual knowledge (HJA, DM, and SRB here), or in central semantic knowledge (KS, GA, and SP). Within the HIT approach, combined effects of perceptual and semantic similarity can be expected since, based on the idea of cascaded activation between processing levels (cf. Humphreys et al., 1988), both factors will directly influence the number of competitors for discrimination at a semantic or name selection level. The present results, on discrimination within previously known sets of items, match data reported by Arguin et al. (1996) on the learning of new stimulus–response associations by a patient with a category-specific deficit for living things. They found that learning was particularly difficult when stimuli (abstract patterns) varied along two dimensions (so that a value on a particular dimension could not be used for identification) and when the names referred to items for which the patient had a semantic impairment. In this case, the complexity of the visual learning task interacted with the semantic properties of the objects. Here we found that perceptual overlap was particularly detrimental for living things, that also shared semantic properties.

## GENERAL DISCUSSION

The data reported in Experiments 1–8 demonstrate differences as well as similarities between the present patients. As a group, the patients are impaired at:

1. Naming drawings of objects from categories with structurally similar members (Experiment 1).
2. Naming animals, fruits, vegetables, and musical instruments (Experiment 3).
3. Making object decisions to stimuli drawn from categories of living things (Experiment 5).
4. Naming definitions that stress the visual/perceptual properties of objects (Experiment 6).
5. Discriminating between perceptually similar living things relative to other classes of stimulus (perceptually dissimilar living and nonliving things, perceptually similar nonliving things).

There were also significant differences between the patients:

1. In the cases of HJA and DW, the problems in accessing stored knowledge about stimuli were much worse from vision than from audition, when they were given the names of objects. These patients did not have difficulty in retrieving verbal/functional knowledge about living things.
2. In contrast, KS, GA, and SP all had problems in retrieving verbal/functional information about structurally similar living things (Experiment 6), and in accessing item-specific semantic knowledge about the affected categories from their names (Experiment 4). The magnitude of these deficits was greater for GA and SP than for KS.
3. Unlike all the other patients, DM and SRB performed well on forced-choice semantic decisions. These patients (along with KS) also made substantial numbers of circumlocution responses when they were unable to name pictures (Tables 2 and 3).
4. Despite (3), patients HJA, DW, DM, and SRB, in particular, showed abnormally strong effects of masking on picture naming (Experiment 7).

### Differences between patients

We begin by discussing the differences between the patients.

[7] The higher semantic similarity between perceptually similar living relative to nonliving things was almost inevitable, as it is difficult to produce pairs of perceptually similar living things that are not also similar in terms of their function.

The differences between the three sets of patients can be understood in terms of them having functional difficulties at contrasting stages of object naming. HJA and DW have a deficit in early stages of vision, which disrupts their visual access to stored knowledge about objects. Consequently these patients perform better when they have to access semantic knowledge from words than when it is accessed from pictures (Experiments 2 and 4). In both HJA and DW we have also documented some change in their stored knowledge about the visual attributes of objects across time (Riddoch et al., 1999; Thomas et al., 2002). This suggests that there is an interaction between high-level visual perception and stored visual knowledge, with intact high-level perception being required to help maintain long-term visual knowledge about objects. Consequently, some problems in retrieving long-term visual knowledge can be apparent in such patients. DW, for instance, was first tested some 3 years after his lesion and it is possible that there was already some deterioration in his long-term visual knowledge (cf. Experiment 6 here). We also propose that both HJA and DW tend to identify objects in a piecemeal fashion, from their local parts (see Riddoch & Humphreys, 1987b; Thomas et al., 2002, for evidence). This may make it difficult for them to identify structurally similar objects, many of which have common parts. Any further loss of stored knowledge may also affect these items more than objects that are more distinctive within their category, since there will already be more overlap for structurally similar items within a perceptual knowledge store (see Riddoch et al., 1999, for direct evidence on this).

KS, GA, and SP, on the other hand, all had some difficulty in accessing item-specific semantic knowledge even from names (Experiment 4), and they all had deficits for verbal/functional as well as for visual/perceptual information about structurally similar, living things. These deficits for verbal/functional knowledge about living things have been noted previously in several patients (Caramazza & Shelton, 1998; Laiacona et al., 1993a; Samson et al., 1998; Sheridan & Humphreys, 1993). We have discussed at least two accounts of the deficit. One is in terms of domain-specific semantic knowledge (Caramazza & Shelton, 1998). These patients may have lost domain-specific semantic knowledge about living things, so impairing their ability even to answer functional questions concerning these stimuli. An alternative is that there is a core deficit in visual/perceptual knowledge (cf. Warrington & Shallice, 1984) and, for living things, this knowledge must be drawn-on to at least some degree to support the retrieval of functional knowledge (Farah & McClelland, 1991; Thompson-Schill, Aguirre, D'Esposito, & Farah, 1999). Our data present some problems for this last account, since the other patients who were impaired at retrieving visual/perceptual knowledge about objects performed at control levels when required to retrieve verbal/functional knowledge from object names (whereas at least a minor deficit might be expected). Indeed, KS tended to be better at forced-choice discrimination based on a visual/perceptual definition of an animal than DW, yet she showed a greater cost on discriminations based on verbal/functional information for animals (Experiment 6). This suggests that the deficit on verbal/functional knowledge cannot simply be attributed to a greater loss of knowledge all round, for some patients.

The final two patients, DM and SRB, were relatively good at all the semantic tests whilst being impaired at naming. Was this a lexical deficit, as has been argued for some patients with apparent category-specific naming problems in the literature (e.g., Farah & Wallace, 1992; Hart et al., 1985)? We have two points to make here. The first is that the argument for a naming deficit has previously been made on the basis of patients being able to categorise the stimuli they fail to name (e.g., sorting into fruits and vegetables). However, note that KS here performed at ceiling on this kind of superordinate categorisation (Experiment 2), yet she was impaired when semantic knowledge was tested at a finer-grained level (Experiment 4). Superordinate categorisation, then, is not a strong test of intact access to semantic knowledge. The second point is that DM and SRB were both impaired when required to make discriminations based on visual/perceptual information (e.g., the object decision test in Experiment 5). To account for this pattern of data, we reiterate arguments that have been made previously about DM and SRB (Forde et al., 1997; Humphreys et al., 1997), and which are further supported by the data presented here. We suggest that DM and SRB have relatively mild deficits in their stored visual/perceptual knowledge about objects; these deficits are sufficient to disrupt naming but not sufficient to prevent access to considerable semantic information about the objects they attempt to name. Additional converging evidence for this comes from the data on masking (Experiment 7), where the apparent naming deficit was increased when the stimuli were masked, where deficits were again apparent even though naming was not required. In general, patients with a mild deficit in stored perceptual knowledge may exhibit a greater deficit on naming than on semantic classification tasks because visual/ perceptual knowledge must be interrogated more to support correct naming than semantic classification. Also, living things may be more difficult than nonliving things for these patients because there is increased overlap in stored perceptual and semantic representations for living items. We discuss this last point below.

## Similarities between patients: The HIT account

Although, as we have pointed out, the patients seem to be impaired at different levels of object processing, there were a number of common effects. In naming tasks there were effects of structural similarity (Experiment 1) and category (Experiment 3) for all patients, and all patients showed a tendency for these effects to interact (Experiment 8). We propose that the above data can be accounted for in terms of the HIT framework put forward by Humphreys and Forde (2001), which stresses the "knock on" effects of visual processing (and damage to visual access procedures) on subsequent stages of object naming. It is a natural consequence of this account that we should expect forms of interaction between perceptual and semantic similarity on discrimination, even if patients have deficits at different processing levels. This would not necessarily follow in other accounts, which do not stress the nature of object processing in addition to the nature of object representation. For example, in terms of a domain-specific semantic deficit, we might predict that, in Experiment 8, there would be a deficit for living things across the board, or even that perceptually dissimilar items would be more difficult than perceptually similar items given that semantic similarity tended to be higher for the perceptually dissimilar pairs. On the other hand, if effects of perceptual overlap are carried through to a semantic level, as proposed by HIT, then it is the combination of perceptual and semantic similarity that should render performance most difficult.

The HIT account is also comfortable with the idea that category-specific deficits can arise from damage at several levels of processing. As we have noted, it is difficult to explain the contrasting patterns of deficit across the current group of patients if the only cause of category-specific impairment were a loss of domain-specific semantic knowledge, since there was little evidence for any loss of verbal/ functional knowledge in four of the cases (HJA, DW, DM, and SRB). It is also difficult to account for the substantial problems in functional knowledge in some of the patients (KS, GA, and SP) if there were a loss of only sensory-perceptual knowledge (Warrington & Shallice, 1984). In addition, even in the cases where there was a clear loss of functional knowledge, there was also an impairment for musical instruments, which held even when potential confounding factors were covaried out (Experiment 3). It is possible that the deficit with musical instruments reflects some additional associated impairment, caused by the overlap in the neural areas supporting the recognition of living things and musical instruments (see Humphreys & Price, 2001, for a recent discussion of such "associated" impairments). However, this is tantamount to proposing that there is domain-specific semantic knowledge for musical instruments that is isolatable from semantic knowledge for other nonliving things (which was relatively preserved in the current patients). This is difficult to justify on evolutionary grounds and is relatively unparsimonious. In contrast, the HIT approach holds that there can be damage to pre-semantic as well as to semantic stages of object naming, all of which can bring about a category-specific deficit for living things and musical instruments, given relatively high levels of perceptual similarity between these items (Gale et al., 2001).

Since the HIT approach supposes that category-specific deficits can emerge at different stages of object processing, it can also capture other patterns of dissociation in the literature. For example, patient SB, reported by Sheridan and Humphreys (1993), performed object decisions at a high level with fruits, vegetables, and fruit–vegetable nonobjects, despite being impaired at retrieving both perceptual and verbal/functional knowledge for these items from their names. This is unlike all of the current patients who were impaired at object decision, even though they were not necessarily impaired at retrieving verbal/functional knowledge (e.g., patients HJA, DW, DM, and SRB). That is, there can be a double dissociation between visual access to stored visual/perceptual knowledge about affected categories (intact in SB, impaired in HJA, DW, DM, and SRB here) and access to verbal/functional information from the names of objects in the same categories (impaired in SB and relatively spared in HJA, DW, DM, and SRB in the present study). This is difficult for some theories of category-deficits to account for. For example, the "distributed semantics" account explains double dissociations between categories in terms of the degree of damage to the system (Tyler & Moss, 2001), but it has little to say about dissociations based on different access processes. On the other hand, HIT provides a straightforward explanation. In a patient such as SB (Sheridan & Humphreys, 1993) there can be good visual access to stored perceptual knowledge, along with impaired functional knowledge at a semantic level. The semantic deficit also prevents access to stored perceptual knowledge from object names. In contrast, patients such as HJA, DW, DM, and SRB have impaired visual access to stored perceptual knowledge along with relatively intact verbal/functional knowledge, at a semantic level.

What about patterns of dissociation within the broad categories of living and nonliving things, such as between fruit and vegetables on the one hand and animals on the other (cf. Caramazza & Shelton, 1998, with Farah & Wallace, 1992)? As we noted in the Introduction, this dissociation seems more straightforward to explain in terms of domain-specific semantic knowledge rather than a simple loss of sensory/perceptual knowledge or the detrimental effect of any single factor (such as structural similarity) on performance. Other accounts of differential deficits within living things emphasise the role of particular types of perceptual knowledge, such as colour, for the identification of fruits and vegetables rather than animals. According to such accounts, deficits in accessing colour knowledge may selectively disrupt fruits and vegetables; loss of other forms of perceptual knowledge (shape, patterns of movement) may generate difficulties with animals (see Humphreys & Forde, 2001, for discussion). A further possibility is that factors such as gender-specific familiarity are contributory factors (cf. Laiacona, Barbarotto, & Capitani, 1998). Note that we found that familiarity was a reliable predictor of naming in Experiment 1 in addition to any effects of within-category perceptual similarity. More work is needed to assess how such finer-grained dissociations may arise.

## Relations to evidence from functional brain imaging

We suggest that the HIT account is also consistent with the general pattern of findings emerging from studies of functional brain imaging. The most frequently studied contrast in imaging studies is between living things and tools. When tools are identified there is substantial evidence for activation in the posterior region of the middle temporal gyrus and inferior frontal regions of the left hemisphere (Devlin et al., 2003; Grabowski et al., 1998; Martin et al., 1996). This is consistent with action-related associations being important for these items (Humphreys et al., 2002; Warrington & Shallice, 1984), since (e.g.) similar regions are activated when action words must be retrieved (Martin, Haxby, Lalande, Wiggs, & Ungerleider, 1995). In contrast, regions of extra-striate cortex, ventral occipito-temporal cortex and anterior temporal cortex have been selectively activated for living things relative to tools (Chao et al., 1999; Gerlach, Law, Gade, & Paulson, 1999; Martin et al., 1996;

Moore & Price, 1999; Perani et al., 1995). At least some of these latter regions are linked to high-level visual processing, suggesting that retrieval of visual/perceptual knowledge may play a strong role in the identification of living things.

However, one of the difficulties in interpreting these data in terms of category-specific effects has been in trying to tie down the critical variables, and the processing stages, at which differences arise. For example, Moore and Price (1999) conducted an orthogonal manipulation of category and pictorial complexity, contrasting simple and complex living things (fruit and animals) with simple and complex nonliving things (tools and vehicles). They replicated prior evidence for activation of the posterior left middle temporal gyrus by tools. However, the main category-specific activation for living things was confined to anterior temporal cortex. Excitation in more posterior regions (e.g., medial extrastriate cortex) was increased for complex relative to simple stimuli. This links activation in medial extra-striate areas to detailed perceptual processing, but not necessarily to the distinction between living and nonliving things. Moore and Price (1999; see also Devlin et al., 2003) instead propose that the "true" category-based activation for living things is found only within the anterior temporal cortex, and this is associated with the retrieval of semantic rather than visual/perceptual knowledge. It remains unclear, however, whether this activation is linked to domain-specific semantic knowledge or to the greater need to integrate perceptual with other forms of information when living things are identified (consistent with the strong weighting of perceptual information for living things). Nevertheless, this evidence from imaging is consistent with our neuropsychological data. In particular we have noted that damage to the anterior temporal regions in patients KS, GA, and SP, was linked to impaired semantic knowledge about living things

Gerlach et al. (1999) also reported that there was increased activation in posterior, inferior temporal cortex (particularly in the right hemisphere) when participants carried out difficult relative to easy object decision tasks. Moore and Price (1999) reported increased activation in similar areas when participants identified line drawings relative to coloured drawings of living things. We presume that coloured drawings require less extensive visual processing to be identified, and that easy object decisions similarly involve less extensive visual processing in order to access stored perceptual knowledge (relative to when nonobjects are more similar to real objects). It follows that there is increased recruitment of regions in the posterior temporal lobe under conditions in which competing stimuli have to be differentiated to access stored perceptual knowledge. Behaviourally, living things appear to place greater demands on perceptual differentiation than nonliving things (see Gerlach et al., 1999, for evidence), so that damage to the processes (and neural regions supporting) the perceptual differentiation of object representations could generate one additional form of category-specific impairment. This impairment should be most apparent in tasks that stress perceptual differentiation, such as making object decisions between stimuli drawn from the same, structurally similar categories, and object naming. This is consistent with the more posterior lesions present in HJA, DW, DM, and SRB, and with their problems being most pronounced in difficult object decision and naming (Experiments 1, 3, and 5).

We also found that problems in perceptual differentiation (in DM and SRB), and in semantic access (in KS), emerged even with unilateral left-hemisphere lesions. It follows that, though imaging studies demonstrate that activation can be pronounced in the right hemisphere (Gerlach et al., 1999; Moore & Price, 1999), this does not seem sufficient for access to fine-grained visual/perceptual or semantic knowledge. The lesion data suggest that some activation of left-hemispheric structures remains necessary in order to individuate objects at these different levels.

Finally we also note other imaging evidence that suggests that areas of the left inferior and posterior temporal lobe are particularly active during name retrieval for objects. Price et al. (1996), for example, found that there was increased activation in this region when object names rather than colour names had to be retrieved to coloured, nonobject stimuli (relative to baselines in which participants simply said "yes" to each stimulus type). These posterior temporal regions may support the increased perceptual differentiation needed to achieve object naming rather than recognition (which presumably operated in both the naming and baseline conditions), as proposed by the HIT account. As indicated by the cases of DM and SRB here, damage to these regions can also generate a disorder that produces a more pronounced effect on object naming than on object recognition.

## REFERENCES


Allport, D. A. (1985). Distributed memory, modular systems and dysphasia. In S. K. Newman & R. Epstein (Eds.), *Current perspectives in dysphasia*. Edinburgh, UK: Churchill Livingstone.

Arguin, M., Bub, D., & Dudek, G. (1996). Shape integration for visual object recognition and its implication in category-specific visual agnosia. *Visual Cognition, 3*, 221–275.

Barbarotto, R., Capitani, E., & Laiacona, M. (2001). Living musical instruments and inanimate body parts? *Neuropsychologia, 39*, 358–363.

Borgo, F., & Shallice, T. (2001). When living things and other "sensory quality" categories behave in the same fashion: A novel category specificity effect. *Neurocase, 7*, 201–220.

Burgess, P. W., & Shallice, T. (1997). *The Hayling and Brixton Tests*. Bury St. Edmunds, UK: Thames Valley Test Co.

Caramazza, A. (1998). The interpretation of semantic category-specific deficits: What do they reveal about the organisation of conceptual knowledge in the brain? *Neurocase, 4*, 265–272.

Caramazza, A., & Shelton, J. R. (1998). Domain specific knowledge systems in the brain: The animate-inanimate distinction. *Journal of Cognitive Neuroscience, 10*, 1–34.

Chainay, H., & Humphreys, G. W. (2001). The real-object advantage in agnosia: Evidence for a role of surface and depth information in object recognition. *Cognitive Neuropsychology, 18*, 175–190.

Chao, L. L., Haxby, J. V., & Martin, A. (1999). Attribute-based neural substrates in posterior temporal cortex for perceiving and knowing about objects. *Nature Neuroscience, 2*, 913–919.

Coslett, B., & Saffran, E. (1992). Optic aphasia and the right hemisphere: A replication and extension. *Brain and Language, 43*, 148–161.

Devlin, J., Gonnerman, L., Anderson, E., & Seidenberg, M. (1998). Category-specific deficits in focal and widespread damage: A computational account. *Journal of Cognitive Neuroscience, 10*, 77–94.

Devlin, J., Moore, C. J., Mummery, C. J., Gorno-Tempini, M., Phillips, J. A., Nopenney, U., & Price, C. J. (2003). *Anatomic constraints on cognitive theories of category specificity*. Manuscript submitted for publication.

Devlin, J., Russell, R. P., Davis, M. H., Price, C. J., Moss, H. E., Fadili, M. J., & Tyler, L. K. (2002). Is there an anatomical basis for category-specificity? Semantic memory studies in PET and fMRI. *Neuropsychologia, 40*, 54–75.

Durrant-Peatfield, M. R., Tyler, L. K., Moss, H. E., & Levy, J. P. (1997). *The distinctiveness of form and function in category structure: A connectionist model*. Proceedings of the 19th Annual Cognitive Science Conference, University of Stanford, USA.

Farah, M. J., & McClelland, J. L. (1991). A computational model of semantic memory impairment: Modality specificity and emergent category specificity. *Psychological Review, 120*, 339–357.

Farah, M. J., Meyer, M. M., & McMullan, P. A. (1996). The living/nonliving dissociation is not an artifact: Giving an a priori implausible hypothesis a strong test. *Cognitive Neuropsychology, 13*, 137–154.

Farah, M. J., & Wallace, M. A. (1992). Semantically bounded anomia: Implications for the neural implementation of naming. *Neuropsychologia, 30*, 609–621.

Forde, E. M. E., Francis, D., Riddoch, M. J., Rumiati, R., & Humphreys, G. W. (1997). On the links between visual knowledge and naming: A single case study of a patient with a category-specific impairment for living things. *Cognitive Neuropsychology, 14*, 403–458.

Forde, E. M. E., & Humphreys, G. W. (1999). Category-specific recognition impairments: A review of important case studies and influential theories. *Aphasiology, 13*, 169–193.

Funnell, E., & Sheridan, J. (1992). Categories of knowledge? Unfamiliar aspects of living and nonliving things. *Cognitive Neuropsychology, 9*, 135–153.

Gado, M., Hanaway, J., & Frank, R. (1979). Functional anatomy of the cerebral cortex by computed tomography. *Journal of Computer Assisted Tomography, 3*, 1–19.

Gainotti, G., Silveri, M. C., Daniele, A., & Giustolisi, L. (1995). Neuroanatomical correlates of category-specific semantic disorders: A critical survey. *Memory, 3*, 247–264.

Gale, T. M., Done, D. J., & Frank, R. J. (2001). Visual crowding and category specific deficits for pictorial stimuli: A neural network model. *Cognitive Neuropsychology, 18*, 509–550.

Garrard, P., Lambon Ralph, M. A., & Hodges, J. R. (2002). Semantic dementia: A category specific paradox. In E. M. E. Forde & G. W. Humphreys (Eds.), *Category specificity in brain and mind* (pp. 149-180). Hove, UK: Psychology Press.

Garrard, P., Patterson, K., Watson, P. C., & Hodges, J. (1998). Category specific semantic loss in dementia of Alzheimer's type: Functional-anatomical correlations from cross-sectional analyses. *Brain, 121*, 633–646.

Gerlach, C. (2001). Structural similarity causes different category-effects depending on task characteristics. *Neuropsychologia, 39*, 895–900

Gerlach, C., Law, I., Gade, A., & Paulson, O. (1999). Perceptual differentiation and category effects in normal object recognition: A PET study. *Brain, 122*, 2159–2170.

Giersch, A., Humphreys, G. W., Boucart, M., & Kovacs, I. (2000). The computation of occluded contours in visual agnosia: Evidence for early computation prior to shape binding and figure-ground coding. *Cognitive Neuropsychology, 17*, 731–760.

Gonnerman, L. M., Anderson, E. S., Devlin, J. T., Kempler, D., & Seidenberg, M. S. (1997). Double dissociation of semantic categories in Alzheimer's disease. *Brain and Language, 57*, 254–279.

Grabowski, T. J., Damasio, H., & Damasio, A. R. (1998). Premotor and prefrontal correlates of category-related lexical retrieval. *Neurimage, 7*, 232–243.

Hart, J., Berndt, R. S., & Caramazza, A. (1985). Category-specific naming deficit following cerebral infarction. *Nature, 316*, 439–440.

Heaton, R. K., Chelune, G. J., Talley, J. L., Kay, G. G., & Curtiss, G. (1993). *Wisconsin Card Sorting Test manual.* Odessa, FL: Psychological Assessment Resources.

Hillis, A. E., & Caramazza, A. (1991). Category-specific naming and comprehension impairment: A double dissociation. *Brain, 114*, 2081–2094.

Hillis, A. E., & Caramazza, A. (1995). Constraining claims about theories of semantic memory: More on unitary versus multiple semantics. *Cognitive Neuropsychology, 12*, 175–186.

Hodges, J. J., Salmon, D. P., & Butters, N. (1991). The nature of the naming deficit in Alzheimer's and Huntington's disease. *Brain, 114*, 1547–1558.

Howard, D., & Patterson, K. E. (1992). *The Pyramids and Palm Trees Test.* Bury St Edmunds, UK: Thames Valley Test Co.

Humphreys, G. W., & Forde, E. M. E. (2001). Hierarchies, similarity, and interactivity in object recognition: 'Category-specific' neuropsychological deficits. *Behavioral and Brain Sciences, 24*, 453–509.

Humphreys, G. W., & Price, C. J. (2001). Cognitive neuropsychology and functional brain imaging: Implications for functional and anatomical models of cognition. *Acta Psychologica, 107*, 119–153.

Humphreys, G. W., Price, C., & Riddoch, M. J. (1999). From objects to names: A cognitive neuroscience approach. *Psychological Research, 62*, 118–130.

Humphreys, G. W., & Riddoch, M. J. (1987). *To see but not to see: A case study of visual agnosia.* Hove, UK: Lawrence Erlbaum Associates Ltd.

Humphreys, G. W., Riddoch, M. J., & Forde, E. M. E. (2002). The principle of target–competitor differentiation in object recognition and naming (and its role in category effects in normality and pathology). In E. M. E. Forde & G. W. Humphreys (Eds.), *Category specificity in brain and mind* (pp. 51–84). Hove, UK: Psychology Press.

Humphreys, G. W., Riddoch, M. J., & Price, C. (1997). Top-down processes in object identification: Evidence from experimental psychology, neuropsychology and functional anatomy. *Proceedings for the Royal Society, Series B, 352*, 1275–1282.

Humphreys, G. W., Riddoch, M. J., & Quinlan, P. T. (1988). Cascade processes in picture identification. *Cognitive Neuropsychology, 5*, 67–103.

Kay, J., Lesser, R., & Coltheart, M. (1992). *PALPA.* Hove, UK: Psychology Press.

Kiefer, M. (2001). Perceptual and semantic sources of category-specific effects in object categorization: Event-related potentials during picture and word categorization. *Memory and Cognition, 29*, 100–116.

Kuçera, H., & Francis, W. N. (1967). *Computational analysis of present-day American English.* Providence, RI: Brown University Press.

Laiacona, M., Barbarotto, R., & Capitani, E. (1993a). Perceptual and associative knowledge in category specific impairment of semantic memory: A study of two cases. *Cortex, 29*, 727–740.

Laiacona, M., Barbarotto, R., & Capitani, E. (1998). Semantic category dissociations in naming: Is there a gender effect in Alzheimer's disease? *Neuropsychologia, 36*, 407–419.

Laiacona, M., Barbarotto, R., Trivelli, C., & Capitani, E. (1993b). Dissociazioni semantiche intercategoriali: Descrizione di una batteria standardizzata e dati normativi. *Archivio di Psicologia, Neurologia e Psichiatria, 53*, 113–154.

Laiacona, M., & Capitani, E. (2001). A case of prevailing deficit of nonliving things or a case of prevailing sparing of living categories? *Cognitive Neuropsychology, 18*, 39–70.

Laiacona, M., Capitani, E., & Caramazza, A. (in press). Category-specific semantic deficits do not reflect the sensory/functional organization of the brain: A test of the "sensory quality" hypothesis. *Neurocase.*

Lloyd-Jones, T., & Humphreys, G. W. (1997). Perceptual differentiation as a source of contour effects in object processing: evidence from naming and object decision. *Memory and Cognition, 25*, 18–35.

Martin, A., Haxby, J. V., Lalonde, F. M., Wiggs, C. L., & Ungerleider, L. G. (1995). Discrete cortical regions associated with knowledge of color and knowledge of action. *Science, 270*, 102–105.

Martin, A., Wiggs, C. L., Ungerleider, L. G., & Haxby, J. V. (1996). Neural correlates of category-specific knowledge. *Nature, 379*, 649–652.

McCarthy, R., & Warrington, E. K. (1986). Visual associative agnosia: A clinico-anatomical study of a single case. *Journal of Neurological and Neurosurgical Psychiatry, 49*, 1233–1240.

McRae, K., & Cree, G. S. (2002). Factors underlying category-specific semantic deficits. In E. M. E. Forde & G. W. Humphreys (Eds.), *Category specificity in brain and mind* (pp. 211–250). Hove, UK: Psychology Press.

McRae, K., De Sa, V. R., & Seidenberg, M. S. (1997). On the nature and scope of featural representations of word meaning. *Journal of Experimental Psychology: General, 126*, 99–130.

Moore, C. J., & Price, C. J. (1999). A functional neuroimaging study of the variables that generate category-specific object processing differences. *Brain, 122*, 943–962.

Moss, H. E., Tyler, L. K., & Devlin, J. T. (2002). The emergence of category-specific deficits in a distributed semantic system. In E. M. E. Forde & G. W. Humphreys (Eds.), *Category-specificity in brain and mind* (pp. 115–148). Hove, UK: Psychology Press.

Moss, H. E., Tyler, L. K., & Jennings, F. (1997). When leopards lose their spots: Knowledge of visual properties in category-specific deficits for living things. *Cognitive Neuropsychology, 14*, 901–950.

Moss, H. E., Tyler, L. K., Durrant-Peatfield, M. R., & Bunn, E. M. (1998). "Two eyes of a see-through": impaired and intact semantic knowledge in a case of a selective deficit for living things. *Neurocase, 4*, 291–310.

Osswald, K., Humphreys, G. W., & Olson, A. (2002). Words are more than the sum of their parts: Evidence for detrimental effects of word-level information in alexia. *Cognitive Neuropsychology, 19*, 675–695.

Perani, D., Cappa, S. F., Bettinardi, V., Bressi, S, Gorno-Tempini, Matarrese, M., & Fazio, F. (1995). Different neural systems for the recognition of animals and man-made tools. *Neuroreport, 6*, 1637–1641.

Perani, D., Schnur, T., Tettamanti, M., Gorno-Tempini, M., Cappa, S. F., & Fazio, F. (1999). Word and picture matching: A PET study of semantic category effects. *Neuropsychologia, 37*, 293–306.

Price, C. J., & Friston, K. J. (2002). Functional imaging studies of category specificity. In E. M. E. Forde & G. W. Humphreys (Eds.), *Category specificity in brain and mind* (pp. 427–448). Hove, UK: Psychology Press.

Price, C. J., Moore, C. J., Humphreys, G. W., Frackowiak, R. S. J., & Friston, K. J. (1996). The neural regions sustaining object recognition and naming. *Proceedings of the Royal Society of London, B263*, 1501–1507.

Riddoch, M. J., & Humphreys, G. W. (1987a). Picture naming. In G. W. Humphreys & M. J. Riddoch (Eds.), *Visual object processing: A cognitive neuropsychological approach.* Hove, UK: Lawrence Erlbaum Associates Ltd.

Riddoch, M. J., & Humphreys, G. W. (1987b). A case of integrative visual agnosia. *Brain, 110*, 1431–1462.

Riddoch, M. J., & Humphreys, G. W. (1987c). Visual object processing in optic aphasia: A case of semantic access agnosia. *Cognitive Neuropsychology, 4*, 131–185.

Riddoch, M. J., & Humphreys, G. W. (1993). *The Birmingham Object Recognition Battery (BORB).* Hove, UK: Psychology Press.

Riddoch, M. J., Humphreys, G. W., Coltheart, M., & Funnell, E. (1988). Semantic system or systems? Neuropsychological evidence re-examined. *Cognitive Neuropsychology, 5*, 3–25.

Riddoch, M. J., Humphreys, G. W., Gannon, T., Blott, W., & Jones, V. (1999). Memories are made of this: The effects of time on stored visual knowledge in a case of visual agnosia. *Brain, 122*, 537–559.

Rumiati, R. I., & Humphreys, G. W. (1997). Visual object agnosia without alexia or prosopagnosia: Arguments for separate knowledge stores. *Visual Cognition, 4*, 207–218.

Samson, D., Pillon, A., & De Wilde, V. (1998). Impaired knowledge of visual *and* nonvisual attributes in a patient with a semantic impairment for living entities: A case of a true category-specific deficit. *Neurocase, 4,* 273–290.

Santos, L. R., & Caramazza, A. (2002). The domain-specific hypothesis: A developmental and comparative perspective on category-specific deficits. In E. M. E. Forde & G. W. Humphreys (Eds.), *Category specificity in brain and mind* (pp. 1–24). Hove, UK: Psychology Press.

Sartori, G., Miozzo, M., & Job, R. (1993). Category-specific naming impairments? Yes. *Quarterly Journal of Experimental Psychology, 46A,* 489–504.

Shelton, J. R., Fouch, E., & Caramazza, A. (1998). The selective sparing of body part knowledge: A case study. *Neurocase, 4,* 339–351.

Sheridan, J., & Humphreys, G. W. (1993). A verbal-semantic category-specific recognition impairment. *Cognitive Neuropsychology, 10,* 143–184.

Silveri, M. C., Daniele, A., Giustolisi, L., & Gainotti, G. (1991). Dissociation between knowledge of living and nonliving things in dementia of the Alzheimer type. *Neurology, 41,* 545–546.

Silveri, M. C., & Gainotti, G. (1988). Interaction between vision and language in category-specific semantic impairment. *Cognitive Neuropsychology, 5,* 677–709.

Snodgrass, J. G., & Vanderwart, M. (1980). A standardised set of 260 pictures: Norms for name agreement, image agreement, familiarity and visual complexity. *Journal of Experimental Psychology: Human Learning and Memory, 6,* 174–215.

Snodgrass, J. G., & Yuditsky, T. (1996). Naming times for the Snodgrass and Vanderwart pictures. *Behavior Research Methods, Instruments and Computers, 28,* 516–536.

Spitzer, M., Kishka, U., Guckel, F., Belleman, M., Kammer, T., Seyyedi, S., Weisbrod, M., Schwartz, A., & Brix, G. (1999). Functional magnetic resonance imaging of category-specific cortical activation: Evidence for semantic maps. *Cognitive Brain Research, 6,* 309–319.

Stewart, F., Parkin, A. J., & Hunkin, N. M. (1992). Naming impairments following recovery from herpes simplex encephalitis. *Quarterly Journal of Experimental Psychology, 44A,* 261–284.

Suzuki, K., Yamadori, A., & Fujii, T. (1997). Category specific comprehension deficit restricted to body parts. *Neurocase, 3,* 193–200.

Thomas, R. M., Forde, E. M. E., Humphreys, G. W., & Graham, K. S. (2002). The effects of passage of time on a patient with a category-specific agnosia. *Neurocase, 8,* 466–479.

Thompson-Schill, S. L., Aguirre, G. K., D'Esposito, M., & Farah, M. J. (1999). A neural basis for category and modality specificity of semantic knowledge. *Neuropsychologia, 37,* 671–676.

Tyler, L., & Moss, H. (1997). Functional properties of concepts: Studies of normal and brain-damaged patients. *Cognitive Neuropsychology, 14,* 511–545.

Tyler, L., & Moss, H. E. (2001). Towards a distributed account of conceptual knowledge. *Trends in Cognitive Sciences, 5,* 244–252.

Warrington, E. K. (1984). *Recognition Memory Test.* Windsor, UK: NFER-Nelson.

Warrington, E. K., & McCarthy, R. (1987). Categories of knowledge: Further fractionations and an attempted integration. *Brain, 110,* 1273–1296.

Warrington, E. K., & Shallice, T. (1984). Category-specific semantic impairment. *Brain, 107,* 829–854.

# APPENDIX A

## Stimuli used for the item-specific associative matching test in Experiment 4

| *Stimuli to be chosen from* | *Associate* |
|---|---|
| *Vegetables* | |
| CORN lettuce pepper tomato celery | butter |
| asparagas artichoke carrot mushroom ONION | tears |
| asparagus artichoke CARROT onion mushroom | rabbit |
| corn lettuce pepper TOMATO celery | sauce bottle |
| artichoke LETTUCE corn pepper onion | mayonnaise |
| lettuce MUSHROOM pepper celery asparagas | woods |
| *Fruit* | |
| strawberry melon apple PINEAPPLE lemon | palm tree |
| LEMON grapes strawberry banana melon | pancake |
| cherry pineapple orange melon GRAPES | wine glass |
| pineapple orange BANANA cherry pineapple | monkey |
| pineapple ORANGE banana cherry grapes | juice squeezer |
| pear melon apple STRAWBERRY grapes | cream |
| *Animals* | |
| cow frog ostrich mouse HEN | egg cups |
| hen ostrich giraffe CAMEL caterpillar | pyramid |
| MOUSE caterpillar giraffe ostrich butterfly | skirting board |
| frog mouse swan butterfly COW | milk bottle |
| cow FROG ostrich mouse hen | tadpole |
| caterpillar camel SWAN butterfly giraffe | lake |
| *Body parts* | |
| hand leg arm ear HAIR | hat |
| hand LEG arm ear hair | trousers |
| FINGER foot nose eye lips | ring |
| Finger foot nose EYE lips | glasses |
| Eye lips HAND foot hair | mitten |
| hand nose eye ear FOOT | boot |
| *Vehicles* | |
| yacht TRAIN car bus helicopter | railtrack |
| lorry bicycle SLEDGE motorbike airplane | snowman |
| lorry MOTORBIKE bicycle sledge airplane | crash helmet |
| lorry motorbike bicycle sledge AIRPLANE | runway |
| bicycle lorry CAR helicopter airplane | garage |
| bicycle lorry car HELICOPTER airplane | launchpad |
| *Furniture* | |
| rockingchair lamp CHEST-OF-DRAWERS bed stool | shirt |
| chair DESK settee vase table | worklight |
| BED rockingchair desk stool vase | pillow |
| lamp bed desk settee CHAIR | table |
| bed desk settee LAMP chair | bulb |
| table SETTEE chest-of-drawers lamp chair | cushion |
| *Tools* | |
| chisel hammer nail scissors SAW | logs |
| screw chisel HAMMER saw pliers | nail |
| hammer chisel spanner SCISSORS screw | paper |
| AXE screwdriver spanner nail scissors | tree |
| hammer chisel spanner SCREW scissors | screwdriver |
| NAIL screwdriver axe saw pliers | hammer |
| Musical instrument | |
| flute BELL guitar harp violin | church |
| bell GUITAR piano horn flute | plectrum |
| accordian trumpet piano DRUM horn | sticks |
| harp bell guitar accordian HORN | trumpet |
| VIOLIN bell flute guitar harp | bow |
| accordian piano TRUMPET harp flute | horn |

# APPENDIX B

## Stimuli used in Experiment 8

| *Stimuli* | | *Related probe* | |
|---|---|---|---|
| | | *Living, perceptually similar* | |
| Kangaroo | Squirrel | From Australia | Lives in trees |
| Pepper | Pumpkin | Green, red or yellow eaten in salads | Halloween |
| Pear | Aubergine | Green summer fruit | Purple vegetable |
| Banana | Pea pod | From a palm tree | You shell this |
| Ox | Camel | Works on farms pulling loads | In desert |
| Peanut | Lemon | Eat before meal with drinks | Used on pancakes |
| Potato | Orange | Used for chips | Squeeze for breakfast |
| Garlic | Apricot | Used to keep vampires away | Fruit with hairy skin |
| Goat | Deer | Used for milk | Male called a stag |
| Strawberry | Artichoke | Eat with cream | Eat its petals |
| | | *Living, perceptually dissimilar* | |
| Squirrel | Deer | Lives in trees | Male called a stag |
| Goat | Ox | Used for milk | Works on farms pulling loads |
| Kangaroo | Camel | From Australia | Found in desert |
| Orange | Banana | Squeeze for breakfast | From a palm tree |
| Potato | Pea pod | Used for chips | You shell this |
| Peanut | Garlic | Eat before meals with drinks | Used to keep vampires away |
| Lemon | Strawberry | Used on pancakes | Eat with cream |
| Apricot | Pear | Fruit with hairy skin | Green summer fruit |
| Pumpkin | Aubergine | Halloween | Purple vegetable |
| Pepper | Artichoke | Red, green, yellow eat with salad | Eat its petals |
| | | *Nonliving, perceptually similar* | |
| Spade | Screwdriver | For digging | To tighten a screw |
| Lock | Earring | Open with a key | Worn in the ear |
| Kettle | Watering can | To boil water | To water gardens |
| Rolling pin | Baseball bat | For pastry | For hitting a home run |
| Necklace | Chain | Jewellery round your neck | Used to secure an anchor |
| Comb | Fence | To tidy your hair | Goes around your garden |
| Flag | Axe | Flies from a building | Used to chop wood |
| Mirror | Paintbrush | To admire yourself | For painting |
| Frying pan | Tennis racket | For cooking bacon | To serve a ball |
| Pencil | Knife | For writing | For cutting fruit |
| | | *Nonliving, perceptually dissimilar* | |
| Baseball bat | Tennis racket | For hitting a home run | To serve a ball |
| Frying pan | Rolling pin | For cooking bacon | For pastry |
| Axe | Screwdriver | For cutting wood | To secure a screw |
| Earring | Necklace | Worn in your ear | Jewellery around your neck |
| Fence | Flag | Goes around your garden | Flies from a building |
| Comb | Mirror | To tidy your hair | To admire yourself |
| Kettle | Knife | For boiling water | For cutting fruit |
| Watering can | Spade | For watering ardens | For digging |
| Lock | Chain | Open with key | Used to secure an anchor |
| Paintbrush | Pencil | For painting | For writing |

COGNITIVE NEUROPSYCHOLOGY, 2003, 20 (3/4/5/6), 307–326

# SEMANTIC DEMENTIA WITH CATEGORY SPECIFICITY: A COMPARATIVE CASE-SERIES STUDY

Matthew A. Lambon Ralph
*University of Manchester, UK*

Karalyn Patterson
*MRC Cognition and Brain Sciences Unit, Cambridge, UK*

Peter Garrard
*Institute of Cognitive Neuroscience, London, UK*

John R. Hodges
*MRC Cognition and Brain Sciences Unit, Cambridge, UK*

Patients with semantic dementia, the temporal variant of frontotemporal dementia, are relevant to both the neuroanatomical and neuropsychological debates in the category-specific literature. These patients present with a selective and progressive semantic deficit consequent on circumscribed atrophy of the inferolateral polar temporal lobes bilaterally, including the inferotemporal gyrus. In this study, a patient KH with a significant advantage for artefacts over living things was compared to five other semantic dementia patients with commensurate levels of semantic impairment. KH demonstrated a consistent category difference in favour of artefacts across all the expressive and receptive semantic tests. This difference was reliable even when familiarity, frequency, and other potential confounding factors were controlled. While KH demonstrated an association between poor knowledge of sensory attributes and a consistently greater impairment on living things than artefacts, the other patients did not. As observed in a number of previous studies, all five of the patients, contrasted to KH, exhibited an advantage for functional/associative over sensory attributes but without demonstrating the category-specific deficit that the sensory-functional theory (and the locus of their atrophy) might predict.

The results of this and other studies are discussed in relation to four accounts of category specificity: the sensory-functional theory, domain-specific knowledge systems, intercorrelated features, and individual differences.

## INTRODUCTION

Since the publication of Warrington and Shallice's (1984) seminal paper on the topic, more than 100 patients with category-specific semantic impairment have been described in the literature, predominantly in the form of single-case studies. The term "category specificity" is actually something of a misnomer, as no patient has been reported with an entirely selective impairment for one domain of

Requests for reprints should be addressed to Prof M. A. Lambon Ralph, Department of Psychology, University of Manchester, Oxford Road, Manchester, M13 9PL, UK. (Tel: +44 (0) 161 275 2551; Fax: +44 (0) 0161 275 2588; Email: matt.lambon-ralph@man.ac.uk).

We would like to thank Jo Drake for her assistance with the significant amount of data collection required for this study. Likewise we thank the patients for their continued assistance with our research. This work was supported by grants from the Medical Research Council (UK) and the National Institute of Mental Health (USA).



http://www.tandf.co.uk/journals/pp/02643294.html
DOI:10.1080/02643290244000301

knowledge. We will, however, continue to use this term as it is so solidly established in the literature. The majority of these cases have *relatively* spared performance for nonliving or man-made objects but significantly poorer scores on the same tests when contrasted with living or animate kinds. This pattern is traditionally associated with patients who have suffered from herpes simplex virus encephalitis (HSVE: e.g., Borgo & Shallice, 2001; Gainotti & Silveri, 1996; Sartori & Job, 1988; Warrington & Shallice, 1984) although it has also been reported after head injury (e.g., Farah, Hammond, Mehta, & Ratcliff, 1989; Laiacona, Barbarotto, & Capitani, 1993), cerebrovascular accidents (CVA: e.g., Caramazza & Shelton, 1998; Forde, Francis, Riddoch, Rumiati, & Humphreys, 1997), and dementia of Alzheimer's type (DAT: e.g., Garrard, Patterson, Watson, & Hodges, 1998; Gonnerman, Andersen, Devlin, Kempler, & Seidenberg, 1997). The opposite dissociation, relatively better performance for living than nonliving kinds, has been reported in only a handful of studies, most often as a consequence of CVA (Hillis & Caramazza, 1991; Sacchett & Humphreys, 1992; Warrington & McCarthy, 1987) in addition to a single patient with progressive atrophy of the left temporal and inferior parietal lobes (Silveri, Gainotti, Perani, Capelletti, Carbone, & Fazio, 1997) and occasionally in patients with DAT (Garrard et al., 1998; Gonnerman et al., 1997). The purpose of the present study was to investigate the relationship between category-specific semantic impairments and semantic dementia. Patients with semantic dementia are relevant to two key themes in the category-specific literature: (1) the sensory-functional theory, and (2) critical neuroanatomical regions. Each of these topics is briefly reviewed below.

## The sensory-functional theory

Although the literature contains many different cognitive and neuroanatomical accounts of category-specific differences (for recent reviews of the neuropsychological and functional neuroimaging literature, see Caramazza & Shelton, 1998; Devlin et al., 2002b; Humphreys & Forde, 2001; Lambon Ralph, Howard, Nightingale, & Ellis, 1998b), the sensory-functional theory is still, perhaps, the most dominant and influential. Warrington and Shallice (1984) were the first to suggest that man-made objects are primarily differentiated by their functional properties whereas animals are distinguished on the basis of their visual appearance. As a consequence, successful differentiation of one exemplar from another for man-made items should require preserved knowledge of functional features whereas the same process for animate kinds would depend on intact perceptual information. If brain damage disrupts perceptual knowledge, then exemplars of living categories should tend to suffer more; if there is degraded functional knowledge, then the opposite dissociation should result. Warrington and Shallice suggested that a division along perceptual/functional lines was preferable to an explanation based on a genuine category basis for these phenomena, because the former account provided an explanation for the fate of concepts that tend not to follow the living/nonliving distinction. For instance, Warrington and Shallice noted that their patients with relatively poor knowledge of animals were also impaired with respect to types of cloth and precious stone (which have only one generic function and are differentiated primarily by colour or texture) but not with respect to body parts (which have very different functions).

The sensory-functional theory has been taken up by a number of other researchers. Farah and McClelland (1991) described a computational model of semantic memory in which living and nonliving items were coded across differing numbers of visual or functional units. They demonstrated that category-specific deficits emerged after selective "lesions" to either the visual or functional units, in line with Warrington and Shallice's original hypothesis. The model was able to explain why there are no truly selective category-specific deficits by suggesting that both living and nonliving concepts rely on the integrity of both perceptual and functional features, the difference being one of degree. The model also predicted and demonstrated that impoverished perceptual knowledge can be accompanied by a mild deficit for functional features: The interactive nature of the semantic system means that with sufficient damage to the visual semantic units, there is insufficient "critical mass" for the remaining functional semantic units to operate normally. Other studies have supported the sensory-functional theory with the observation that some patients impaired for living categories tend to exhibit poor knowledge about visual but not functional/associative properties of items (e.g., De Renzi & Lucchelli, 1994). In other words there is an interaction between category and attribute type resulting in relatively poor performance on tasks tapping visual knowledge about animate objects. The patient reported by Gainotti and Silveri (1996), for example, when tested on naming to definition, was significantly less likely to provide the appropriate label to a living thing than to a man-made object when the verbal definition stressed perceptual attributes. If the definitions stressed functional information, there was no significant difference between categories—the patient was equally anomic for the animate and inanimate kinds (it should, perhaps, be noted here that these results have been criticised on methodological grounds in that the living and nonliving concepts were not matched for familiarity: Caramazza & Shelton, 1998). In a thorough analysis of patient SRB, Forde et al. (1997) gathered evidence favouring the hypothesis that SRB was impaired on any task that required fine perceptual differentiation. They showed that in addition to exhibiting a category-specific deficit for living things, SRB was also impaired when required to name faces and subordinate categories such as types of car. When asked to put names to definitions containing either functional-associative or visual-perceptual information, SRB was only impaired for the latter type.

Despite these forms of support for the sensory-functional theory, at least seven recent studies have reported patients with a living things deficit without the predicted differential impairment of perceptual knowledge (Caramazza & Shelton, 1998; Funnell & De Mornay Davies, 1996; Laiacona, Barbarotto, & Capitani, 1993; Lambon Ralph et al., 1998b; Moss, Tyler, Durrant-Peatfield, & Bunn, 1998; Samson, De Wilde, & Pillon, 1998; Sheridan & Humphreys, 1993). Perhaps the most memorable of these, because of the historical irony, is a reassessment of patient JBR, originally reported by Warrington and Shallice (1984). Funnell and De Mornay Davies replicated JBR's relatively poor performance for living things even with improved balance of confounding psycholinguistic factors. They found, however, that JBR performed equally well for visual and associative knowledge on a semantic feature questionnaire.

The nature of conceptual impairment in semantic dementia is germane to any potential link between poor perceptual knowledge and category-specific deficits for living things. Patients with semantic dementia (SD) suffer from a progressive deterioration of knowledge about the meanings of words, objects, and concepts (Hodges, Patterson, Oxbury, & Funnell, 1992; Snowden, Goulding, & Neary, 1989). The semantic deficit applies to all modalities of input and output and is accompanied by a profound anomia (Bozeat, Lambon Ralph, Patterson, Garrard, & Hodges, 2000; Lambon Ralph, McClelland, Patterson, Galton, & Hodges, 2001; Snowden, Neary, & Mann, 1996b). These patients are particularly relevant to the category-specific debate because there is accumulating evidence that their semantic deficit is characterised by relatively poor knowledge of perceptual relative to functional/associative information. Patient TOB with SD (McCarthy & Warrington, 1988; Parkin, 1993), for example, produced definitions of objects that contained considerable functional content with little sensory information; and detailed analyses of word and picture definitions provided by nine other SD patients have confirmed this finding (Lambon Ralph, Graham, Patterson, & Hodges, 1999). Cardebat, Demonet, Celsis, and Puel (1996) reported that their SD patient was able to produce some semantic features regarding function but was unable to draw either animals or objects. Patient DM (Breedin, Saffran, & Coslett, 1994b; Srinivas, Breedin, Coslett, & Saffran, 1997) exhibited a relative preservation of functional over perceptual attributes and a similar dissociation has been shown for patient NV (Basso, Capitani, & Laiacona, 1988). This pattern has been demonstrated not only in verbal output tasks such as definition but also in receptive tasks such as definition-to-word matching and semantic priming (Lambon

Ralph et al., 1998b; Moss, Tyler, Hodges, & Patterson, 1995; Tyler & Moss, 1998).

The problem for the sensory-functional theory is that there is rather little evidence to suggest that this poor visual knowledge in SD leads to category-specific effects. The single-case study by Cardebat et al. (1996) did report a category effect both in naming and word-picture matching but it is unclear if the items were matched for any of the relevant cognitive and psycholinguistic variables. In a group study of nine patients, Hodges, Garrard, and Patterson (1998) obtained a significant category effect in word-to-picture matching (with items balanced for familiarity only) but not in naming. TOB (McCarthy & Warrington, 1988) was reported to have a category effect in verbal definition, and NV (Basso et al., 1988) for verbal comprehension and naming, although in both papers the items were controlled for frequency alone. TOB's naming was assessed by Parkin (1993), who found no category effect when the stimuli were controlled for frequency and familiarity. Breedin et al. (Breedin, Martin, & Saffran, 1994a; Breedin et al., 1994b) reported a significant advantage in DM's comprehension for tools over animals with items matched for frequency. A closer look at the data reveals, however, that DM was impaired on many other man-made categories (e.g., vehicles) and he only exhibited the effect in two out of the three administrations. In addition, on the visual vs. associative attribute test referred to above (which was matched for frequency and familiarity), DM showed a significant difference between attribute types but no difference between living and nonliving categories. In an analysis of the factors that predict naming accuracy in semantic dementia, Lambon Ralph, Graham, Ellis, and Hodges (1998a) found consistent effects of frequency, familiarity, and age of acquisition across the nine patients and for the group as a whole. Only one out of the nine cases, however, demonstrated a significant effect of category over and above the influence of the other variables.

The most convincing report of a category-specific deficit in a case of semantic dementia to date is patient MF studied by Barbarotto, Capitani, Spinnler, and Trivelli (1995). In word-to-picture matching, naming, and answering semantic attribute questions, MF exhibited significantly poorer performance for living categories even when other factors were accounted for, including familiarity, frequency, and item difficulty. In fact for the first two testing sessions in the longitudinal study, MF's scores for the nonliving categories remained in the normal range (i.e., there was a classical dissociation between the two sets). His drawing from memory also indicated a strong category effect. Even this dramatic effect, however, is problematic for the sensory-functional theory because, unlike most other semantic dementia patients, MF failed to show a significant difference between perceptual and associative knowledge on the semantic feature questionnaire.

## Critical neuroanatomical regions

Category-specific deficits for living things tend to be associated with temporal lesions typically involving medial and inferior temporal areas (Gainotti & Silveri, 1996; Gainotti, Silveri, Daniele, & Giustolisi, 1995; Saffran & Schwartz, 1994), although there are some notable exceptions (e.g., Caramazza & Shelton, 1998). The majority of deficits affecting man-made items in particular co-occur with lesions to frontoparietal regions (Breedin et al., 1994a; Garrard et al., 1998; Hillis, Rapp, Romani, & Caramazza, 1990; Sacchett & Humphreys, 1992; Warrington & McCarthy, 1983), although sometimes with temporal involvement as well (Silveri et al., 1997; Warrington & McCarthy, 1987, 1994) or occasionally just with temporal atrophy (Hillis & Caramazza, 1991; Tippett, Glosser, & Farah, 1996). Although it is imperative to treat extrapolations from neuroanatomical nonhuman primate data with great caution (Gloor, 1997), these neural substrates are of particular interest because they coincide with the ventral and dorsal visual pathways identified in studies of monkeys (Ungerleider & Mishkin, 1982). This opens up the intriguing possibility of linking neuroanatomy with a cognitive model in the form of the sensory-functional theory: A lesion to the inferior temporal lobe should lead to impaired high-level visual processing and, in turn, to relatively poor performance for animate kinds.

Patients with semantic dementia are also relevant to this aspect of the category-specific literature. The disorder is associated with progressive atrophy of the anterior and inferior temporal lobes bilaterally (Hodges et al., 1992; Mummery, Patterson, Price, Ashburner, Frackowiak, & Hodges, 2000). As noted above, this pattern of atrophy is associated with relatively greater degradation of sensory relative to functional-associative knowledge, but with sparse evidence that this leads, in turn, to a category-specific pattern for living things.

In addition to highlighting the potential importance of the inferior temporal structures, recent neuroanatomical reviews have noted that many of the published category-specific cases for living things have had damage to medial as well as neocortical temporal areas (Gainotti et al., 1995). Likewise a recent meta-analysis of seven PET studies of word retrieval and semantic decision tasks found evidence for activation of bilateral medial temporal poles (Devlin et al., 2002a). Two possibilities arise, therefore: (1) that it is the medial temporal region specifically that is the critical area for this category-specific pattern, or (2) that there is a critical combination of medial and inferolateral damage that leads to poor knowledge for living things. Although recent neuroanatomical investigations have in fact uncovered atrophy to the medial temporal area in patients with semantic dementia (Galton et al., 2001), the balance of atrophy is weighted towards the inferolateral regions (Hodges, 2001). Such a pattern is the reverse of that found in Alzheimer's disease, in which atrophy is most pronounced in the medial temporal lobe (Galton et al., 2001). There are some hints in the current semantic dementia literature that medial areas might be critical to deficits for living things (Garrard, Lambon Ralph, & Hodges, 2002). As noted above, patients with semantic dementia generally have more prominent lateral than medial temporal lobe damage and tend not to have a category-specific semantic impairment. The one case with a clear category effect is different (MF: Barbarotto et al., 1995). MF's temporal lobe atrophy involved medial structures including the hippocampus and parahippocampal gyrus to a much greater extent than that normally seen in semantic dementia. It is also worth noting that MF had greater atrophy in the right than the left temporal lobe. Although recent studies have highlighted bilateral involvement in all but the mildest cases (Mummery et al., 2000), the atrophy is typically asymmetrical and tends to affect the left side more often than the right. The laterality of temporal lobe atrophy and its relationship with category-specific impairments is investigated further in this study.

In this paper, we present case-series data of six patients with semantic dementia. The study was prompted by clinical neuropsychological data that had highlighted an emerging category-specific pattern in one of the cases (patient KH). Assessed three times over a period of 1 year from first presentation, KH's performance on a 64-item naming test remained relatively constant for the 32 man-made items (session 1: 91%; session 2: 91%; session 3: 81%) but dropped steadily for the 32 living items (session 1: 75%; session 2: 63%; session 3: 50%). The same pattern was found for the identical items in a word–picture matching test—man-made (session 1: 100%; session 2: 100%; session 3: 97%) vs. living (session 1: 94%; session 2: 81%; session 3: 63%). At the third testing round, KH was assessed in more detail along with five other patients with mild-to-moderate semantic impairment. This allowed for a direct neuropsychological comparison between semantically impaired patients, with the same aetiology, who varied on whether or not they demonstrated a clear category-specific deficit. Given that patients with semantic dementia are typically homogeneous with respect to both neuroanatomical and neuropsychological profiles, the within-group comparison might provide a revealing method of testing various assumptions regarding category-specific deficits.

## STUDY

### Patients

The six patients were identified through the Memory and Cognitive Disorders Clinic at Addenbrooke's Hospital, Cambridge, UK, where they were seen by a senior neurologist (JRH), a senior psychiatrist, and a clinical neuropsychologist. In addition to clinical assessment, all patients were given a number of standard psychiatric rating scales to exclude major functional disorders such as depression and schizophrenia. They all underwent MRI scanning together with the usual battery of screening blood tests to exclude treatable causes of dementia.

All six patients fulfilled previously proposed neuropsychological and neuroanatomical criteria for semantic dementia (Hodges, 2001; Hodges et al., 1992; Snowden, Griffiths, & Neary, 1996a): progressive loss of vocabulary affecting expressive and receptive language plus impairments on nonverbal tests of semantic knowledge in the context of relative preservation of phonology, syntax, visuospatial skills, and day-to-day memory. As noted above, longitudinal neuropsychological assessment had revealed an emerging category-specific difference in KH's performance on word–picture matching and picture naming. The five other patients with semantic dementia were selected using both neuropsychological and neuroanatomical criteria; their mild-to-moderate levels of semantic impairment and anomia were roughly commensurate with those for KH. It was important to exclude very severely anomic cases because a number of the planned assessments relevant to the category-specific theories require verbal responses (e.g., picture naming and the production of definitions). In terms of neuroanatomical factors, KH presented with bilateral atrophy with greater damage in the right than the left temporal lobe. This right-sided distribution tends to be less common clinically, but we were able to include one other patient with right-sided atrophy (patient CS). The remaining four cases either had atrophy largely limited to the left temporal lobe (patient AN) or bilateral involvement with a left-sided distribution (patients MA, AT, and SL).

### Background neuropsychology

Background neuropsychological results are shown in Table 1. This and all subsequent tables order the patients in the following way. For ease of comparison, KH is always placed last and the remaining five patients are ordered left to right in terms of the severity of their semantic impairment (as measured by their naming and word–picture matching scores—see Table 2). At this time, patient AN was at the very early stages of semantic dementia, such that his mild semantic impairment did not lead to an impairment on all of the semantic assessments included here. His results are included in this study in order to span a range of semantic severity. On the Mini-Mental State Examination (MMSE: Folstein, Folstein, & McHugh, 1975) two patients achieved excellent scores (AN and MA) while the rest fell below normal control performance. Typically patients with semantic dementia pass the orientation questions but fail at those requiring expressive and receptive language skills. Like other SD patients reported in the literature, the four cases who were tested on the Raven's Coloured Progressive Matrices—a test of nonverbal problem solving (Raven, 1962)—performed very well. With the exception of CS, the remaining five patients achieved normal scores on digit span (on both forward and backward subtests from the Weschler Memory Scale-Revised: Wechsler, 1987). On other measures of recall and recognition memory (the Rey-Osterrieth figure delayed copy: Osterrieth, 1944; the Recognition Memory Test: Warrington, 1984), CS again performed poorly. AN, MA, and SL produced scores within the normal range. KH's and AT's recognition scores were relatively weak. CS's immediate copy of the Rey figure was also impaired. On the perceptual and spatial subtests (VOSP: Warrington & James, 1991), all patients demonstrated the typical pattern of good scores with the exception of silhouette identification, which requires access to semantic memory.

Table 1. *Background neuropsychology*

| | | | Patient | | | | | | |
|---|---|---|---|---|---|---|---|---|---|
| *Test* | *Subtest* | *Max* | *AN*[a] *63 yrs* | *CS*[b] *64 yrs* | *MA*[a] *63 yrs* | *AT*[a] *65 yrs* | *SL*[a] *52 yrs* | *KH*[b] *59 yrs* | *Controls*[c] |
| MMSE | | 30 | 30 | 15 | 29 | 25 | 24 | 22 | 28.8 (0.5) |
| RCPM | | %tiles | 36 | NT | 75th | 90–95th | 90–95th | 95th | |
| Digit span | Forward | | 7 | 4 | 6 | 8 | 5 | 6 | 6.8 (0.9) |
| | Backward | | 7 | 2 | 3 | 5 | 4 | 5 | 4.7 (1.2) |
| RMT | Word | %tiles | 50–75 | <5 | 50 | 25 | <25 | <5 | |
| | Faces | %tiles | 75–95 | <5 | 25 | <5 | 50–75 | <5 | |
| Rey Figure | Immediate | 36 | 36 | 21 | 36 | 36 | 30 | 29.5 | 34.0 (2.9) |
| | Delayed | 36 | 27 | 0 | 6.5 | 24 | 14 | 12.5 | 15.2 (7.4) |
| VOSP | Letters | 20 | 19 | 18 | 19 | 20 | 20 | 19 | 16–20 |
| | Silhouettes | 30 | 17 | 9 | 7 | 7 | NT | NT | 15–30 |
| | Object decision | 20 | 20 | 15 | 16 | 19 | 13 | 18 | 14–20 |
| | Dot count | 10 | 10 | 10 | 10 | 10 | 9 | 10 | 8–10 |
| | Position discrimination | 20 | 20 | 19 | 20 | 20 | NT | NT | 18-20 |
| | Number location | 10 | 9 | 9 | 10 | 9 | NT | NT | 7–10 |
| | Cube analysis | 10 | 10 | 8 | 10 | 10 | 10 | 9 | 6–10 |

MMSE: Mini-Mental State Examination. RCPM: Raven's Coloured Progressive Matrices. RMT: Recognition Memory Test. VOSP: Visual Object and Space Perception Battery. NT: Not tested.
[a]Left greater than right temporal lobe atrophy.
[b]Right greater than left temporal lobe damage.
[c]Given as Mean (*SD*) or range.

## Assessments of semantic memory

The performance of the patients on a set of semantic and name production tasks is shown in Table 2. On the Pyramids and Palm Trees test of associative semantics (Howard & Patterson, 1992), all patients' scores fell below the control range [pictures: mean = 51.1, *SD* = 1.1; words: mean = 51.2, *SD* = 1.4]. Their pronounced anomia gave rise to poor letter and category fluency scores [data of 38 age- and education-matched controls: letter fluency: mean = 44.2, *SD* = 11.2; category fluency for four animal categories: mean = 60.3, *SD* = 12.6; for four man-made categories: mean = 54.8, *SD* = 10.3]. As a group, the patients showed no significant difference in the number of exemplars produced for the living and manmade domains. In the 64-item naming and word–picture matching tests, both CS and KH exhibited a statistically reliable difference between living and man-made items. As a group the patients tended to perform slightly better on the man-made items, although the small differences only reached borderline significance in word–picture matching (this replicates the pattern found previously by Hodges et al., 1998).

The 64-item semantic battery was designed to form part of a general neuropsychological assessment for all patients presenting to the Memory and Cognitive Disorders clinic. By using this same battery on all patients, both cross-sectionally and longitudinally, clinical and theoretical insights about the status and nature of conceptual knowledge have been gleaned (e.g., Bozeat et al., 2000; Garrard, Lambon Ralph, Watson, Powis, Patterson, & Hodges, 2001b; Hodges & Patterson, 1995). Indeed, it was the use of this battery that highlighted KH's emerging category-specific deficit. One drawback, however, is that the full subsets of 32 living and 32 man-made items are not matched for concept familiarity. Many previous studies have demonstrated that the accuracy of patients with semantic dementia is influenced by familiarity (e.g., Bozeat et al., 2000; Lambon Ralph et al., 1998a), and this variable is known to vary

**Table 2.** *Background semantic and naming assessments*

| | | | *Patient* | | | | | | |
|---|---|---|---|---|---|---|---|---|---|
| *Test* | *Subtest* | *Max* | *AN* | *CS* | *MA* | *AT* | *SL* | *KH* | *Mean* |
| PPT | Pictures | 52 | NT | 41 | 41 | 47 | 44 | 42 | – |
| | Words | 52 | NT | 39 | 42 | 45 | 38 | 40 | – |
| Fluency | Letters (FAS) | N/A | 40 | 14 | 9 | 20 | 30 | 13 | – |
| | Man-made[a] | N/A | 34 | 25 | 8 | 18 | 7 | 14 | 17.7 |
| | Living[a] | N/A | 47 | 13 | 7 | 14 | 12 | 8 | 16.8 |
| | | | | | | | | | $t$ = 0.23 |
| | | | | | | | | | $p$ = .83 |
| 64 naming | Man-made | 32 | 32 | 28 | 5 | 12 | 7 | 26 | 18.3 |
| | Living | 32 | 32 | 19 | 8 | 5 | 11 | 16 | 15.2 |
| | $\chi^2$ | | – | 5.13 | 0.39 | 2.88 | 0.70 | 5.61 | $t$ = 1.24 |
| | $p$ | | – | *.02* | .53 | .09 | .40 | *.02* | $p$ = .27 |
| 64 word-picture matching | Man-made | 32 | 32 | 29 | 30 | 30 | 24 | 31 | 29.3 |
| | Living | 32 | 32 | 22 | 27 | 27 | 24 | 20 | 25.3 |
| | $\chi^2$ | | – | 3.48 | 0.64 | 0.64 | 0 | 9.65 | $t$ = 2.28 |
| | $p$ | | – | .06 | .42 | .42 | 1 | *.002* | $p$ = .07 |
| Controlled set naming | Man-made | 30 | 28 | 15 | 7 | 11 | 10 | 24 | 15.8 |
| | Living | 30 | 30 | 14 | 17 | 6 | 13 | 17 | 16.2 |
| | $\chi^2$ | | 0.52 | 0.07 | 6.94 | 2.05 | 0.64 | 3.77 | $t$ = 0.13 |
| | $p$ | | n.s. | n.s. | *.008* | .15 | n.s. | *.05* | n.s. |

[a]4 categories.

across living and nonliving domains (on average animals are less familiar than artefacts: Funnell & Sheridan, 1992). We administered, therefore, three additional assessments designed to test for category differences over and above the influence of familiarity and other potential confounding factors. The first contrasts 30 animal–man-made pairs that are closely matched on a variety of psycholinguistic factors including familiarity, frequency, length, and imageability (taken from Lambon Ralph et al., 1998b). On this naming test (shown in the bottom row of Table 2), CS's previous category difference disappeared while KH's better naming for man-made things remained and was statistically reliable. The other patients continued to show no difference between the two domains except for patient MA, who was significantly more accurate for the living things. Overall the patients' performance for this test was very similar for living and nonliving domains.

In addition to the controlled naming test, we also administered naming and word–picture matching tests based on the full Snodgrass and Vanderwart picture set (1980). For picture naming, the patients were simply asked to provide the name of each item. In the word–picture matching test, the name of each picture was spoken by the experimenter and the patient was required to point to the correct item from a choice of four within-category exemplars. Given the large number of pictures, it is possible to test for an effect of domain whilst controlling for a series of other possible confounding factors (logistic regression for individual data and multiple regression for overall, by-item data). Values for rated familiarity, objective age-of-acquisition (AoA), rated imageability, name agreement, phoneme length, rated visual complexity, and Celex frequency are available for 221 of the 260 pictures (taken from Morrison, Chappell, & Ellis, 1997). The patients' raw scores on the two tests for this subset of items and the results of the regression analyses are shown in Tables 3a and 3b.

Table 3a shows the results from the word–picture matching test. In terms of raw scores, three patients were significantly less accurate for living than nonliving items. CS and MA exhibited a 10% difference between the two domains while a greater differential was observed in KH (18%). A by-subjects *t*-test with KH included reached borderline significance, with better performance overall for the man-made domain. With KH excluded, the reduced domain difference failed to reach any level of statistical significance. The lower half of Table 3a lists the *p* values obtained for each patient's logistic regression analysis plus two multiple regressions based on the by-items data. The multiple regression was repeated with KH included and excluded to test whether the overall result was changed by his

**Table 3a.** *Analysis of factors affecting word-to-picture matching*

| | | *Patient* | | | | | | *Average with KH* | *Average without KH* |
|---|---|---|---|---|---|---|---|---|---|
| | *N* | *AN* | *CS* | *MA* | *AT* | *SL* | *KH* | | |
| Domain | | | | | | | | | |
| Man-made | 138 | 136 (99%) | 135 (98%) | 127 (92%) | 134 (97%) | 121 (88%) | 131 (95%) | 94.8% | 94.8% |
| Living | 83 | 82 (99%) | 74 (89%) | 67 (81%) | 78 (94%) | 75 (90%) | 64 (77%) | 88.3% | 90.6% |
| $\chi^2$ | | 0 | 5.99 | 6.18 | 0.62 | 0.37 | 15.9 | $t = 2.11$ | $t = 1.67$ |
| *p* | | n.s. | .01 | .01 | n.s. | n.s. | <.001 | $p = .09$ | n.s. |
| Regression factor | | | | | | | | | |
| Domain | | n.s. | n.s. | n.s. | n.s. | n.s. | .001 | .007 | n.s. |
| Familiarity | | n.s. | n.s. | n.s. | n.s. | n.s. | n.s. | n.s. | n.s. |
| Objective AoA | | n.s. | n.s. | .05 | n.s. | n.s. | n.s. | <.001 | <.001 |
| Imageability | | n.s. | n.s. | n.s. | n.s. | n.s. | n.s. | n.s. | n.s. |
| Name agreement | | n.s. | n.s. | n.s. | n.s. | n.s. | n.s. | n.s. | n.s. |
| Phoneme length | | n.s. | n.s. | n.s. | n.s. | n.s. | n.s. | n.s. | n.s. |
| Visual complexity | | n.s. | n.s. | n.s. | n.s. | n.s. | n.s. | n.s. | n.s. |
| Celex frequency | | n.s. | n.s. | n.s. | n.s. | n.s. | n.s. | n.s. | n.s. |

**Table 3b.** *Analysis of factors affecting naming*

| | | *Patient* | | | | | | *Average with KH* | *Average without KH* |
|---|---|---|---|---|---|---|---|---|---|
| | *N* | *AN* | *CS* | *MA* | *AT* | *SL* | *KH* | | |
| Domain | | | | | | | | | |
| Man-made | 138 | 127 (94%) | 93 (67%) | 66 (48%) | 69 (50%) | 52 (38%) | 102 (74%) | 61.8% | 59.4% |
| Living | 83 | 77 (93%) | 47 (57%) | 40 (48%) | 22 (27%) | 31 (37%) | 39 (47%) | 51.5% | 52.4% |
| $\chi^2$ | | 0.15 | 2.59 | 0 | 11.8 | 0 | 16.3 | $t = 2.11$ | $t = 1.60$ |
| *p* | | n.s. | n.s. | n.s. | .001 | n.s. | <.001 | $p = .09$ | n.s. |
| Regression factor | | | | | | | | | |
| Domain | | n.s. | n.s. | n.s. | .03 | n.s. | <.001 | n.s. | n.s. |
| Familiarity | | n.s. | .008 | .001 | <.001 | <.001 | <.001 | <.001 | <.001 |
| Objective AoA | | .002 | .001 | .001 | n.s. | .001 | .003 | <.001 | <.001 |
| Imageability | | n.s. | n.s. | n.s. | n.s. | n.s. | n.s. | .009 | .02 |
| Name agreement | | n.s. | n.s. | n.s. | n.s. | .01 | n.s. | n.s. | n.s. |
| Phoneme length | | n.s. | n.s. | n.s. | n.s. | n.s. | n.s. | n.s. | .05[a] |
| Visual complexity | | n.s. | .02 | n.s. | n.s. | n.s. | n.s. | n.s. | n.s. |
| Celex frequency | | n.s. | n.s. | n.s. | .001 | n.s. | n.s. | n.s. | n.s. |

[a]Better performance for longer than for shorter words.

data specifically. Once other confounding variables were controlled in this way, neither CS nor MA exhibited a significant independent effect of domain. Likewise, no domain effect emerged for any of the cases who had failed to show a domain effect in their raw data (AN, AT, and SL). In contrast, even with these other factors controlled, the effect of domain remained significant for KH, with no other variables reaching significance. In the overall by-items regression analysis with KH included, both domain and age-of-acquisition were significant. While the effect of AoA remained even if KH was excluded, domain became nonsignificant. This suggests that it was KH's data, specifically, which gave rise to the domain effect in the overall data.

The analyses of the naming data are summarised in Table 3b. In terms of raw scores only AT (who had not shown a domain effect in word–picture matching) and KH demonstrated a significant domain difference. Again the overall by-subjects *t*-test only reached borderline significance if KH's data were included. In the regression analyses most of the patients were affected by familiarity and object AoA (replicating the results found previously for a different group of semantic dementia patients: Lambon Ralph et al., 1998a). In addition, the domain effect remained significant for AT and KH individually, though in the overall by-items regression, only effects of familiarity, AoA, and imageability were found.

## Assessment of attribute knowledge

The patients' knowledge of specific types of semantic attribute was assessed using three tasks. The first two were naming to description and description-to-picture matching. In both tests, patients were presented with a definition for each of the 64 items used in the basic naming and word–picture matching tasks described above. For each item two definitions were prepared, one that emphasised sensory information and another that utilised functional-associative attributes. In naming to description, the definition was simply read by the experimenter and the patient was required to give the name of the concept described. The matching version of this task was prepared in an attempt to circumvent any floor effects that might have arisen due to the pronounced anomia of patients with semantic dementia. In this task, after listening to the description, instead of attempting to name it, the patient was asked to pick the correct picture from an array of within-category exemplars (the same arrays as those used in the 64 word–picture matching test).

The results for naming to description and description-to-picture matching are shown in Tables 4a and 4b. In each table, the upper half shows the patients' accuracy split by attribute type while the lower half divides their data by domain. When split by attribute type a clear pattern emerged for the patients—all were numerically better when presented with associative-functional rather than sensory definitions. For the naming task, this difference was statistically significant for four of the six cases (MA, AT, SL, and KH) and was reliable overall in the by-subjects analysis. Despite their relatively poor ability to name in response to the sensory definitions, it was only KH who demonstrated a clear and significant domain difference. The overall by-subject analysis was also nonsignificant. Although the patients were substantially more accurate with the matching version of this task, the same basic pattern emerged. Despite being presented with pictures of the target item, all patients were numerically worse at the sensory definitions. Though the differences were small, the effect was reliable for SL individually, and in the overall by-subjects analysis. Again there was no clear pattern when the data were split by domain. Only KH exhibited a clear domain difference and the overall by-subjects analysis was nonsignificant.

The third assessment elicited verbal definitions to test the patients' attribute knowledge. The 6 patients were compared with 10 age-matched controls. The subjects were asked to give definitions for each of the 64 concepts included in the various semantic assessments described above. Specifically, the participants were given the spoken name of a concept and were asked to provide as much information as they could about that item. General prompts (e.g., "What does it look like?", "What does it do?", "Where would you find it?", "What

Table 4a. *Naming to description*

| | | *Patient* | | | | | | |
|---|---|---|---|---|---|---|---|---|
| | | *AN* | *CS* | *MA* | *AT* | *SL* | *KH* | *Mean* |
| Definition type | | | | | | | | |
| Functional | /64 | 48 | 21 | 37 | 18 | 24 | 37 | 30.8 |
| Sensory | /64 | 42 | 15 | 27 | 8 | 13 | 16 | 20.2 |
| $\chi^2$ | | 1.35 | 1.39 | 3.13 | 4.83 | 3.87 | 14.2 | $t$ = 4.75 |
| $p$ | | n.s. | n.s. | .08 | .03 | .05 | <.001 | .005 |
| Domain | | | | | | | | |
| Nonliving | /64 | 41 | 21 | 35 | 12 | 16 | 33 | 26.3 |
| Living | /64 | 49 | 15 | 29 | 14 | 21 | 20 | 24.6 |
| $\chi^2$ | | 2.4 | 1.4 | 1.13 | 0.19 | 0.95 | 5.4 | $t$ = 0.5 |
| $p$ | | n.s. | n.s. | n.s. | n.s. | n.s. | .02 | n.s. |

Table 4b. *Description-to-picture matching*

| | | *Patient* | | | | | | |
|---|---|---|---|---|---|---|---|---|
| | | *AN* | *CS* | *MA* | *AT* | *SL* | *KH* | *Mean* |
| Definition type | | | | | | | | |
| Functional | /64 | 62 | 48 | 47 | 55 | 24 | 49 | 47.5 |
| Sensory | /64 | 61 | 41 | 38 | 53 | 13 | 43 | 41.5 |
| $\chi^2$ | | 0 | 1.81 | 2.84 | 0.24 | 4.6 | 1.39 | $t$ = 3.77 |
| $p$ | | n.s. | n.s. | n.s. | n.s. | .03 | n.s. | .01 |
| Domain | | | | | | | | |
| Nonliving | /64 | 63 | 46 | 42 | 56 | 16 | 53 | 46 |
| Living | /64 | 60 | 43 | 43 | 52 | 21 | 39 | 43 |
| $\chi^2$ | | 0.83 | 0.33 | 0.04 | 0.95 | 0.95 | 7.58 | $t$ = 1.16 |
| $p$ | | n.s. | n.s. | n.s. | n.s. | n.s. | .006 | n.s. |

else do you know about it?") were used repeatedly with patients and controls to encourage information regarding each object's perceptual features, function, and other encyclopaedic-associative facts. Definitions were collected over two or three sessions for the patients because the process was very time-consuming and arduous for them. The definition naming and matching tests, reported above, were administered during other testing sessions to minimise any likelihood of priming or cueing effects. The elicited definitions were broken down into individual features and each was classified into five main types: sensory, functional, encyclopaedic, superordinate, and errors (using the same criteria as Garrard, Lambon Ralph, Hodges, & Patterson, 2001a). Classifications were made by one scorer (JD) and then double-checked (by MALR). The upper half of Table 5 shows the number of each type of feature produced by each patient individually, the patient and control means plus the performance of the worst control (i.e., the least information produced by a control for that feature type). The results for the patients were consistent across individuals and replicated the pattern found in the naming to description task—the patients' definitions were generally impoverished in comparison to the controls' and were dominated by functional and encyclopaedic attributes. Like the controls, the patients produced a relatively low rate of superordinate classifications and incorrect features. As in previous analyses of definitions produced by patients with semantic dementia, there is a striking contrast between the proportions of sensory and functional information given. In this study the ratio of sensory to functional attributes in the patients' definitions (35%: 41%) was the reverse of that

**Table 5.** *Analysis of the rate and type of attributes produced in verbal definition*

| *Attribute type* | *AN* | *CS* | *MA* | *AT* | *SL* | *KH* | *Patient mean* | *Control mean* | *Worst control* |
|---|---|---|---|---|---|---|---|---|---|
| | | | | *Number of attributes given (Percentage of own total production)* | | | | | |
| Sensory | 158 (40%) | 39 (21%) | 53 (37%) | 91 (35%) | 59 (34%) | 103 (38%) | **83.8 (35%)** | **512.5 (57%)** | 351 (55%) |
| Functional | 154 (39%) | 81 (45%) | 62 (44%) | 113 (43%) | 75 (43%) | 106 (39%) | **98.5 (41%)** | **196.8 (22%)** | 152 (24%) |
| Encyclopaedic | 68 (17%) | 39 (21%) | 26 (18%) | 35 (13%) | 20 (12%) | 36 (13%) | **37.3 (15%)** | **125 (14%)** | 91 (14%) |
| Superordinate | 44 (11%) | 23 (13%) | 1 (1%) | 18 (7%) | 19 (11%) | 13 (5%) | **19.7 (8%)** | **62.7 (7%)** | 44 (7%) |
| Errors | 0 (0%) | 0 (0%) | 0 (0%) | 5 (2%) | 0 (0%) | 11 (4%) | **2.7 (1%)** | **0 (0%)** | 0 (0%) |
| Total | 424 | 182 | 142 | 262 | 173 | 269 | **242** | **897** | 638 |
| | | | | *Percentage of control mean performance* | | | | | |
| Sensory | 31% | 8% | 10% | 18% | 12% | 20% | 16% | | |
| Functional | 78% | 41% | 32% | 57% | 38% | 54% | 50% | | |
| Encyclopaedic | 54% | 31% | 21% | 28% | 16% | 29% | 30% | | |
| Superordinate | 70% | 38% | 20% | 29% | 30% | 21% | 20% | | |
| Total | 47% | 20% | 16% | 29% | 19% | 30% | 27% | | |

found for the control subjects (57%: 22%). A 2 (subject group) × 2 (feature type: sensory vs. functional) ANOVA confirmed that this crossover interaction was significant, $F(1, 14) = 90.8, p < .001$. Post-hoc *t*-tests revealed that the feature type difference for controls was significant and for patients it approached significant albeit in the opposite direction [semantic dementia: $t_{(5)} = 2.2$, $p = .08$; controls: $t(9) = -12.1, p < .001$].

The lower half of Table 5 summarises the patients' definitions in a different way. The number of attributes of each type is expressed as a proportion of the mean control performance. This confirms two key aspects of the patients' definitions. First, the patients produced a much smaller number of features than the control subjects. Overall, the patients gave only 27% of the number of features that control subjects did. The rate was low even for the mildest SD patient (AN: 47%). The average rate of sensory features was lowest (16%). The rate of encyclopaedic and superordinate attributes dropped moderately (encyclopaedic: 30%; superordinate: 31%). In contrast, although the rate of functional features reduced considerably, the proportion (50%) was twice that of the other attribute types.

To finish this section, we will consider another control dataset against which the patients' performance can be compared. A growing number of studies, using a variety of verbal and nonverbal tasks, have found that semantic dementia patients are relatively more likely to produce attributes shared by many concepts (e.g., has legs, moves, is found in the UK) than features specific to a few (e.g., has long ears, burrows, was introduced into the UK by the Romans: Hodges, Graham, & Patterson, 1995). This pattern is true of the definitions collected for these and other patients with semantic dementia. It is important, therefore, to rule out the possibility that the change in the sensory:functional ratio is not merely an artefact of the patients' definitions becoming increasingly dominated by shared attributes. We can do this by comparing the present data against the detailed analyses of normal feature-listing performance provided by Garrard and colleagues (2001a). In that study, Garrard et al. split the attributes both by type and by their relative distinctiveness: i.e., into those that were shared by at least half of the concepts within a category versus those that were true for only a small number of exemplars (less than half the concepts in a category). One possible analysis of the semantic dementia data is, therefore, to compare the patients' rate of production not against the total number of features produced by control subjects but instead against the rate of relatively shared features. If the patients' poor knowledge of sensory features is simply an artefact of their definitions becoming increasingly dominated by the shared features, then the shared attributes produced by control subjects should mimic the patient's results. Even for these features, however, Garrard et al.'s normative data show that the rate of shared sensory features for the 64 concepts was twice that found for shared functional and encyclopaedic facts (see Figure 6 in Garrard et al., 2001a). It seems, therefore, that in addition to the general finding that distinctive features are particularly vulnerable in this form of semantic impairment, the loss of conceptual knowledge in patients with semantic dementia is characterised by a relative preservation of functional information.

## DISCUSSION

This study investigated the issue of category-specific semantic differences with reference to neuropsychological data of patients with semantic dementia. Six patients with mild to moderate semantic impairment were studied. One of the six (patient KH) had presented an emerging category-specific advantage for man-made over living concepts. A battery of neuropsychological tasks was used to compare KH directly with the other semantic dementia patients and to test various accounts of category-specificity. KH demonstrated a consistent domain difference across all semantic tests both for receptive tasks (word–picture matching and definition-to-picture matching) and expressive tasks (various picture naming tests, and naming to definition). The difference between living and nonliving concepts remained even when other possible confounding factors such as familiarity and frequency were controlled. In contrast, none of the remaining patients exhibited a *consistent* category-specific difference. A patient would occasionally demonstrate a difference on one test that either was removed when confounding variables were controlled or failed to be replicated with another test even of the same type—e.g., on two picture naming tasks. In other aspects, all six patients, including KH, produced homogeneous results. As in previous investigations of factors that affect semantic performance (Bozeat et al., 2000; Funnell, 1995; Lambon Ralph et al., 1998a), each individual and the group as a whole were affected by concept familiarity. In addition, all patients exhibited a relative preservation of functional over sensory features when asked to provide verbal definitions, name to definition, and match definitions to pictures.

Along with one other patient in the literature (patient MF: Barbarotto et al., 1995), KH represents one of the clearest cases of category-specificity in semantic dementia. As we will discuss further below, the combination of semantic dementia and category specificity is something of a rarity. This study aimed to compare KH with a series of other semantic dementia patients and, with this potentially powerful case-series design, to reveal any underlying neuropsychological or neuroanatomical factors that might underpin the category-specific difference. Four factors can be considered. First KH, like MF (Barbarotto et al., 1995), presented with bilateral temporal lobe atrophy with an asymmetric distribution weighted towards greater atrophy of the right temporal lobe. Unlike patient MF, KH had the usual SD pattern of greater atrophy of the inferopolar regions than of the medial temporal lobe. Although the opposite, left-distributed pattern of atrophy tends to be the most common in the clinic (Hodges, 2001; Mummery et al., 2000), the case-series studied here included one other patient with greater right than left temporal lobe damage (CS). There was little evidence for a category effect in CS and thus it seems unlikely that the left–right distribution of temporal lobe atrophy is the critical factor.

A second possibility relates to the severity of the semantic impairment. It is possible that category differences might only arise in patients with a certain degree of semantic impairment (indeed, this is a prediction of those theories that explain category specificity in terms of intercorrelated features, see below). The case-series was selected, however, with the criterion that the patients should be roughly commensurate with KH in terms of semantic severity. Although patient AN was milder than KH, the other four cases produced very similar scores across the range of semantic assessments (see Table 2). It would seem, therefore, that the severity of semantic impairment is not a critical factor in KH's category-specific pattern.

The third factor relates to the possibility that category-specific impairments arise when a semantic impairment combines with some other cognitive deficit. For example, reviews of the category-specific literature have noted that patients often have the combination of semantic impairment and a dense amnesia (e.g., those patients with category-specific deficits in the context of the medial and inferolateral temporal damage observed in HSVE: Gainotti et al., 1995). There is existing evidence that this combination is not critical: Patients with Alzheimer's disease normally have amnesia combined with semantic impairment without a category-specific pattern (also in the context of medial and inferolateral temporal damage: Garrard et al., 1998, 2001b) and patients with category-specific impairments for living things following middle-cerebral artery stroke do not have dense amnesia (e.g., Caramazza & Shelton, 1998; Hillis & Caramazza, 1991). In addition, there is no evidence that KH's semantic impairment was accompanied by any additional neuropsychological impairment that the other SD cases did not also have. For example, although KH's scores on the recognition memory tests were relatively weak (see Table 1), patient CS, unusually for patients with mild SD, had a much more pronounced amnesia than KH but without the category-specific pattern. The other background neuropsychological assessments also failed to highlight any other critical impairment.

The final possibility relates to the pattern of semantic breakdown itself. For example, KH's category-specific impairment might have occurred in the context of a pattern with other unusual semantic characteristics. Our fairly extensive semantic assessment, which included relatively rich sources of data such as verbal definitions, failed to highlight any obvious differences. Just like the other five patients, KH's semantic degradation was characterised by relatively impoverished concepts in which distinctive properties are the most vulnerable and, although significantly reduced too, functional features are less affected than sensory attributes. In summary, KH's neuroanatomical and neuropsychological profile matched the other five semantic dementia patients included in this case-series in all respects save for the fact that, over and above this typical SD profile, KH had some unspecified additional impairment which produced relatively poor performance for living things.

The basis of the sensory-functional theory is that concepts in the living domain are more reliant on sensory features while man-made items are strongly represented in terms of functional attributes. The performance of the patients described here replicates that reported before (Lambon Ralph et al., 1998b, 1999): When SD patients define object concepts, they provide significantly fewer sensory attributes than for functional features. With the exception of patient KH, the remaining five SD patients plus the others reported previously failed to show the predicted disadvantage for living things. The combination of relatively poor sensory knowledge without an emergent category-specific pattern would appear problematic for the sensory-functional theory. There are, however, at least two possible counterarguments that can be considered in the light of the comparative data provided by KH. First, these patients do not have a classical dissociation for functional over sensory attributes—their overall feature knowledge is greatly impoverished relative to normal controls for *all* types of feature. The possibility arises, therefore, that the difference between functional and sensory information is insufficiently large to produce a category difference (Lambon Ralph et al., 1998b, 1999). KH's comparative data would seem to make this counterargument less likely: his performance on the feature-based tasks (naming to definition, definition matching, and verbal definitions) was indistinguishable from the other five patients. If the difference between sensory and functional knowledge was sufficient to produce a category effect in KH, it should have also done so with the other five cases.

The second, related counterargument relates to the strong familiarity-frequency effects observed for comprehension and production in semantic dementia (Funnell, 1995; Lambon Ralph et al., 1998a). Borgo and Shallice (2001) have argued that a previously described patient's poor sensory knowledge in receptive and expressive tasks (patient IW: Lambon Ralph et al., 1998b) might have been due to a potential confound with frequency—if the perceptual terms were relatively low-frequency words. Again KH's comparative data are illuminating here. KH's pattern is compatible with the sensory-functional theory: Poor sensory knowledge is paired with a category-specific deficit for living things. The remaining patients' data could be explained using the Borgo and Shallice hypothesis if psycholinguistic factors such as word frequency artificially suppressed the patients' performance for sensory attributes when, in fact, there was parity between sensory and functional knowledge and thus there should have been no category effect. The two arguments are *not* mutually compatible, however, because the same materials were used for all six patients. This means either that poor sensory knowledge resulted in no emergent category effect in the majority of cases, or else that KH's category effect was not meaningfully related to his relatively poor sensory knowledge. Both results are incongruent with the sensory-functional hypothesis.

The category-specific literature contains a relatively large number of explanations of which the sensory-functional theory is only one. We will conclude this paper by considering three other proposals: domain-specific knowledge systems, intercorrelated features, and individual differences.

Domain-specific knowledge systems are based on the idea that semantic memory is divided into subsystems for each broad domain (animals, vegetation, and artefacts) either through evolutionary pressures (Caramazza & Shelton, 1998) or by the learning process itself (Ritter & Kohonen, 1989). Under these proposals, category-specific deficits really do reflect dissociations between separable, domain-specific neural systems or processes. Under this hypothesis, for the majority of semantic dementia patients, all domains/semantic subsystems are affected equally by the progressive disease. KH, on the other hand, had an uneven distribution of damage to the three domains such that the artefact domain was relatively preserved. The major problem with this approach is that it is little more than a redescription of the data and lacks any form of neuroanatomical or neuropsychological explanatory power (although it does predict that there is no causal relationship between feature type and category knowledge, which is supported by the semantic dementia data). Although Caramazza and Shelton (1998) do not link any of the domain-specific knowledge systems to any particular neural regions, it is implicit in the theory that each domain must be neurally separable from each other in order to produce neuropsychological double dissociations. There is no evidence, however, that KH's temporal lobe atrophy was any different to the other cases included in this series or reported elsewhere. In general, the lack of independent, a priori, neuroanatomical or neuropsychological predictors of which domain should become impaired significantly limits the appeal of domain-specific proposals (more detailed critiques of these theories can be found elsewhere: Borgo & Shallice, 2001; Lambon Ralph et al., 1998b).

Recent studies have tried to explain category specificity in terms of the distribution and effect of intercorrelation between constituent semantic features (Devlin, Gonnerman, Anderson, & Seidenberg, 1998; Gonnerman et al., 1997; McRae & Cree, 2002; Tyler, Moss, Durrant-Peatfield, & Levy, 2000). There are two separate theories based on intercorrelated features, which produce opposite predictions regarding the impact of disease severity. The first theory (Devlin et al., 1998; Gonnerman et al., 1997) notes that the constituent features of living concepts are significantly more intercorrelated than the features for nonliving items (McRae, De Sa, & Seidenberg, 1997). When this pattern is coded within a computational model of semantic memory, a double dissociation can be produced without selective lesioning of one type of attribute over another (which was the basis of Farah and McClelland's model, 1991). Intercorrelated features are relatively robust to mild levels of semantic impairment and, therefore, at this level of damage concepts for living things are better preserved than for nonliving things. At greater degrees of semantic impairment the intercorrelation leads to a catastrophic loss of information underpinning living concepts and in these circumstances the category-specific pattern is reversed (nonliving > living). The second form of these theories highlights a different pattern of intercorrelated features. Moss et al. (1998) and Tyler et al. (2000) argue that for living things the intercorrelated features are also those shared across exemplars within a category (e.g., eyes, ears, sees, hears), whereas for nonliving things there is a subset of form–function intercorrelations that are relatively specific to each exemplar (e.g., saw blade and cutting). The direction of category difference with respect to the severity of the semantic impairment is reversed in this theory: Living concepts suffer initially from not having highly intercorrelated distinctive features but they become relatively preserved at more extreme levels of semantic impairment because they are somewhat protected by their intercorrelated shared features. Although the basis of both theories has been questioned on various grounds including feature norms (Garrard et al., 2001a), computational modelling (Perry, 1999), and neuropsychological data (Garrard et al., 1998, 2001b; Hillis & Caramazza, 1991), the critical prediction for the semantic dementia data presented here is that the direction of the category difference should depend on the degree of the semantic impairment. The patients selected for this study were in the mild–moderate range of semantic impairments. KH, the patient with relatively poor performance for living things, fell into the middle of this group. Neither the milder (e.g., patient AN) nor more severely impaired patients (e.g., patient SL) demonstrated the same pattern as KH. Likewise a previous investigation of factors affecting naming in patients with semantic dementia failed to find category-specific differences in much more severely impaired cases (whilst also controlled for confounding psycholinguistic factors: Lambon Ralph et al., 1998a). Although models of conceptual knowledge based on the statistical co-occurrence of object properties provide important insights about semantic memory in general, the SD patients provide little positive evidence for the intercorrelated feature theories of category differences specifically (see also McRae & Cree, 2002).

The final possibility we shall consider is the influence of individual differences. One of the limitations of single-case methodology is that individual fluctuations in performance are hard to detect and to control. Thus it can be difficult to know when a significant effect in performance (e.g., artefacts better than living) truly reflects a stable characteristic of the underlying cognitive architecture, random fluctuations in test performance, or a premorbid individual difference that alters the functioning of the cognitive process (Lambon Ralph, Moriarty, & Sage, 2002; Plaut, 1997). The case-series approach, including multiple assessments of each task (e.g., several naming tests), suffers less from this drawback because each patient can be compared not only with normal performance but also with the other patients of the same type and even with himself or herself. Fluctuations in test scores leading to Type I statistical errors were observed in this study—occasionally an individual patient would exhibit a difference between the two domains of knowledge on a specific test. It was only KH, however, who demonstrated a consistent pattern across essentially all tests requiring semantic memory. Random fluctuation in test scores does not explain KH's category-specific impairment, therefore; but individual differences could do so.

There is clear evidence for significant individual differences in conceptual knowledge within the normal population. Analyses of control performance have identified individual variation in knowledge for animate, plant, and artefact domains (Funnell & De Mornay Davies, 1996). Male–female differences for knowledge of praxic objects, animals, and edible substances have also been found in psychometrically graded tests (McKenna, 1997). If a person happened to have considerable experience of artefacts, or a lack of experience with animals, then it would not be surprising if a generalised semantic impairment produced differences between living and nonliving domains for that patient. The underlying mechanism for this effect is the same as for the role of familiarity: PDP models clearly demonstrate that frequent presentation during training makes representations more robust to damage (e.g., Plaut, McClelland, Seidenberg, & Patterson, 1996). Without some form of independent measure of premorbid individual differences, however, this explanation suffers from the same criticism as that noted above for domain-specific knowledge theories—that it is simply a redescription of the data: Patients with no category difference are assumed to have had equivalent premorbid knowledge of each domain while KH's premorbid knowledge of animals was weak.

An individual differences explanation is made more plausible, at least for semantic dementia, if we consider the prevalence of category-specificity within that disorder. Over the last decade, approximately 40 SD patients, presenting to the Memory and Cognitive Disorders Clinic at Addenbrooke's Hospital, have been given a neuropsychological clinical battery including the 64-item naming and word–picture matching tasks reported here. Of these 40 patients, KH is the only one to have demonstrated a clear difference in favour of artefacts. If we combine the current patients with those reported in three recent papers (Lambon Ralph et al., 1998a, 1998b, 1999), then there are 18 cases who have been assessed in more detail whilst controlling for confounding psycholinguistic factors. KH is once again the only patient to have presented with significant and reliably worse performance for living things. Of course, if there are individual differences then the majority of cases should fall into the middle ground (i.e., show no category effect) while a small number should fall to *both* ends of the distribution. It is important to note, therefore, that while KH was the only case with poorer performance for living things, another 1 of the 18 demonstrated a small but consistent difference in the opposite direction, which persisted over the course of her progressive illness (patient IW: Lambon Ralph & Howard, 2000; Lambon Ralph et al., 1998b).

This proposal begs the obvious question of whether individual differences provide an explanation for category-specific deficits in semantic dementia alone or for other patients as well. It is possible that at least some of the other reported single cases could have arisen from premorbid differences in knowledge. Future case-series or group studies are required to rule out individual differences as a general explanation for category specificity. If a certain category-specific pattern is consistently associated with a certain disease type, underlying distribution of neurological damage, or pattern of cognitive deficits, then an account on the basis of individual differences would not be plausible. In any event, an explanation in terms of individual differences will continue to feel under constrained and unsatisfying unless and until there is some independent basis on which to predict who should fall where in the distribution. At present, however, it remains a leading contender for explaining an otherwise puzzling set of patterns in the domain of category specificity.

## REFERENCES


Barbarotto, R., Capitani, E., Spinnler, H., & Trivelli, C. (1995). Slowly progressive semantic impairment with category specificity. *Neurocase, 1*, 107–119.

Basso, A., Capitani, E., & Laiacona, M. (1988). Progressive language impairment without dementia: A case with isolated category specific semantic defect. *Journal of Neurology, Neurosurgery and Psychiatry, 51*, 1201–1207.

Borgo, F., & Shallice, T. (2001). When living things and other "sensory quality" categories behave in the same fashion: A novel category specificity effect. *Neurocase, 7*, 201–220.

Bozeat, S., Lambon Ralph, M. A., Patterson, K., Garrard, P., & Hodges, J. R. (2000). Nonverbal semantic impairment in semantic dementia. *Neuropsychologia, 38*, 1207–1215.

Breedin, S. D., Martin, N., & Saffran, E. M. (1994a). Category-specific semantic impairments: An infrequent occurrence. *Brain and Language, 47*, 383–386.

Breedin, S. D., Saffran, E. M., & Coslett, H. B. (1994b). Reversal of the concreteness effect in a patient with semantic dementia. *Cognitive Neuropsychology, 11*, 617–660.

Caramazza, A., & Shelton, J. R. (1998). Domain-specific knowledge systems in the brain: The animate–inanimate distinction. *Journal of Cognitive Neuroscience, 10*, 1–34.

Cardebat, D., Demonet, J. F., Celsis, P., & Puel, M. (1996). Living/nonliving dissociation in a case of semantic dementia: A SPECT activation study. *Neuropsychologia, 34*, 1175–1179.

De Renzi, E., & Lucchelli, F. (1994). Are semantic systems separately represented in the brain? The case of living category impairment. *Cortex, 30*, 3–25.

Devlin, J. T., Gonnerman, L. M., Anderson, E. S., & Seidenberg, M. S. (1998). Category-specific semantic deficits in focal and widespread brain damage: A computational account. *Journal of Cognitive Neuroscience, 10*, 77–94.

Devlin, J. T., Moore, C. J., Mummery, C. J., Gorno-Tempini, M. L., Phillips, J. A., Noppeney, U., Frackowiak, R. S. J., Friston, K. J., & Price, C. J. (2002a). Anatomic constraints on cognitive theories of category specificity. *Neuroimage, 15*, 675–685.

Devlin, J. T., Russell, R. P., Davis, M. H., Price, C. J., Moss, H. E., Fadili, M. J., & Tyler, L. K. (2002b). Is there an anatomical basis for category-specificity? Semantic memory studies in PET and fMRI. *Neuropsychologia, 40*, 54–75.

Farah, M. J., Hammond, K. M., Mehta, Z., & Ratcliff, G. (1989). Category-specificity and modality-specificity in semantic memory. *Neuropsychologia, 27*, 193–200.

Farah, M. J., & McClelland, J. L. (1991). A computational model of semantic memory impairment: Modality specificity and emergent category specificity. *Journal of Experimental Psychology: General, 120*, 339–357.

Folstein, M. F., Folstein, S. E., & McHugh, P. R. (1975). Mini-mental state: A practical method for grading the cognitive state of patients for the clinician. *Journal of Psychiatric Research, 12*, 189–198.

Forde, E. M. E., Francis, D., Riddoch, M. J., Rumiati, R. I., & Humphreys, G. W. (1997). On the links between visual knowledge and naming: A single case study of a patient with a category-specific impairment for living things. *Cognitive Neuropsychology, 14*, 403–458.

Funnell, E. (1995). Objects and properties: A study of the breakdown of semantic memory. *Memory, 3*, 497–518.

Funnell, E., & De Mornay Davies, P. (1996). JBR: A reassessment of concept familiarity and a category-specific disorder for living things. *Neurocase, 2*, 461–474.

Funnell, E., & Sheridan, J. (1992). Categories of knowledge? Unfamiliar aspects of living and nonliving things. *Cognitive Neuropsychology, 9*, 135–153.

Gainotti, G., & Silveri, M. C. (1996). Cognitive and anatomical locus of lesion in a patient with a category-specific semantic impairment for living beings. *Cognitive Neuropsychology, 13*, 357–390.

Gainotti, G., Silveri, M. C., Daniele, A., & Giustolisi, L. (1995). Neuroanatomical correlates of category-specific semantic disorders: A critical survey. *Memory, 3*, 247–264.

Galton, C. J., Patterson, K., Graham, K., Lambon Ralph, M. A., Williams, G., Antoun, N., Sahakian, B. J., & Hodges, J. R. (2001). Differing patterns of temporal atrophy in Alzheimer's disease and semantic dementia. *Neurology, 57*, 216–225.

Garrard, P., Lambon Ralph, M. A., & Hodges, J. R. (2002). Semantic dementia: A category-specific paradox. In E. M. E. Forde & G. W. Humphreys (Eds.), *Category-specificity in brain and mind.* Hove, UK: Psychology Press.

Garrard, P., Lambon Ralph, M. A., Hodges, J. R., & Patterson, K. (2001a). Prototypicality, distinctiveness and intercorrelation: Analyses of the semantic attributes of living and nonliving concepts. *Cognitive Neuropsychology, 18*, 125–174.

Garrard, P., Lambon Ralph, M. A., Watson, P., Powis, J., Patterson, K., & Hodges, J. R. (2001b). Longitudinal profiles of semantic impairment for living and nonliving concepts in dementia of Alzheimer's type. *Journal of Cognitive Neuroscience, 13*, 892–909.

Garrard, P., Patterson, K., Watson, P. C., & Hodges, J. R. (1998). Category-specific semantic loss in dementia of Alzheimer's type. *Brain, 121*, 633–646.

Gloor, P. (1997). *The temporal lobe and the limbic system.* Oxford: Oxford University Press.

Gonnerman, L. M., Andersen, E. S., Devlin, J. T., Kempler, D., & Seidenberg, M. S. (1997). Double dissociation of semantic categories in Alzheimer's disease. *Brain and Language, 57*, 254–279.

Hillis, A. E., & Caramazza, A. (1991). Category-specific naming and comprehension impairment: A double dissociation. *Brain, 114*, 2081–2094.

Hillis, A. E., Rapp, B., Romani, C., & Caramazza, A. (1990). Selective impairment of semantics in lexical processing. *Cognitive Neuropsychology, 7*, 191–243.

Hodges, J. R. (2001). Frontotemporal dementia (Pick's disease): Clinical features and assessment. *Neurology, 56*, S6–S10.

Hodges, J. R., Garrard, P., & Patterson, K. (1998). Semantic dementia. In A. Kertesz & D. G. Munoz (Eds.), *Pick's disease and Pick complex.* New York: Wylie-Liss.

Hodges, J. R., Graham, N., & Patterson, K. (1995). Charting the progression of semantic dementia: Implications for the organisation of semantic memory. *Memory, 3*, 463–495.

Hodges, J. R., & Patterson, K. (1995). Is semantic memory consistently impaired early in the course of Alzheimer's disease? Neuroanatomical and diagnostic implications. *Neuropsychologia, 33*, 441–459.

Hodges, J. R., Patterson, K., Oxbury, S., & Funnell, E. (1992). Semantic dementia: Progressive fluent aphasia with temporal lobe atrophy. *Brain, 115*, 1783–1806.

Howard, D., & Patterson, K. (1992). *The Pyramids and Palm Trees Test: A test of semantic access from words and pictures.* Bury St Edmunds, UK: Thames Valley Test Company.

Humphreys, G. W., & Forde, E. M. E. (2001). Hierarchies, similarity, and interactivity in object recognition: "Category-specific" neuropsychological deficits. *Brain and Behavioural Sciences, 24*, 453–496.

Laiacona, M., Barbarotto, R., & Capitani, E. (1993). Perceptual and associative knowledge in category specific impairment of semantic memory: A study of two cases. *Cortex, 29*, 727–740.

Lambon Ralph, M. A., Graham, K. S., Ellis, A. W., & Hodges, J. R. (1998a). Naming in semantic dementia—what matters? *Neuropsychologia, 36*, 775–784.

Lambon Ralph, M. A., Graham, K. S., Patterson, K., & Hodges, J. R. (1999). Is a picture worth a thousand words? Evidence from concept definitions by patients with semantic dementia. *Brain and Language, 70*, 309–335.

Lambon Ralph, M. A., & Howard, D. (2000). Gogi aphasia or semantic dementia? Simulating and assessing poor verbal comprehension in a case of progressive fluent aphasia. *Cognitive Neuropsychology, 17*, 437–466.

Lambon Ralph, M. A., Howard, D., Nightingale, G., & Ellis, A. W. (1998b). Are living and nonliving category-specific deficits causally linked to impaired perceptual or associative knowledge? Evidence from a category-specific double dissociation. *Neurocase, 4*, 311–338.

Lambon Ralph, M. A., McClelland, J. L., Patterson, K., Galton, C. J., & Hodges, J. R. (2001). No right to speak? The relationship between object naming and semantic impairment: Neuropsychological evidence and a computational model. *Journal of Cognitive Neuroscience, 13*, 341–356.

Lambon Ralph, M. A., Moriarty, L., & Sage, K. (2002). Anomia is simply a reflection of semantic and phonological impairments: Evidence from a case-series study. *Aphasiology, 16*, 56–82.

McCarthy, R. A., & Warrington, E. K. (1988). Evidence for modality-specific meaning systems in the brain. *Nature, 334*, 428–430.

McKenna, P. (1997). *Category Specific Names Test.* Hove, UK: Psychology Press.

McRae, K., & Cree, G. S. (2002). Factors underlying category-specific semantic deficits. In E. M. E. Forde & G. W. Humphreys (Eds.), *Category-specificity in brain and mind.* Hove, UK: Psychology Press.

McRae, K., De Sa, V. R., & Seidenberg, M. S. (1997). On the nature and scope of featural representation of word meaning. *Journal of Experimental Psychology: General, 126*, 99–130.

Morrison, C. M., Chappell, T. D., & Ellis, A. W. (1997). Age of acquisition norms for a large set of object names and their relation to adult estimates and other variables. *Quarterly Journal of Experimental Psychology, 50A*, 528–559.

Moss, H. E., Tyler, L. K., Durrant-Peatfield, M., & Bunn, E. M. (1998). Two eyes of a see-through: Impaired and intact semantic knowledge in a case of selective deficit for living things. *Neurocase, 4*, 291–310.

Moss, H. E., Tyler, L. K., Hodges, J. R., & Patterson, K. (1995). Exploring the loss of semantic memory in semantic dementia: Evidence from a primed monitoring study. *Neuropsychology, 9*, 16–26.

Mummery, C. J., Patterson, K., Price, C. J., Ashburner, J., Frackowiak, R. S. J., & Hodges, J. R. (2000). A voxel based morphometry study of semantic dementia: The relation of temporal lobe atrophy to cognitive deficit. *Annals of Neurology, 47*, 36–45.

Osterrieth, P. (1944). Le test de copie d'une figure complexe. *Archives de Psychologie, 30*, 205–550.

Parkin, A. J. (1993). Progressive aphasia without dementia: A clinical and cognitive neuropsychological analysis. *Brain and Language, 44*, 201–220.

Perry, C. (1999). Testing a computational account of category-specific deficits. *Journal of Cognitive Neuroscience, 11*, 312–320.

Plaut, D. C. (1997). Structure and function in the lexical system: Insights from distributed models of word reading and lexical decision. *Language and Cognitive Processes, 12*, 765–805.

Plaut, D. C., McClelland, J. L., Seidenberg, M. S., & Patterson, K. (1996). Understanding normal and impaired word reading: Computational principles in quasi-regular domains. *Psychological Review, 103*, 56–115.

Raven, J. C. (1962). *Coloured Progressive Matrices: Sets A, AB, B.* London: H. K. Lewis.

Ritter, H., & Kohonen, T. (1989). Self-organizing semantic maps. *Biological Cybernetics, 61*, 241–254.

Sacchett, C., & Humphreys, G. W. (1992). Calling a squirrel a squirrel but a canoe a wigwam: A category-specific deficit for artefactual objects and body parts. *Cognitive Neuropsychology, 9*, 73–86.

Saffran, E. M., & Schwartz, M. F. (1994). Of cabbages and things: Semantic memory from a neuropsychological perspective: A tutorial review. *Attention and Performance, 25*, 507–536.

Samson, D., De Wilde, V., & Pillon, A. (1998). Impaired knowledge of visual and nonvisual attributes in a patient with a naming impairment for living entities: A case of a true category-specific deficit. *Neurocase, 4*, 273–290.

Sartori, G., & Job, R. (1988). The oyster with four legs: A neuropsychological study on the interaction of visual and semantic information. *Cognitive Neuropsychology, 5*, 105–132.

Sheridan, J., & Humphreys, G. W. (1993). A verbal-semantic category-specific recognition impairment. *Cognitive Neuropsychology, 10*, 143–184.

Silveri, M. C., Gainotti, G., Perani, D., Cappelletti, J. Y., Carbone, G., & Fazio, F. (1997). Naming deficit for nonliving items: Neuropsychological and PET study. *Neuropsychologia, 35*, 359–367.

Snodgrass, J. G., & Vanderwart, M. (1980). A standardised set of 260 pictures: Norms for name agreement, image agreement, familiarity, and visual complexity. *Journal of Experimental Psychology: Human Learning and Memory, 6*, 174–215.

Snowden, J. S., Goulding, P. J., & Neary, D. (1989). Semantic dementia: A form of circumscribed cerebral atrophy. *Behavioural Neurology, 2*, 167–182.

Snowden, J. S., Griffiths, H. L., & Neary, D. (1996a). Progressive language disorder associated with frontal lobe degeneration. *Neurocase, 2*, 429–440.

Snowden, J. S., Neary, D., & Mann, D. M. A. (1996b). *Frontotemporal lobar degeneration: Frontotemporal dementia, progressive aphasia, semantic dementia.* London: Churchill Livingstone.

Srinivas, K., Breedin, S. D., Coslett, H. B., & Saffran, E. M. (1997). Intact perceptual priming in a patient with damage to the anterior inferior temporal lobes. *Journal of Cognitive Neuroscience, 9*, 490–511.

Tippett, L. J., Glosser, G., & Farah, M. J. (1996). A category-specific naming impairment after temporal lobectomy. *Neuropsychologia, 34*, 139–146.

Tyler, L. K., & Moss, H. E. (1998). Going, going, gone? . . . Implicit and explicit tests of conceptual knowledge in longitudinal study of semantic dementia. *Neuropsychologia, 36*, 1313–1323.

Tyler, L. K., Moss, H. E., Durrant-Peatfield, M. R., & Levy, J. P. (2000). Conceptual structure and the structure of concepts: A distributed account of category-specific deficits. *Brain and Language, 75*, 195–231.

Ungerleider, L. G., & Mishkin, M. (1982). Two cortical visual systems. In D. J. Ingle, M. A. Goodale, & R. J. W. Mansfield (Eds.), *Analysis of visual behaviour.* Cambridge, MA: MIT Press.

Warrington, E. K. (1984). *Recognition Memory Test.* Windsor, UK: NFER-Nelson.

Warrington, E. K., & James, M. (1991). *The Visual Object and Space Perception Battery.* Bury St Edmunds, UK: Thames Valley Test Company.

Warrington, E. K., & McCarthy, R. (1983). Category specific access dysphasia. *Brain, 106*, 859–878.

Warrington, E. K., & McCarthy, R. (1987). Categories of knowledge: Further fractionations and an attempted integration. *Brain, 110*, 1273–1296.

Warrington, E. K., & McCarthy, R. A. (1994). Multiple meaning systems in the brain: A case for visual semantics. *Neuropsychologia, 32*, 1465–1473.

Warrington, E. K., & Shallice, T. (1984). Category specific semantic impairments. *Brain, 107*, 829–854.

Wechsler, D. A. (1987). *Wechsler Memory Scale-Revised.* San Antonio, TX: Psychological Corporation.

COGNITIVE NEUROPSYCHOLOGY, 2003, 20 (3/4/5/6), 327–353

# CATEGORY SPECIFICITY AND FEATURE KNOWLEDGE: EVIDENCE FROM NEW SENSORY-QUALITY CATEGORIES

**Francesca Borgo**
*Neuroscience Programme SISSA-ISAS and University of Trieste, Italy*

**Tim Shallice**
*University College London, UK and Neuroscience Programme SISSA-ISAS, Trieste, Italy*

Category-specific deficits and their relation to types of feature knowledge are addressed with respect to three semantic domains: artefacts, living things, and mass-kinds. The performance of a herpes encephalitic patient with a classic category-specific pattern of knowledge, MU, was compared to that of the other HSE patients and normal subjects. In a feature verification task involving over 4000 questions, MU showed a severe impairment with the mass-kind category, where his sensory features knowledge was at chance and much worse than his functional knowledge. In the feature production task, however, MU was grossly impaired with respect to sensory relative to functional features across all categories. Control experiments suggest that the deficits were of knowledge. Overall, these findings give some support to the sensory-functional theory, and are difficult to explain on the domain-specific knowledge theory. However, an account is still needed of the differences observed in MU's performance between the two paradigms.

## INTRODUCTION

A large number of studies of brain-damaged patients have been reported in the neuropsychological literature, concerning deficits selectively affecting the knowledge of concepts belonging to either one of two distinct conceptual domains, living things and artefacts. Although impairments restricted just to the input or the output side of processing have been also described, these so-called category-specific deficits have generally been reported to affect both the semantic comprehension and verbal production of concepts associated to living things or artefacts.

Analysis of these category-specific deficits has led to a long-lasting debate on the nature of the organisation of concepts within the semantic memory system. From a broad perspective, two main types of theories have been put forward to account for category-specific deficits. One theoretical approach assumes a featural organisation of semantic memory, and that correlation among features accounts for category-specificity effects. Different categories are held to be differentially susceptible to impairment according to the way that the features of different exemplars of the category are intercorrelated (Caramazza, Hillis, Rapp, & Romani, 1990; Devlin, Gonnerman, Andersen, &

Requests for reprints should be addressed to Professor Tim Shallice, Institute of Cognitive Neuroscience, University College London, Alexandra House, 17 Queen Square, London WC1N 3AR, UK (Email: t.shallice@ucl.ac.uk or shallice@sissa.it).

We would like to thank Dr Peter Garrard (ICN, University College London, UK) for making available to us extensive material from his battery before publication for use in this work, and also Prof Vito Toso and Dr Teresa Maria Sgaramella (Neurology Department, Vicenza Hospital, Italy) for their collaboration and support throughout this study.



http://www.tandf.co.uk/journals/pp/02643294.html
DOI:10.1080/02643290244000310

Seidenberg, 1998; Tyler, Moss, Durrant-Peatfield, & Levy, 2000).

Thus, the OUCH (Organized Unitary Content Hypothesis) model has been proposed by Caramazza et al. (1990; Hillis, Rapp, & Caramazza, 1995; Rapp, Hillis, & Caramazza, 1993). On this approach, both the living thing and artefact classes are held to be organised in terms of conceptual properties, which are highly intercorrelated and represented in a nonhomogenous fashion within a multidimensional space. As members of the living things category share far more intercorrelated features than artefacts, it is held that "the denser regions represent concept domains characterized by highly correlated properties, with the densest regions most likely corresponding to natural kind concepts" (Caramazza & Shelton, 1998). Therefore focal damage is likely to affect the living things category more than artefacts. More importantly, highly intercorrelated features are held to involve both sensory and functional properties of a given concept, so that a category-specific deficit is claimed to be *independent* of the disproportionate impairment of visual/functional properties.

There have been two main implementations of this type of approach. For Devlin et al. (1998; see also Gonnerman, Andersen, Devlin, Kempler, & Seidenberg, 1997) some features are held to occur almost exclusively for individual items within a category, therefore allowing the differentiation of a concept from related ones (distinguishing features); this is more typical of artefacts. From this it is predicted that in degenerative diseases a different pattern of conceptual loss will occur across the two types of category: Artefact knowledge will decrease linearly during time, while a cross-over will be observed with living things: Initially, living things are better preserved than artefacts, whereas over time, knowledge of them declines more rapidly than that concerning artefacts.

On the view of Tyler et al. (2000), however, artefacts are characterised by strong links between their form (perceptual features) and their function. The functions of artefacts tend to be highly specific, and are therefore associated to "distinctive" perceptual properties. On the other hand, living things are held to be highly characterised by "shared" perceptual properties, which are closely related to common biological functions. Since highly correlated features are held to be more resistant to damage than weakly correlated properties, "distinctive perceptual attributes for artefacts and shared features for biological kinds will be correlated with functional information and will be the most resistant to damage." Their model predicts a qualitatively different pattern of decline compared with that of Gonnerman et al. (1997) and Devlin et al. (1998). However, studies of semantic dementia patients provide no support for either set of predictions (Garrard, Patterson, Watson, & Hodges, 1998). Moreover, there is no explanation as to why selective damage to the living things category so frequently occurs from herpes simplex encephalitis while the complementary syndrome has not been reported with this aetiology (see Gainotti, 2000; Warrington & Shallice, 1984). Finally, none of these models accounts for deficits co-occurring for living things and different types of materials, as observed in early reports of category-specific effects (Warrington & Shallice, 1984) and in a more recent and systematic study (Borgo & Shallice, 2001).

A second broad approach to category-specific effects focuses on the idea of hardware specialisation for different types of concept within the semantic memory system. On this type of theory some properties of the macro-organisation of the nervous system determine the structure of semantic organisation. Two main groups of theories have been proposed, which are based on a "hardware" account of category-specificity phenomena. One group is often called the sensory-functional theory (SFT). This was originally proposed by Warrington and Shallice (1984) for the living things deficit often found in herpes encephalitis, and by Warrington and McCarthy (1983, 1987) for the relative sparing of living things found in certain global aphasic patients. A somewhat related theory, although more oriented to the object-form level, has been developed by Chao, Haxby, and Martin (1999) to account for functional imaging evidence on recognition of different classes of visual stimuli within the general context of the different properties of the ventral and dorsal routes, or of ventral occipito-temporal cortex and lateral temporal cortex in particular. The position of Humphreys and Forde (2001)—their hierarchical interactive theory—also has some similarities to these accounts, but in this case has more links with the overall perspective of Warrington and McCarthy.

In their original work, Warrington and Shallice described four HSE patients who all had predominantly bilateral temporal damage. Despite differences in the degree of their global impairment, their comprehension and identification abilities for artefacts were relatively preserved, but they all showed gross deficits when required to identify living things and foods. After this first account of this type of category-specific deficit, a considerable number of patients with herpes simplex encephalitis have been investigated who show a similar pattern. By 2001 at least 22 cases with this pattern had been described in the literature (see Borgo, 2001; Gainotti, 2000). In most if not quite all (see Capitani, Laiacona, Mahon, & Caramazza, 2003-this issue) of the patients, the impairment involves knowledge of animals, plants, and foods, although the testing of foods was often limited to fruit and vegetables. We will treat this pattern as a "putative functional syndrome" using the approach of Plaut and Shallice (1993). MU, the patient investigated, behaved in an analogous fashion to the patients of Warrington and Shallice (1984).

An alternative type of hardware account was put forward by Caramazza and Shelton (1998). They proposed the domain-specific account of category-specific deficits, assuming that evolutionary pressures have been responsible for the categorical organisation of semantic knowledge in producing two specific systems, one holding knowledge of potential predators and foods (animals), and the other of sources of food (plants). These authors held that in terms of neural and functional mechanisms, the relevant adaptations might consist, respectively, of dedicated neural circuits—or specialised cognitive processes—for processing information about animals and plants. Thus the categories of animals and plants would segregate, and could both be separated from the representation of other categories, such as utensils. One line of evidence they used was of patients showing fractionations within the living things class (e.g., Caramazza & Shelton, 1998; Hart, Berndt, & Caramazza, 1985; Hillis & Caramazza, 1991). The authors' predictions were met in the description of the performance of their category-specific patient EW, who had a lesion, due to a left cerebral vascular accident, involving the left posterior frontal and parietal lobes. The patient had an impairment affecting both production and comprehension of knowledge of animals relative to other living things, such as fruits and vegetables, and relative to other categories tested, including musical instruments and vehicles. Furthermore EW had a second characteristic that presented problems for the SFT: She performed equally poorly with functional/associative and visual property judgments of animals.

Caramazza and Shelton (1998) argued that additional evidence problematic for the SFT comes from observations that category-specific deficits are not necessarily associated with a difficulty in the analysis of either sensory or functional properties, as in EW. For instance, Laiacona, Barbarotto, and Capitani (1993a) described the selective disruption of the knowledge of living things in two patients (FM and RG) who had suffered from brain injury. Patient FM had lesions in the left posterior parietal areas; furthermore, the patient had a deep cortical atrophy, involving the frontal lobes bilaterally and the left temporal lobe. Patient RG showed diffuse compromising of the left hemisphere with specific involvement of the left frontal and left posterior temporal parts. Both patients showed an equal performance with respect to functional/associative and perceptual properties in a semantic questionnaire. A selective deficit for living entities was also recently reported by Samson, Pillon, and De Wilde (1998), who described a patient, JEN, with an atrophy in the posterior part of the left hemisphere and hypodensity in the left frontal paramedian areas. The patient's knowledge of both visual and nonvisual attributes of living things was impaired overall, while in the case of artefacts both types of properties were found to be spared. Furthermore, Lambon Ralph, Howard, Nightingale, and Ellis (1998) described an Alzheimer's disease patient, DB, with a category-specific deficit that affected living things in naming and comprehension tasks; she did not show any difference between attribute type (perceptual vs. functional-associative) when her knowledge about living things and artefacts was assessed (but for criticisms, see Borgo & Shallice, 2001). Moreover, Caramazza and Shelton point out that in only one patient is there a statistically defensible and theoretically critical interaction of type of knowledge by category, namely in patient Michelangelo (Sartori & Job, 1988; Sartori, Miozzo, & Job, 1993).

There are three types of approach on the SFT to the problems the performance of these patients poses. First, Farah and McClelland (1991) developed a connectionist model in which the semantic system is separated into a visual and a functional component. Living things are held to be much more dependent on visual features than functional, whilst the opposite is characteristic of artefacts representation. In the learning process, access to the functional aspects of living thing becomes partly dependent on the mediation of the activity of set of visual units, which is larger and overall more critical. For this category, through the learning process, activity in the visual units, comes to support the knowledge of the functional aspects. For artefacts the situation is somewhat complementary with the functional units supporting knowledge of visual aspects.

The predictions of the theory of Farah and McClelland depend upon the assumption that different types of semantic category differ substantially in the ratio of functional-to-sensory features. In their original account Warrington and Shallice (1984, p. 849) used the term "function" in a narrow sense: "Inanimate objects unlike, say, most animals and plants have clearly defined functions. The evolutionary development of tool using has led to finer and finer functional differentiations of artefacts for an increasing range of purposes. . . . We would suggest that identification of an inanimate object crucially depends on determination of its functional significance, but that is irrelevant for identification of living things. . . . We would therefore speculate that a semantic system based on functional specifications might have evolved for the identification of inanimate objects." This system was held to have a particular pattern of associative links to the systems underlying action and intention.

On this approach the assumptions of Farah and McClelland concerning the relative number of functional and sensory quality features across the living things and artefact categories are entirely appropriate. However, in empirical work they tried to operationalise the theory in terms of an actual number of different types of features for particular items. They defined "functional descriptions" as "what an item does or what it is for" (p. 342), which is somewhat broader than the Warrington and Shallice definition since it includes, for instance, characteristic movements of animals (e.g., monkey: *"can swing"*).

Caramazza and Shelton (1998) criticised the Farah and McClelland procedure because it "will not provide a fair estimate of the *nonsensory properties* known for living things" (p. 18). This is correct but if *nonsensory properties* are treated as the relevant contrast for *sensory properties* then the theory being tested is not the SFT as originally put forward. Different estimates of the ratio of "functional" or "functional/associative" to "sensory" features have then been produced depending on the definition of function used (see also Garrard, Lambon Ralph, Hodges, & Patterson, 2001; Cree & McRae, 2001).

A second way of dealing with the existence of more selective dissociations per se is that adopted by Warrington and McCarthy (1987) and Humphreys and Forde (2001): subdividing the basic sensory-quality and functional routes. Warrington and McCarthy suggest that fine-grained fractionations *within* a semantic domain, such as the one described in their patient YOT, might be better explained by taking into account the contribution of differing weighting values for semantic information depending on sensory/motor modalities and, within each modality, on specialised channels for particular semantic attributes, for example colour or texture in the case of a sensory channel (but see Miceli, Fouch, Capasso, Shelton, Tomaiuolo, & Caramazza, 2001, for potentially conflicting evidence that may create problems for this approach). This does not, however, deal with Caramazza and Shelton's (1998) objection that in most of the published literature it is categories that are generally affected rather than type of information within a category. Humphreys and Forde present a more complex perspective, involving stored structural descriptions, stored functional and interobject association information, and name representations. They see information as "cascading" between these levels. Moreover, included levels can be subdivided into a number of subsystems in a related fashion to the position of Warrington and McCarthy. They refer to some simulations that may be relevant with regard to Caramazza and Shelton's critique of the Warrington and McCarthy theory. However, they are unpublished.

There is, however, a third response to the overall critique of the SFT presented by Caramazza and Shelton (1998). They comment that the existence of very narrow category-specific deficits is "undermining the expectation derived from the SFT that the categories should be damaged together" (p. 17), as the originally described disorder "fractionates" into more specific ones. This is presented as the primary evidence for the "refutation" of the theory. This argument of Caramazza and Shelton is based on the implicit premise that the category-specific deficits of all patients can be explained by damage to the same system. This sounds appropriate but it is entirely possible that damage to different subsystems of the overall system can give rise to category-specific effects. In this case to try to explain the properties of all the cases by the same theory would be very dangerous. To use a simple analogy, inferences to the operation of an early stage of the visual system that can be derived from the phenomenon that recognition of all types of object are affected by retinal disease are in no way invalidated by the existence of more specific category-specific effects affecting only a limited range of objects; these latter effects arise from damage to a quite different part of the overall system.

Is there any evidence that this hypothetical possibility might be the case? One obvious line of evidence concerns the localisation of the different putative subsystems. We will make the additional assumptions that cognitive subsystems are isolable and fairly specifically localised (see Shallice, 1981, for discussion). Thus, if an argument based on fractionation is to be used against SFT, one type of lesion site—that involving the more specific disorder—should at the very least overlap the other functionally wider impairment. However, as Gainotti (2000) has pointed out, the more general living things deficit observed in herpes simplex encephalitis (HSE) has a well defined neuroanatomical location, namely the bilateral (particularly left) anterior mesial inferior temporal lobes. Moreover, the temporal lobe location of the wider impairment is amply supported by an analysis of Capitani et al. (2003-this issue), which is a more thorough review on the cognitive level (see also Laiacona, Capitani, & Barbarotto, 1997). However, on Gainotti's analysis this type of specificity is not found for the more selective disorders. Gainotti finds no clear localisation for them. Indeed, the most critical patient of this type, EW, has a parieto-frontal lesion site, quite distinct from those of the broader living things deficit. Thus on the most straightforward view of localisation of function contained in the above assumption, which Paulesu, Shallice, Frackowiak, and Frith (2003) term the "canonical view," the properties of EW's disorder would be irrelevant for understanding the operation of the systems involved in the general living things deficit, the category-specific disorder found most frequently in HSE. Complementarily, none of the findings obtained with patients with temporal lobe lesions would be relevant to any interpretation of EW's disorders.

The SFT can be tested in another way. One can ask which categories other than that of living things should be affected by any deficit of this type. In an earlier investigation, Borgo and Shallice (2001) followed De Renzi and Lucchelli (1994) and Tyler and Moss (1997), who have argued that it is the form of an artefact that constrains its function and that function is also linked to form through the affordances it provides for action. In addition, Buxbaum and Saffran (1998) had claimed that manipulability—knowledge of the action schema with which a tool is used—can be selectively impaired in patients with fronto-parietal lesions. Thus manipulability may be a more critical variable than the related but more abstract variable "function." In fact this had already been suggested by

Warrington and McCarthy (1987) on the basis of their patient YOT, who was selectively impaired on the identification of small manipulable objects. YOT had the complementary category-specific syndrome to that of the HSE patients.

On these bases Borgo and Shallice investigated mass-kind categories such as materials, edible substances, and drinks. As they lack a consistent form they would be particularly impaired on this extension of SFT. We found a clear parallel between living things and mass-kinds in a group of five patients with HSE. A selective deficit of both types of categories was found in the critical patient MU. However, a parallel level of impairment for the mass-kinds categories and the living things class was shown in the performance of each patient, and this pattern differed qualitatively from their performance with artefacts. Moreover, in their early study of HSE patients Warrington and Shallice (1984) found that their patient JBR performed very poorly at giving verbal characteristics of *metals* and *cloth*, and Warrington and McCarthy (1987) had found the opposite pattern of intact performance on fabrics in their patient who showed an artefact impairment, YOT.

It is critical on the SFT that the generalisation from a living things deficit to a mass-kinds deficit should be of the same general type, namely a semantic one. Borgo and Shallice (2001) showed that MU was significantly worse than the control group for word–picture matching and picture–word matching for both living things and the mass–kind categories (see Borgo, 2001) but not for artefacts. More critically, he was tested on a procedure based on that used by Laiacona, Barbarotto, Trivelli, and Capitani (1993b) on knowledge of both functional and sensory attributes. He was significantly below the controls on both types of knowledge for living things, substances, and materials.

In the light of the critique by Caramazza and Shelton (1998) of other studies comparing knowledge of functional and sensory knowledge in patients with a living things deficit, and the theoretical importance that had been given to semantic distinctiveness by Devlin et al. (1998) and Tyler et al. (2000), it is necessary to carry out a more methodologically sophisticated and detailed investigation. Recently, Garrard et al. (2001) have developed a very detailed procedure for the investigation of different attributes of living things and artefacts. Twenty normal controls generated features for 64 items, half living and half artefacts. Four different types of property (categorical, encyclopaedic, functional, and sensory) were induced by the use of different sentence frames. Generated features were then rated for dominance—whether there were many participants generating the feature—and distinctiveness—how often the feature was generated for other items in the set.

Garrard (2000) applied this procedure to Alzheimer's disease and semantic dementia patients. In this paper we apply it to MU and control subjects, and in addition produce a set of features for the mass-kind categories, which are obtained using the procedure developed by Garrard et al. (2001).

## EXPERIMENTAL INVESTIGATION

From the perspective of Borgo and Shallice (2001), it seemed to be fundamental to examine HSE patients who show large categorical effects. This investigation therefore concentrates on MU, the patient studied in that paper. However, the adoption, where possible, of HSE patients who do not show the classical category-specific effect, but are matched in performance to critical patients with respect to performance on artefacts, will help to control confounding factors more than the use of normal controls, given the ceiling performance that is often observed in relevant tasks in normal subjects when used as controls for the performance of patients.

The experimental work involved the use of two different paradigms, both using verbally presented stimuli. First, the ability to specify different types of featural knowledge (feature verification task) related to members of the categories of living things, artefacts, and mass-kinds was examined in MU and essentially in the HSE patient group previously described by Borgo and Shallice (2001). Second, the ability to produce semantic attributes of concepts belonging to the three critical categories has been examined (feature production task). Both paradigms were developed on the lines proposed by Garrard et al. (2001).

## Case report

A detailed description of the neurological damage and the general neuropsychological assessment of HSE patients who are subjects (patients MU and, as controls, BAR, BAI, MIO, SAR) are reported in Borgo and Shallice (2001); see also Tables 1 and 2, for an account of their cognitive profile. MU, the critical patient, has a bilateral lesion affecting the infero-medial parts of the temporal lobes, the medial frontal regions, and the medial right occipital areas.

A new patient, CAL, not a subject in Borgo and Shallice's (2001) investigation, was included in the patient control group for the current study. CAL was 59 years old and had had 8 years of education; before his illness, he was a clerk employed by the local council. On admission to hospital in October 1996 he was feverish and confused. A diagnosis of encephalitis of probable herpetic origin was made, and he was treated with Acyclovir, showing a rapid recovery after its administration. Unfortunately, PCR (polymerase chain reaction) was not performed, and the viral origin of his illness was not clear from other cytological exams. An EEG performed after admission to the hospital showed an abnormal diffuse encephalitic signal, characterised by theta and delta waves, along with other more regular but slower rhythms, in fronto-bilateral areas, principally on the right side; these were considered compatible with a viral encephalitis. An EEG performed 2 months later showed resting activity characterised by a basal bilateral rhythm of 10 Hz, considered within normal limits, and showed clear signs of recovery from the acute phase of the illness. The CT scan was negative. The MRI scan showed a lesion localised in the left frontal lobe at the boundaries between cortical and subcortical layers. The typical onset of his disease, the prompt recovery after Acyclovir treatment, the pattern shown by the first EEG, and the lesion site demonstrated by the MRI were all considered compatible with the diagnosis of probable encephalitis of herpes viral origin.

On neuropsychological assessment CAL had slight problems in some WAIS subtests; however, in some general intelligence tasks (see Table 1) he was well within the normal range for his age and education. Both his verbal and categorical fluencies were in the normal range. His ability to perform visual search and other attentional tests was generally well preserved. Verbal reasoning was normal. When memory functions were assessed, his short-term memory was just within the average range. On the Weschler Memory Scale he showed some problems in orientation and information, and he could not learn paired associates. He was just within the normal range in story recall. His spontaneous language production was good and, although he showed initial difficulties in the Token Test, his comprehension skills recovered quickly. In perceptual tests (see Table 2) CAL was within normal limits on Benton's Line Orientation Judgement and Benton's Face Recognition test, but was severely impaired on the Hooper Visual Organization test and on Street's Visual Completion test. On the VOSP battery CAL was completely correct on the majority of tasks, with the exception of Silhouettes and Object Decision tasks. On the BORB subtests, CAL was below normal controls only in the two versions of the Object Decision tasks (easy version 22/32; hard version 17/32). He was impaired in naming colours, but had no deficits in colour identification.

## Experiment 1: Feature verification task

The feature verification task was aimed at assessing patients' knowledge of the semantic properties of living things, artefacts, and mass-kind stimuli. Two parallel versions of the task were devised, aimed at assessing patients' knowledge of a large series of semantic properties related to either artefacts and living things (Experiment 1a), or three mass-kinds categories, namely, edible substances, drinks, and materials (Experiment 1b). The two experiments were administered in two separate sessions. For the artefacts vs. living things set (Experiment 1a) the performance of MU was compared with patient

**Table 1.** *Performance of HSE patients on general neuropsychological assessment*

| | *MU* | *Bai* | *Bar* | *Cal* | *Mio* | *Sar* |
|---|---|---|---|---|---|---|
| *WAIS*[c] (Wechsler, 1986) | | | | | | |
| Picture completion | 10 | 14 | 14 | 9 | 14 | 7 |
| Block design | 10 | 9 | 9 | 11 | 14 | 9 |
| Picture arrangement | 8 | 11 | 12 | 8 | 12 | 13 |
| Object assembly | 7[e] | 10 | 19 | 6 | 13 | 7 |
| Performance IQ | 91 | 112 | 126 | 107 | 126 | 92 |
| *Perceptual maze test*[a] (Spinnler & Tognoni, 1987) | 9.50[d] | 11.75[e] | 16.55 | 18.00 | 15.75 | 18.00 |
| *Progressive coloured matrices*[b] (Raven, 1962) | 31.50 | 18.50[e] | 36.25 | 30.50 | 41.50 | 30.50 |
| *Verbal reasoning*[b] (Spinnler & Tognoni, 1987) | 30.25[d] | – | 45.75[e] | 55.00 | 24.00[d] | 47.25 |
| *Verbal fluency (FAS)*[b] (Ghidoni et al., 1995) | 2.80[d] | 51.30 | 26.30[e] | 28.80 | 24.40 | 24.80 |
| *Categorical fluency*[b] (Spinnler & Tognoni, 1987) | 3.50[d] | 17.00 | 11.50[e] | 12.25[e] | 12.00 | 57.00 |
| *Visual search*[a] (Spinnler & Tognoni, 1987) | 42.25[e] | 51.00 | 42.25[e] | 51.50 | 44.00 | 33.75[e] |
| Trail making test (Giovagnoli et al., 1996) | | | | | | |
| A[a] | 38" | 45" | 64"[f] | 58" | 240"[f] | 63"[f] |
| B[a] | 105" | with help | with help | 135" | 360"[f] | 127" |
| *Wechsler Memory Scale*[c] (Wechsler, 1981) | | | | | | |
| Information | 2[d] | 1[d] | 2[d] | 4[d] | 2[d] | 6 |
| Orientation | 5 | 5 | 3[d] | 3[d] | 3[d] | 5 |
| Mental control | 2[d] | 6 | 6 | 9 | 2[d] | 7 |
| Logic memory | 0.50[d] | 2.50[d] | 0.00[d] | 5.50 | 0.00[d] | 7.00 |
| Learning paired associates | 7[d] | 7[d] | 5[d] | 0.00[d] | 3[d] | 13 |
| Digit span forward | 6.50 | 4.75 | 4.75 | 4.75 | 4.50 | 6.00 |
| Digit span backward | 4[e] | 3[e] | 3[e] | 3[e] | 2[d] | 4[e] |
| *Word span*[b] (Spinnler & Tognoni, 1987) | 4.50 | – | 2.75[d] | 3.75 | 3.50 | 4.00 |
| *Corsi's span*[a] (Spinnler & Tognoni, 1987) | 5.50 | – | 2.50[d] | 4.75 | 4.25 | 3.75[e] |
| *Story recall*[b] (Spinnler & Tognoni, 1987) | 2[d] | 9.75 | 5.75[e] | 10.30 | 1.25[d] | 8.10 |
| *Token test (errors)*[a] (Luzatti et al., 1991) | 17[g] | 11[g] | 9[g] | 16[g] | 3[h] | 3[h] |

[a]The scores are scaled by age, sex and education; [b]the scores are scaled by age and education; [c]the scores are scaled by age.
[d]Score 2 *SD* below normal mean; [e]score <1 *SD* below normal mean; [f]score below upper limits for the normal range; [g]mild level of impairment; [h]normal performance.

controls (BAI, CAL, MIO, SAR) using analogous type of controls to Borgo and Shallice (2001). However, in the case of mass-kinds (Experiment 1b) the performance of patient MU was compared with that of a group of five normal subjects, matched to him according to sex (all males), age (mean = 30.2; range 28–33), and years of schooling (13), as the HSE patient control group was no longer available when the testing was carried out.

*Method: Stimuli and procedure*

The first experiment (1a, see Table 3) comprised 30 living things and 32 artefacts; in the second experiment (1b, see Table 3) a set of 40 items was

Table 2. *Performance of HSE patients on visual perception tasks*

| | *MU* | *Bai* | *Bar* | *Cal* | *Mio* | *Sar* |
|---|---|---|---|---|---|---|
| *Visual organization test* [d] (Hooper, 1985) | 10/30[g] | – | 16/30[g] | 13/30[g] | 13/30[g] | 10/30[g] |
| *Completion test* [a] (Spinnler & Tognoni, 1987) | 5.00[f] | – | 2.25[e] | 3.00[e] | 6.75 | 4.75[f] |
| *Line orientation judgement* [c] (Benton et al., 1990) | 20 | – | 19 | 26 | 19 | 21[g] |
| *Face recognition test* [b] (Benton et al., 1992) | 25[g] | – | – | 43 | 38[g] | 35[g] |
| *BORB* [d] (Riddoch & Humphreys, 1993) | | | | | | |
| Foreshortened view | 23/25 | 24/25 | 25/25 | 22/25 | 23/25 | 24/25 |
| Minimal features | 24/25 | 25/25 | 25/25 | 24/25 | 24/25 | 23/25 |
| Item match | 30/32 | 32/32 | 31/32 | 31/32 | 32/32 | 32/32 |
| Object decision (hard version) | 16/32[e] | 27/32 | 27/32 | 17/32[e] | 21/32[e] | 19/32[e] |
| Object decision (easy version) | 16/32[e] | 30/32 | 28/32 | 22/32[e] | 25/32[e] | 26/32[e] |
| *VOSP* [c] (Warrington & James, 1991) | | | | | | |
| Screening test | 20/20 | 20/20 | 19/20 | 20/20 | 20/20 | 20/20 |
| Incomplete letters | 14/20[h] | 18/20 | 17/20 | 17/20 | 16/20 | 16/20 |
| Silhouettes | 5/30[h] | 20/30 | 22/30 | 11/30[h] | 4/30[h] | 16/30 |
| Object decision | 14/20[h] | 18/20 | 15/20 | 11/20[h] | 17/20 | 18/20 |
| Progressive silhouettes | 16[h] | 6 | 13 | 13 | 17[h] | 13 |
| Dot counting | 10/10 | 10/10 | 10/10 | 10/10 | 10/10 | 9/10 |
| Position discrimination | 19/20 | 20/20 | 19/20 | 20/20 | 19/20 | 15/20[h] |
| Number location | 9/10 | 10/10 | 9/10 | 10/10 | 8/10 | 10/10 |
| Cube analysis | 8/10 | 6/10[h] | 10/10 | 10/10 | 9/10 | 9/10 |
| *Test for colour perception* [a] (De Vreese et al., 1994) | | | | | | |
| Colour naming | 8.20[f] | 9.70 | 5.30[e] | 7.40[e] | 5.70[e] | 7.50[e] |
| Colour identification | 8.01[e] | 9.80 | 5.30[e] | 10.20 | 7.20[e] | 10.30 |

[a]The scores are scaled by age, sex and education; [b]the scores are scaled by age and education; [c]the scores are scaled by age; [d]the scores are not scaled.

[e]Score 2 *SD* below normal mean; [f]score <1 *SD* below normal mean; [g]score below range for normal controls; [h]score below 5% cut-off score.

employed, taken from a larger set of 118 stimuli used in the feature production task (Experiment 3b).

*Experiment 1a: Living things and artefacts.* The featural database developed by Garrard et al. (2001) was employed. A subset of item–feature pairs related to each of the 62 items was selected (32 artefacts and 30 living things). Table 4 gives the mean and standard deviation of the distinctiveness/sharedness index—the extent to which a feature allows a particular concept to be distinguished from other members of the same category (Garrard et al., 2001)—which were broadly comparable between the two semantic domains for the two key semantic information types, functional and sensory information. Category information refers to the broader or narrower semantic domain to which a concept belongs (e.g., *cow*: animal; *bus*: vehicle). For the encyclopaedic information type there is an almost necessary difference between artefacts and living things. (Much encyclopaedic information, which at a first sight may seem to be distinctive of a concept, may generalise over a considerable number of living things—e.g., many animals live in Africa; but in the case of artefacts this type of property tends not to be shared over a large group of objects—thus utensils can be bought in many different types of shop.) The need to select from Garrard et al.'s (2001) database, which provides balanced subsets of shared/distinctive encyclopaedic features for living things and

**Table 3.** *Mean and standard deviation (SD) values for relevant factors characterising living things, artefacts, and mass-kind stimuli*

| Semantic category | No. of items: Exp. 1 | No. of items: Exp. 3 | Frequency | Familiarity | Visual complexity | Name agreement |
|---|---|---|---|---|---|---|
| *Experiments 1a and 3a* | | | | | | |
| Artefacts | 32 | 32 | 2.09 (1.36) | 1.24 (0.23) | 1.02 (0.29) | 0.46 (0.50) |
| Living things | 30 | 30 | 1.98 (1.41) | 0.97 (0.31) | 1.16 (0.36) | 0.33 (0.36) |
| *Experiments 1b and 3b* | | | | | | |
| Whole set | 40 | 118 | 1.83 (1.58) | 1.16 (0.27) | – | – |
| Edible substances | 16 | 52 | 1.61 (1.49) | 1.25 (0.24) | – | – |
| Liquids | 8 | 27 | 2.08 (1.74) | 1.18 (0.27) | – | – |
| Materials | 16 | 39 | 1.93 (1.55) | 1.04 (0.27) | – | – |

Experiments 1a and 3a: Word frequency means were calculated from the values presented in the *Dizionario di Frequenza della Lingua Italiana*, CNR, Roma (1989). Picture familiarity and visual complexity are calculated from the mean values given by subjects to pictures on a 5-point scale. Name agreement score is calculated through the information statistic H on the basis of the number of different names given to each picture and the proportion of subjects giving each name. The H value ranges from 0 (perfect name agreement) to 1 (same frequency of, say, two different names relative to the same picture). Familiarity, visual complexity, and name agreement values are taken from Snodgrass and Vanderwart (1980). Experiments 1b and 3b: Familiarity and frequency normative data were transformed into natural log, in order ensure their joint use in further analysis. Frequency norms for Italian written words were taken from the *Dizionario di Frequenza della Lingua Italiana*, CNR, Roma (1989); familiarity norms were collected from a group of Italian 10 normal subjects (see Experiment 3b). The frequency and familiarity values are given for Experiment 1b.

artefacts, meant that we could not have many examples of the subset shared encyclopedic information for artefacts; this subset was therefore not used for this category. The selected set of semantic features was translated into Italian and item–feature pairs were transformed into single very simple questions, which require a yes/no answer; finally, each feature relating to an item was coupled with another conceivable one, comparable in terms of the distinctiveness/sharedness characteristic, which was plausible but not pertinent to that item (e.g., category: *"Is an eagle a bird?"* / *"Is a saw a vehicle?"*; encyclopaedic: *"Are monkeys found in Africa?"* / *"Is a hammer found in a grocery shop?"*; functional: *"Can a frog jump?"* / *"Can a screwdriver be used for watering plants?"*; sensory: *"Is a banana yellow?"* / *"Is a fork very heavy?"*). This procedure was adopted in order to present patients with a series of questions that led

**Table 4.** *Experiment 1a: Distribution of shared and distinctive properties over the four types of semantic features*

| Properties | Category | Encyclopaedic | Functional | Sensory |
|---|---|---|---|---|
| *Artefacts* (*n* = 32) | | | | |
| Shared | 1 (0) | – | 0.66 (0.16) | 0.81 (0.11) |
| No. of items | 120 | – | 60 | 60 |
| Distinctive | 0.21 (0.17) | 0.15 (0.09) | 0.13 (0.06) | 0.31 (0.27) |
| No. of items | 60 | 180 | 180 | 180 |
| *Living* (*n* = 30) | | | | |
| Shared | 0.96 (0.06) | 0.60 (0.12) | 0.75 (0.14) | 0.76 (0.18) |
| No. of items | 180 | 180 | 120 | 116 |
| Distinctive | – | 0.18 (0.08) | 0.24 (0.12) | 0.20 (0.11) |
| No. of items | – | 180 | 120 | 156 |

Data drawn from Garrard et al. (2001). Table shows the mean and standard deviation (in parentheses) of the distinctiveness index; the number of items for living things and artefacts over semantic feature types is provided.

to the same chance probability of answering with yes or no (chance level: 50%). Information on the number and type of questions (mean and *SD* of the distinctiveness index) and number of questions in the two general domains of living things and artefacts and for four different types of semantic information is given in Table 4.

*Experiment 1b: Mass-kinds.* A featural database was collected on 118 items from 15 normal Italian subjects, all matched to MU for age, sex, and education (see Experiment 3b), following exactly the procedure adopted by Garrard and colleagues (2001) for artefacts and living things. From the original set, a reduced featural database related to 40 item was selected: edible substances, 16 items: 8 sauces (4 powdery, e.g., *paprika*, and 4 creamy, e.g., *mayonnaise*) and 8 foods (4 meats, e.g., *boiled ham*, and 4 cheeses, e.g., *gorgonzola cheese*); drinks, 8 items: 4 alcoholic (e.g., *beer*) and 4 nonalcoholic (e.g., *coke*); materials, 16 items: 4 metals (e.g., *gold*) and 4 precious stones (e.g., *sapphire*), 4 textiles (e.g., *wool*) and 4 "other kinds of materials" (e.g., *wood*). From the 40-item database, two indexes of semantic relatedness to the three main categories were computed with the same procedure as that followed by Garrard et al. (2001): dominance (proportion of subjects who generated each attribute) and distinctiveness (the extent to which a feature allows a particular concept to be distinguished from other members of the same category).

A subset of features related to the 40 items was selected, with the same procedure as for the artefacts and living things set. Items were made into "yes" questions, and a set of "no" questions was generated (e.g., category: *"Is mayonnaise a sauce? / Is mayonnaise a material?"*; encyclopaedic: *"Does mineral water contain gas? / Is mineral water found in jewellery shops?"*; functional: *"Can wood be cut? / Can wood be eaten?"*; sensory: *"Is coarse salt white? / Is coarse salt reddish?"*). Table 5 provides basic information on the distribution of distinctive and shared features (mean and *SD* of the distinctiveness index; number of questions) over (1) both the whole questionnaire and the three subsets of mass-kinds, and (2) the four different types of semantic information.

**Table 5.** *Experiment 1b: Distribution of shared and distinctive properties over the four types of semantic features*

| *Properties* | *Category* | *Encyclopaedic* | *Functional* | *Sensory* |
|---|---|---|---|---|
| *Whole set* (*n* = 40) | | | | |
| Shared | 0.68 (0.05) | 0.70 (0.17) | 0.57 (0.08) | 0.56 (0.06) |
| No. of items | 70 | 50 | 58 | 54 |
| Distinctive | 0.28 (0.09) | 0.14 (0.11) | 0.14 (0.09) | 0.16 (0.10) |
| No. of items | 36 | 788 | 584 | 586 |
| *Edible substances* (*n* = 16) | | | | |
| Shared | 0.73 (0.01) | – | – | – |
| No. of items | 32 | – | – | – |
| Distinctive | 0.32 (0) | 0.14 (0.11) | 0.14 (0.10) | 0.13 (0.08) |
| No. of items | 8 | 380 | 264 | 234 |
| *Drinks* (*n* = 8) | | | | |
| Shared | 0.65 (0) | 0.84 (0.08) | 0.55 (0.10) | 0.67 (0.03) |
| No. of items | 8 | 16 | 22 | 14 |
| Distinctive | 0.21 (0.08) | 0.13 (0.10) | 0.16 (0.07) | 0.22 (0.12) |
| No. of items | 4 | 194 | 88 | 94 |
| *Materials* (*n* = 16) | | | | |
| Shared | 0.63 (0.01) | 0.53 (0.05) | 0.60 (0) | 0.52 (0.01) |
| No. of items | 30 | 34 | 36 | 40 |
| Distinctive | 0.30 (0.10) | 0.14 (0.12) | 0.14 (0.09) | 0.17 (0.11) |
| No. of items | 24 | 214 | 232 | 258 |

The table shows the mean and standard deviation (in parentheses) of the distinctiveness index; the number of items for both the whole set of mass-kinds and the three subsets over semantic feature types is provided.

Given the large number of questions, 1892 in Experiment 1a and 2226 in Experiment 1b, the tests were administered to HSE patients in about 7–8 (Experiment 1a) or 10 (Experiment 1b) sessions. In Experiment 1b about four sessions were sufficient for normal subjects in order to complete the test. In both experiments the question sets were presented orally in a random sequence to subjects. Since, in the case of patients, and in MU's case in particular, responses to questions were often characterised by don't know answers, and they refused to guess, the responses were divided into three categories: *correct*, *don't know*, and *wrong*. Therefore, computations have been made with MU's correct answers considered equal to 1, don't know answers equal to .5, and wrong answers equal to 0. The comparison of MU's performance across different conditions uses nonparametric trend tests.

### *Results*

*Experiment 1a.* With the general domains of artefacts and living things (see Table 6), when MU's performance was evaluated in contrast to the mean percentage of patient controls a deficit was found to affect the living things domain, where he was about 32% worse than the patient controls; his performance was, however, comparable to that of patient controls with respect to artefacts. The patient control group was slightly better on living things than on artefacts. However, when a comparison was carried out over items the difference was not significant (Mann-Whitney test: U(n = 62) = 363, $p > .50$, two-tailed). However, MU's performance was strikingly different, being significantly better on artefacts (Jonckheere-Terpstra test (n = 1892) = −15.40, $p < .0001$).

Table 7 shows performance across different question types. MU showed a significant superiority of artefacts over living things on all of the category (Jonckheere-Terpstra test (n = 360) = −4.65, $p < .0001$), encyclopaedic (Jonckheere-Terpstra test (n = 544) = −6.84, $p < .0001$), functional (Jonckheere-Terpstra test (n = 483) = −8.63, $p < .0001$), and sensory (Jonckheere-Terpstra test: (n = 516) = −8.67, $p < .0001$) type of questions. Controls showed a trend towards performing better on living things than on artefacts (which was significant for category information (Mann-Whitney test over items: U(n = 62) = 18.50, $p < .001$), except for functional questions, where they were significantly better for artefacts (Mann-Whitney test over items: U(n = 62) = 289, $p < .01$).

In a second analysis, the different types of questions about features were collapsed together into four sets, concerning categorical, encyclopaedic, functional, and sensory information respectively.

**Table 6.** *Experiments 1a and 1b: Knowledge of five semantic domains*

| | *Experiment 1a* | | *Experiment 1b* | | |
|---|---|---|---|---|---|
| | *Artefacts* | *Living* | *Edible substances* | *Drinks* | *Materials* |
| *MU* | | | | | |
| Correct | 88.20 | 57.20 | 53.10 | 54.70 | 52.10 |
| DK | 10.40 | 28.40 | 21.60 | 31.40 | 24.90 |
| Wrong | 1.40 | 15.10 | 25.10 | 14.90 | 22.60 |
| *Controls*[a] | | | | | |
| Correct | 86.40 | 89.80 | 91.80 | 93.80 | 91.90 |
| (*SD*) | (12.90) | (5.50) | (6.30) | (4.40) | (4.80) |
| *MU–control comparison*[b] | | | | | |
| *z* | +0.10 | −6 | −6.14 | −8.89 | −8.29 |
| *p* | >.10 | <.0001 | <.0001 | <.0001 | <.0001 |

MU's performance in different conditions is represented as percentage of correct, "don't know" (DK) and wrong answers. Controls' score is given as mean percentage (*SD*) correct.

[a]HSE patients were used as control group to MU's performance in Experiment 1a; normal subjects were used as control group in Experiment 1b.

[b]*z* refers to the comparison of correct results (the other subjects did not produce "don't know" responses).

Table 7. *Experiments 1a and 1b: Knowledge of different feature types across semantic domains*

| | *Experiment 1a* | | *Experiment 1b* | | |
|---|---|---|---|---|---|
| *Feature types* | *Artefacts* | *Living* | *Edible substances* | *Drinks* | *Materials* |
| *Category* | | | | | |
| MU | | | | | |
| Correct | 99.40 | 87.20 | 87.50 | 80 | 36 |
| DK | 0.55 | 10 | 0 | 7.50 | 37.90 |
| Wrong | 0 | 2.78 | 12.50 | 12.50 | 26.10 |
| Controls[a] | | | | | |
| Correct | 85.40 | 98.60 | 97.50 | 98 | 90.40 |
| (*SD*) | (12.40) | (1.30) | (5.50) | (4.50) | (10.80) |
| MU–control comparison[b] | | | | | |
| $z$ | +1.10 | −8.80 | −1.82 | −4 | −5.04 |
| $p$ | >.10 | <.0001 | <.05 | <.0001 | <.0001 |
| *Encyclopaedic* | | | | | |
| MU | | | | | |
| Correct | 75 | 48.60 | 54.70 | 59.80 | 56.30 |
| DK | 24.40 | 32.50 | 20.30 | 29.40 | 28.80 |
| Wrong | 0.56 | 19.40 | 25 | 10.80 | 14.40 |
| Controls[a] | | | | | |
| Correct | 81.10 | 88.20 | 91.60 | 94.10 | 90.50 |
| *SD* | (16.60) | (8.90) | (10.50) | (2.70) | (4.50) |
| MU–control comparison[b] | | | | | |
| $z$ | −0.4 | −4.50 | −3.51 | −12.70 | −7.60 |
| $p$ | >.10 | <.0001 | <.0005 | <.0001 | <.0001 |
| *Functional* | | | | | |
| MU | | | | | |
| Correct | 94.60 | 60 | 67.90 | 64.40 | 65.40 |
| DK | 3.75 | 21.70 | 11.20 | 23.30 | 16.30 |
| Wrong | 1.67 | 18.30 | 20.90 | 13.30 | 18.20 |
| Controls[a] | | | | | |
| Correct | 92.10 | 86 | 91.60 | 93.20 | 95.10 |
| (*SD*) | (7.50) | (6.30) | (7.60) | (5.60) | (3.30) |
| MU–control comparison[b] | | | | | |
| $z$ | +0.33 | −8.44 | −3.12 | −5.14 | −9 |
| $p$ | >.10 | <.0001 | <.001 | <.0001 | <.0001 |
| *Sensory* | | | | | |
| MU | | | | | |
| Correct | 83.30 | 48.80 | 29 | 28 | 33.90 |
| DK | 13.70 | 41.20 | 38.80 | 50 | 29.03 |
| Wrong | 2.90 | 10 | 31.90 | 22 | 37.10 |
| Controls[a] | | | | | |
| Correct | 85.60 | 89.30 | 91.40 | 93.20 | 89.80 |
| *SD* | (4.90) | (2.80) | (9.20) | (7.60) | (6.80) |
| MU–control comparison[b] | | | | | |
| $z$ | −0.50 | −14.60 | −6.78 | −8.59 | −8.22 |
| $p$ | >.10 | <.0001 | <.0001 | <.0001 | <.0001 |

MU's performance in different conditions is represented as a percentage of correct, "don't know" (DK), and wrong answers. Controls' score is given as mean percentage (*SD*) correct.

[a]HSE patients were used as control group to MU's performance in Experiment 1a; normal subjects were used as control group in Experiment 1b.

[b]$z$ refers to the comparison of correct results (the other subjects did not produce "don't know" responses).

For artefacts MU did not differ from the patient controls on *any* of the question types in the number of correct answers he gave. However, for living things he differed significantly from controls on each of the question types in terms of the number of correct answers given (see Table 7). There was no essential difference in his performance on functional and sensory questions.

*Experiment 1b.* MU's knowledge of the mass-kinds domain was very impaired in comparison to the performance of the group of normal subjects (Table 6). For all feature types he was significantly worse than the control group for all of the three categories of edible substances, drinks, and materials (see Table 7). The critical comparison concerned knowledge of different question types (see Table 7). MU was well above chance on all question types except one. The one exception was on sensory questions, where he was very slightly and insignificantly below chance for all categories, in the sense that his "wrong" score was slightly higher than the "correct" one. Moreover his performance on sensory questions was significantly worse than for functional features (edible substances: Jonckheere-Terpstra test ($n = 251$) $= -5.08$, $p < .0001$; drinks: Jonckheere-Terpstra test ($n = 110$) $= -3.31$, $p < .001$; materials: Jonckheere-Terpstra test ($n = 283$) $= -5.11$, $p < .0001$; whole set: Jonckheere-Terpstra test ($n = 644$) $= -7.94$, $p < .0001$). Normal controls were above 89% for all question types for all of mass categories. In addition, except for a small but significant difference on materials (Mann-Whitney test over items: $U(n = 283) = 8230$, $p < .001$), but absolutely no difference for edible substances and drinks, their performance was virtually identical for functional and sensory questions (see Table 7 and Figure 1).

*Discussion*

MU's ability to verify the appropriateness of different feature types was characterised by a sparing of both functional and sensory information for artefacts. With mass-kinds, the patient showed a complete loss of sensory properties, while functional features were significantly better preserved across all the three subsets. For edible substances and drinks controls showed no difference between the two types of knowledge. For materials the difference between functional and sensory knowledge was much greater for MU than for normal controls (25.14% vs. 5.3%). However, his performance with living things did not show a significant difference between the two types of critical feature, although he was somewhat poorer with sensory properties relative to functional.

One possible explanation of MU's poor performance with auditory presented sensory features of mass-kinds is that it arises from an inability to access the concept underlying sensory feature terms given verbal input. Thus he might have lost the

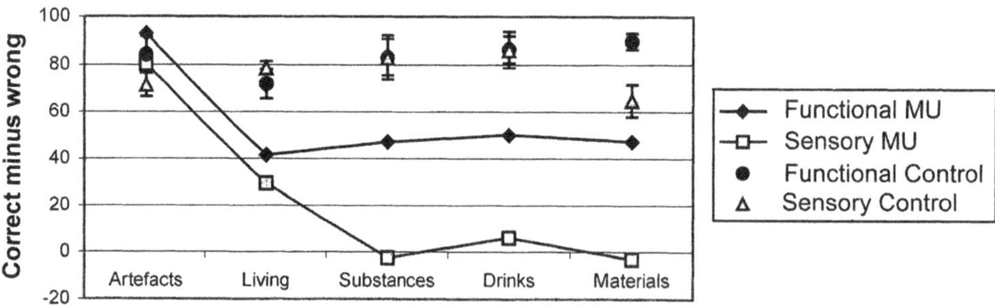


**Figure 1.** *Experiments 1a and 1b: Interaction between knowledge of features and semantic domains: comparison between functional and sensory information in MU and control groups. Please note that data are represented as correct* minus *wrong answers. HSE patients were used as control group to MU's performance in Experiment 1a; normal subjects were used as control group in Experiment 1b.*

meaning of a concept like "red" or "hard," or have difficulty accessing them from verbal input.

## Experiment 2: Feature comprehension control tasks

Could MU's problem arise from an inability to comprehend the questions about sensory feature properties or to access sensory features from the verbal modality? In order to ascertain MU's ability to deal with the meaning of different types of property tested in Experiment 1, a series of control tasks was devised that involved a modality of presentation for the stimulus itself that was different from the auditory one. Two conditions were used. In one the information requested in the auditory question has to be obtained from the subject's knowledge of the item. In the second it is directly available from perception of the item itself. If the patient has a real problem in knowledge, performance in the two conditions will differ.

### *Method: Stimuli and procedure*

In this experiment, a verbal property (e.g., *"Is this thing smooth?"*) is given to the patient when an item is presented. The patient's task is to judge whether the property is appropriate for the presented item. Properties were again selected from the mass-kinds database adopted in Experiment 1b. The same number of features was used in both types of presentation (353 functional and 291 sensory). In the first condition, which is broadly equivalent to the previous experiment except that the input was primarily visual, actual mass-kind items were presented to the patient. The patient was only allowed to inspect them visually, since some sensory information cannot be derived from a visually presented object any more than from the verbal labels used in Experiment 1b (e.g., visual presentation of wood: *"Is it hard?"*). In the second condition, a multimodal presentation was used. The actual item is presented and the patient is allowed to inspect it in any way he wants, including manipulating and smelling it. Clearly this type of presentation is not practicable with living things. Stimuli were administered in random order to the patient. Eight sessions (once weekly, 1 hour per session) were necessary in the case of mass-kinds and the patient was allowed to stop whenever he needed. He insisted on responding "yes," "no," "don't know."

### *Results*

MU's ability to comprehend the meaning of functional and sensory features of mass-kinds proved to be highly sensitive to the type of presentation adopted (see Table 8). With visual presentation MU's performance was similar to that observed in Experiment 1b. An advantage in favour of functional features relative to sensory features characterised MU's performance for edible substances

**Table 8.** *Experiment 2: MU's ability to judge functional and sensory features related to stimuli with different types of presentation*

| | *Functional* | | | *Sensory* | | | *F–S difference* |
|---|---|---|---|---|---|---|---|
| *Categories* | *Correct* | *DK* | *Wrong* | *Correct* | *DK* | *Wrong* | *Correct* |
| *Visual presentation* | | | | | | | |
| Whole set | 67.40 | 26.60 | 5.90 | 41.90 | 46.40 | 11.70 | 25.50 |
| Drinks | 76.70 | 18.30 | 5.00 | 60.00 | 26.00 | 14.00 | 16.70 |
| Edible substances | 59.70 | 30.60 | 9.70 | 39.30 | 51.30 | 9.40 | 20.40 |
| Materials | 70.40 | 26.40 | 3.10 | 37.10 | 50.00 | 12.90 | 33.30 |
| *Multi-modal presentation* | | | | | | | |
| Whole set | 79.30 | 16.70 | 4.00 | 76.60 | 13.00 | 10.30 | 2.69 |
| Drinks | 85.00 | 11.70 | 3.30 | 84.00 | 12.00 | 4.00 | 1.00 |
| Edible substances | 73.90 | 20.10 | 6.00 | 67.50 | 21.40 | 11.10 | 6.40 |
| Materials | 81.80 | 15.70 | 2.50 | 82.20 | 5.60 | 12.10 | -0.40 |

Performance is expressed as mean percentage of correct, "don't know" (DK) and wrong answers: (1) visual and (2) multi-modal presentation of actual mass-kind stimuli.

(Jonckheere-Terpstra test (n = 251) = −2.78, $p < .01$), for drinks (Jonckheere-Terpstra test (n = 110) = −1.99, $p < .05$), for materials (Jonckheere-Terpstra test (n = 283) = −5.76, $p < .001$), and for the whole mass-kinds set (Jonckheere-Terpstra test (n = 644) = −6.40, $p < .001$).

However, when MU was allowed to explore mass-kind stimuli through many modalities, his performance was much better (see Figure 2). Moreover the difference between functional and sensory features is no longer present when he is allowed to explore the real thing. This finding was confirmed by the comparison of MU's behaviour with the two types of features; no difference was observed for any of the mass-kind sets (drinks: Jonckheere-Terpstra test (n = 110) = −0.15, $p > .50$; edible substances: Jonckheere-Terpstra test (n = 251) = −1.26, $p > .10$; materials: Jonckheere-Terpstra test (n = 283) = −0.27, $p > .50$; whole mass-kinds set: Jonckheere-Terpstra test: (n = 644) = −1.18, $p > .10$).

Did the improvement that MU showed in the multimodal test for sensory-quality types of information occur only as a result of sensory attributes for which manipulation, or a richer visual representation, produced a direct answer (e.g., *wood*: *"Is the surface smooth?"*)? Or did the effect also occur for features that are not helped by the enhanced quality of the input (e.g., *wood*: *"Is it transparent?"*)? A further inspection of MU's performance with mass-kinds showed that the first possibility was the case (see Table 9). With sensory features of mass-kinds that could be directly helped by manipulation and detailed inspection (items = 175), he was far poorer in the first modality of presentation, but his performance was dramatically enhanced when he was allowed to manipulate. In contrast, with mass-kinds sensory features that could not be further helped by manipulation and detailed inspection (items = 116), MU had a similar level of performance in the two conditions. Therefore, with the mass-kinds MU's performance (correct plus "50% don't know" answers) benefited much more for sensory features that could be directly explored by manipulation (25.43% vs. 6.90% difference).

*Discussion*

In the control experiment it was shown that MU's impairment in the verification task on knowing the sensory features of mass-kinds did not arise from a general difficulty in comprehending the meaning of the questions from auditory input. With all categories he had a comparable level of performance with sensory and functional features if an enriched sensory input was provided (i.e., if he was allowed to explore an actual object).

By contrast, MU showed a much poorer performance on all mass-kind categories when the modality of presentation was constrained to the

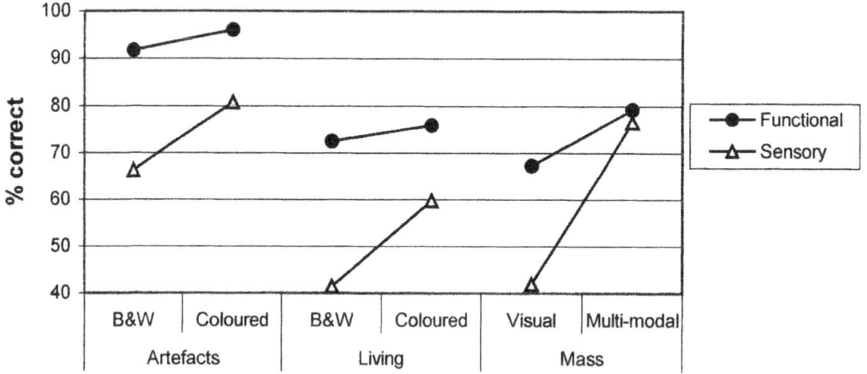


**Figure 2.** *Experiment 2: MU's correct judgements about item–feature pairs in (a) visual and (b) multi-modal presentation of actual mass-kind stimuli; (c) black-&-white and (d) coloured presentation of living things and artefact drawings.*

**Table 9.** *Experiment 2: Effect of different types of presentation on sensory features that can or cannot be directly checked on the stimulus*

| | *Sensory features* | | | | | | *Difference between presentation types* | |
|---|---|---|---|---|---|---|---|---|
| | *Direct available* | | | *No direct available* | | | | |
| *Presentation* | *Correct* | *DK* | *Wrong* | *Correct* | *DK* | *Wrong* | *Direct available* | *No direct available* |
| *Mass-kinds* | | | | | | | | |
| Visual | 43 (57.71) | 116 | 16 | 79 (76.29) | 19 | 18 | 25.43 | 6.9 |
| Multi-modal | 131 (83.14) | 29 | 15 | 92 (83.19) | 9 | 15 | | |

Raw data are given for correct, "don't know" (DK), and wrong answers. Percentage of correct *and* "0.5 don't know" answers are in parentheses. The percentage difference on correct answers between the two types of presentation is presented in the last two columns for sensory features that can or cannot be directly determined from the stimulus.

simple inspection of an actual stimulus. Finally, his improvement in the richer input conditions was not a generalised effect of using multiple modalities of input, but was instead specific for the sensory features that could be directly checked on the stimulus in the multimodal condition.

## Experiment 3: Feature production task

The spontaneous production of semantic information about a large number of living things, artefacts (Experiment 3a), and mass-kinds (Experiment 3b) was investigated through the adoption of an attribute generation procedure. In this task, patients were presented with a series of words referring to artefacts, living things, and mass-kind categories.

### *Method: Stimuli and procedure for Experiments 3a and 3b*

In Experiment 3a the stimulus set comprised the same set of 30 living things and 32 artefacts (see Table 3) used in Experiment 1a. In Experiment 3b a set of 118 stimuli, subdivided into 52 edible substances, 27 drinkable and nondrinkable liquids, and 39 materials was used (see Table 3). The set of mass-kinds was presented to 10 normal subjects who had to rate the familiarity of each item on a 5-point scale.

In Experiment 3a, MU's performance was compared to that of three HSE patient controls (CAL, SAR, and BAI), since the fourth patient, MIO, refused to complete the task. In Experiment 3b, since HSE patient controls were not available at the time testing was performed, the 15 male normal subjects, matched to MU in terms of their age (mean = 29.2 years; range = 26–33) and education (13 years), from whom the database (also used in Experiment 1b as a reduced version) was collected, were treated as control group.

All participants had unlimited time to describe each of the items as exhaustively as they could, and were allowed to rearrange or change their definitions until they were satisfied. In Experiment 3a patients' production of semantic details was constantly encouraged by a standard procedure, because they often tended to provide highly sketchy descriptions of the stimuli. This involved four questions: *"What is the general category of this item?"*; *"This item can . . ."*; *"This item has . . ."*; *"This item is . . ."*. The spoken responses were recorded by the examiner. Furthermore, a range of three–four sessions of testing was necessary for each patient, in order to prevent responses becoming stereotyped and to avoid losing their collaboration. Patients were tested weekly for an hour per session, and were allowed to stop roughly every 10 min.

In Experiment 3b, a featural database for mass-kinds was collected from normal subjects, following exactly the same procedure adopted by Garrard et al. (2001), where participants were asked to answer in the written modality. For MU, six testing sessions were necessary. The patient was tested in the auditory modality weekly, for an hour per session, and was allowed to stop about every 10 min in order to prevent stereotyped responses.

In both Experiments 3a and 3b, the semantic attributes production was classified by two independent judges as pertaining to four classes of semantic information, namely, category, encyclopaedic, functional, and sensory information, on the basis of the criteria developed by Garrard et al. (2001). Only the semantic properties that were classified by both of two judges as belonging to a given type of semantic information were included in the subsequent analyses. Since the number of features produced by each participant was different, the raw scores related to each condition were recomputed in terms of proportions with respect to the total number of features generated by each of the subjects.

*Results*

*Experiment 3a.* The overall ability to produce information related to each of the five semantic domains was examined in MU and in the patient controls. MU's performance with living things was much reduced with respect to the performance of patient controls; a similar trend was also observed in the case of artefacts. As can be seen in Table 10, the ratio of functional-to-sensory information produced by MU was much greater than that of the controls for both artefacts ($z = 5.79, p < .001$) and living things ($z = 6.35, p < .001$).

*Experiment 3b.* MU produced many fewer features overall than the normal controls. However, as can be seen from Table 10, the ratio of functional-to-sensory features produced by MU was again much greater than that of normal controls. This was the case for all the types of mass-kinds (edible substances: $z = 14.20, p < .001$; liquids: $z = 4.14, p < .001$), except for materials ($z = 0.47, p > .10$).

*Discussion*

MU's production of features related to different semantic classes was in general poor. However, while his performance with living things and artefacts was comparable to patient controls (Experiment 3a), he showed a significant difference with the three categories of mass-kinds in comparison to normal subjects (Experiment 3b). As his performance is being compared to different types of controls, this difference between types of semantic domain is not interpretable. What is critical is that for four of the semantic categories he produced a higher ratio of functional-to-sensory features than did controls.

As can be observed in Figure 3, even when the scores of MU and the two control groups related to all five semantic categories are collapsed across different types of features, the crossover interaction between functional and sensory features is observed. It should be noted that encyclopaedic properties show a similar pattern to functional features both in MU and the controls. Therefore the patient's knowledge of associative and contextual information about different semantic domains is relatively intact. This is of relevance with respect to previous studies, where these types of information were often included under the "functional" label. As far as category information is concerned, MU's performance is closely comparable to that of controls. It can be concluded that his knowledge of superordinate information is well preserved.

*Experiment 4: Feature explanation control tasks*

In order to rule out the possibility that MU's performance with functional and sensory attributes in the feature production task was due to an inability to know the appropriate type of feature information rather than lack of knowledge of the items themselves, a feature explanation task was devised for patient MU only.

*Method: Stimuli and procedure*

As far as living things and artefacts were concerned, the test comprised a total number of 58 functional and 80 sensory features. In the case of mass-kinds, the patient was asked to deal with 160 functional and 108 sensory features. All features were selected from the two databases used in Experiments 1a and 1b. Since a large number of identical features, used in the two databases, could apply to a variety of stimuli belonging to any of the semantic categories being investigated (e.g., *black* can be appropriate for *"tyre," "panther," "crow," "aubergine," "petroleum,"*

Table 10. *Experiments 3a and 3b: Feature production for five categories (z and p refer to proportions of different feature types)*

| | | *Experiment 3a* | | *Experiment 3b* | | |
|---|---|---|---|---|---|---|
| | | *Artefacts* | *Living* | *Edible substances* | *Liquids* | *Materials* |
| *Category* | MU | | | | | |
| | Raw | 4 | 18 | 8 | 8 | 6 |
| | Proportion | 3.01 | 16.70 | 3.52 | 7.14 | 6.06 |
| | Controls[a] | | | | | |
| | Raw mean | 15.30 | 25.30 | 42.00 | 24.10 | 29.50 |
| | Proportion | 6.49 | 12.60 | 6.96 | 8.37 | 7.01 |
| | (*SD*) | (2.30) | (4.20) | (1.73) | (1.75) | (2.40) |
| | MU–control comparison | | | | | |
| | *z* | −1.49 | +0.96 | −1.99 | −1.70 | −0.39 |
| | *p* | >.05 | >.10 | <.05 | <.05 | >.10 |
| *Encyclopaedic* | MU | | | | | |
| | Raw | 50 | 29 | 96 | 50 | 42 |
| | Proportion | 37.60 | 26.80 | 42.29 | 44.60 | 42.40 |
| | Controls[a] | | | | | |
| | Raw mean | 63.30 | 73.30 | 242.40 | 123.30 | 132.00 |
| | Proportion | 27.60 | 35.20 | 37.90 | 41.00 | 30.00 |
| | (*SD*) | (9.40) | (15.00) | (5.00) | (5.50) | (3.50) |
| | MU–control comparison | | | | | |
| | *z* | +1.07 | −0.56 | +0.89 | +0.66 | +3.50 |
| | *p* | >.10 | >.10 | >.10 | >.10 | <.0005 |
| *Functional* | MU | | | | | |
| | Raw | 56 | 44 | 93 | 39 | 30 |
| | Proportion | 42.10 | 40.70 | 40.97 | 34.80 | 30.30 |
| | Controls[a] | | | | | |
| | Raw mean | 73.00 | 55.00 | 186.70 | 97.10 | 156.80 |
| | Proportion | 32.80 | 24.03 | 29.02 | 31.80 | 35.50 |
| | (*SD*) | (6.50) | (8.40) | (4.60) | (5.10) | (4.70) |
| | MU–control comparison | | | | | |
| | *z* | +1.43 | +1.99 | +2.57 | +0.58 | −1.10 |
| | *p* | >.05 | <.05 | <.01 | >.10 | >.10 |
| *Sensory* | MU | | | | | |
| | Raw | 23 | 17 | 30 | 15 | 21 |
| | Proportion | 17.30 | 15.70 | 13.20 | 13.40 | 21.20 |
| | Controls[a] | | | | | |
| | Raw mean | 71.30 | 59.30 | 160.60 | 56.00 | 120.20 |
| | Proportion | 33.10 | 28.10 | 26.10 | 18.80 | 27.50 |
| | (*SD*) | (5.20) | (12.50)[b] | (4.23) | (2.80) | (2.58) |
| | MU–control comparison | | | | | |
| | *z* | −3.04 | −0.99 | −3.05 | −1.94 | −2.44 |
| | *p* | <.0005 | >.10 | <.0005 | <.05 | <.01 |
| *Ratio F/S* | MU | | | | | |
| | Raw | 56/23 | 44/17 | 93/30 | 39/15 | 30/21 |
| | Proportion | 2.43 | 2.59 | 3.10 | 2.60 | 1.43 |
| | Controls | | | | | |
| | Raw mean | 73/71.30 | 55/59.30 | 186.7/160.60 | 97.1/56 | 156.8/120.20 |
| | Proportion | 1.00 | 0.90 | 1.11 | 1.69 | 1.29 |
| | (*SD*) | (0.24) | (0.26) | (0.14) | (0.22) | (0.30) |
| | MU–control comparison | | | | | |
| | *z* | +5.79 | +6.35 | +14.20 | +4.14 | +0.47 |
| | *p* | <.00001 | <.00001 | <.00001 | <.00001 | >.10 |

For patient MU raw data are provided; the performance of the controls is expressed as a mean of the individual subjects. In the lower part of the table the comparison between MU and controls' performance on the critical variables is expressed as ratio of functional (F) and sensory (S) features.

[a]HSE patients were used as control group to MU's performance in Experiment 3a; normal subjects were used as control group in Experiment 3b.

[b]Task insensitive: The patient controls range is such that MU cannot perform 2 *SD* below the controls mean.

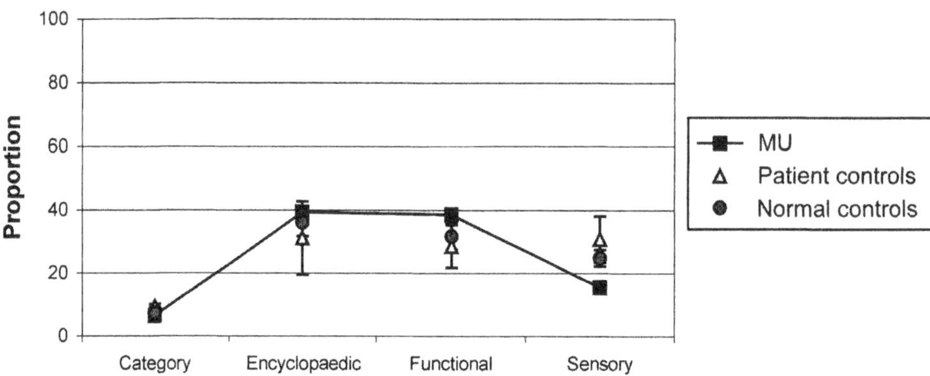


**Figure 3.** *Experiments 3a and 3b: Production of different feature types in MU and two control groups. HSE patients were used as control group to MU's performance in Experiment 3a; normal subjects were used as control group in Experiment 3b.*

*"liquorice," "coal"*), care was taken in the feature selection not to repeat the same property twice.

In this task, a verbal property was given to the patient, who had to provide a description or examples of things that have that attribute (e.g., *"Tell me the meaning of something having spots, or give me an example of something having spots"* or *"Tell me the meaning of something being soft, or give me an example of something soft"*). The task was administered verbally, and the features to be explained were given in random order; for living things and artefacts, about three sessions (occurring weekly, 1 hour per session) were needed to collect the data. For mass-kinds, the task was carried out in about four sessions (occurring weekly, 1 hour per session). In both tasks the patient was allowed to stop whenever he needed to. MU's answers were classified by two independent judges as appropriate for the item (correct description or example), inappropriate (wrong description or example), or omission if he refused to answer ("don't know"). The answers that were not classified in the same fashion by the two blind judges were discarded. The statistical analysis was again carried out on MU's correct answers.

### *Results*

MU's ability to provide appropriate descriptions or examples of sensory and functional features was found to be comparable for all the semantic domains considered (see Table 11). In the case of living things, he could provide correct explanations of both types of features, and no significant difference was observed (Jonckheere-Terpstra test (n = 63) = −1.17, $p > .10$). The same pattern was also found for artefacts (Jonckheere-Terpstra test (n = 76) = −1.50, $p > .10$). With the three mass-kind sets,

**Table 11.** *Experiment 4: Comprehension of two types of features: MU's mean percentage for living things, artefacts, and mass-kinds*

| | *Functional* | | | *Sensory* | | | *F–S* |
|---|---|---|---|---|---|---|---|
| | *Correct* | *DK* | *Wrong* | *Correct* | *DK* | *Wrong* | *difference* |
| *Living* | 79.20 | 12.50 | 8.30 | 64.10 | 25.60 | 10.20 | 15.10 |
| *Artefacts* | 97.00 | 2.90 | 0.00 | 82.90 | 9.70 | 7.30 | 14.10 |
| *Drinks* | 70.40 | 14.80 | 14.80 | 81.80 | 4.50 | 13.60 | −11.40 |
| *Edible substances* | 75.00 | 5.30 | 19.60 | 68.20 | 6.80 | 25.00 | 6.80 |
| *Materials* | 77.90 | 13.00 | 9.10 | 83.30 | 12.00 | 4.80 | −5.40 |

although he was somehow better with sensory than functional features in the case of drinks and materials, MU did not show significant differences in providing explanations of the two types of features (drinks: Jonckheere-Terpstra test (n = 40) = 0.80, $p > .10$; edible substances: Jonckheere-Terpstra test (n = 100) = −0.74, $p > .10$; materials: Jonckheere-Terpstra test (n = 119) = 0.76, $p > .10$).

Then, his behaviour across semantic domains was analysed with respect to functional and sensory features considered separately. Examining MU's performance on functional features across all five semantic domains, no significant difference was observed between his performance on the five sets (Jonckheere-Terpstra test (n = 219) = −0.90, $p > .10$). Similarly, in the case of sensory features MU did not show a significant difference in performance across the five categories (Jonckheere-Terpstra test (n = 188) = 0.97, $p > .10$).

### *Discussion*

In this experiment there was no significant difference in MU's ability to explain functional and sensory features in any of the five categories. Thus his poor performance in producing sensory features (Experiments 3a and 3b) cannot be attributed to the lack of knowledge of the features per se. In fact, MU's explanations of feature meaning were characterized by definitions or examples mostly related to artefacts (e.g., *something hard*: *"The table is hard"*).

## GENERAL DISCUSSION

MU is a herpes encephalitic patient whose knowledge of a set of categories we have previously investigated (Borgo & Shallice, 2001). He had the selective problem with comprehension and naming of living things previously found in over 20 patients with this aetiology (Borgo, 2001; Capitani et al., 2003-this issue; Gainotti, 2000; Warrington & Shallice, 1984). We showed, however, that his impairment also extended to three additional categories—edible and nonedible substances, drinkable and nondrinkable liquids, and materials—which we called collectively mass-kinds. Difficulty with mass-kind categories had also been reported by Warrington and Shallice (1984) in one of their original herpes category-specific patients, JBR.

In the current paper we used an approach developed by Garrard et al. (2001) to investigate in detail MU's knowledge of the functional and sensory characteristics of artefacts, living things, and mass-kinds. The approach involves the use of large data sets of features rated for frequency, familiarity, distinctiveness, and dominance. Two different procedures were then adopted. The first involved questions concerning specific features. In all, MU answered 4118 questions. The second involved production of information about items in the categories elicited by particular probe questions. The assumption also needs to be made that all categories lend themselves equally well to the linguistic specification of their critical properties.

The first type of procedure produced clear results for the mass-kind categories and for artefacts. For the mass-kind categories MU's performance was very similar across the three categories. He was worse than controls on knowledge of functional aspects of mass-kind categories but well above chance. However, in tests of his knowledge of the sensory aspects of three categories, he performed no better than chance. Moreover, a control condition showed that the difficulty that MU had in decisions about the sensory features of mass-kinds could not be attributed to any lack of understanding of the concepts used in the questions. When the same questions were asked but with the object itself being present the patient could generally answer it. In this condition his performance on sensory categories was much improved and now showed no difference from his knowledge of the functional properties of these categories. This implies that he had no sensory knowledge of items in mass-kind categories when it was not physically apparent to him from the stimulus. By contrast his knowledge of artefacts was good for all types of question. For living things his performance was significantly below normal controls but well above chance for all types of question. As for a number of patients discussed by Caramazza and Shelton (1998), who we refer to in the Introduction, he was only marginally, and not significantly, better on knowledge of functional than sensory aspects of living things.

The results of Experiment 1 are quite similar to those reported in Borgo and Shallice (2001), where MU was tested with the three-alternatives questionnaires on living things and artefacts devised by Laiacona et al. (1993b) and on a similar mass-kinds one. In this earlier work, MU was worse than controls on living things and mass-kinds, while comparable to controls on artefacts; moreover, though no difference was observed between functional and sensory knowledge in the case of artefacts and living things, a clear difference between feature types was obtained for mass-kinds (functional vs. sensory over all mass-kind categories: 81% vs. 58% correct; 24% difference). It should be noted that Laiacona et al.'s questionnaire controls only for properties of individual stimuli, such as frequency, and not for cross-stimuli properties like distinctiveness. Critically, however, the current Experiment 1 is based on a much larger set of items and, being a two-alternatives task, is also simpler than Laiacona et al.'s questionnaire. With this task a clear difference is observed in MU's feature type knowledge (see Figure 1), with small functional/sensory differences in the case of artefacts (11.30%) and living things (11.20%), but a much larger one for the mass-kinds categories (overall 35.90% difference). In addition, in Experiment 2 performance on the sensory features of mass-kinds is very much improved if a richer sensory input is provided.

The second procedure also produced clear results suggesting a loss of sensory quality knowledge, but it was somewhat different in pattern to the findings from the first procedure. MU was—across the board, for all categories—less able to produce information on sensory characteristics than functional ones in comparison to controls, except, rather oddly, for the materials category. Again we showed that this effect could not be attributed to loss of knowledge of the features per se as, when asked to indicate what the features meant, he was equally able to do so for sensory and functional features.

Why should the pattern be different when using the two types of method? A possible explanation of MU's difficulty in producing sensory features spontaneously in Experiment 3 could be because of an inability to generate mental images, which would result in a generalised difficulty in inspecting and so producing the visual characteristics of the stimuli. It should, however, be noted that in Experiment 4, where he produces examples of particular concepts (e.g., *"soft"*), he virtually always gives an example from an artefact (e.g., *"pillow"*). This pattern is somewhat difficult to explain if a problem in imagery is the only relevant factor.

The feature elicitation task also clearly has characteristics in common with the fluency tasks used to study supervisory and executive functions. As a task, it has more processing components than the feature knowledge probe task. One possibility is therefore that certain of the systems, other than those responsible for knowledge of attributes, are producing a biasing effect with respect to the feature type × category interaction. This possibility cannot be ruled out but, given that the feature elicitation procedure produces a quite different pattern from the feature knowledge procedure, such a biasing must be complex. An alternative possibility is that relatively fragile sensory representations of living things and artefacts can be "supported" on Farah and McClelland's theory by functional representations (for categories where they are well represented) for the simple task of direct feature knowledge testing but are insufficient to allow spontaneous generation to occur in the feature elicitation task.

If we restrict consideration to the simpler procedure—the feature knowledge task—we are faced with a second set of questions. MU's performance on sensory knowledge of mass-kinds clearly supports the SFT, since in the categories where his naming deficit is most clearly manifested he is at chance on the sensory questions. However, three questions remain.

1. Why is he less good than controls on the functional questions for mass-kinds?
2. Why is he intact on sensory knowledge of artefacts?
3. Why is his performance on living things not more like that on mass-kinds?

A definitive answer cannot be given to these questions with the present set of findings. However, three *nonexclusive* possibilities need to be considered.

The first is that a Farah and McClelland type of theory applies and the strong functional representation for artefacts "supports" the degraded sensory representation. It is not clear on this account, however, why the functional attributes of living things are only insignificantly better than the sensory ones.

A second possibility is that the four-fold differentiation of type of knowledge is insufficiently fine-grained. Thus the sensory features that are properties of artefacts are often very strongly linked to functional knowledge. This approach would combine De Renzi and Lucchelli (1994) and Tyler et al.'s (2000) position on the form–function relation for artefacts with the SFT to explain the preservation of sensory knowledge of artefacts. As Cree and McRae (2001) have pointed out, a typical sensory feature tested for artefacts is a part, and parts of artefacts characteristically have a subfunction with respect to the whole artefact. This is not typical of the sensory features of materials; thus the colour of, say, mayonnaise or coal is not obviously related to their being added to dishes of cold salmon or being burnable.

Why, on this perspective, should there be a difference between living things and mass-kinds? Cree and McRae (2001), who also refer to relevant unpublished work by Wu and Barsalou, have argued in this type of context that a finer-grain analysis of feature types may be useful. The sensory attribute questions for living things in Garrard et al.'s battery which we used contains questions like *"Is a turtle brown?"* and *"Does a peacock make a noise?"*, which relate to sensory quality aspects but also ones concerned with body parts *"Does a turtle have a shell?"* or size *"Is a peacock large?"* or actions *"Can a peacock fan its tail?"*. The sensory attribute questions for mass-kinds were nearly all of the first type that were not related to parts or size or movements.

We accordingly reanalysed the living things findings in Experiment 1 using a finer grain analysis of features. The results are shown in Table 12. There is a significant difference across feature subtypes, $\chi^2(8) = 38.81$, $p < .0001$. Moreover performance is better with the more shape-related features, $\chi^2(1) = 11.50$, $p < .001$. This suggests that there is a deficit in sensory quality information for living things compared with functional information, but that this is masked by a relative sparing of shape-related information. As mass-kinds lack this latter type of information, MU's deficit is clearer in these categories. As far as we know, no such detailed investigation of knowledge of living things has been carried out in any other patient with a "broad living things" impairment, and in particular not in the theoretically problematic patients of this type discussed by Caramazza and Shelton in their review.

**Table 12.** *Reanalysis of sensory features of living things used in Experiment 1 into subtypes*

| | *MU's* | |
|---|---|---|
| *Subtype of features* | *raw score* | *% correct* |
| *Shape-related* | | |
| Body parts | 11/18 | 61.10 |
| Details of body | 41/102 | 40.20 |
| Dimension/shape | 56/88 | 63.60 |
| External parts | 9/22 | 40.90 |
| Internal parts | 15/27 | 55.60 |
| Total score | 132/257 | 51.40 |
| *Not shape-related* | | |
| Auditory | 17/29 | 58.60 |
| Colour | 4/36 | 11.10 |
| Tactile | 8/23 | 34.80 |
| Taste | 4/16 | 25.00 |
| Total score | 33/104 | 31.73 |

The third possibility, Warrington and McCarthy's position, that the different types of knowledge within the sensory and functional domains may be subdivisible, clearly fits closely with this last analysis. Living things, as just discussed, contain shape and size and movement information, which are generally lacking for the mass-kinds category. If they were generally more preserved in MU than, say, knowledge of texture, colour, pattern, smell, taste, and so on this could explain the relative advantage of the sensory quality aspects of living thing performance in MU by comparison with these aspects in mass-kinds. What is required is a more intensive investigation of different specific feature types in patients like MU. This too would address the problem of the differing definitions of "function," which was raised in the Introduction.

From the perspective of Caramazza and Shelton's theory, the data obtained with the feature verification task in Experiment 1 seems to fit well with their predictions when only living things and artefacts are considered, ignoring the finer-grain analysis of sensory quality information across living things. MU shows an advantage for artefacts over living things, without an interaction with functional and sensory features. However, contrary to assumptions that all aspects of a category will be affected in the same way, a large advantage of functional features relative to sensory ones was observed for all the three mass-kind categories. Moreover, sensory features were also demonstrated to be highly sensitive to the provision of an enriched sensory input in the control Experiment 2, so that the difference between sensory and functional features was one of knowledge.

Mass-kinds are not specifically considered on Caramazza and Shelton's theory. However, the more detailed analysis on living things also presents some difficulties for their position. Complementarily, as they point out findings on highly selective categorical deficits, in turn they potentially provide a major problem for the SFT. However, as discussed in the Introduction, these patients do not yet form a clear functional syndrome. We will consider two, EW (Caramazza & Shelton, 1998), with a selective loss of knowledge of animals, and JJ (Hillis & Caramazza, 1991), with selective preservation of this category.

EW's lesion site is very different from that of MU and those patients, typically with herpes simplex encephalitis, who show larger generalised living things impairments. EW had a fronto-parietal lesion. If one makes the assumption that the information-processing systems that one needs to postulate to account for neuropsychological data are relatively localised, a commonly assumed but rarely tested position (see Paulesu et al., 2003), then the gross difference in the lesion sites of MU and EW suggests that different subsystems are impaired. If this is the case then the fact that they exhibit category specificity as a behaviour is no more a reason for trying to explain them with the same type of account than it would be for any other single manifestation of behaviour, such as, say, exhibiting letter-by-letter reading. Indeed, the characteristics of the two types of disorder, both in terms of the categories impaired and the relative role of sensory and functional features, means that it would be an error to attempt to force them into the same theoretical mould.

JJ, by contrast, had a vascular lesion involving some part of the left temporal lobe (and the basal ganglia) and yet has selective *preservation* of animal naming (91% vs. 20% in other categories *including* fruit and vegetables at an early stage of the illness). However, somewhat later the contrast between animals on the one hand and other categories seemed to be predominantly one of naming, not storage, since only 15% of his definitions of nonanimal names were clearly wrong, with another 8% being "ambiguous." Moreover, in defining 70 nouns of animals and vegetables only 16% were wrong, while 70 names of other categories were all correctly defined (at an earlier stage such a test was not carried out). Again, one appears to have qualitatively a very different type of disorder from that of MU, quite apart from the categories affected. Assessment of the theoretical consequences of such patients awaits more detailed investigations of both their neurology as well as their neuropsychology.

The relation between the current results and the hierarchical interactive theory (HIT) is unclear. The HIT model contains three types of knowledge.

1. Stored structural descriptions.
2. Stored functional and inter-object association information.
3. Name representations.

Humphreys and Forde (2001), referring to the model of Humphreys, Lamote, and Lloyd-Jones (1995), describe "stored structural descriptions" as representing information about the shape of objects. It is not therefore clear in the model where colour, texture, and pattern information are stored. However, from the representation of their current model in Figure 3 of Humphreys and Forde (2001), it would appear that a position similar to that of Warrington and McCarthy (1987) is held. The results would presumably therefore be compatible with the HIT.

Overall, then, this investigation supports the conclusion of Borgo and Shallice (2001) that the sensory functional theory can be used to predict deficits in categories other than living things by showing that the impairments in these new categories mass-kinds are particularly linked with loss of sensory-information. A number of more specific questions about MU's performance need, however, to be addressed, as critically it remains to be seen whether these findings can be replicated in other patients with the same functional syndrome and in particular those with the prototypic aetiology for the impairment.

## REFERENCES

Benton, A. L., Silvan, A. B., Hamsher, K. de S., Varney, N. R., & Spreen, O. (1990). *Judgement of line orientation, form H.* Firenze, Italy: Organizzazioni Speciali.

Benton, A. L., Silvan, A. B., Hamsher, K. de S., Varney, N. R., & Spreen, O. (1992). *Facial recognition.* Firenze, Italy: Organizzazioni Speciali.

Borgo, F. (2001). *When panthers are really pink and diamonds are black. Living things and "mass" kinds knowledge in Herpes Simplex Virus Encephalitis: New evidence for a theoretical redefinition of category specific effects.* Doctoral dissertation, SISSA-ISAS, Trieste, Italy.

Borgo, F., & Shallice, T. (2001). When living things and other "sensory-quality" categories behave in the same fashion: A novel category-specificity effect. *Neurocase, 7*, 201–220.

Buxbaum, L., & Saffran, E. M. (1998). Knowing "how" vs. "what for": A new dissociation. *Brain and Language, 65*, 73–76.

Capitani, E., Laiacona, M., Mahon, B., & Caramazza, A. (2003). What are the facts of semantic category-specific deficits? A critical review of the clinical evidence. *Cognitive Neuropsychology, 20*, 213–261.

Caramazza, A., Hillis, A. E., Rapp, B. C., & Romani C. (1990). The multiple semantics hypothesis: Multiple confusion? *Cognitive Neuropsychology, 7*, 161–189.

Caramazza, A., & Shelton, J. R. (1998). Domain-specific knowledge systems in the brain: The animate-inanimate distinction. *Journal of Cognitive Neuroscience, 10*, 1–34.

Chao, L. L., Haxby, J. V., & Martin, A. (1999). Attribute-based neural substrates in temporal cortex for perceiving and knowing about objects. *Nature Neuroscience, 2*, 913–919.

Consiglio Nazionale delle Ricerche. (unpublished). *Dizionario di Frequenza della Lingua Italiana.* Unpublished. Roma, Italy.

Cree, G. S., & McRae, K. (2001). Beyond the sensory/functional dichotomy. *Behavioral and Brain Sciences, 24*, 480–481.

De Renzi, E., & Lucchelli, F. (1994). Are semantic systems separately represented in the brain? The case of living category impairment. *Cortex, 30*, 3–25.

Devlin, J. T., Gonnerman, L. M., Andersen, E. S., & Seidenberg, M. S. (1998). Category-specific semantic deficits in focal and widespread brain damage: A computational account. *Journal of Cognitive Neuroscience, 10*, 77–94.

De Vreese, L. P., Faglioni, P., & Agnetti, V. (1994). A battery of colour tests. *Archivio di Psicologia, Neurologia e Psichiatria, 55*, 742–790.

Farah, M. J., & McClelland, J. L. (1991). A computational model of semantic memory impairment: Modality specificity and emergent category specificity. *Journal of Experimental Psychology: General, 120*, 339–357.

Gainotti, G. (2000). What the locus of a brain lesion tells us about the nature of the cognitive defect underlying category-specific disorders: A review. *Cortex, 36*, 539–559.

Garrard, P. (2000). *Organisation of semantic memory.* Doctoral dissertation, University of Cambridge, UK.

Garrard, P., Lambon Ralph, M. A., Hodges, J. R., & Patterson, K. (2001). Prototypicality, distinctiveness and intercorrelation: Analyses of the semantic attributes of living and nonliving concepts. *Cognitive Neuropsychology, 18*, 125–174.

Garrard, P., Patterson, K., Watson, P. C., & Hodges, J. R. (1998). Category-specific semantic loss in dementia of Alzheimer's type: Functional-anatomical correlations from cross-sectional analyses. *Brain, 121*, 633–646.

Ghidoni, E., Poletti, M., & Bondavalli, M. (1995). An Italian standardization test for autobiographical memory. *Archivio di Psicologia, Neurologia e Psichiatria, 56*, 428–443.

Giovagnoli, A. R., Del Pesce, M., Mascheroni, S., Simonelli, M., Laiacona, M., & Capitani, E. (1996). Trail making test: Normative values from 287 normal adult controls. *Italian Journal of Neurological Sciences, 17*, 305–309.

Gonnerman, L. M., Andersen, E. S., Devlin, J. T., Kempler, D., & Seidenberg, M. S. (1997). Double dissociation of semantic categories in Alzheimer's disease. *Brain and Language*, *57*, 254–279.

Hart, J., Berndt, R. S., & Caramazza, A. (1985). Category-specific naming deficit following cerebral infarction. *Nature*, *316*, 439–440.

Hillis, A. E., & Caramazza, A. (1991). Category-specific naming and comprehension impairment: A double dissociation. *Brain*, *114*, 2081–2094.

Hillis, A. E., Rapp, B. C., & Caramazza, A. (1995). Constraining claims about theories of semantic memory: More on unitary versus multiple semantics. *Cognitive Neuropsychology*, *12*, 175–186.

Hooper, E. (1985). *The Hooper visual organization test*. Los Angeles: Western Psychological Services.

Humphreys, G. W., & Forde, E. M. E. (2001). Hierarchies, similarity, and interactivity in object recognition: "Category-specific" neuropsychological deficits. *Behavioral and Brain Sciences*, *24*, 453–476.

Humphreys, G. W., Lamote, C., & Lloyd-Jones, T. J. (1995). An interactive activation approach to object processing: Effects of structural similarity, name frequency and task in normality and pathology. *Memory*, *3*, 535–586.

Laiacona, M., Barbarotto, R., & Capitani, E. (1993a). Perceptual and associative knowledge in category specific impairment of semantic memory: A study of two cases. *Cortex*, *29*, 727–740.

Laiacona, M., Barbarotto, R., Trivelli, C., & Capitani, E. (1993b). Dissociazioni semantiche intercategoriali: Descrizione di una batteria standardizzata e dati normativi. *Archivio di Psicologia, Neurologia e Psichiatria*, *54*, 209–248.

Laiacona, M., Capitani, E., & Barbarotto, R. (1997). Semantic category dissociations: A longitudinal study of two cases. *Cortex*, *33*, 441–461.

Lambon Ralph, M. A., Howard, D., Nightingale, G., & Ellis, A. W. (1998). Are living and nonliving category-specific deficits causally linked to impaired perceptual or associative knowledge? Evidence from a category-specific double dissociation. *Neurocase*, *4*, 311–338.

Luzzatti, C., Willmes, K., & De Bleser, R. (1991). *Aachener Aphasie Test (AAT)*. Firenze, Italy: Organizzazioni Speciali.

Miceli, G., Fouch, E., Capasso, R., Shelton, J. R., Tomaiuolo, F., & Caramazza, A. (2001). The dissociation of color from form and function knowledge. *Nature Neuroscience*, *4*, 662–667.

Paulesu, E., Shallice, T., Frackowiak, R. S. J., & Frith, C. D. (2003). *Anatomical modularity of working memory: Evidence from a much studied patient*. Manuscript submitted for publication.

Plaut, D. C., & Shallice, T. (1993). Deep dyslexia: A case study of connectionist neuropsychology. *Cognitive Neuropsychology*, *10*, 377–500.

Rapp, B. C., Hillis, A. E., & Caramazza, A. (1993). The role of representations in cognitive theory: More on multiple semantics and the agnosias. *Cognitive Neuropsychology*, *10*, 235–249.

Raven, J. C. *Coloured progressive matrices: Sets A, Ab, B*. (1962). London: H.K. Lewis.

Riddoch, M. J., & Humphreys, G. W. (1993). *Birmingham Object Recognition Battery*. Hove, UK: Lawrence Erlbaum Associates Ltd.

Samson, D., Pillon, A., & De Wilde, V. (1998). Impaired knowledge of visual and non-visual attributes in a patient with a semantic impairment for living entities: A case of a true category-specific deficit. *Neurocase*, *4*, 273–290.

Sartori, G., & Job, R. (1988). The oyster with four legs: A neuropsychological study on the interaction of visual and semantic information. *Cognitive Neuropsychology*, *5*, 105–132.

Sartori, G., Miozzo, M., & Job, R. (1993). Category-specific impairments? Yes. *Quarterly Journal of Experimental Psychology*, *46A*, 489–504.

Shallice, T. (1981). Neurological impairment of cognitive processes. *British Medical Bulletin*, *37*, 187–92.

Snodgrass, J., & Vanderwart, M. (1980). A standardized set of 260 pictures: Norms for name agreement, familiarity and visual complexity. *Journal of Experimental Psychology: General*, *6*, 174–215.

Spinnler, H., & Tognoni, G. (1987). Standardizzazione e taratura italiana di test neuropsicologici. *The Italian Journal of Neurological Sciences*, *8*, 1–120.

Tyler, L. K., & Moss, H. E. (1997). Functional properties of concepts: Studies of normal and brain-damaged patients. *Cognitive Neuropsychology*, *14*, 511–545.

Tyler, L. K., Moss, H. E., Durrant-Peatfield, M. R., & Levy, J. P. (2000). Conceptual structure and the structure of concepts: A distributed account of category-specific deficits. *Brain and Language*, *72*, 195–231.

Warrington, E. K., & James, M. (1991). *The Visual Object and Space Perception Battery*. Bury St Edmunds, UK: Thames Valley Test Company.

Warrington, E. K., & McCarthy, R. A. (1983). Category specific access dysphasia. *Brain*, *106*, 859–878.

Warrington, E. K., & McCarthy, R. A. (1987). Categories of knowledge: Further fractionations and an attempted integration. *Brain, 110*, 1273–1296.

Warrington, E. K., & Shallice, T. (1984). Category specific semantic impairments. *Brain, 107*, 829–854.

Wechsler, D. (1981). *Wechsler Memory Scale, forma 1*. Firenze, Italy: Organizzazioni Speciali.

Wechsler, D. (1986). *Scala d'intelligenza Wechsler per adulti (WAIS)*. Firenze, Italy: Organizzazioni Speciali.

COGNITIVE NEUROPSYCHOLOGY, 2003, 20 (3/4/5/6), 355–372

# THE SELECTIVE IMPAIRMENT OF FRUIT AND VEGETABLE KNOWLEDGE: A MULTIPLE PROCESSING CHANNELS ACCOUNT OF FINE-GRAIN CATEGORY SPECIFICITY

Sebastian J. Crutch
*University College and Imperial College, London, UK*

Elizabeth K. Warrington
*University College, London, UK*

We report the case of a gentleman, FAV, who developed a grave anomia and selective comprehension deficit following a left temporo-occipital infarction. His word retrieval abilities were significantly more impaired for living things than for man-made artefacts. There was no difference between his performance when naming to confrontation and naming to verbal description. However, further assessment revealed a more fine-grain deficit at the level of comprehension. FAV had significantly more difficulty with fruit and vegetables than animals or nonliving foods on a number of tests probing semantic knowledge. These results are discussed within the context of current theories of the organisation of conceptual knowledge. We conclude that this pattern of performance and other fine-grain category effects within the realms of living and nonliving things are best explained by a multiple processing pathways account.

## INTRODUCTION

Long vaunted by philosophers as a possibly exhaustive set of classes among which all things might be distributed, "categories" were hardly considered as a potential principle of neural organisation until the concept of semantic memory was defined and elucidated in the original works of Tulving (1973) and Warrington (1975). Since that time, a large number of studies have reported broad category-specific effects in comprehension of verbal and visual stimuli. The most thoroughly debated category effect is that of the selective impairment of semantic knowledge for living things (e.g., De Renzi & Lucchelli, 1994; Silveri & Gainotti, 1988; Warrington & Shallice, 1984). The reverse dissociation between preserved living things and relatively impaired man-made artefacts has also been observed, albeit less frequently (e.g., Hillis & Caramazza, 1991; McKenna & Parry, 1994; Warrington & McCarthy, 1987).

Within such broad classes of information, more closely delimited effects may be evident; not all of these are encompassed within the broad living/nonliving dichotomy. Colour agnosia and autotopagnosia, which were originally described in the

Requests for reprints should be addressed to Sebastian Crutch, Dementia Research Group, The National Hospital for Neurology and Neurosurgery, 8–11 Queen Square, London WC1N 3BG, UK (Email: s.crutch@dementia.ion.ucl.ac.uk).

We would like to thank Prof Narinder Kapur for referring FAV to us and for kindly providing neuropsychological assessment data. We wish to thank Dr John Stevens for his detailed assessment of the neuroimaging data. We are also extremely grateful to FAV for his generous help and patience.





http://www.tandf.co.uk/journals/pp/02643294.html

DOI:10.1080/02643290244000220

neurological literature 100 years ago, can now be reasonably viewed as examples of fine-grain category comprehension deficits. Indeed, there are now a multitude of category-specific phenomena; the preserved and impaired comprehension of concrete and abstract concepts and nouns and verbs are both well established (McCarthy & Warrington, 1985, 1986; Warrington, 1975). More recently, there have been many examples of fine-grain category effects within the broad categories of nonliving things and proper names. For example, dissociations between manipulable and nonmanipulable objects and between people's names and place names have been observed (McKenna & Warrington, 1980; Warrington & McCarthy, 1987).

However, in this paper we limit our account to dissociations within the broad category of living things. Hart, Berndt, and Caramazza (1985) were the first to report a dissociation within this broad category. The patient had significantly more difficulty in naming pictures of fruit and vegetables than any other subcategory of pictureable nouns. Although this patient had some difficulties in categorising pictures, he was not reported to have a deficit at the level of comprehending the spoken word. This pattern of naming performance has been replicated (Farah & Wallace, 1992), whilst the reverse dissociation has also been documented (Hart & Gordon, 1992). In addition, Hillis and Caramazza (1991) have reported a case, JJ, who showed selective sparing of animals relative to both fruit and vegetables and also, notably, to foods. Complementing these investigations, McKenna and Parry (1994) were the first to describe a selective deficit for fruit and vegetables at the level of comprehension. They compared both spoken and written word comprehension of fruit and vegetables with animals, manipulable objects, and nonmanipulable objects and, in a series of 28 left-hemisphere patients, found 2 cases in which the deficit was highly selective for fruit and vegetables. It seems unlikely that fruit and vegetables are more difficult as a class, in that the double dissociation has been described; Caramazza and Shelton (1998) reported the case EW in whom knowledge of animals was impaired while knowledge of fruit and vegetables was intact.

The original descriptions of category specificity described the double dissociation between what were termed living and nonliving things. In these original studies, the broad category of foods was also assessed and was found to be preserved or impaired along with the living things. After all, fruit and vegetables are not only living things but also foods. Nonliving foods (e.g., bread, spaghetti, bacon) are also an interesting category in that the ratio of the living component to the man-made artefact component is greatly varied. In the present study, we include the broad category of foods within our discussion of dissociations between living things.

In the context of so many apparent dissociations between categories, it should be noted nonetheless that what constitutes a category is still a matter of debate. As we shall see in the discussion of the cognitive theories of conceptual organisation, it has been posited that processing modalities, commonality of features and attributes, and evolutionary pressures are just a few of the potential principles. Furthermore, the delineation of boundaries between categories can sometimes be rather unclear. Many researchers have considered category membership to be determined by the presence or absence of a number of core features. However there are at least two problematic issues when such an approach is considered. First, the representations of some items may have reasonably been allocated to more than one category. For example, in the verbal modality, "lamb" can be classified both as an animal and as a food. It is possible that such multiple classification may require the double representation of some lexical items. Second, descriptions of category distinctions may require refinement. For example, category effects that were originally attributed to a dissociation between indoor and outdoor objects may be more easily captured by the manipulable/nonmanipulable distinction (Warrington & McCarthy, 1987; Yamadori & Albert, 1973). In this case, refining category membership requirements can resolve problems in classifying items (e.g., a bucket) that might otherwise have straddled two supposedly opposing categories (indoor and outdoor objects). Further problems or inconsistencies in the width of categories referred to in the literature may partly derive from the methodologies used to assess such deficits. For example, failure to distinguish between semantically close and distant control items in comparison to a selectively impaired or preserved category can make it difficult to draw firm conclusions over the exact width of the category in question (Shallice, 1988).

## Cognitive theories of conceptual organisation

The first attempt to give a principled account of category specificity was the introduction of the concept that items can be classified by their sensory or functional attributes (Warrington & McCarthy, 1983; Warrington & Shallice, 1984). Patients were described who appeared to have grave difficulties in identifying living items together with preservation of man-made artefacts. However, more detailed probing of a wider range of items uncovered some exceptions to this broad dichotomy. For example, knowledge of body parts was preserved while types of metal were impaired. It was these anomalies that motivated the attempt to express the observed category effect in terms of the sensory-functional theory (SFT). Living things were considered to be highly dependent on their perceptual features for identification while, by contrast, man-made objects were more dependent on detection of their functional attributes. The sensory–functional distinction has been misconstrued as equating to the proposal of separate verbal and visual semantic stores (e.g., Caramazza & Shelton, 1998; Hart & Gordon, 1992). This verbal–visual split is in fact orthogonal to the sensory–functional debate, as reiterated by Warrington, McCarthy, and Shallice, because the split refers to the nature of the input stimulus and not the nature of the central representations.

Further evidence for the SFT comes from a recent investigation by Borgo and Shallice (2001). In this study, the authors focussed upon the broad category of food. They argue that despite being man-made, nonliving foods (e.g., steak, milk) tend to be more dependent on sensory qualities for their identification because they lack a characteristic shape. As a result, they tend to behave in a similar manner to other living things rather than to man-made artefacts.

A number of other views are not wholly dissimilar from those above. For example, De Renzi and Lucchelli (1994) stress the importance of the relationships between such contrasting sensory and functional features. For example, man-made artefacts enjoy a close relationship between form and function, whereas living things do not. Any damage that leads to a distancing of the relationship between such features might lead to a disproportionate problem with living things. Tyler and Moss (1997) also emphasise the importance of the relationship between sensory and functional features, although the principles governing the strength of the relationship are conceived rather differently.

As an alternative to either of these accounts, Caramazza and Shelton (1998) have forwarded the domain-specific hypothesis (DSH), which states that evolutionary pressures have led to a categorical organisation of the conceptual system. In particular, semantic knowledge develops through the acquisition of properties that characterise a category-exemplar. As the categorical distinction rather than the perceptual–functional property distinction is fundamental, knowledge of perceptual and functional properties should be equally impaired in any category-specific deficit. They propose a tripartite semantic structure, with animals (potential predators and food) and plants (including fruit and vegetables; sources of food and medicine) represented in separate semantic domains. A third domain is loosely ascribed to "tools" but more broadly to all items not included in the animal or plant domains. Consequently, the authors suggest that the only pure category-specific effects will involve animals or plants and man-made artefacts. Finer-grain dissociations should not be observed. It is also stated that damage that affects the categories of animals or fruit and vegetables is likely (but not necessarily) to affect the semantic category of foods.

Warrington and McCarthy (1987) were dissatisfied with the original sensory–functional distinction in that it failed to account for more fine-grain dissociations within the broad bands of living things and man-made artefacts. However, the significance of the difference between the original 1983 and 1984 accounts and this developed account has perhaps not been fully appreciated. For example, they reported a patient who exhibited greater difficulty with, as they termed them, manipulable objects than nonmanipulable objects. They proposed an elaboration of the sensory–functional distinction, in which they attached importance to the fact that there are multiple specialised channels of processing within both the motor and sensory modalities. It is such activation during the process of acquisition that is claimed to lay the foundations for category specificity. Other accounts also stress the importance of these channels of processing, but at the stage of concept retrieval and not initial concept acquisition (e.g., A. R. Damasio, 1990; Humphreys & Forde, 2001). Taking the sensory modality of vision as an example, the occurrence of such channels of processing at the level of semantics may be related to the early separation of processing for the form, colour, and movement of a visual stimulus. Therefore they proposed that rather than items from different categories merely being differentiated by the relative balance of input information from the major motor and sensory modalities, they also receive differently weighted input from the more specialised channels within each modality. These different weighting values permit all the relevant channels to make a relative contribution to processes supporting the acquisition and subsequent comprehension of different categories of knowledge. As such, the differential weightings could be a possible basis for the categorical organisation of semantic knowledge systems.

In the present study, we investigate the case of a gentleman with a selective impairment of knowledge for fruit and vegetables. His performance on various tests of word and picture comprehension and knowledge of item attributes and associations is compared to his ability to retrieve the names of the same stimuli. We discuss the implications of these results for current theories of conceptual organisation.

## CASE HISTORY

FAV is a 78-year-old retired businessman (born in August 1923). In May 2000 he suffered a left posterior artery haemorrhagic infarct, following which he developed a right homonymous hemianopia and episodic memory difficulties. He was able to remember very little of the first week of his stay in hospital. An MRI scan shortly after the stroke revealed damage to the left posterior cerebral territory including the primary visual cortex and the inferior temporal region. The hippocampus, posterior parahippocampal gyrus, and medial and superior temporal gyri were unaffected, as was part of the anterior temporal lobe (see Figure 1). He made a good recovery and 18 months later at the time of this experimental investigation, he had a residual language impairment (described in more detail below) and a persisting right homonymous hemianopia.

### Neuropsychological background

FAV was assessed on selected formal neuropsychological tests between May and July 2000. At this time he had a selective verbal memory deficit. He scored below the 5th percentile (17/25) on the verbal version of the Camden Recognition Memory Test and above the 75th percentile (24/25) on the visual version. He obtained a pass score on all six subtests of the Visual Object and Space Perception battery that he attempted (VOSP; Warrington & James, 1991). His literacy skills were intact. He read the Schonell Graded Reading Test with only one error (99/100). His prepositional speech was fluent and the content well expressed, with only occasional episodes of word-finding difficulty. By contrast, his naming to confrontation was quite impaired. He failed to name any items on the Graded Naming Test (GNT 0/30; McKenna & Warrington, 1983). On the much easier Oldfield Naming Test he scored 5/30. His total score on a category naming test of very high-frequency items was 34/50, with most difficulty naming colours and animals (5/10 and 5/10, respectively). On frequency matched sets he was able to name 39/40 verbs but only 24/40 pictureable nouns.

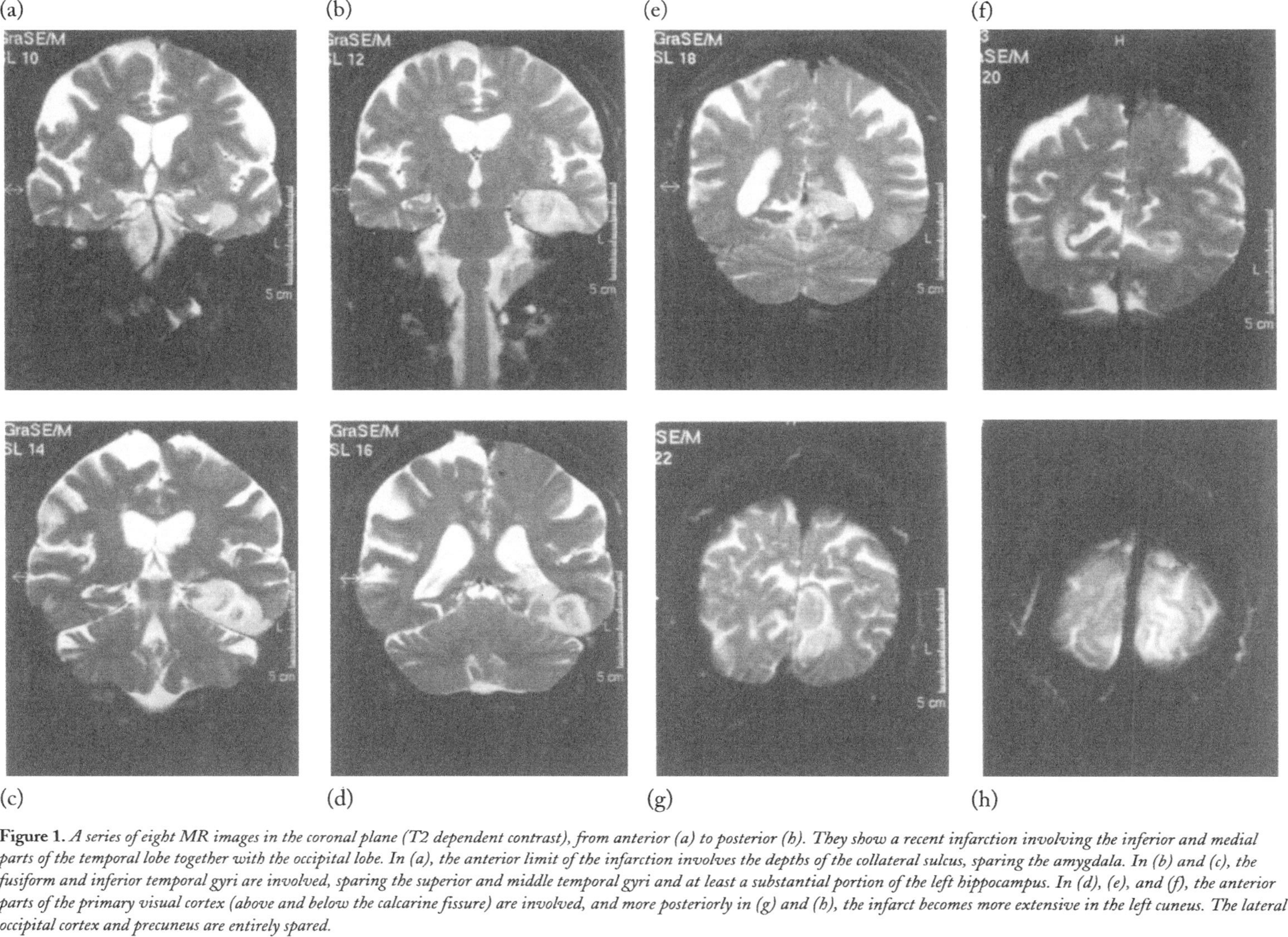


**Figure 1.** *A series of eight MR images in the coronal plane (T2 dependent contrast), from anterior (a) to posterior (h). They show a recent infarction involving the inferior and medial parts of the temporal lobe together with the occipital lobe. In (a), the anterior limit of the infarction involves the depths of the collateral sulcus, sparing the amygdala. In (b) and (c), the fusiform and inferior temporal gyri are involved, sparing the superior and middle temporal gyri and at least a substantial portion of the left hippocampus. In (d), (e), and (f), the anterior parts of the primary visual cortex (above and below the calcarine fissure) are involved, and more posteriorly in (g) and (h), the infarct becomes more extensive in the left cuneus. The lateral occipital cortex and precuneus are entirely spared.*

## Documentation of language skills

The investigations reported in this paper were conducted between June and December 2001. FAV was still gravely anomic and at this time was only able to score 2/30 on the GNT. He attempted to name the majority of items drawn from the Snodgrass and Vanderwart (1980) corpus, on which he scored 105/246. In this context, it is worth noting that only 31% of items in the Snodgrass corpus are drawn from the category of living things. By contrast FAV's comprehension appeared to be intact. His comprehension at the sentence level was entirely satisfactory, scoring without error on a test probing word order and function words (Schwartz, Saffran, & Marin, 1980). In contrast with his very poor naming skills, FAV scored at a very high level on a graded two-choice synonym test for both concrete and abstract nouns (24/25 and 22/25, respectively; Warrington et al., 1998). This was comparable to his high score on a stringent test assessing comprehension of concrete and abstract verbs (37/39 and 39/42, respectively; Manning & Warrington, 1996). He also obtained a very satisfactory score on a word–picture matching test that probed abstract and emotion words in addition to concrete words, scoring 18/21, 9/10, and 18/19 respectively (Shallice & McGill, unpublished). When we required FAV to provide a spoken definition of a number of frequency-matched concrete and abstract nouns, his definitions of the majority of abstract and nonliving concrete nouns were of the highest order. However, his responses to several living items were rather vague and nonspecific. It was this observation that led to the present investigation.

## Comparison cases

To ensure that any category effects evident in our experimental investigations were not merely the result of a task difficulty artefact, two patients with moderately impaired verbal comprehension skills were selected as comparison cases.

Comparison case 1 (C1) is a 75-year-old retired businessman who reports a 7-year history of insidious onset memory impairment, initially affecting memory for appointments, conversations, and object placement. He has also got lost on occasion. MRI revealed quite striking mesial temporal atrophy, which was reasonably symmetrical. No other regionally definable atrophy, was present. Ischaemic lesion load was relatively light. Altogether, these findings were considered more compatible with Alzheimer's disease than frontotemporal degeneration or vascular dementia. A brief neuropsychological assessment revealed significant word-retrieval difficulties, with the patient able to name only 3/30 items on the GNT. He also showed evidence of a verbal comprehension deficit, achieving a score of 26/32 on the short form of the British Picture Vocabulary Scale (BPVS; Dunn, Dunn, Whetton, & Pintilie, 1982). On the more difficult synonyms test, there was some indication of a discrepancy between his concrete *and* abstract word knowledge (13/25, 1st percentile and 19/25, 25th percentile, respectively).

Comparison case 2 (C2) is a 65-year-old right-handed man who experienced an episode of viral encephalitis in 1972, resulting in left-hemispheric damage. An MRI scan 3 years prior to these investigations provided evidence of mature damage of the left temporal lobe. This patient exhibits significant word retrieval difficulties, correctly naming only one item on the GNT. He also shows a mild semantic impairment, scoring 28/32 on the short form of the BPVS. On the synonyms test he achieved creditable scores on both the concrete and abstract word versions (17/25, 10th percentile and 18/25, 10–25th percentile respectively).

C1 was assessed on all the comprehension components of Experiments 2–4. C2 was assessed only on the comprehension test in Experiment 3.

# EXPERIMENTAL INVESTIGATIONS

## Experiment 1—Comparison of picture naming with naming from verbal description

The clinical assessment of FAV's language abilities established that he had a grave anomia in the context of apparently preserved comprehension. However, his word-retrieval skills were assessed entirely by naming to confrontation. It was therefore pertinent to examine whether he had a modality-selective naming impairment. At this stage, no attempt was made to examine any possible *category*-specific effects. Our aim in this experiment was to compare picture naming with naming from verbal description.

*Methods*
The stimuli consisted of 80 concrete nouns, the majority belonging to the categories of living things, man-made artefacts, or body parts. They were randomly divided into four sets of 20 items. Each set was presented once as a spoken description and once as a simple line drawing in an ABAB BABA design. Spoken descriptions of each item were based upon simple dictionary definitions (e.g., "What do we call the heavy, lockable, metal box used for keeping valuable goods?": *Safe*. "What do we call the salad vegetable which is long and thin with a dark green skin?": *Cucumber*). Picture stimuli were presented individually on 10 × 15 cm cards.

*Results*
FAV correctly named 42/80 items when provided with a spoken description and 39/80 items when shown picture stimuli. A Sign test reveals this difference to be not significant ($N = 15$, $x = 6$, $p > .3$). An item-by-item analysis of FAV's responses also shows his performance to be consistent across the modalities, not conforming to the Binomial distribution, $\chi^2 = 31.3$, $p < .001$. The majority of FAV's errors were either circumlocutions (e.g., *strawberry*: "We eat them, popular, seasonal now") or close semantic approximations that the subject did not accept (e.g., *ladle*: "Not spoon, not shovel, I can see it but I can't tell you the word").

*Comment*
These results establish that the picture-naming impairment observed in our patient is not the result of a modality-specific input deficit (e.g., an optic aphasia). The levels of performance between naming from pictures and from spoken description are very closely matched. Combined with FAV's satisfactory performance on formal tests of visuoperceptual function, this indicates there is no perceptual deficit that might otherwise have invalidated the use of pictorial stimuli for further investigation of FAV's word-retrieval deficit.

## Experiment 2—Category naming task and semantic probe test

As noted in the documentation of FAV's language skills, there was a suggestion that he might exhibit an advantage for defining man-made artefacts over living things. There was also a hint that he may have even more difficulty with flora than fauna. In this experiment we explored both the issues of category specificity and the locus of his deficit by comparing his naming and comprehension of man-made artefacts, flora, and fauna.

*Methods*
The stimuli consisted of 120 items: 40 man-made artefacts (including manipulable and non-manipulable objects), 40 items of flora (including fruit, vegetables, flowers), and 40 items of fauna (including mammals, birds, and invertebrates). The three sets were matched for word frequency using Thorndike–Lorge ratings (Thorndike & Lorge, 1942; G count). These ratings were used in preference to the Kuçera and Francis set, which were only able to provide frequency data for 73% of the chosen pictureable items. Age of acquisition and visual complexity ratings were not available for this corpus. The experiment was conducted in two distinct parts.

*Comprehension task.* A series of written multiple-choice questions probing conceptual knowledge of each item was devised. FAV was asked to choose between the target and two semantically related distractor items. The questions probed either attribute (e.g., *apple*: <u>pips</u>, stone, segments) or associative knowledge (e.g., *ostrich*: <u>walk</u>, swim, fly). The proportion of attribute questions to association questions for flora and fauna items was identical (15 vs. 25 for both). All bar three of the questions about man-made artefacts probed associative knowledge. An effort was also made to match the probe words themselves for word frequency (Kuçera & Francis, 1967). In particular, the probe words for fauna and

Table 1. *Number and percentage correct responses on the naming and semantic probe tasks*

| | | | *Semantic probe task* | | | |
|---|---|---|---|---|---|---|
| | *Naming* | | *Pictorial presentation* | | *Auditory verbal presentation* | |
| *Category* | *N correct* | *% correct* | *N correct* | *% correct* | *N correct* | *% correct* |
| Artefacts ($N$ = 40) | 29 | 73 | 39 | 98 | 39 | 98 |
| Flora ($N$ = 40) | 7 | 18 | 25 | 63 | 28 | 70 |
| Fauna ($N$ = 40) | 7 | 18 | 38 | 95 | 38 | 95 |

flora items were well matched (fauna: mean = 56.3, $SD$ = 104.1, 88% data available; flora: mean = 49.3, $SD$ = 75.0, 87% data available; man-made artefacts: mean = 97.2, $SD$ = 109.7, 96% data available).

*Naming task.* The stimuli consisted of detailed colour photographs displayed on a high resolution PC monitor.

The stimuli were divided into two matched halves, each containing 20 artefacts, 20 flora items, and 20 fauna items. The experiment was conducted over two sessions, 1 week apart. In Session 1, only semantic probe questions were administered. Half the items were presented in the pictorial form and the other half in the auditory verbal form. In Session 2, all items were presented in pictorial form for naming to confrontation. Subsequently, the semantic probe questions were readministered with stimuli presented either in auditory verbal or pictorial form, in a pattern complimentary to that of Session 1. Thus over the two sessions, all items were probed in both auditory verbal and pictorial form, in a split AB BA design.

To ensure that the probe questions from all three categories were of equivalent difficulty, comparison case C1 was presented with the auditory verbal form of the comprehension task. He was not assessed on the pictorial form or on the naming task.

### Results

The number and percentage correct naming responses for each category are shown in Table 1. There was a highly significant difference in naming performance between categories, $\chi^2(2) = 35.12, p < .001$. More detailed analysis revealed FAV was able to retrieve the names of man-made artefacts significantly more accurately than either the names of flora or fauna items, $\chi^2(1) = 22.27, p < .001$, both.

On the probe test of comprehension, a different pattern of results was found. The number and percentage correct responses on the visual and verbal presentation conditions of the probe test are also shown in Table 1. FAV's accuracy was significantly different between the three categories in both the visual and auditory verbal presentation conditions, $\chi^2(2) = 23.93, p < .001$; $\chi^2(2) = 16.92, p < .001$, respectively. However, in both the visual and verbal conditions, these differences reflected the fact that FAV's accuracy was significantly worse for flora items than for either man-made artefacts, $\chi^2(1) = 13.2, p < .001$; $\chi^2(1) = 9.18, p < .01$, respectively, or fauna items, $\chi^2(1) = 10.76, p < .01$; $\chi^2(1) = 7.01, p < .01$. As with the word-retrieval data from Experiment 1, though, there was no evidence of any significant effect of presentation modality upon the overall accuracy of response in the comprehension task (Sign test, $N$ = 10, $x$ = 3, $p$ > .15).

This category effect cannot be due to an artefact of task difficulty, as C1 was not significantly worse

Table 2. *Number and percentage correct responses made by C1 on the single level semantic probe task with auditory verbal presentation*

| | *C1—Auditory verbal presentation* | |
|---|---|---|
| *Category* | *N correct* | *% correct* |
| Artefacts ($N$ = 40) | 37 | 93 |
| Flora ($N$ = 40) | 23 | 58 |
| Fauna ($N$ = 40) | 29 | 73 |

with flora items than fauna items, $\chi^2 = 1.98, p > .1$ (see Table 2).

*Comment*

The results of the naming test provide strong evidence of weaker word retrieval for living things than for man-made artefacts in FAV. However, as seen in this experiment and with the Snodgrass and Vanderwart corpus, FAV's naming of nonliving things is also seriously compromised. As noted previously, his naming of concrete items is also inferior to his retrieval of abstract words (e.g., verbs). Thus the broad category effect shown here is observed in the context of a global anomia, which may show a concrete–abstract gradient of severity.

The pattern of this naming deficit, though, does not appear to be mirrored in our patient's word and picture comprehension skills, where the deficit appears more selective for flora items. Thus it would appear that FAV's naming deficit for flora is underpinned by a comprehension deficit, but this does not appear to be the case for man-made artefacts and fauna. This evidence for a fine-grain category-specific comprehension deficit, we would argue, cannot be attributed to task difficulty as our control subject had equal difficulty with flora and fauna. It should also be noted that the flora items in this experiment included a number of flowers and plants. Despite being a keen gardener, FAV had more difficulty with these items than comparison case C1, who has only ever once had a garden with which he did not involve himself. Nonetheless, flowers and plants, unlike common fruits and vegetables, are likely to represent a form of specialist knowledge developed by only a small proportion of the population. Thus flower items were omitted from the design of subsequent experiments.

## Experiment 3—Multiple-level semantic category probe test

The discrepancy in the effect of categories observed in naming and comprehension prompted us to further examine FAV's ability to retrieve and comprehend the names of living things. The relatively high percentage of correct responses on fauna items in the probe test suggests that FAV may have been approaching some form of ceiling effect. Thus we attempted to design a more demanding test of comprehension for these fine-grain categories.

Following recent investigations (e.g., Borgo & Shallice, 2001) of the relationship between living things and other so-called "sensory quality" categories, we also included the category of nonliving foods. Sensory quality in this case refers to edible liquids and solids that tend not to have a specific perceptual form, and which may rely rather more upon taste and texture for identification.

*Methods*

A pool of 85 items (not included in previous experiments) was drawn from the categories of animals, fruit and vegetables, and nonliving foods. Item selection was partly guided by previous attempts to explain category-specific deficits on the basis of differences in item familiarity within categories (Funnell & Sheridan, 1992). In the present case, 10 age-matched male control subjects (mean age = 73.4 yrs, *SD* = 6 yrs) were requested to rate item familiarity on a scale from 1–5, according to the instructions used by Snodgrass and Vanderwart (1980). From this pool of items, 20 animals, 20 fruit and vegetables, and 20 foods were selected, which were matched for familiarity and word frequency where possible (Thorndike & Lorge, 1942; L count). Again, Thorndike–Lorge ratings were employed in preference to Kuçera–Francis as they provided data for a higher proportion of the animal, fruit, and vegetable items selected (animal data: 90% and 75% respectively; fruit and vegetables: 90% and 70% respectively). The familiarity and frequency means and standard deviations for each category are shown in Table 3.

**Table 3.** *Mean (and standard deviation) item familiarity and word frequency ratings*

| | *Item familiarity* | | *Word frequency* | |
|---|---|---|---|---|
| Animals | 3.7 | (0.6) | 569.5 | (556.4) |
| Fruits and vegetables | 3.7 | (0.6) | 510.0 | (401.1) |
| Foods | 3.9 | (0.5) | N/A | |

N/A: data not available.

Two procedures, conducted in the following order, were adopted to assess knowledge of these stimuli.

*Multiple-level probe test.* Three written multiple-choice questions, of the type described in Experiment 2, were devised to probe conceptual knowledge of each item. The formulation of the probes was guided by data from 20 male age-matched control subjects who were asked to produce three distinctive features or characteristics for each item. The frequency of occurrence of each feature or attribute in the total control sample was calculated.

The probe questions were then ranked into three levels on the basis of rated difficulty. All items were presented to a further eight control subjects. These subjects were asked to rank the three probe questions relating to each stimulus for difficulty on a scale from 1–3. All probe questions were allocated to Level I, II, or III on the basis of their mean difficulty rating. Level I probes assessed highly distinctive knowledge about the target item, whilst Level II and III probes required an increasingly in-depth knowledge of an item's attributes and associations. No attempt was made to balance associative probes with attribute probes. Two sets of example probes are given below.

| | | |
|---|---|---|
| *Hippo* | Level I | *river*, sea, field |
| | Level II | fur, *hide*, scales |
| | Level III | *fierce*, friendly, clever |
| *Plum* | Level I | pips, *stone*, segments |
| | Level II | plant, bush, *tree* |
| | Level III | thick skin, *thin skin*, no skin |

Three lists were prepared, each containing the stimulus words in the same random order. In each list there was a mixture of Level I, II, and III probes. Thus Level I, II, and III probes occurred approximately equally often in each of the three lists. All questions and response choices were spoken and repeated if necessary.

Again, to ensure that the probe questions in each category were of equivalent difficulty, comparison cases C1 and C2 were tested on the multiple semantic probes task.

*Naming task.* Pictorial stimuli were presented in the same item order as used in the preceding multiple-level probe test. As before, the pictorial stimuli were detailed colour photographs displayed on a high resolution PC monitor.

### *Results*

The number and percentage correct responses made by FAV for each category for each semantic level probe are shown in Table 4. Summing across the three levels of probes, there was a significant difference in accuracy between categories, $\chi^2(2) = 18.26$, $p < .001$. FAV correctly answered significantly more questions about animals and foods than about fruit and vegetables, $\chi^2(1) = 10.7$, $p < .01$, both. Although FAV's performance on all levels of probes revealed an advantage for animals and foods over fruit and vegetables, not all differences were significant. On Level I probes alone, there was no significant difference among the three categories, $\chi^2(2) = 2.35$, $p > .3$. However, significant performance differences between categories were found

**Table 4.** *Number and percentage correct responses on the multiple level semantic probe task*

| | *Number (and percentage) correct responses* | | | | | | | | | | | |
|---|---|---|---|---|---|---|---|---|---|---|---|---|
| | *Level I probes* | | | *Level II probes* | | | *Level III probes* | | | *Sum of all probes* | | |
| *Category* | *FAV* | *C1* | *C2* | *FAV* | *C1* | *C2* | *FAV* | *C1* | *C2* | *FAV* | *C1* | *C2* |
| Animals | 18 | 6 | 12 | 18 | 9 | 10 | 16 | 8 | 12 | 52 | 23 | 34 |
| ($N$ = 20) | (90%) | (30%) | (60%) | (90%) | (45%) | (50%) | (80%) | (40%) | (60%) | (87%) | (38%) | (57%) |
| Fruits and vegetables | 15 | 14 | 11 | 9 | 11 | 13 | 11 | 10 | 8 | 35 | 35 | 32 |
| ($N$ = 20) | (75%) | (70%) | (55%) | (45%) | (55%) | (65%) | (55%) | (50%) | (40%) | (58%) | (58%) | (53%) |
| Foods | 18 | 18 | 12 | 16 | 12 | 11 | 18 | 15 | 12 | 52 | 45 | 35 |
| ($N$ = 20) | (90%) | (90%) | (60%) | (80%) | (60%) | (55%) | (90%) | (75%) | (60%) | (87%) | (75%) | (58%) |

on both Level II and III probes, $\chi^2(2) = 10.96, p < .01$; $\chi^2(2) = 6.94, p < .05$, respectively.

The results of comparison cases C1 and C2 are also shown in Table 4. Summing across all levels, C1 showed a significant difference between categories, $\chi^2(2) = 16.51, p < .001$. Indeed C1 showed the reverse pattern to FAV, correctly answering more questions about fruit and vegetables than about animals, $\chi^2(1) = 4.06, p < .05$. C1 also showed better performance with foods than fruit and vegetables, but this difference was not significant, $\chi^2(1) = 3.04$, $p > .05$. On each individual level, C1 showed a performance gradient with knowledge of foods better than fruit and vegetables better than animals, but the only significant difference was that between fruit and vegetables and animals on Level I, $\chi^2(1) = 4.9, p < .05$.

In contrast to both FAV and C1, comparison case C2 showed no significant difference between any of the three categories, $\chi^2(2) = 0.32, p > .8$. C2 also showed no significant differences between categories on any of the individual levels of probes.

Naming to confrontation performance was extremely poor on this set of stimuli. FAV managed to name only 1/20 animals, 1/20 foods, and 0/20 fruit and vegetables. This was despite FAV commenting for the majority of items that he recalled they had been discussed earlier in the session (during the probe test).

### *Comment*

More detailed probing of knowledge for living things has confirmed that FAV has a selective fine-grain semantic impairment for fruit and vegetables that dissociates from his relatively preserved knowledge for animals. In addition, knowledge for the sensory quality group of nonliving foods appears to also be relatively well preserved and well matched to knowledge of animal names. The performances of our comparison cases are also salient, with FAV and C1 providing evidence of a double dissociation between knowledge for fruits and vegetables and knowledge for animals. Furthermore, our second comparison case C2 showed no significant differences in performance between categories. These findings indicate that the probes were balanced for overall task difficulty across categories.

Despite good comprehension of animal and food names, retrieval of the same names to confrontation was extremely impaired. Indeed, naming accuracy for these two categories was no better than for fruit and vegetables. Whilst this may reflect a floor effect with the current stimulus set, taken together with the analysis of naming data from Experiment 2 the results indicate that word retrieval skills for animals and fruit and vegetables are equally impaired, as compared to man-made artefacts. Thus these findings provide further evidence that FAV's word-retrieval deficit for fruit and vegetable items is underpinned by a loss of conceptual knowledge. Furthermore, such an explanation does not appear to account for his anomia for animals. Given this situation, one must propose that FAV's poor animal naming skills are the consequence of an additional impairment, which has a post-semantic locus.

## Experiment 4—Word–picture matching task

In Experiment 3, we showed that FAV's knowledge of fruit and vegetables was significantly worse than his knowledge of animals and foods. Our aim in this experiment was to find corroborative evidence of this category-specific deficit using an alternative methodology that was less likely to be subject to confounding factors.

### *Methods*

The stimuli consisted of the same familiarity- and frequency-matched items used in Experiment 3; namely 20 animals, 20 fruit and vegetables, and 20 foods. The patient was requested to match spoken item names to their pictorial forms. The pictures were displayed in arrays of 10 items, each comprising 5 targets from the same category and 5 semantically and perceptually related distractors. The 10 items were arranged randomly on a PC monitor. Comparison case C1 was also assessed on this word–picture matching task.

### *Results*

The number and percentage correct responses made by FAV for each category on the word–pic-

**Table 5.** *Number and percentage correct responses on the word–picture matching task*

| | Correct responses | | | |
|---|---|---|---|---|
| | FAV | | C1 | |
| Category | N | % | N | % |
| Animals ($N$ = 20) | 19 | 95 | 7 | 35 |
| Fruits and vegetables ($N$ = 20) | 11 | 55 | 10 | 50 |
| Foods ($N$ = 20) | 19 | 95 | 12 | 60 |

ture matching task are shown in Table 5. As with the summed correct probe scores in Experiment 3, there was a significant between-categories effect, $\chi^2(2) = 14.15$, $p < .001$, which was explained by FAV's significantly higher accuracy with both animals and foods than with fruit and vegetables, $\chi^2(1) = 6.53$, $p < .02$, both. There was no difference between animal and food matching performance. The results of case C1 are also shown in Table 5. C1 correctly matched food items better than fruit and vegetables, and fruit and vegetables better than animals, but this between-categories effect was not significant, $\chi^2(2) = 2.54$, $p > .02$.

*Comment*

This experiment provides corroborative evidence for the claim that FAV has a fine-grain category-specific deficit for fruit and vegetables, by demonstrating the same dissociative effect as was observed in Experiment 3. As with previous experiments, the result is not an artefact of task difficulty as comparison case C1 showed no significant performance differences across categories.

## DISCUSSION

The understanding of category-specific effects within the conceptual knowledge system has evolved from the broad dichotomy between living and nonliving things. More narrowly delimited dissociations provide the opportunity for detailed hypotheses regarding the cerebral organisation of conceptual knowledge. We have described a patient with a marked selective impairment of knowledge for fruit and vegetables. His scores on a range of tests probing knowledge of both verbal and visual stimuli were significantly worse with fruit and vegetables than with animals or foods. Indeed, for both animals and foods there was only a very minor deficit on our probe tasks. Although FAV's comprehension deficit was selective for fruit and vegetables, this was not the case for word retrieval, for which all three categories were equally and markedly impaired. This was observed in the context of a global anomia. Furthermore, there appeared to be no difference in his performance whether word retrieval was elicited by naming to confrontation or naming to verbal description. We report the first case of a fine-grain category-specific deficit of knowledge of fruit and vegetables to both verbal and visual presentation.

Before going on to consider FAV's categorical semantic impairment, it is important to comment upon the disparity between his comprehension and naming skills. In addition to the fine-grain semantic loss, which we believe accounts for his poor naming of fruit and vegetables, we assume he has a supplementary, less category-specific deficit in word retrieval that has a post-semantic locus. This second deficit is most likely to be responsible for the apparent graded nature of FAV's anomia, with verb naming relatively preserved in comparison to impaired object naming and even worse retrieval of living things and foods. We also have no reason to believe that this anomia reflects poor premorbid knowledge of the categories in question. Our patient was an educated and very well-travelled gentleman. He had a beautiful garden in which he took a keen interest and he greatly enjoyed eating out in restaurants. Furthermore, in deference to the fact that some gentlemen of this or any other age are relatively unfamiliar with the names of most varieties of flowers, no such items were included in the stimuli employed in Experiments 3 and 4.

Returning to our main discussion, we will first consider whether the domain-specific hypothesis or the sensory-functional theory can account for our data of a fine-grain category-specific effect. Second, we will examine whether we can give an alternative principled account of the genesis of such categorical effects and how they relate to the neural substrate in the brain. Finally, we will consider lesion and functional imaging data that speak to the loci of such deficits.

The domain-specific hypothesis (DSH) of Caramazza and Shelton (1998) predicts that "the only true category specific deficits are those involving categories of knowledge for which evolutionary pressures have led to the development of specialised neural mechanisms for their perceptual and conceptual distinction" (p. 9). In this sense, the category-specific deficit of knowledge for fruit and vegetables described in the current study is compatible with the DSH account, unlike observations of fine-grain category effects observed outside the realm of living things. However, the DSH makes only a very weak prediction about the place of knowledge of foods within a categorically organised brain: ". . . damage to neural structures that affect the categories of animals or fruit and vegetables are also likely (though not necessarily) to result in impairment of the category of foods, even though many members of the latter category are more properly considered artefacts." Admittedly, nonliving foods can be derived from animals (e.g., bacon from a pig) and from plants (e.g., bread from ground wheat), and hence may share some quasi-perceptual and functional features with these representations of these categories of knowledge. Indeed, their account makes no claims about the organisation of semantic knowledge within a domain. But the issue surrounding foods is one of categorisation, not perceptual or functional properties. In the original account of the double dissociation between living and nonliving things, foods were treated as a separate category, which was in both instances associated with the preservation or impairment of living things. There is no evidence that a selective impairment of animals or fruit and vegetables leads to particular difficulties with their relative derivatives. In the present case, there is a clear dissociation between fruit and vegetables and other foods. In the case of Caramazza and Shelton's patient, EW, there was a dissociation between animate items and other stimuli. Although foods were not directly examined, we assume that the author's use of the term "animate" was literal. With dissociative evidence suggesting a degree of independence for nonliving foods, the absence of a prediction in the DSH regarding whether foods are represented within the animal, plant, or artefact domains somewhat weakens the theory. Given the evolutionary principles that Caramazza and Shelton claim have guided this domain-specific organisation of conceptual knowledge, it is difficult to imagine why nonliving foods would represent a domain (as defined) of their own.

The classical sensory-functional theory (SFT) also struggles to account for FAV's pattern of deficit. Borgo and Shallice (2001) have published evidence that classes of items that do not have a distinctive form (edible substances, liquids, and materials) closely follow living things in terms of a subject's performance on tasks probing naming and semantic knowledge. Indeed, the authors claim that their results strongly advocate the SFT because the test items were generated on the basis of the sensory–functional distinction. However, it is clear from this claim that Borgo and Shallice would not predict such different patterns of performance on fruit and vegetables as compared to animals as was observed in FAV. Furthermore, the dissociation between fruit and vegetables and nonliving foods would also be unaccounted for. According to the SFT, these dissociations should not occur as the categories are all primarily defined by their sensory properties.

## An account of category specificity in terms of multiple processing channels

Our preferred account of these data is most in line with Warrington and McCarthy's (1987) multiple processing channels theory, which was described previously. The essential tenets of this theory stress the importance of specialised channels of processing within the broad sensory and motor channels during the acquisition phase. Items from diverse categories receive differentially weighted inputs from these channels. The result could be an organisation of conceptual space in which category membership reflects a particular pattern of input contributions from a range of specialised channels. Subsequent damage to a semantic system organised in this way might result in a loss of knowledge for items whose positions in the organisational framework have a similar origin. The theory has the advantage of not only suggesting *why* conceptual knowledge has a categorical cerebral organisation (cf. DSH), but also *how* that principled organisation has evolved. All first-hand experience of the world must be conveyed, accommodated, and assimilated by a combination of these sensory and motor processes. In this regard, we would concur that these channels of information might be bound together in topographically distinct "convergence zones" (A. R. Damasio, 1990). However, the relative sharpness of zone boundaries and the degree to which such zones might overlap remain issues for empirical debate.

With regard to the fine-grain category effect observed in this paper, it is proposed that fruit and vegetables, animals, and nonliving foods are also differentially dependent upon specific sensory and motor subchannels for their acquisition and, consequently, comprehension. Fruit and vegetables are often critically distinguished by their colour, with other important sensory inputs including their taste and their visual/tactile form. By comparison, animals are less dependent upon their colour and taste, tending to rely more upon form and movement information. In contrast to fruit, vegetables, and animals, nonliving foods tend to be less dependent upon their form for identification (as pointed out by Borgo & Shallice, 2001). Instead, information about their taste and oral texture is more likely to be highly weighted in any representation.

It should be noted that such an explanation is equally appropriate when considering the organisation of nonliving and living things. This is best exemplified by the differentiation of minimal semantic pairs. For example, a pair of scissors, a knife, a lighthouse, and a windmill would all be more dependent upon functional attributes for recognition than animals or flowers, say. However, different constellations of the more specialised channels within the sensory or motor modalities are invoked in the acquisition of these items. Differentiation of the scissors and knife places a greater reliance upon proximal finger movement information whereas differentiation of a lighthouse and a windmill relies more heavily upon visual form information.

Several possible shortcomings of the revised account proposed by Warrington and McCarthy (1987) have been put forward. Caramazza and Shelton (1998) have questioned the absence of evidence that the distinction between members of different semantic categories depends differentially on colour, shape, or other sensory features. In this regard, it is worth noting that Warrington and McCarthy (1987) suggested that, ". . . category specific deficits may be an emergent property of the acquisition of competence in such processing" (p. 1292). The multiple processing channels theory outlined here represents a hypothesis that is testable using a neural network model. If the principles of acquisition outlined in the account were to be instantiated as learning parameters in such a model, a direct comparison would be possible between the results of lesioning the network and the patterns of deficits observed in many of the patients reported as having category-specific effects.

Caramazza and Shelton also claim the theory is weakened by the lack of reported associations between the impairment of particular semantic categories and special difficulties for specific types of sensory information, quoting the example of "greater difficulty processing color in patients with selective damage to the categories of fruit and vegetables." However, this may be based on a misunderstanding. The Warrington and McCarthy position is based on the claim that this information is only important in setting up the central representation and not in subsequent access to it. Thus they would attach no significance to either an association or a dissociation between colour and fruit and vegetables.

An attempt to portray the multiple processing channels account in diagram form is shown in Figure 2. It should be emphasised that the number of specialised channels, living and nonliving categories, and multi-sensory inputs in the diagram are not in any way an exhaustive depiction of conceptual knowledge. Instead, the diagram aims to illus-

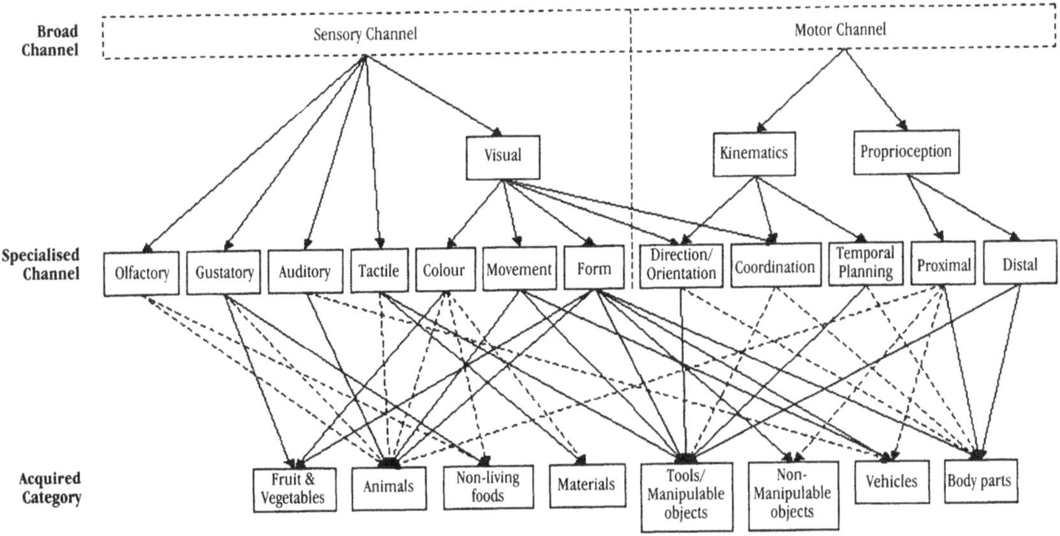


**Figure 2.** *An illustration of the multiple processing channels account.*

trate the notion of relative input weightings, with solid lines representing relatively important processing channels and dotted lines less important channels. The diagram is also an attempt to emphasise the importance of overlap between sensory and motor/functional inputs for various living and nonliving categories of knowledge. For example, several specialised channels of sensory processing, such as visual movement and tactile stimulation information, are shown as contributing to categories of items typically defined by their functional properties, such as tools. Conceptualising the types of information required to appreciate and take advantage of an object's properties in this way may help to achieve the improved specification of the term "function" which has been recognised as necessary by some authors (e.g., Borgo & Shallice, p. 218). It should also be noted that, on the whole, this scheme does not prejudge the issue over whether there are modality-specific semantic systems. Whether such a scheme applies to the organisation of a unimodal knowledge base or whether it is developed primarily in the visual domain, which then subsequently provides the blueprint for a verbal knowledge base, remains subject to debate.

## The nature of the damage underlying category-specific effects

Lesion data from patients with category-specific effects has been varied but reveals two general trends. The first trend relates to the breadth of the deficit. An analysis by Goodglass and Boudin (1988) found that highly delimited category effects tended to be associated with focal brain lesions, while impairments of broader categories usually resulted from diffuse lesions (within this latter group one would include the category effects observed in most herpes simplex encephalitis patients; e.g., Capitani, Laiacona, Barbarotto, & Trivelli, 1994; Laiacona, Capitani, & Barbarotto, 1997; Sartori & Job, 1988; Warrington & Shallice, 1984). The present report of a patient with a finely delimited category deficit is consistent with Goodglass and Boudin's analysis, in that MRI data reveals FAV's lesion to be focal (albeit large) in nature. Indeed, highly selective effects following focal brain damage are likely to be rare. The second trend concerns the neuroanatomical bases of living and nonliving category effects. Deficits for living things are often associated with predominantly left temporal lobe damage, although frontal and inferior parietal areas may also be involved. Given that FAV has a mainly occipital lesion, one might speculate that knowledge for the category of fruit and vegetables has a relatively posterior locus.

Functional imaging studies into category effects in the brain have also been conducted (Cappa, Perani, Schnur, Tettamanti, & Fazio, 1998; H. Damasio, Grabowski, Tranel, Hichwa, & Damasio, 1996; Gorno-Tempini, Cipolotti, & Price, 2000; Martin, Wiggs, Ungerleider, & Haxby, 1996; Perani et al., 1995, 1999). Most studies have indicated the role of left inferior temporal lobe in semantic processing, particularly for animals, but some studies have failed to detect significant semantic category effects. There has also been some debate recently as to why bilateral occipital activation is greater for pictures of living than nonliving stimuli (Martin et al., 1996; Moore & Price, 1999; Perani et al., 1995).

Attempts have also been made to highlight discrete cortical regions that support representations of more fine-grain categories. Several such efforts have followed the notion that neurons supporting objects within a category may be finely tuned to features shared by objects within that category. For example, tools have been reported to elicit greater activity in the left posterior middle temporal gyrus than other object categories (e.g., Chao, Haxby, & Martin, 1999; Martin et al., 1996). The proximity of this region to areas associated with the processing of visual motion information has led to speculation that these neurons are tuned to motion information associated with different objects (see Martin & Chao, 2001, for a review).

In the current case, some might draw significance from the fact that much of the inferior temporal lobe is subsumed within FAV's large lesion. This area has been found to be activated by the retrieval of information about object colour (Chao & Martin, 1999), information that is considered to be particularly relevant to fruit and vegetable knowledge. However, this study concluded that retrieving previously acquired information about an object's colour does not require the reactivation of colour regions that subserve perception. In the same vein, the current multiple processing channels theory claims that such colour information is only criticial for the acquisition of these concepts, and not necessarily their subsequent activation. This theoretical discrepancy, taken together with the locus and extent of the lesion in our patient, means that our data are relatively neutral with regard to the localisation of fruit and vegetable conceptual knowledge within the occipito-temporal cortex. Nonetheless, we would predict that such fine-grain effects as observed in the present study will in due course be mapped to very localised anatomical regions.

## REFERENCES


Baxter, D. M., & Warrington, E. K. (1994). Measuring dysgraphia: A graded-difficulty spelling test. *Behavioural Neurology*, *7*, 107–116.

Borgo, F., & Shallice, T. (2001). When living things and other "sensory quality" categories behave in the same fashion: A novel category specificity effect. *Neurocase*, *7*, 201–220.

Capitani, E., Laiacona, M., Barbarotto, R., & Trivelli, C. (1994). Living and nonliving categories. Is there a "normal" asymmetry? *Neuropsychologia*, *32*, 1453–1463.

Cappa, S. F., Perani, D., Schnur, T., Tettamanti, M., & Fazio, F. (1998). The effects of semantic category and knowledge type upon lexical-semantic access: A PET study. *NeuroImage*, *8*, 350–359.

Caramazza, A., & Shelton, J. R. (1998). Domain-specific knowledge systems in the brain: The animate-inanimate distinction. *Journal of Cognitive Neuroscience*, *10*, 1–34.

Chao, L. L., Haxby, J. V., & Martin, A. (1999). Attribute-based neural substrates in temporal cortex for perceiving and knowing about objects. *Nature Neuroscience*, *2*, 913–919.

Chao, L. L., & Martin, A. (1999). Cortical representation of perception, naming and knowing about color. *Journal of Cognitive Neuroscience*, *11*, 25–35.

Coughlan, A., & Hollows, S. E. (1985). *The Adult Memory and Information Processing Battery.* Leeds, UK: St James University Hospital.

Damasio, A. R. (1990). Category-related recognition defects as a clue to the neural substrates of knowledge. *Trends in Neurosciences*, *13*, 95–98.

Damasio, H., Grabowski, T. J., Tranel, D., Hichwa, R. D., & Damasio, A. R. (1996). A neural basis for lexical retrieval. *Nature*, *380*, 499–505.

De Renzi, E., & Lucchelli, F. (1994). Are semantic systems separately represented in the brain? The case of living category impairment. *Cortex, 30*, 3–25.

Dunn, L. M., Dunn, L. M., Whetton, C., & Pintilie, D. (1982). *British Picture Vocabulary Scale.* Windsor, UK: NFER-Nelson.

Farah, M. J., & Wallace, M. A. (1992). Semantically-bounded anomia: Implications for the neural implementation of naming. *Neuropsychologia, 29*, 185–193.

Funnell, E., & Sheridan, J. (1992). Categories of knowledge? Unfamiliar aspects of living and nonliving things. *Cognitive Neuropsychology, 9*, 135–153.

Goodglass, H., & Boudin, C. (1988). Category and modality specific dissociations in word comprehension and concurrent phonological dyslexia. A case report. *Neuropsychologia, 26*, 67–78.

Gorno Tempini, M. L., Cipolotti, L., & Price, C. J. (2000). Category differences in brain activation studies: Where do they come from? *Proceedings of the Royal Society, London B, 267*, 1253–1258.

Hart, J. Jr, Berndt, R. S., & Caramazza, A. (1985). Category specific naming deficit following cerebral infarction. *Nature, 316*, 439–440.

Hart, J. Jr, & Gordon, B. (1992). Neural subsystems for object knowledge. *Nature, 359*, 60–64.

Hillis, A. E., & Caramazza, A. (1991). A category specific naming and comprehension impairment: A double dissociation. *Brain, 114*, 2081–2094.

Humphreys, G. W., & Forde, E. M. E. (2001). Hierarchies, similarity, and interactivity in object recognition: "Category-specific" neuropsychological deficits. *Behavioral and Brain Sciences, 24*, 453–509.

Kucera, H., & Francis, W. N. (1967). *Computational analysis of present-day American English.* Providence, RI: Brown University Press.

Laiacona, M., Capitani, E., & Barbarotto, R. (1997). Semantic category dissociations: A longitudinal study of two cases. *Cortex, 33*, 441–461.

Manning, L., & Warrington, E. K. (1996). Two routes to naming: A case study. *Neuropsychologia, 34*, 809–817.

Martin, A., & Chao, L. L. (2001). Semantic memory and the brain: Structure and processes. *Current Opinion in Neurobiology, 11*, 194–201.

Martin, A., Wiggs, C. L., Ungerleider, L. G., & Haxby, J. V. (1996). Neural correlates of category-specific knowledge. *Nature, 379*, 649–652.

McCarthy, R. A., & Warrington, E. K. (1985). Category specificity in an agrammatic patient: The relative impairment of verbal retrieval and comprehension. *Neuropsychologia, 23*, 709–727.

McCarthy, R. A., & Warrington, E. K. (1986). Visual associative agnosia: A clinico-anatomical study of a single case. *Journal of Neurology, Neurosurgery and Psychiatry, 49*, 1233–1240.

McKenna, P., & Parry, R. (1994). Category and modality deficits of semantic memory in patients with left hemisphere pathology. *Neuropsychological Rehabilitation, 4*, 283–305.

McKenna, P., & Warrington, E. K. (1980). Testing for nominal dysphasia. *Journal of Neurology, Neurosurgery and Psychiatry, 43*, 781–788.

McKenna, P., & Warrington, E. K. (1983). *The Graded Naming Test.* Windsor, UK: NFER-Nelson.

Moore, C. J., & Price, C. J. (1999). A functional neuroimaging study of the variables that generate category-specific object processing differences. *Brain, 122*, 943–962.

Perani, D., Cappa, S. F., Bettinardi, V., Bressi, S., Gorno Tempini, M. L., Matarrese, M., & Fazio, F. (1995). Different neural networks for the recognition of biological and man-made entities. *Neuroreport, 6*, 1637–1641.

Perani, D., Schnur, T., Tettamanti, M., Gorno Tempini, M. L., Cappa, S. F., & Fazio, F. (1999). Word and picture matching: A PET study of semantic category effects. *Neuropsychologia, 37*, 293–306.

Sartori, G., & Job, R. (1988). The oyster with four legs: A neuropsychological study on the interaction of visual and semantic information. *Cognitive Neuropsychology, 5*, 105–132.

Schonell, F. J. (1942). *Backwardness in basic subjects.* Edinburgh: Oliver & Boyd.

Schwartz, M. F., Saffran, E. M., & Marin, O. S. M. (1980). The word order problem in agrammatism. 1. Comprehension. *Brain and Language, 10*, 249–262.

Shallice, T. (1988). *From neuropsychology to mental structure.* Cambridge: Cambridge University Press.

Silveri, M. C., & Gainotti, G. B. (1988). Interaction between vision and language in category specific semantic impairment. *Cognitive Neuropsychology, 5*, 677–709.

Snodgrass, J., & Vanderwart, M. (1980). A standardized set of 260 pictures: Norms for name agreement, familiarity and visual complexity. *Journal of Experimental Psychology: General, 6*, 174–215.

Thorndike, E. L., & Lorge, I. (1942). *The teacher's word book of 30,000 words.* New York: Teachers College, Columbia University.

Tulving, E. (1973). Episodic and semantic memory. In E. Tulving & W. Donaldson (Eds.), *Organisation of memory* (pp. 382–403). New York: Academic Press.

Tyler, L. K., & Moss, H. E. (1997). Functional properties of concepts: Studies of normal and brain-damaged patients. *Cognitive Neuropsychology*, *14*, 511–545.

Warrington, E. K. (1975). The selective impairment of semantic memory. *Quarterly Journal of Experimental Psychology*, *27*, 635–657.

Warrington, E. K. (1984). *Recognition Memory Test.* Windsor, UK: NFER-Nelson.

Warrington, E. K., & James, M. (1991). *The visual object and space perception battery*. Bury St. Edmunds, UK: Thames Valley Test Company.

Warrington, E. K., & McCarthy, R. A. (1983). Category specific access dysphasia. *Brain*, *106*, 859–878.

Warrington, E. K., & McCarthy, R. A. (1987). Categories of knowledge. Further fractionations and an attempted integration. *Brain*, *110*, 1273–1296.

Warrington, E. K., McKenna, P., & Orpwood, L. (1998). Single word comprehension: A concrete and abstract word synonym test. *Neuropsychological Rehabilitation*, *8*, 143–154.

Warrington, E. K., & Shallice, T. (1984). Category specific semantic impairments. *Brain*, *107*, 829–853.

Yamadori, A., & Albert, M. L. (1973). Word category aphasia. *Cortex*, *9*, 112–125.

COGNITIVE NEUROPSYCHOLOGY, 2003, 20 (3/4/5/6), 373–400

# A CASE OF IMPAIRED KNOWLEDGE FOR FRUIT AND VEGETABLES

**Dana Samson and Agnesa Pillon**
*Université catholique de Louvain, Louvain-la-Neuve, Belgium*

In this paper, we report the case of RS, a brain-damaged patient presenting with a disproportionate conceptual impairment for fruit and vegetables in comparison to animals and artefacts. We argue that such a finer-grained category-specific deficit than the living/nonliving dichotomy provides a source of critical evidence for assessing current alternative theories of conceptual organisation in the brain. The case study was designed to evaluate distinct expectations derived from the categorical and the knowledge-specific accounts for category-specific semantic deficits. In particular, the integrity of object-colour knowledge has been assessed in order to determine whether the patient's deficit for fruit and vegetables was associated with a deficit for that kind of knowledge, which has been claimed to be highly diagnostic for fruit and vegetables. The results showed that the patient's pattern of performance is consistent with theories assuming a topographical category-like organisation of conceptual knowledge in the brain.

## INTRODUCTION

The fact that brain damage can impair conceptual knowledge for some categories of entities while leaving knowledge of other categories relatively spared has found widespread empirical support in the last 20 years. The most often-reported pattern (e.g., Forde, Francis, Riddoch, Rumiati, & Humphreys, 1997; Laiacona, Capitani, & Barbarotto, 1997; Lambon Ralph, Howard, Nightingale, & Ellis, 1998; Moss, Tyler, Durrant-Peatfield, & Bunn, 1998; Samson, Pillon, & De Wilde, 1998) is certainly that of patients showing a loss of conceptual knowledge for living entities (animals, fruit and vegetables, flowers) in the face of relatively spared knowledge for nonliving ones (tools, vehicles, furniture), but there is now an increasing number of case reports of patients showing the reverse pattern of dissociation (e.g., Cappa, Frugoni, Pasquali, Perani, & Zorat, 1998; Gaillard, Auzou, Miret, Ozsancak, & Hannequin, 1998; Laiacona & Capitani, 2001; Moss & Tyler, 2000; Sacchett & Humphreys, 1992; Silveri, Gainotti, Perani, Cappelletti, Carbone, & Fazio, 1997; Warrington & McCarthy, 1983, 1987).

Such patterns of conceptual impairment have been used to inform theories of the organisation of conceptual knowledge in the brain/mind. Given the prevalence of selective or disproportionate deficits for either living or nonliving entities, current theoretical proposals and debates mainly focused on the issue of which organising principle of conceptual knowledge could be responsible for patterns of deficits conforming to the living/non-

Requests for reprints should be addressed to Agnesa Pillon, Unité de neurosciences cognitives, Faculté de psychologie et des sciences de l'éducation, Université catholique de Louvain, 10, place du Cardinal Mercier, B-1348 Louvain-la-Neuve, Belgium (Email: Agnesa.Pillon@psp.ucl.ac.be).

We especially thank RS for his willing participation in this study. We also thank Marie-Pierre de Partz for referring RS to us, Valérie Cornil for her help in preparing the object-colour knowledge tasks, and Adrian Ivanoiu for providing us the details of the MR scan. We are also grateful to the two anonymous reviewers for their useful comments on an earlier version of this paper.



http://www.tandf.co.uk/journals/pp/02643294.html DOI:10.1080/02643290244000329

living distinction (see Caramazza, 1998; Forde & Humphreys, 1999, for a review). However, there is some evidence suggesting that the living/nonliving dimension is not the relevant one to account for the occurrence of category-specific deficits. Patients have been reported who were impaired in some but not all living categories. Thus, in several cases, the body part category has been found to be spared relative to the animal and fruit and vegetable categories (e.g., De Renzi & Lucchelli, 1994; Forde et al., 1997; Shelton, Fouch, & Caramazza, 1998; Silveri & Gainotti, 1988). In other cases, the animal category appeared to be more impaired than the fruit and vegetable category (e.g., Caramazza & Shelton, 1998; De Renzi & Lucchelli, 1994; Gainotti & Silveri, 1996; Hart & Gordon, 1992), while, in some others, fruit and vegetables were more impaired than animals (e.g., Farah & Wallace, 1992; Forde et al., 1997; Hart, Berndt, & Caramazza, 1985; Hillis & Caramazza, 1991; Pietrini, Nertempi, Vaglia, Revello, Pinna, & Ferro-Miloni, 1988).

In this paper, we will report an additional case of a brain-damaged patient presenting with a pattern of dissociation within the living category, namely, a disproportionate conceptual impairment for fruit and vegetables in comparison to animals and artefacts, and we will argue that such a finer-grained category-specific semantic deficit than the living/nonliving dichotomy provides a source of critical evidence for assessing current alternative theories of conceptual organisation in the brain/mind.

Among the previous case reports suggesting that all categories of living things are not necessarily equally impaired in case of a living things impairment, those of EW (Caramazza & Shelton, 1998), KR (Hart & Gordon, 1992), MD (Hart et al., 1985), TU (Farah & Wallace, 1992), and JJ (Hillis & Caramazza, 1991) present the clearest evidence that the animal category, on the one hand, and the fruit and vegetable category, on the other hand, can be damaged independently from each other. EW and KR both showed marked difficulty in naming animals, while they performed at ceiling when naming fruit and vegetables as well as manufactured objects. This pattern of dissociation was further observed in semantic tasks that did not require the production of the name of the object. Thus, in attribute verification tasks, EW performed very poorly with animals whether visual or nonvisual attributes were tested, but normally with inanimate objects, which comprised fruit and vegetables and artefacts. Likewise, KR performed at ceiling in attribute verification tasks both for fruit and vegetables and artefacts while his performance for animals was clearly impaired (the deficit was, however, confined to the retrieval of visual attributes). Hence, in both cases, the pattern of performance indicated a dissociation *within* the living things category, with impaired conceptual knowledge for animals and spared conceptual knowledge for fruit and vegetables.

On the other hand, the patients MD (Hart et al., 1985) and TU (Farah & Wallace, 1992) showed a selective impairment for fruit and vegetables, which appeared, however, to be restricted to naming. Thus, MD showed selective difficulty for fruit and vegetables as compared to other items in picture naming, naming from a verbal description, and verbal fluency tasks. He nevertheless showed quite good scores for fruit and vegetables in word categorisation, word/picture matching, and attribute verification tasks. The only task not requiring the production of the object's name, and for which MD showed a mild selective impairment for fruit and vegetables as compared to other items, was a picture categorisation task. TU's pattern of performance was quite similar. This patient was selectively impaired with fruit and vegetables in naming (from a picture or from a verbal description) and verbal fluency tasks. However, he performed well for fruit and vegetables in a word/picture matching task and could accurately define fruit and vegetables from a spoken name. Hence, in MD and TU, the selective difficulties in processing the category of fruit and vegetables seemed to be located at the name retrieval processing level.[1] Although there is no evidence in these cases that retrieving conceptual knowledge for fruit and vegetables is impaired per

[1] In the case of MD, an additional impairment at the visual recognition level cannot be excluded.

se, the selective naming difficulties might suggest that entries in the output lexicon are addressed by semantically categorised information in such a way that access to the name of fruit and vegetables from semantics can be selectively disrupted.

Finally, JJ (Hillis & Caramazza, 1991) showed marked difficulty with fruit and vegetables as well as manufactured objects in a picture naming task, while he was relatively accurate in naming animals. JJ also showed difficulties with nonanimal items when asked to provide definitions of them from spoken words, a pattern suggesting that semantic knowledge was impaired for these items. However, no separate scores were provided for fruit and vegetables and manufactured objects in this task, so that the extent to which semantic knowledge for fruit and vegetables was impaired relative to other item categories is unknown.

How could current theories of conceptual knowledge organisation explain that the animal and the fruit and vegetable categories can jointly be impaired (or spared) but, in some cases, can also selectively be impaired (or spared)? Current theories advanced to account for category-specific semantic deficits can be broadly classified into three classes.

The first class of theories assumes that category-specific semantic deficits reflect a topographical category-like organisation of conceptual knowledge within the brain: Conceptual knowledge associated with objects belonging to a particular category would be grouped in specific brain regions. Three proposals have been advanced within this framework, each of them making different assumptions as to the organising principle that would have led to such a topographical organisation of conceptual knowledge in the brain. The first proposal, the OUCH model (Caramazza, Hillis, Rapp, & Romani, 1990), adopts the view of a unitary semantic system whose internal organisation is determined by the strength of association between the various semantic properties. It is assumed that properties that are highly correlated tend to be represented in close proximity within the "semantic space." Given that members of a given category share many properties in common that are highly intercorrelated, the semantic properties of objects belonging to a given category tend to cluster together within the "semantic space." Selective semantic deficits for either animals or fruit and vegetables can hence be accounted for by assuming that the semantic properties associated with fruit and vegetables, on the one hand, and the semantic properties associated with animals, on the other hand, form two distinct clusters within the semantic space. Brain damage could then disrupt processing of both categories or only one of them, depending on the regions of the semantic space that happened to be damaged.

The second proposal assuming a topographical category-like organisation of knowledge is the one put forward by Damasio and his collaborators (e.g., Damasio, 1990; Tranel, Damasio, & Damasio, 1997). According to these authors, the retrieval of conceptual knowledge is achieved by "convergence zones" within the brain. These "convergence zones" are dedicated to reconstructing the various object properties that were pertinently associated in experience, which are represented across multiple sensory and motor cortices. Stemming from the assumption that the object properties that were pertinently associated in experience differ in kind across the various categories, the authors propose that the retrieval of conceptual knowledge associated with the various categories of objects is achieved by partially segregated convergence zones. Each of these convergence zones would indeed be located in the best suited anatomical region to permit the most effective interactions with those brain areas which represent the object properties they were designed to integrate. Although the empirical evidence advanced in support of this proposal mainly focused on the animal/tool/familiar person distinction (Tranel et al., 1997; Tranel, Logan, Frank, & Damasio, 1997), it could be extrapolated that the retrieval of conceptual knowledge for fruit and vegetables also relies on the activation of specific convergence zones. Thus, processing animals or fruit and vegetables or both categories could be impaired, depending on the particular brain region that is damaged.

The third proposal related to the notion that conceptual knowledge for the various categories of objects is represented and processed in distinct brain areas is known as the domain-specific knowledge hypothesis (Caramazza & Shelton, 1998). Within this hypothesis, the driving force leading to such a topographical organisation is believed to be an evolutionary one. The organisation of conceptual knowledge in the brain would reflect neural adaptations in response to evolutionary pressures for the rapid and successful identification of evolutionary salient categories of objects. These were identified as animals, plant life, and conspecifics. From this point of view, category-specific deficits reflect either a defect to one (or several) of the specialised neural systems (i.e., the systems sustaining knowledge about animals, plant life, or conspecifics) or a selective preservation of these neural systems in the case of a category-specific deficit for nonliving things. This third proposal is certainly the one that most explicitly expects a dissociation between the animal and the fruit and vegetable categories.

The second class of theories also takes category-specific semantic deficits as evidence for a topographical structuration of conceptual knowledge in the brain. However, semantic properties would not be grouped within the brain according to the category of object they are associated with, but rather on the basis of the kind of object properties to which they refer. Initially, it has been proposed that the semantic system is subdivided into a visual and a functional subsystem, storing knowledge about visual and functional properties of objects, respectively (Farah & McClelland, 1991; Warrington & Shallice, 1984). Stemming from the assumption that the distinction between objects from the various semantic categories covaries with the kind of semantic properties that are the most diagnostic for these objects, category-specific deficits were attributed to selective damage either to the visual or the functional semantic subsystem. Thus, as living things were assumed to be primarily defined by visual properties, category-specific deficits for living things were seen as resulting from damage to the visual semantic subsystem. Conversely, as the semantic representation of nonliving things was assumed to be highly weighted on functional properties, category-specific deficits for nonliving things would result from damage to the functional semantic subsystem. This account could only explain category-specific deficits that conform to the living/nonliving distinction. However, subsequently, other authors enlarged the visual vs. functional dichotomy and proposed that conceptual knowledge is stored across more distributed knowledge stores (Humphreys & Forde, 2001; Warrington & McCarthy, 1987). Thus, visual knowledge would be represented across distinct shape, colour, and texture knowledge stores, other sensory knowledge across distinct auditory, tactile, and olfactory knowledge stores, and functional knowledge across encyclopaedic and action-related knowledge stores. This modified theoretical framework leaves room to explain finer-grained dissociation within the broad living and nonliving categories. According to this "knowledge-specific" account, a selective deficit for animals or a selective deficit for fruit and vegetables would result from selective damage to the knowledge store representing information assumed to have high weighting in the representation of animals or fruit and vegetables, i.e., the shape or the colour knowledge store, respectively (Humphreys & Forde, 2001; Warrington & McCarthy, 1987).

A third class of accounts attributes category-specific deficits to some object or concept properties that systematically covary with semantic category. The most frequently invoked properties are structural similarity (Gaffan & Heywood, 1993; Humphreys, Riddoch, & Quinlan, 1988) and the structure of correlations among the concept's features (Devlin, Gonnerman, Andersen, & Seidenberg, 1998; Tyler, Moss, Durrant-Peatfield, & Levy, 2000). Up to now, these accounts were mainly articulated in relation to category-specific deficits for living or nonliving things; they are nevertheless based on assumptions that might be extended to account for finer-grained specific deficits.

The structural similarity account highlighted the fact that exemplars belonging to living categories are more structurally similar than exemplars belonging to nonliving categories, so that more competition needs to be resolved throughout the identification processes of living things. Accordingly, living things would be more vulnerable to brain damage than nonliving things. The hypothesis of greater structural similarity between living than nonliving things found empirical support in a study by Humphreys et al. (1988), which also found that fruit and vegetables were slightly more structurally similar than animals. Thus, the structural similarity account could explain why brain damage impairs fruit and vegetables more than animals. However, the reverse pattern, that is, a selective impairment for animals with spared knowledge for fruit and vegetables, could not find an explanation within this framework.

The correlational structure account is based on the assumption that concepts are represented as patterns of activation over many semantic features within a unitary distributed conceptual system and that category-specific deficits emerge as a result of differences in the internal structure of concepts across categories. The internal structure of concepts is determined by the set of features activated and the degree of correlations among these features, which reflect the extent to which they co-occur together in concepts (for example, the feature "having a head" and "having eyes" are very strongly correlated as they always occur together). Feature correlations are thought to have significant consequences in the condition of brain damage. It is assumed that correlated features support each other with mutual activation, so that strongly correlated features should be more resilient to damage within the semantic system than features that are more weakly correlated. One of the variants of the correlational account, that of Devlin et al. (1998), proposes that features of the concepts in the living category are more strongly intercorrelated than those in the nonliving category so that living concepts should be more resilient to mild damage within the semantic system than nonliving ones. As the level of damage increases, however, the intercorrelated features would collapse en masse so that living concepts would be far more impaired than nonliving concepts. The variant of the correlational account proposed by Tyler and her colleagues (Moss et al., 1998; Tyler et al., 2000; Tyler & Moss, 2001) makes the reverse prediction, namely, living concepts should be less robust to damage than nonliving ones; nonliving deficits will only be seen when damage to the semantic system is particularly severe (Moss & Tyler, 2000; Tyler et al., 2000). This expectation derives from the additional notion that successfully identifying an individual concept relies heavily on activating its *distinctive* features, i.e., those features that are necessary for accurate discrimination among similar members of a category. Thus, individual concepts will be preserved, following brain damage, insofar as they have strong correlations among their more distinctive properties. It is further claimed that concepts of living things have distinctive properties that tend to be weakly correlated, or not correlated at all, with other properties and so are particularly vulnerable to damage. In contrast, because artefacts have distinctive forms that are consistently associated with the distinctive functions for which they were created, concepts of artefacts are characterised by strong correlations between their distinctive properties, which makes the individual concepts of artefacts more resistant to damage than those of living things.

In principle, correlational structure accounts could be able to explain finer-grained category-specific impairments, such as a specific impairment for fruit and vegetables or a specific impairment for animals, on the basis of the additional assumption that the internal structure of both these kinds of living thing concepts differs in a systematic way. The available empirical estimates of feature relations do reveal some differences within the living thing category. Thus, estimates by Devlin et al. (1998) indicate that concepts of fruit and vegetables have a higher number of correlated features than animals. Under the Devlin et al. approach, such a pattern should make the concepts of fruit and vegetables more robust to damage than the concepts of animals. This implies that fruit and vegetables should be spared in case of mild damage and, furthermore, when fruit and vegetables are impaired, animals should be impaired too. As regards the pattern of correlations among distinctive features, the available data seem less consistent.

Tyler and Moss (2001; Moss, Tyler, & Devlin, 2002) stated that fruit and vegetables have very few, poorly correlated distinctive features. On this basis, the authors predict that concepts in the category of fruit and vegetables will be the most vulnerable at all levels of damage. However, estimates by McRae and Cree (2002) indicate that fruit and vegetables tend to have more, rather than fewer, distinctive features than animals, and a similar, if not a higher, number of correlated features. Unfortunately, the degree of intercorrelation among distinctive features is not provided in this study. Thus it appears that one must wait for more complete estimates of feature relations before being able to draw firm predictions concerning finer category-specific deficits within the correlational structure accounts. It is worth underlining, however, that even if the results of these estimates supported the notion that the concepts of fruit and vegetables systematically differ from the concepts of animals in their internal structure, both variants of the correlational structure account would still have great difficulty accounting for a pattern of a *double* dissociation between animals and fruit and vegetables reported in the context of a *mild* semantic impairment.

From this brief overview of the main theoretical accounts for category-specific deficits, it appears that the first two classes of accounts, the topographical category-like and knowledge-specific organisation accounts, provide a theoretical framework that most naturally explains the deficits affecting selectively either the animal or the fruit and vegetable category. It also appears that the inspection of the kind of semantic properties that are impaired in such cases might be a basis on which both types of accounts can be put to the test. The accounts assuming a category-like organisation of knowledge predict that all kinds of semantic properties associated with objects from the impaired category should be impaired while all kinds of semantic properties associated with objects from the spared categories should be spared. In contrast, the accounts assuming an organisation of knowledge by kind of semantic properties predicts that a selective impairment of a given category should be associated with a selective impairment in retrieving knowledge that is particularly diagnostic for that impaired category, namely, shape knowledge for animals and colour knowledge for fruit and vegetables, as proposed by the defenders of the knowledge-specific accounts (Humphreys & Forde, 2001; Warrington & McCarthy, 1987). Moreover, this particular kind of knowledge should be impaired across all categories (but see Humphreys & Forde, 2001, for a challenge of this latter prediction, and Pillon & Samson, 2001, for a discussion).

The previous case studies of patients presenting with a selective deficit for either the animal or the fruit and vegetables category provide little, if any, evidence with respect to these expectations. Among the case studies of patients presenting with a selective deficit for animals (EW: Caramazza & Shelton, 1998; KR: Hart & Gordon, 1992), only the KR study provided data relative to the patient's ability to retrieve the specific kind of visual knowledge that would be particularly diagnostic for animals, such as shape as opposed to colour information. It was found that KR was impaired at retrieving both shape and colour knowledge about animals, with her performance being nevertheless better for shape than colour knowledge probes (scoring 74% and 47% correct, respectively). In contrast, KR's performance was perfect when asked to retrieve both shape and colour knowledge about fruit and vegetables, as well as shape knowledge about vehicles. This pattern is inconsistent with the one expected in case of a selective loss of shape knowledge, which should lead to impaired retrieval of shape knowledge and spared retrieval of colour knowledge for all categories of items. However, the shape attributes that were probed in this study only related to very general shape properties, such as having or not having four legs for the animal items and having or not having wheels for the vehicle items. (The type of shape questions probed for fruit and vegetables was not specified.) Had the patient's knowledge been assessed with more specific or distinctive shape properties of objects, this study would have provided stronger evidence against the knowledge-specific accounts for category-specific deficits. As for the case studies of patients presenting with a selective deficit for fruit and vegetables

(JJ: Hillis & Caramazza, 1991; TU: Farah & Wallace, 1992; MD: Hart et al., 1985), the ability to retrieve different kinds of properties has been assessed only in the case of MD. MD was asked to give judgements about size, colour, shape, and texture for the eight fruit and vegetables he had previously misnamed and for four animals. His responses were 100% accurate for all the properties, which suggests spared access to both shape and colour knowledge. However, the item set used to probe the different kinds of objects' properties was very limited in size and the relevance of these data for the theories of conceptual knowledge organisation might be questioned on the grounds that MD appeared to suffer from a name-retrieval rather than a conceptual impairment for fruit and vegetables.

Other cases are potentially informative about the actual relationship between processing fruit and vegetables and object-colour information. These are cases of patients presenting with a deficit in retrieving object-colour knowledge (Della Sala, Kinnear, Spinnler, & Stangalino, 2000; Luzzatti & Davidoff, 1994; Miceli, Fouch, Capasso, Shelton, Tomaiuolo, & Caramazza, 2001). Within the framework of the knowledge-specific accounts, such a deficit should result in disproportionate difficulties in identifying and naming fruit and vegetables in comparison to other categories. Luzzatti and Davidoff (1994) reported the case of two patients, GG and AV, having difficulties in retrieving the colour of objects. The patients were presented with a picture naming task including natural and manufactured objects, with the natural items set comprising fruit and vegetables items (12 items among 44). GG was slightly more impaired with natural (61% correct) than manufactured objects (70% correct), whereas AV showed no category effect (86% and 88% correct for natural and manufactured items, respectively). Unfortunately, no separate scores were provided for the fruit and vegetables items within the natural set and it is thus unclear whether naming of fruit and vegetables was spared or not in these patients. More recently, Della Sala et al. (2000) investigated the retrieval of object-colour knowledge in a group of 33 patients with probable Alzheimer's disease. Among them, three patients were found to be impaired in retrieving the colour of objects pictured as black and white drawings, while being perfectly able to name the same objects as well as colours. The small number of items used in this study (i.e., nine items, among which were four fruit and vegetable items) does not allow us to draw a firm conclusion from this finding. However, it is worth noting that these patients failed to retrieve the colour of at least two of the fruit and vegetables they were able to name. This suggests that impaired access to object-colour knowledge does not necessarily result in impaired identification and naming of items from the fruit and vegetable category. Additional evidence pointing to that conclusion comes from the study of Miceli et al. (2001). The authors reported the case of a patient, IOC, who had impaired knowledge of the colour of objects in face of spared knowledge of other objects' properties like form, size, and function. This selective impairment of object-colour knowledge was not associated with disproportionate impairment in processing the meaning of fruit and vegetables items in comparison to other item categories like animals and artefacts. Thus, in a word-to-picture verification task, the patient scored 63% for animals, 69% for artefacts, and 75% for fruit and vegetables (Shelton et al., 1998), a pattern that is clearly inconsistent with what is expected under the knowledge-specific account for category-specific deficits.

In sum, the previous case studies of patients presenting with a disproportionate deficit for either the animal or the fruit and vegetable category, or with a deficit in retrieving object-colour knowledge, did not investigate in a systematic way the issue of the particular association of deficits predicted by the knowledge-specific account for category-specific deficits, namely the association of a selective deficit in retrieving a particular kind of object's knowledge (shape vs. colour knowledge) with a selective or disproportionate deficit in processing a particular category of objects (animals vs. fruit and vegetables). Some of these studies (Della Sala et al., 2000; Hart & Gordon, 1992; Miceli et al., 2001) nevertheless provide some indirect evidence that seem inconsistent with this expectation. The main purpose of the following case study was to seek for more direct evidence pertaining to that issue. In particular, the integrity of object-colour knowledge has been assessed in a patient presenting with a category-specific deficit for fruit and vegetables, in order to determine whether this deficit was associated with a deficit for that particular kind of knowledge.

The following study had two additional purposes. The first one was to show that brain damage could result in *conceptual* knowledge of fruit and vegetables being disproportionately impaired in comparison to knowledge of animals. As we have previously mentioned, there was no evidence that conceptual knowledge for fruit and vegetables was impaired in the cases of selective naming deficit for fruit and vegetables reported so far (MD: Hart et al., 1985; TU: Farah & Wallace, 1992; and JJ: Hillis & Caramazza, 1991), which makes unclear the significance of such patterns for theories of conceptual knowledge organisation. The second additional purpose of this case study was to ascertain that the dissociation in the patient's performance could not be caused by potentially confounding factors, such as word frequency and, more particularly, concept familiarity. In the cases of JJ (Hillis & Caramazza, 1991) and MD (Hart et al., 1985), the items from the various categories were not controlled for factors such as word frequency and concept familiarity. At first sight, concept familiarity alone could not explain the patients' disproportionate deficit for fruit and vegetables since, arguably, fruit and vegetables are much more familiar in our daily life than animals. However, personal or gender-specific experience must also be taken into consideration. For instance, Hart et al. reported that MD confessed "to knowing little about cooking or food in general". Studies with normal subjects found that males rated fruit and vegetables as less familiar than did females (Albanese, Capitani, Barbarotto, & Laiacona, 2000) and that, with fruit and vegetables, males perform worse than females in naming (McKenna & Parry, 1994) and verbal fluency tasks (Capitani, Laiacona, & Barbarotto, 1999). Strikingly, the two patients who were reported to have a selective impairment for animals (EW: Caramazza & Shelton, 1998; and KR: Hart & Gordon, 1992) were both females, whereas TU (Farah & Wallace, 1992), MD (Hart et al., 1985) and JJ (Hillis & Caramazza, 1991), who showed an impairment for fruit and vegetables, were all males. Accordingly, the dissociation along the animal/fruit and vegetable distinction reported so far might be an artefact of gender-specific familiarity. Given that the present report also concerns a male patient, an attempt was made to control for personal and gender-specific familiarity in assessing the patient's knowledge about fruit and vegetables.

## CASE REPORT

RS is a right-handed and French-speaking civil engineer, who worked as General Secretary in an international company. In December 1997, at the age of 63, he suffered from an ischaemic stroke in the territory of the left posterior cerebral artery (PCA). Clinically, he showed a right homonymous hemianopia as well as some mild sensitive deficit on the right side of the body. The brain MR performed 24 hours after the onset of troubles showed a recent ischaemic-type lesion involving the whole arterial territory of PCA: the medial and inferior temporal lobe (hippocampus, parahippocampal gyrus, fusiform and lingual gyrus), the occipital lobe on its medial side, the left side of the splenium, as well as part of the left thalamus (see Figure 1).

Neuropsychological disorders were confined to the language area. On evaluation at 2 to 3 months post-stroke, RS's spontaneous speech was grammatical and fluent, without articulatory difficulties, but suggested a mild anomia. Anomia was also evidenced in a picture naming task (Bachy-Langedoc, 1988), in which the patient named only 22 of the 41 items correctly. The patient was impaired in a word-to-picture matching task (*LEXIS*: De Partz, Bilocq, De Wilde, Seron, & Pillon, 2001), scoring 63/80 (controls' mean = 79.3, *SD* = 0.46). However, his performance was within the normal range in a semantic matching task where he had to choose which of two pictures of object was semantically

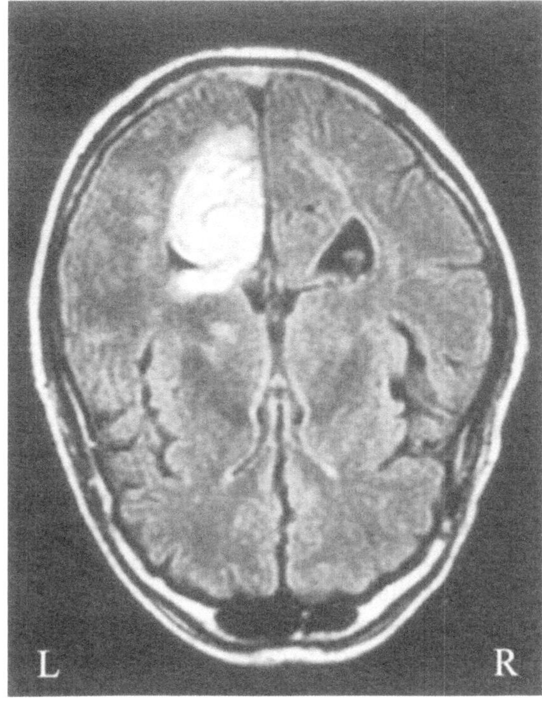


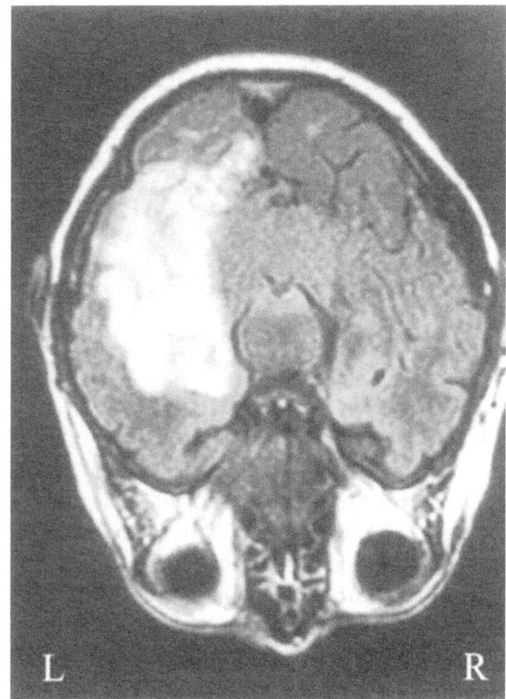


**Figure 1.** *MRI scan of RS, 24 hours post-onset.*

related to a target picture (*LEXIS*) and in a synonym matching task with concrete and abstract words (*Batterie d'épreuves évaluant la reconnaissance, la compréhension et la production de verbes et substantifs concrets et abstraits*, Pillon, Samson, & Gilmont, 1995). The reading and writing assessment revealed an alexia without agraphia for letters and words but not for numbers. Finally, at the BORB battery (Riddoch & Humphreys, 1993), RS performed within the normal range in the length, size, orientation, and position in gap matching tasks. His performance was also within the normal range on the different view matching tasks as well as in the object decision task.

RS was aware of his word-finding problems and appeared to be particularly dismayed by his difficulty in handling fruit, vegetables, and food items. He reported, for instance, that he never knew what he would find on his plate when ordering a meal in a restaurant. This apparently specific difficulty in identifying fruit and vegetables as well as food items was the focus of the study reported here. All the tests reported in this paper were carried out between March and December 1998.

## EXPERIMENTAL INVESTIGATION

### General assessment of RS's category-specific deficit

#### *Test 1. Naming the items of the living/nonliving battery*

*Method.* RS was presented with the living/nonliving battery (Samson et al., 1998), which includes 72 items: 18 animals, 18 fruit and vegetables, 18 implements, and 18 means of transport. The mean word frequency across all four categories did not differ significantly, but the mean rated concept familiarity and visual complexity (for the pictures) differed across the different semantic categories (see Samson et al., 1998, for more details and Table

**Table 1.** *RS's number and percentage of correct responses in naming tasks*

| | Mean familiarity[a] | Mean male familiarity[a] | Mean visual complexity[b] | Mean word frequency[c] | Oral picture naming | | Oral naming to description | |
|---|---|---|---|---|---|---|---|---|
| | | | | | *N* | % | *N* | % |
| Fruit and vegetables | 3.64 | 3.48 | 2.16 | 430 | 3/18 | 17 | 7/18 | 39 |
| Animals | 1.65 | 1.67 | 3.55 | 1249 | 5/18 | 28 | 10/18 | 56 |
| Implements | 3.35 | 3.34 | 2.34 | 648 | 16/18 | 89 | 13/18 | 72 |
| Transport | 2.57 | 2.65 | 3.51 | 2516 | 17/18 | 94 | 14/18 | 78 |

[a]Familiarity as rated on a 5-point scale (1 = low familiarity; 5 = high familiarity).
[b]Visual complexity as rated on a 5-point scale (1 = low visual complexity; 5 = high visual complexity).
[c]Frequency value per $100 \times 10^6$ taken from Content, Mousty, and Radeau (1990).

1 for the mean values). Importantly, however, fruit and vegetables had the highest mean value of concept familiarity and the lowest mean value of visual complexity. Note that familiarity was rated by a group of 15 normal subjects, 6 of whom were males. When taking into account the ratings of the male subjects only (cf. the gender-specific familiarity effect, Albanese et al., 2000; Capitani et al., 1999), the fruit and vegetable category was still the most familiar category of items (see Table 1). The 72 items were presented in two naming conditions: oral picture naming and oral naming to verbal description. The verbal descriptions provided information about category-membership of the target, its physical appearance and functional properties, as well as encyclopaedic information.

*Results.* RS's scores in the two naming conditions are displayed in Table 1. Strikingly, despite the fruit and vegetable category being both the most familiar and the less visually complex category of items, RS's score was the lowest for that category in both naming conditions. It is therefore unlikely that concept familiarity (either general or gender-specific) and visual complexity alone could explain RS's low performance in naming fruit and vegetables. However, although the four item categories did not significantly differ in word frequency, fruit and vegetable items appeared to have the lowest word frequency values. A logistic regression analysis was therefore performed in order to control for this potentially confounding factor. Another aim of this analysis was to evaluate the significance of RS's poor performance in naming animals, by controlling for the factors of visual complexity and concept familiarity. Both these factors could indeed make animal items more difficult to name than the items of the other categories since animal items were the less familiar and among the most visually complex items used in the battery.

The performances in the two naming tasks were analysed separately by means of a logistic regression analysis with the number of correct responses in each naming condition as the dependent variable and category (animals/fruit and vegetables/implements/means of transport), concept familiarity (either general familiarity, i.e., obtained from both male and female judges, or gender-specific familiarity), word frequency, and visual complexity (this latter factor being added for the picture naming condition only) as the independant variables. For the picture naming task, the analysis showed no significant effect of word frequency or visual complexity (both $\chi^2 < 1$); the effect of concept familiarity did not reach significance (general familiarity: $\chi^2 = 2.94$, $p = .09$; gender-specific familiarity: $\chi^2 = 2.10$, $p = .15$). However, the analysis showed a highly significant category effect once the three potentially confounded factors were controlled for (with general familiarity: $\chi^2 = 40.41$, $p < .001$; with gender-specific familiarity: $\chi^2 = 38.63$, $p < .001$). Planned contrasts showed that naming accuracy was significantly lower for fruit and vegetables as compared to the two nonliving categories (with general familiarity: $\chi^2 = 27.27$, $p < .001$; with gender-specific familiarity: $\chi^2 = 27.12$, $p < .001$). Naming accuracy was also significantly lower for animals as compared to the two nonliving categories (with general familiarity: $\chi^2$ = 4.51, $p$ < .04; with gender-specific familiarity: $\chi^2$ = 4.88, $p$ < .03). However, despite RS's naming accuracy for fruit and vegetables being lower than that for animals, this difference failed to reach significance (with general familiarity: $\chi^2$ = 3.58, $p$ = .06; with gender-specific familiarity: $\chi^2$ = 2.79, $p$ = .09).

For the naming to description task, the analysis revealed a significant effect of concept familiarity (general familiarity: $\chi^2$ = 4.59, $p$ < .04; gender-specific familiarity: $\chi^2$ = 4.96, $p$ < .03) but no significant effect of word frequency ($\chi^2$ < 1). The category effect was again significant once concept familiarity and word frequency were controlled for (with general familiarity: $\chi^2$ = 10.20, $p$ < .02; with gender-specific familiarity: $\chi^2$ = 10.13, $p$ < .02). Planned contrasts showed that RS's score for fruit and vegetables was significantly lower than his score for the two nonliving categories (with general familiarity: $\chi^2$ = 10.08, $p$ < .01; with gender-specific familiarity: $\chi^2$ = 9.90, $p$ < .01) and significantly lower than his score for animals (with general familiarity: $\chi^2$ = 5.06, $p$ < .03; with gender-specific familiarity: $\chi^2$ = 5.30, $p$ < .03). In contrast, RS's performance for animals was not significantly different from his score for the two nonliving categories (with general familiarity: $\chi^2$ <1; with gender-specific familiarity: $\chi^2$ < 1).

As regards the nature of RS's errors in both naming tasks, they were nonresponses (81% and 68% of the errors in the picture naming and naming to description tasks, respectively) and semantic errors (19% and 32% of the errors, respectively). Semantic errors all consisted of providing a semantic coordinate of the target, e.g., *girafe* (giraffe) → *zèbre* (zebra); *fraise* (strawberry) → *orange* (orange); *pioche* (pickaxe) → *bêche* (spade); *mobylette* (motor cycle) → *vélo* (bike). Another striking feature of RS's responses in the picture naming task is that he frequently used verbal and nonverbal self-cueing strategies in order to cope with his word-finding problem. He tried to describe the entity (e.g., for *hippopotamus*, he said "it lives in the south, in a herd, near rivers, its head emerges from the water, it is peaceful"), made pantomimes, attempted to cue the target name by self-generating a sentence context (e.g., for "donkey," he said "stubborn as a . . ."), or by excluding other names (e.g., for "chain saw", he said "not a drill, not a saw . . ."). As can be seen in Table 2, RS mainly used naming approaches for fruit and vegetables, animals, and implements. (For means of transport, his responses were mostly straightforward and correct.) However, the quality of the naming approaches differed according to the category of the target item. Naming approaches more often contained precise and correct semantic information when produced for a target in the implement category than for a target in the animal or fruit and vegetables categories, with the naming

**Table 2.** *Distribution of RS's responses in the picture naming task according to whether they were produced after a naming approach or not*

| | *Fruit and veg* | *Animals* | *Implements* | *Transport* | *Total* |
|---|---|---|---|---|---|
| *Without naming approach* | | | | | |
| Correct response | 2 | 3 | 7 | 14 | 26 (81%) |
| Semantic error | 1 | 1 | 0 | 1 | 3 (9%) |
| Nonresponse | 0 | 3 | 0 | 0 | 3 (9%) |
| *After a naming approach providing precise and correct semantic information*[a] | | | | | |
| Correct response | 1 | 2 | 7 | 2 | 12 (55%) |
| Semantic error | 1 | 0 | 0 | 0 | 1 (5%) |
| Nonresponse | 4 | 4 | 1 | 0 | 9 (41%) |
| *After a naming approach providing only vague and/or incorrect semantic information* | | | | | |
| Correct response | 0 | 0 | 2 | 1 | 3 (17%) |
| Semantic error | 1 | 1 | 0 | 0 | 2 (11%) |
| Nonresponse | 8 | 4 | 1 | 0 | 13 (72%) |

[a]Semantic approaches containing at least one specific semantic property and no false semantic property.

approaches produced for fruit and vegetables containing the least frequently precise and correct semantic information. Moreover, naming approaches led to a successful name retrieval mostly for items in the implement category. For the items in the fruit and vegetable and animal categories, even the few approaches containing some precise/correct information seldom led to a successful name retrieval. These qualitative observations not only suggest that the severity of RS's word-finding difficulties differ across the four categories, they also suggest that, for fruit and vegetables and, to a lesser extent, for animals, RS had additional difficulties in accessing the underlying semantic representations.

*Test 2. Naming fruit and vegetables, manufactured food items, and domestic implements*

In the previous naming tasks, we have shown that RS's poor performance in naming fruit and vegetables could not be explained by a familiarity effect, even when taking into account gender-specific familiarity ratings. Still, the possibility that RS shows a particularly low idiosyncratic familiarity with fruit and vegetables should be considered. RS actually stated that he almost never cooked nor bought food in stores. RS also claimed that he was not familiar with household activities. We therefore explored RS's naming abilities on a second set of items that was aimed at contrasting RS's performance for fruit and vegetables with his performance for domestic implements, i.e., a nonliving category which we believed would match fruit and vegetables more closely in idiosyncratic familiarity. The set of items also included manufactured food items, in order to determine if RS's problem was limited to fruit and vegetables or if it extended to the broader category of food.

*Method.* One hundred and fifty-three photographs depicting fruit and vegetables, manufactured food items, and domestic implements were presented to a group of five normal subjects (three males and two females). The subjects were instructed to name each item and rate on a 5-point scale how familiar the item was in their daily life (we used the same familiarity instructions as those used by Snodgrass & Vanderwart, 1980). From the 153 items, we chose 21 fruit and vegetables, 21 food items, and 21 domestic implements, which were closely matched for familiarity and could be correctly named by the control subjects. The selected items were also presented to a control subject matching RS in gender, age, educational level, and occupation. Note that the control subject also stated he was not expert in cooking and was almost never in charge of household activities.

*Results.* The performance of both RS and the control subject is displayed in Table 3. RS's performance for implements was comparable to that of the control subject (Fisher exact probability = .5); his performance for fruit and vegetables was however significantly lower than that of the control subject (Fisher exact probability = .0002) and the same pattern was found for manufactured food items (Fisher exact probability = .004). RS's deficit thus seemed to extend to the food category. RS's good performance for domestic implements in the face of his low familiarity with household activities is also interesting. It suggests that RS's poor performance for fruit and vegetables as well as for food

**Table 3.** *RS's and the control subject's naming performance (number and percentage of correct responses) for fruit and vegetables, manufactured food items, and domestic implements*

| | *Mean familiarity*[a] | *RS* | | *Control subject* | |
|---|---|---|---|---|---|
| | | *N* | *%* | *N* | *%* |
| Fruit and vegetables | 3.09 | 11/21 | 52 | 21/21 | 100 |
| Food | 3.1 | 14/21 | 67 | 21/21 | 100 |
| Domestic implements | 3.09 | 17/21 | 81 | 18/21 | 86 |

[a]Familiarity as rated on a 5-point scale (1 = low familiarity; 5 = high familiarity).

items did not result simply from his low idiosyncratic familiarity with such items.

*Test 3. Object decision task*

RS's performance in the object decision task of the BORB (Riddoch & Humphreys, 1993) was within the normal range. However, since RS's naming for fruit and vegetables and animals appeared to be slightly more impaired in the picture naming condition than in the naming to description condition, mild damage to the structural processing level could not be dismissed at this stage. Thus, in order to assess further the patient's structural processing abilities, another object decision task, which included items drawn from the four categories tested in the naming tasks, was presented.

*Method.* Seventy-two line drawings were presented. The items belonged to four semantic categories: animals, fruit and vegetables, implements, and means of transport. Half of the line drawings for each semantic category depicted real objects; the other half depicted unreal objects. Unreal objects were a combination of parts of two objects belonging to the same category (see Samson et al., 1998, for more details). RS was presented with the line drawings in a random order and was asked to say, for each line drawing, whether he recognised the entity depicted in the drawing as something that existed in real life.

*Results.* RS performed quite well in this task as he scored 67/72 (93%, a score within the normal range of the young controls used in a previous study, Samson et al., 1998). All errors consisted of accepting unreal objects. Four errors involved fruit and vegetables and one error involved an implement.

*Test 4. Picture and word categorisation*

*Method.* RS was presented with the 72 items of the living/nonliving battery, once as picture stimuli and once as word stimuli, and was asked to classify these items into four broad semantic categories: animals, fruit and vegetables, implements, and means of transport.

*Results.* RS performed this categorisation task easily and faultlessly, both with the pictures and with the words.

*Test 5. Word/picture verification*

*Method.* RS was given the picture of each of the 72 items of the living/nonliving battery simultaneously with a spoken word. He was asked to say if the word was the correct name for the pictured object. Each picture was presented once with the correct word, once with a word that was a "close" coordinate of the correct word (i.e., the picture of a donkey with the word *horse*) and once with a word that was a "far" coordinate of the correct word (i.e., the picture of a donkey with the word *hippopotamus*). An item was scored as correct when for a given picture, RS both accepted the correct word and rejected the two coordinate words.

*Results.* RS's performance was poorer for fruit and vegetables than for animals and the two nonliving categories (see Table 4). Errors in all four categories of items mostly consisted of accepting the close coordinate word (RS only once rejected the correct name of an animal, twice rejected the correct name of an implement, and twice accepted the name of a far coordinate for fruit and vegetables).

A logistic regression analysis with the same factors as those described in Test 1 revealed a significant effect of concept familiarity (general familiarity: $\chi^2 = 11.33$, $p < .001$; gender-specific familiarity: $\chi^2 = 10.23$, $p < .01$) but no significant effect of visual complexity or word frequency (all $\chi^2 < 1$). The category effect was significant even when the three potentially confounded factors were controlled for (with general familiarity: $\chi^2 = 12.41$, $p < .01$; with gender-specific familiarity: $\chi^2 = 11.15$, $p < .02$). Planned contrasts showed that RS's performance for fruit and vegetables was significantly lower than for animals (with general familiarity: $\chi^2 = 11.79$, $p < .001$; with gender-specific familiarity: $\chi^2 = 10.69$, $p < .01$) and the two nonliving categories (with general familiarity: $\chi^2 = 9.75$, $p < .01$; with gender-specific familiarity: $\chi^2 = 8.09$, $p < .01$). In contrast, RS's performance for animals was significantly better than his performance for nonliving

**Table 4.** *RS's number and percentage of correct responses in the word/picture verification and verbal description tasks*

| | *Word/picture verification* | | *Verbal description from a word* | | *Verbal description from a picture* | |
|---|---|---|---|---|---|---|
| | *N* | % | *N* | % | *N* | % |
| Fruit and vegetables | 9/18 | 50 | 8/18 | 44 | 7/18 | 39 |
| Animals | 16/18 | 89 | 13/18 | 72 | 13/18 | 72 |
| Implements | 13/18 | 72 | 14/18 | 78 | 16/18 | 89 |
| Transport | 16/18 | 89 | 18/18 | 100 | 15/18 | 83 |

things (with general familiarity: $\chi^2 = 4.42, p < .04$; with gender-specific familiarity: $\chi^2 = 4.59, p < .04$).

*Test 6. Picture and word description task*

*Method.* RS was given the 72 items of the living/nonliving battery, once as a picture and once as a word, and was asked to describe the object they referred to. Instructions stressed the fact that he should give as much relevant information as possible so that a subject, unaware of the picture RS was looking at or the word he heard, would be able to find out which entity he was defining. All his verbal descriptions were tape-recorded and then transcribed to be submitted to two groups of six independent judges. One group was asked to identify the items described in the "word" condition, and the other group was asked to identify the items described in the "picture" condition. An item was scored as correct if at least one judge had identified it with certainty from the patient's description. The patient's descriptions leading to correct but unsure identifications or for which the judges considered that part of the provided information was wrong were scored as incorrect. In that way, we considered as correct responses the descriptions that contained not only correct, but also sufficiently relevant semantic information to allow one to identify the entity described with certainty.

*Results.* In both the picture and the word description tasks, a similar pattern to that found in the word/picture verification task emerged (see Table 4), with the patient's performance being poorer for fruit and vegetables than animals and the two nonliving categories. Qualitatively, we noted that RS's descriptions of nonliving items as well as animals were strikingly precise (including both visual and nonvisual attributes) as compared to his descriptions of fruit and vegetables. For instance, RS described a camel (from a picture input) as "an exotic animal with two humps on its back; it is used as transport with people sitting between the two humps; it is a peaceful animal widely used by nomads who cross the desert" or a giraffe (from a word input) as "an animal of a big size with a long neck and a handsome head; it lives in a herd and its coat has white and black spots. Its long neck allows it to eat the leaves from the trees, a food it really likes." Similarly, RS described a balloon (from a picture input) as "an air transportation that transports humans but also cameras or other things; it moves in the sky because it is filled with a light gas; its height can be adjusted by changing the proportion of gas" or a screwdriver (from a word input) as "a tool with a handle and an active part which is flat and relatively pointed, it allows to enter into a body through a rotary movement." In contrast, RS's descriptions of fruit and vegetables were more hesitant and less precise. He described a cherry (from a word input) as "a nice fruit, it grows in our country" or a carrot (from a word input) as "a vegetable, longer than large, its colour is gray-green; you cut it into small pieces; it gives taste to the dishes." In the picture condition, RS often only described what he saw on the picture. For instance, in front of the picture of a tomato, he said "it is a vegetable, it has an appendage, an envelope, it is maybe of a kind of rose colour and inside . . . it depends, I think it could be two or three different vegetables" or, for watermelon (the picture shows the internal part of the fruit), he said "it is a condiment, a fruit, surrounded with a shell, it is more or less 20 cm big, it is elongated, inside there is a mixture of seeds and things to eat."

A logistic regression analysis was conducted separately for the picture and word conditions with the same factors as those described earlier (with visual complexity being introduced into the analysis for the picture condition only). For the picture condition, the analysis showed no significant effect of concept familiarity, word frequency or visual complexity ($1.24 < \chi^2 < 0.11$, $0.26 < p < .74$), but a significant category effect once all these three factors were controlled for (with general familiarity: $\chi^2 = 12.05$, $p < .01$; with gender-specific familiarity: $\chi^2 = 11.41$, $p < .01$). Planned contrasts showed that RS's performance was significantly lower for fruit and vegetables than for nonliving items (with general familiarity: $\chi^2 = 9.18$, $p < .01$; with gender-specific familiarity: $\chi^2 = 8.30$, $p < .01$), but the difference between his performance for fruit and vegetables and for animals was not statistically significant (with general familiarity: $\chi^2 = 2.01$, $p = .16$; with gender-specific familiarity: $\chi^2 = 1.10$, $p = .30$). Again, RS's performance for animals was comparable to his performance for nonliving items (with general familiarity: $\chi^2 < 1$; with gender-specific familiarity: $\chi^2 < 1$).

In the word condition, the logistic regression analysis showed a significant effect of concept familiarity (general familiarity: $\chi^2 = 5.11$, $p < .03$; gender-specific familiarity: $\chi^2 = 7.73$, $p < .01$) but no significant effect of word frequency ($\chi^2 < 1$). The category effect was significant once concept familiarity and word frequency were controlled for (with general familiarity: $\chi^2 = 19.16$, $p < .001$; with gender-specific familiarity: $\chi^2 = 21.70$, $p < .001$). Planned contrasts revealed a significant difference between RS's score for fruit and vegetables and his score for nonliving things (with general familiarity: $\chi^2 = 17.91$, $p < .001$; with gender-specific familiarity: $\chi^2 = 19.97$, $p < .001$) as well as a significant difference between RS's score for fruit and vegetables and his score for animals (with general familiarity: $\chi^2 = 7.25$, $p < .01$; with gender-specific familiarity: $\chi^2 = 9.77$, $p < .01$). RS's performance for animals was however not significantly different from his performance for nonliving things (with general familiarity: $\chi^2 < 1$; with gender-specific familiarity: $\chi^2 < 1$).

### *Test 7. Attribute verification task*

The aim of this test was to assess RS's ability to retrieve a set of semantic properties of fruit and vegetables as well as of items from the other categories. Although the task was not designed to properly evaluate possible differences in retrieving visual vs. nonvisual knowledge, both kinds of knowledge were probed, so that it could provide some information on this issue.

*Method.* Fifteen animals, 15 fruit and vegetables, 16 implements, and 16 means of transport were used for this task. These items were a subset of the items used in the naming and other semantic tasks. The name of each of the 62 items was presented in four sentences, two stressing a correct semantic attribute (one visual, one nonvisual) and two stressing a wrong semantic attribute (one visual, one nonvisual). The visual attributes consisted of describing a part of the object, its global appearance or its colour. The nonvisual attributes referred, for animals, to eating habits, moving habits, living environment or human use; for fruit and vegetables, they referred to taste, cooking, or growing environment; for implements, to their functional use; and for means of transport, stated what is transported, the context in which it is used, or the specific place where it is used. False statements were constructed by assigning a true attribute of an item to another item of the same category. The 248 verbal statements were submitted in questionnaire form to 10 control subjects (age 19 to 27 years) who were asked to verify the statements and to rate on a 5-point scale how easy it was to answer (1 = *very easy*; 5 = *very difficult*). The mean rated difficulty was 1.66 ("true" statements) and 2.11 ("false" statements) for fruit and vegetables, 1.92 ("true" statements) and 2.16 ("false" statements) for animals, 1.92 ("true" statements) and 1.97 ("false" statements) for implements, and 1.65 ("true" statements) and 2.00 ("false" statements) for means of transport. False statements were judged more difficult than true statements, $F(1, 240) = 9.00$, $p < .01$, but there was no significant difference in the mean difficulty of statements between the four item categories, $F(3, 240) = 1.03, p = .38$. No significant item category × truth value interaction was found either, $F(3, 240) < 1$. RS was presented with each statement and asked to say if it was true or false.

*Results.* An item was scored as correct when the two true statements were accepted and the two false statements rejected. The performance of RS and the control subjects is displayed in Table 5(a).[2] Similarly to the pattern observed in the word/picture verification and the description tasks, RS's performance was the lowest for fruit and vegetables whereas his performance for animals was close to his performance for the two nonliving categories. In fact, RS performed below the normal range of the control subjects' performance for the fruit and vegetable category only. RS's score was entered in a logistic regression analysis with the same factors as those described earlier (excluding visual complexity). The analysis showed no significant effect of concept familiarity or word frequency ($0.64 < \chi^2 < 3.16$, $0.43 < p < .07$) but a significant effect of category once both these factors were controlled for (with general familiarity: $\chi^2 = 8.80, p < .04$; but with gender-specific familiarity: $\chi^2 = 7.18$, $p = .07$). Planned contrasts showed that RS's score for fruit and vegetables was significantly lower than his score for nonliving things (with general familiarity: $\chi^2 = 6.81, p < .01$; with gender-specific familiarity:

Table 5. *RS's and the controls' number and percentage of correct responses in (a) the attribute verification task and (b) for the visual vs. nonvisual attributes in the attribute verification task*

| | Mean rated difficulty[c] | RS | | Controls | | |
|---|---|---|---|---|---|---|
| | | *N* | *%* | *Mean N* | *Mean %* | *Range* |
| (a) *Attribute verification task*[a] | | | | | | |
| Fruit and vegetables | 1.89 | 7/15 | 47 | 11.9/15 | 79 | 10–14 |
| Animals | 2.04 | 12/15 | 80 | 12/15 | 80 | 10–14 |
| Implements | 1.94 | 14/16 | 88 | 13.8/16 | 86 | 12–15 |
| Transport | 1.82 | 13/16 | 81 | 13.7/16 | 86 | 11–16 |
| (b) *Visual vs. nonvisual attributes in the attribute verification task*[b] | | | | | | |
| *Visual attributes* | | | | | | |
| Fruit and vegetables | 1.72 | 8/15 | 53 | 13/15 | 87 | 12–14 |
| Animals | 1.91 | 12/15 | 80 | 13/15 | 87 | 12–14 |
| Implements | 2.43 | 14/16 | 88 | 14/16 | 88 | 12–16 |
| Transport | 1.88 | 14/16 | 88 | 14.1/16 | 88 | 11–16 |
| Total | 1.99 | 48/62 | 77 | 54.1/62 | 87 | 50–59 |
| *Nonvisual attributes* | | | | | | |
| Fruit and vegetables | 2.05 | 12/15 | 80 | 13.9/15 | 93 | 12–15 |
| Animals | 2.17 | 15/15 | 100 | 13.8/15 | 92 | 13–15 |
| Implements | 1.45 | 16/16 | 100 | 15.7/16 | 98 | 15–16 |
| Transport | 1.77 | 15/16 | 94 | 15.6/16 | 98 | 14–16 |
| Total | 1.85 | 56/62 | 90 | 58.9/62 | 95 | 57–62 |

[a]One item has been scored as correct when a correct response was provided for all the four statements related to it (true and false visual and nonvisual).
[b]One item has been scored as correct when a correct response was provided for both the true and the false statements related to it.
[c]Difficulty as rated on a 5-point scale (1 = very easy; 5 = very difficult).

[2] The data from one of the control subjects had to be excluded because that subject had an overall accuracy score of only 52% (i.e., 5.2 *SD*s below the mean score of the other nine subjects). The subject's score was poor for all four categories: he was 60% correct for fruit and vegetables, 47% for animals, 44% for implements, and 56% for means of transport.

$\chi^2 = 5.13, p < .03$), whereas his score for animals was comparable to his score for nonliving things (both $\chi^2 < 1$). There was also a significant difference between RS's score for fruit and vegetables and his score for animals, which did not, however, reach significance once gender-specific familiarity was controlled for (with general familiarity: $\chi^2 = 4.85$, $p < .03$; with gender-specific familiarity: $\chi^2 = 2.74$, $p = .10$).[3] It is also worth noting that RS's performance was below the range of the controls' performance for the fruit and vegetable category only; his performance for animals and the two categories of nonliving things fell entirely inside the controls' range.

Although the task was not designed to evaluate possible differences in retrieving visual vs. nonvisual knowledge, it could be indicative to also look at RS's pattern of performance for the statements stressing visual vs. nonvisual attributes. Thus, in an additional analysis, we considered separately the statements stressing visual and nonvisual attributes and scored as correct an item for which both the true statement was accepted and the false one rejected. Note, however, that in doing this, the mean rated difficulty of the statements was no longer equated across conditions. While the mean difficulty of the statements did not significantly differ between the four item categories, $F(3, 232) = 1.17$, $p = .32$, nor between visual and nonvisual attributes, $F(1, 232) = 2.29$, $p = .14$, there was a significant attribute type × category interaction effect, $F(3, 232) = 12.73$, $p < .001$. Separate analyses performed for each category showed that, for the implement category, the statements stressing visual attributes were rated as more difficult than the statements stressing nonvisual attributes, $t(47.2) = 6.34$, $p < .001$. An opposite trend was noted for fruit and vegetables, but this difference failed to reach significance, $t(51.3) = 1.92$, $p = .06$. However, there was no significant difference in the mean rated difficulty of the statements stressing visual vs. nonvisual attributes for animals, $t(58) = 1.38$, $p = .17$, and means of transport, $t(62) < 1$.

As can be seen in Table 5(b), RS's performance was worse, on the whole, for the visual than the nonvisual attributes (77% vs. 90% correct, respectively). The logistic regression analysis performed with attribute type (visual/nonvisual), category membership (fruit and vegetables/animals/implements/means of transport) as well as concept familiarity and word frequency as independent variables revealed that this attribute effect was significant (with general familiarity: $\chi^2 = 8.14$, $p < .01$; with gender-specific familiarity: $\chi^2 = 7.99$, $p < .01$) once all the other variables were controlled for. However, a similar trend was noted for the control subjects, whose performance was 87% vs. 95% correct for the visual and nonvisual attributes, respectively. In fact, RS's performance was below the range of controls only for the visual attributes of fruit and vegetables.[4]

Moreover, the results in Table 5(b) once again indicate that, for both visual and nonvisual statements, RS's performance was worse for fruit and vegetables than for any other category, while no similar trend was noted for the control subjects.

[3] Among the visual statements used to assess knowledge of fruit and vegetables, seven of them stressed a colour attribute. RS gave a wrong response to three of them. As we will show later, RS seemed to have lost the link between a colour name and the corresponding colour concept. These three errors could therefore be due to a failure to comprehend the colour name rather than a failure to access the concept or the attribute probed. However, these errors do not by themselves explain RS's lower performance for fruit and vegetables. The three colour statements for which RS made a wrong response related to two items for which he also provided a wrong response to another, noncolour, statement. Given the scoring procedure adopted here (i.e., one item being considered as correct when all four statements were correctly judged), the general score would thus remain unchanged if the three colour statements were excluded from the analysis.

[4] The scoring procedure adopted here does not allow us to examine separately RS's scores for the visual statements stressing colour and noncolour attributes because, for a given item, the "true" and "false" statements did not necessarily stress the same kind (colour vs. noncolour) of attribute. By scoring separately the response accuracy for each individual "true" or "false" statements stressing visual attributes of fruit and vegetables, scores were as follows: for the statements stressing a colour attribute, RS made 4/7 (57%) correct responses (controls' mean score: 6.9/7, 99%; range: 6–7); for the statements stressing a noncolour attribute, RS had 17/23 (74%) correct responses (controls' mean score: 21.1/23, 92%; range: 20–22). Thus, it appears that RS's performance was below the normal range for both the colour and noncolour attributes of fruit and vegetables.

This category effect was significant once all other variables, including attribute type, were controlled for (with general familiarity: $\chi^2 = 11.44$, $p < .01$; with gender-specific familiarity: $\chi^2 = 9.45$, $p < .03$), which indicates that the category effect is not reducible to an attribute type effect. Planned contrast showed that RS's scores for fruit and vegetables were significantly lower than his scores for nonliving items (with general familiarity: $\chi^2 = 9.11$, $p < .01$; with gender-specific familiarity: $\chi^2 = 7.04$, $p < .01$), and significantly lower than his score for animals (with general familiarity: $\chi^2 = 6.04$, $p < .02$; but with gender-specific familiarity: $\chi^2 = 3.43$, $p = .06$). On the other hand, RS's scores for animals were not significantly different from his scores for nonliving things (both $\chi^2 < 1$).

### *Discussion*

In all the naming tasks, RS's lowest scores were for the fruit and vegetable category as compared to the other categories of items. This was particularly striking when RS was asked to name the items of the living/nonliving battery, despite fruit and vegetables being the most familiar (even when only the male familiarity ratings were taken into account) and the less visually complex items. RS's naming impairment also extended to the food category and the animal category. Access to category membership, from a word or from a picture, appeared to be preserved for all the categories of items tested. However, when access to specific semantic attributes was required without necessitating the production of the target word (i.e., word/picture verification, word and picture description, and attribute verification tasks), RS's disproportionate deficit for fruit and vegetables was more apparent than in the naming tasks: RS's scores for fruit and vegetables were indeed lower than his scores for nonliving items *and* for animals but no difference could be observed between the animal category and the two nonliving categories (see Figure 2 for a summary of the results). That RS's impairment for fruit and vegetables appeared in all semantic tasks, whatever the modality in which the items were presented (pictures or words) and even when no name production was required, points to the semantic processing level as the likely locus of RS's deficit for fruit and vegetables.

RS's slightly lower score for animals and fruit and vegetables in the picture naming task relative to the

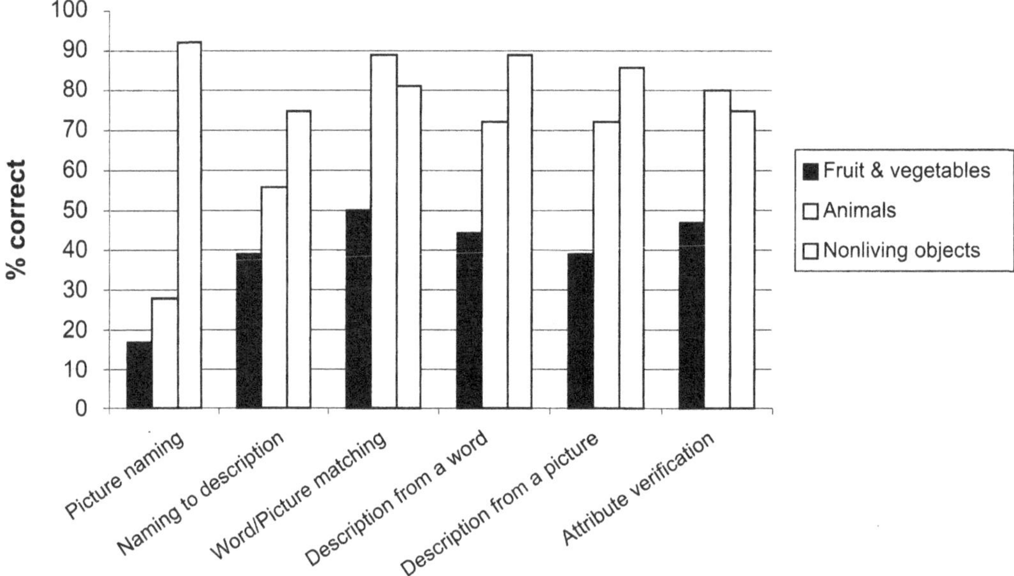


**Figure 2.** *RS's percentage of correct responses in the naming and semantic tasks for the fruit and vegetable, animal, and nonliving object categories.*

naming from description task could suggest greater difficulty in accessing semantic knowledge from a picture than from a verbal input. However, it seems unlikely that the difference resulted from a structural processing impairment, since RS's performance in the two object decision tasks (cf. BORB in Case Report and Test 3) was within the normal range. Nor did the difference seem to result from a disruption of the processes by which the semantic system is accessed from the structural description store, since no similar discrepancy was found when RS had to describe animals and fruit and vegetables from a picture vs. from a spoken word. Therefore, we propose that the discrepancy between RS's score in the picture naming and the naming from description tasks results from differences in the kind and amount of information being provided directly in both tasks. The verbal description of an object by the examiner indeed provides more detailed and selected semantic information (category membership and *only relevant* visual, functional, and encyclopaedic information) than the picture of that object (which yields only structural/visual information directly). Thus verbal descriptions might facilitate semantic processing by enhancing the activation of the relevant semantic properties of the objects within the semantic system.

Finally, the results of the attribute verification task indicated that RS's performance in verifying visual attributes of fruit and vegetables was below the range of the control subjects, while his performance for both visual and nonvisual attributes of the other categories of items was within the normal range. This observation is inconsistent with the hypothesis of a selective deficit in retrieving visual knowledge as a source of RS's difficulties with fruit and vegetables, which should lead to below-normal performance in verifying visual statements for *all* categories of items. Evidence that RS was not impaired in retrieving visual knowledge in general was also found in the picture and word description tasks. For animals and manufactured items, RS's descriptions were very detailed and precise (see earlier), not only as regards the nonvisual attributes, but also the visual appearance of the objects, in spite of the fact that describing the visual appearance of animals, implements or means of transport might be far more difficult than describing their function.

## Assessing object-colour knowledge

The following tests were aimed at testing RS's object-colour knowledge, as colour knowledge has been claimed to be a kind of knowledge that is particularly diagnostic for fruit and vegetables. These tests were designed to contrast RS's object-colour knowledge for fruit and vegetables with object-colour knowledge for another category of items, matched for familiarity with fruit and vegetables and for which RS showed a less marked deficit in naming and semantic tasks.

The criteria chosen for the selection of items was that the objects had a typical colour and that, altogether, they allowed us to cover the widest range of colours in each category. Thus, only fruit and vegetables and manufactured items have been selected in this test. Items from the animal category could not be included due to the difficulty in finding animal items covering a range of different (typical) colours and liable to match fruit and vegetables in terms of familiarity. For the fruit and vegetables category, only 10 out of the 18 items used in the previous tasks were kept and 10 additional items were selected. For the manufactured objects, 20 new items had to be selected, because almost none of those from the living/nonliving battery had a typical colour. These manufactured items were taken from various subcategories, such as cloth, vehicles, sport items, and urban items.

The tasks usually used to assess object-colour knowledge require a colour-related response, either by pointing to a colour patch, colouring a line drawing, choosing among coloured line drawings the one that is correctly coloured, producing the colour name, or pointing to a colour name. Hence, the results of these tasks are informative about object-colour knowledge retrieval provided that the patient can adequately report to the examiner the colour he believes to be associated with a particular object. For instance, a patient might know that a tomato is red, but at the same time, because of a colour anomia, he might be unable to select and produce the word *red*. In order to determine the most reliable response modality that could be used to assess RS's object-colour knowledge, the patient was thus first presented with several tasks assessing his colour perceptual processing and naming. All the tests described below were also presented to RS's matched control subject who participated in Test 2.

*Test 8. Colour discrimination*
RS and the control subject were presented with the Ishihara (1974) plates. Both correctly and easily identified all items.

*Test 9. Colour matching*
*Method.* RS and the control subject were given an array of 11 target colour patches randomly positioned (the colours were: white, yellow, orange, red, purple, green, blue, black, brown, pink, and grey). They were then presented with 38 colour patches consisting of three or four different shades of each target colour, one at a time, and asked to associate these patches with one of the colour patches of the array.

*Results.* Both RS and the control subject scored 35/38 (92%) on this task. All the errors consisted of choosing a closely related colour patch. RS's performance thus indicates that he was able to perceptually categorise colours into the 11 selected basic colours.

*Test 10. Colour naming*
*Method.* RS was presented with 44 colour patches and asked to name each of them. The items consisted of four different shades of each of the 11 basic colours presented in Test 9. The same procedure was used for the control subject.

*Results.* RS scored 28/44 (64%). He made no errors for the different shades of white, green, and yellow, but never provided the correct name for the different shades of purple (which were three times named as pink and once as blue) and orange (which were all named as pink). For all the other colours, he gave the correct name at least twice (errors were the following: black patch → *blue*, *brown*; pink patch → *red*; blue patch → *green*; brown patch → *green*; grey patch → *green*, *green*; red patch → *brown*, *brown*). The patient's performance was significantly lower than the control subject's performance (39/44, 89%; Fisher exact probability = .006). The control subject must also have found it difficult to name the purple patches, as he only provided the correct name once (he twice misnamed it as blue and once as grey). The control subject made also one error for the brown and the pink colour patches, which were misnamed as black and red, respectively.

*Test 11. Spoken word/colour matching*
*Method.* RS was presented with an array of 11 colour patches, each patch corresponding to one of the 11 basic colours. He was asked to point to the colour patch that corresponded to the auditory presented words. The test was performed four times, each time with different shades of the 11 basic colours. The control subject was also tested.

*Results.* RS scored 37/44 (84%), a score again lower than that of the control subject (41/44, 93%), although the difference was not statistically significant (Fisher exact probability = .16). RS made errors when pointing to the colour patch corresponding to the following names: brown (pointing three times to the grey patch), purple (pointing once to the green and once to the brown patches), orange (pointing once to the pink patch), and grey (pointing once to the purple patch). The control subject's errors involved the following colour names: purple (associated with the pink patch), grey (associated with the purple patch), and blue (associated with the purple patch).

*Test 12. Spoken word/colour verification*
*Method.* RS was presented simultaneously with a colour name and a colour patch. He was asked to tell if the word was the correct name for the colour patch. Each colour was presented three times, once with the correct name, once with the name of a closely related colour (e.g., the word "orange" for the yellow colour patch), and once with a less closely related colour (e.g., the word "purple" for the yellow colour patch). An item was scored as correct when, for a given colour patch, the patient both accepted the correct name and rejected the two distractors. The same procedure was used for the control subject.

*Results.* RS scored 7/11 (64%), a performance significantly lower than the control subject's level (11/11; Fisher exact probability = .05). RS made errors for the following colour patches: brown (accepted as purple), blue (accepted as green), purple (rejected as not being purple), and yellow (accepted as orange).

*Test 13. Colour name fluency*
*Method.* RS and the control subject were asked to produce as many colours as possible in 2 min. (This test was administered before all the other tests involving colour processing.)

*Results.* RS provided 17 names (control subject: 22). Both produced the names of the 11 basic colours used in the previous tests.

*Discussion*
RS showed no colour discrimination difficulties and was quite accurate when asked to classify colour patches into the 11 basic colours. He also performed quite well in the colour name fluency task. However, he was not able to correctly associate a given colour with the appropriate name or vice versa. Within current models of colour processing (see, for instance, Davidoff, 1991), RS's pattern of performance suggests a preservation of the internal colour space (as evidenced by his good performance in classifying visually presented colours). However, he seemed to suffer from a disruption of the links between the input verbal lexicon and the internal colour space (as evidenced by his poor performance when asked to match a name with the corresponding colour) and from a disruption of the links between the internal colour space and the output verbal lexicon (as evidenced by his colour naming impairment). As RS seemed to have lost the link between a colour and its name, we avoided the use of the colour names in the tasks assessing object-colour knowledge and instead asked the patient to point to a colour patch.

*Test 14. Retrieval of object-colour knowledge about fruit and vegetables from a visual input*
*Method.* RS was asked to point to the appropriate colour of 20 fruit and vegetables presented as black-and-white drawings. For each item, he had a choice of three patches of colours. All the distractor patches displayed a plausible colour for the fruit and vegetable category. The shade of almost all the correct colour patches differed from the shade of the actual colour of the object. The control subject did the same test.

*Results.* RS scored 17/20 (85%), a performance similar to the control subject's level (16/20).

*Test 15. Retrieval of object-colour knowledge from a verbal input*
*Method.* We used the same 20 fruit and vegetables items and the same colour patches as in Test 14. But instead of being presented with the picture of the target item, RS was given its name. RS was also asked to point to the appropriate colour (among three colour patches) of 20 manufactured objects that have a salient and typical colour (e.g., a pillar box, a golf ball, a tyre). The number of items for a given colour were matched as closely as possible across the two categories of items. All 40 items used in that task were submitted to six control subjects (half of which were males), who were asked to rate on a 5-point scale how familiar the item denoted by the word was to them in daily life (we used the same procedure as the one used by Snodgrass & Vanderwart, 1980). The mean rated familiarity for fruit and vegetables appeared to be slightly higher than the mean rated familiarity for objects (3.08 and 2.63, respectively).

*Results.* RS's score was significantly below the control subject's score for fruit and vegetables (RS: 13/20, control: 19/20, Fisher exact probability = .02) but the difference didn't reach significance for objects (RS: 16/20, control: 19/20, Fisher exact probability = 0.17).[5]

[5] Unfortunately, the testing had been aborted at this stage and there was no opportunity to ask RS to name the items used in that task.

*Discussion*

RS's performance was not perfect when asked to retrieve object-colour knowledge and he appeared to be impaired (as compared to the control subject) when asked to retrieve object-colour knowledge about fruit and vegetables. Interestingly, RS's impairment at retrieving object-colour knowledge about fruit and vegetables disappeared when the fruit and vegetables were presented as picture stimuli, indicating that at least in some conditions (i.e., from a picture) RS could accurately access object-colour knowledge about fruit and vegetables. We will discuss this point in the General Discussion.

## GENERAL DISCUSSION

In this paper, we reported an additional case of a patient, RS, who shows more difficulties in processing fruit and vegetables than other categories of objects. In contrast to previously reported cases of category-specific deficits for fruit and vegetables (Farah & Wallace, 1992; Hart et al., 1985), RS's disproportionate impairment was not confined to the tasks requiring the production of the name of objects, such as picture naming and naming from description tasks. RS also showed a disproportionate impairment for fruit and vegetables in a word-to-picture verification task, when asked to describe them, both from a picture and a spoken name, and in an attribute verification task. Given that RS's deficit for fruit and vegetables was observed in tasks requiring access to semantic knowledge whatever the modality of input (a picture or a word) and even when no name production was needed, the most likely locus of his disproportionate impairment is the semantic processing level. RS's good performance for fruit and vegetables in a picture and word categorisation task further suggests that his semantic impairment only affects the retrieval of specific semantic attributes about fruit and vegetables but not category membership information.

RS's category-specific deficit for fruit and vegetables did not seem to be an artefact of potentially confounding factors, at least as far as word frequency, concept familiarity, or visual complexity are concerned. In a number of tasks, RS was presented with the items of the living/nonliving battery where all categories were equated in word frequency, and where fruit and vegetables had the highest mean familiarity value and the lowest mean visual complexity value. The category effect remained significant when these factors were controlled for in a logistic regression analysis. In the other tasks, fruit and vegetables were matched in familiarity to the other categories of items.

It has recently been claimed that familiarity is modulated by gender and, more particularly, that males are less familiar with fruit and vegetables than females (Albanese et al., 2000). This point appears to be particularly relevant in the face of the striking gender effect observed when examining the patients who have been reported to date with a dissociation along the animal/fruit and vegetable distinction. The patients presenting with a selective sparing of the fruit and vegetable category as compared to the animal category (namely, EW: Caramazza & Shelton, 1998; and KR: Hart & Gordon, 1992) were both females, whereas the three previously reported patients presenting with the reverse pattern (TU: Farah & Wallace, 1992; MD: Hart et al., 1985; and JJ: Hillis & Caramazza, 1991) were males. The present case of RS, a male patient, is consistent with this gender effect. Still, when taking into account the familiarity ratings of the male subjects who participated in the familiarity rating of the items of the living/nonliving battery, fruit and vegetables remained the most familiar category of items in the battery. Furthermore, controlling for gender-specific familiarity (instead of general familiarity) did not modulate the results of our logistic regression analyses (except for one contrast in the attribute verification task, where the difference between RS's score for fruit and vegetables, on the one hand, and animals, on the other hand, failed to reach significance after controlling for gender-specific familiarity).

In order to further investigate the issue of a potential confounding familiarity effect, RS's naming of fruit and vegetables was contrasted with his naming of domestic implements, that is, items belonging to the nonliving category and which we believed would match fruit and vegetables in terms of idiosyncratic familiarity. Indeed, RS stated not only that he was poorly acquainted with cooking activities but also, more generally, that he knew little about household activities. On naming these items, RS was found to be impaired for fruit and vegetables but not for domestic implements as compared to a matched control subject.

Our study, in contrast to the studies of Farah and Wallace (1992) and Hart et al. (1985), also provides direct evidence on the extent to which the performance for fruit and vegetables deviates from the performance for animals. In all the semantic tasks in which access to specific semantic properties were required and in which the items had not to be named (word/picture verification, word and picture description, attribute verification tasks), RS's performance was the lowest for fruit and vegetables while his performance for animals was as good as for nonliving things. The pattern of performance observed in the naming tasks appeared to be slightly different. In the picture naming task, RS was worse at naming both animals and fruit and vegetables as compared to nonliving things. This pattern of impaired naming performance for animals in face of relatively spared performance in the semantic tasks could suggest that RS's naming deficit for animals arises as a consequence of damage to word retrieval processes from spared semantics. However, we found that RS's performance for animals improved in the naming to description task in comparison with the picture naming task. His performance for animals was then not significantly different from his performance for nonliving items, while his performance for fruit and vegetables remained significantly worse than for nonliving items. We suggested earlier that the kind of information provided in the verbal descriptions, by pointing directly to the *relevant* visual and nonvisual semantic properties of the item to be named, could have facilitated access to those semantic properties and, hence, to the item's semantic representation as a whole. That RS's performance in naming animals could have been facilitated when he was provided with *semantic* cues suggests that he had to suffer from a slight impairment in accessing the semantic representations for animals, in addition to his word retrieval impairment. Thus, RS could have suffered from a more subtle semantic deficit for animals than fruit and vegetables; the semantic tasks used in this study may not have been sensitive enough to detect this. Still, even if RS suffered from a semantic deficit for the animal category, his conceptual knowledge about fruit and vegetables appeared to be disproportionately impaired as compared to his conceptual knowledge about animals. So, taken all together, RS's pattern of performance is consistent with previous reports suggesting that a semantic impairment does not necessarily affect all the items from the living things category uniformly, but rather can conform to a finer-grained distinction between animals and fruit and vegetables.

RS's pattern of performance seriously challenges Devlin et al.'s (1998) correlational structure account for category-specific deficits, at least if Devlin et al.'s estimates of feature relations are taken into consideration. On the basis of these estimates, this account predicts that concepts of fruit and vegetables should be the most robust to mild damage. Consequently, in case of mild damage, the concepts of fruit and vegetables should be relatively spared in comparison with the concepts of animals and artefacts. RS has just presented with the reverse pattern—fruit and vegetables were disproportionately impaired in comparison with all other categories—while he did indeed suffer from very mild semantic damage, as shown by his performance at the semantic matching and the synonym matching tasks, for example, which was within the normal range (cf. Case Report). In contrast, RS's pattern fits well with the Tyler and colleagues' claims (Moss et al., 2002; Tyler & Moss, 2001) that the concepts of fruit and vegetables should be more vulnerable to mild damage than the concepts of animals. However, the reverse pattern of dissociation along the animal/fruit and vegetable distinction has also been reported in the patient EW (Caramazza & Shelton, 1998), who presented with a semantic deficit that could also be considered as a mild one, as EW scored 204/250 (82%) when asked to name the Snodgrass and Vanderwart (1980) set of items. EW was, however, impaired in naming animals and in verifying semantic properties of animals while, for fruit and vegetables, her performance was close to perfect.[6] Thus, together with the case of EW, the present case report of a patient being disproportionately impaired in processing fruit and vegetables, and whose pattern of performance strongly suggests a semantic, rather than a purely word-retrieval locus for this category-specific deficit, provides additional neuropsychological data (cf. Garrard, Lambon Ralph, Watson, Powis, Patterson, & Hodges, 2001; Garrard, Patterson, Watson, & Hodges, 1998) that undermines the contribution of the correlational approaches in understanding the occurrence of category-specific deficits.

Two types of account of category-specific deficits could explain a double dissociation along the animal/fruit and vegetable distinction. The first type of account assumes a topographical category-like organisation of semantic knowledge within the brain (Caramazza et al., 1990; Caramazza & Shelton, 1998; Damasio, 1990; Tranel et al., 1997). According to this view, category-specific semantic deficits affecting selectively either the animal or the fruit and vegetable category reflect damage to a particular brain region that sustains the retrieval and processing of all the semantic knowledge associated with animals or with fruit and vegetables, respectively. Thus this account predicts that patients showing a selective deficit for animals or for fruit and vegetables should be impaired at retrieving any kind of semantic knowledge associated with the impaired category while all kinds of semantic knowledge associated with other categories should be spared. In contrast, the second type of account assumes that the topographical organisation of knowledge within the brain is based on the kind of semantic properties that are represented (Humphreys & Forde, 2001; Warrington & McCarthy, 1987; Warrington & Shallice, 1984). Within this framework, category-specific semantic deficits reflect damage to one or several semantic subsystems that store the particular kinds of knowledge that are particularly diagnostic for the impaired category, conceivably shape knowledge for animals and colour knowledge for fruit and vegetables (Humphreys & Forde, 2001; Warrington & McCarthy, 1987). Thus this account predicts that category-specific semantic deficits should be associated with disproportionate difficulty in retrieving specific kinds of object properties across all categories of objects.

RS's pattern of performance in tasks probing the retrieval of object-colour knowledge does not conform to the hypothesis of a loss of object-colour knowledge being at the origin of his deficit in processing fruit and vegetables. First, although RS was unable to name or describe fruit and vegetables from a picture, he could nevertheless accurately retrieve the colour associated with visually presented fruit and vegetables. Thus, at least for visually presented fruit and vegetables, RS's inability to retrieve semantic knowledge was not due to a loss of object-colour knowledge. Second, although RS had difficulty in retrieving object-colour knowledge from a spoken name, both for fruit and vegetables and for manufactured objects, his score was significantly lower than the score of the control subject only for fruit and vegetables. This pattern is inconsistent with the expectation of a general loss of object-colour knowledge in the condition of damage to the colour-knowledge store, which should equally impair colour-knowledge retrieval for fruit and vegetables *and* manufactured objects.

RS's pattern of performance in the object-colour knowledge retrieval tasks also speaks to the issue of the status of object-colour knowledge within a model of object knowledge representation. First, RS was able to retrieve colour-knowledge about visually presented fruit and vegetables despite his semantic impairment for this category of objects. Other patients have been reported with the opposite pattern of performance. For example, Della Sala et al. (2000) reported the case of three patients who could name colours perfectly (which suggests intact colour processing) and name visually

[6] Whatever the actual degree of semantic damage present in a given patient, if the category of fruit and vegetables were the most vulnerable category then, in case of impairment for the concepts of animals, the concepts for fruit and vegetables should be impaired as well (or even more impaired).

presented objects perfectly (which suggests intact structural and semantic knowledge about objects) but could not match visually-presented objects to their corresponding colour. Similarly, IOC, the patient studied by Miceli et al. (2001), was impaired at retrieving the colour of objects but performed close to normal range when asked to retrieve other visual as well as nonvisual semantic attributes about them. Thus, the case of RS, together with the cases reported by Della Sala et al. and Miceli et al., suggest that object-colour knowledge is represented in a segregated way from structural and semantic knowledge (see also Luzzatti & Davidoff, 1994; Price & Humphreys, 1989). Second, although RS was able to retrieve object-colour knowledge about visually-presented fruit and vegetables, he showed impaired performance when asked to retrieve the colour of fruit and vegetables from their spoken name. This pattern suggests that object-colour knowledge can be directly retrieved from the object's structural representation without requiring prior access to the object's semantic representation. In contrast, the retrieval of object-colour knowledge from a spoken name would require prior access to the object's semantic representation, on the basis of which the corresponding object's colour properties could be addressed (see Figure 3).

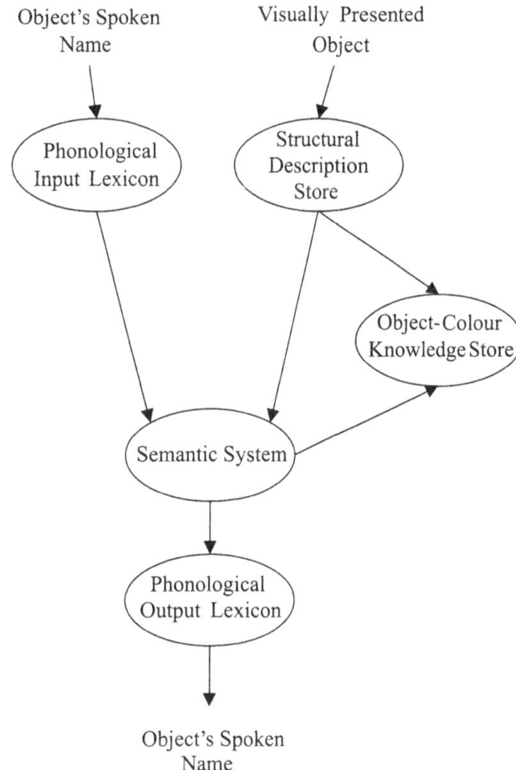


**Figure 3.** *A schematic representation of the stored knowledge systems involved in object-colour processing.*

Within such a model of object-knowledge representation, the various features of RS's performance in the object-colour knowledge retrieval tasks would be accounted for as follows. RS's more marked difficulty at retrieving colour knowledge for fruit and vegetables as compared to manufactured objects when provided with their spoken name results from the semantic representations of fruit and vegetables being disproportionately impaired in comparison with manufactured objects. In contrast, when provided with (black-and-white) drawings of fruit and vegetables, RS could retrieve their corresponding colour because of spared structural knowledge of fruit and vegetables from which (spared) object-colour knowledge could be accessed. Thus, within this model of how processing of an object's colour and its other properties are related, RS's pattern of performance is interpreted as resulting from selective (or disproportionate) damage to the semantic representations of fruit and vegetables in the face of *spared* representations of colour properties of fruit and vegetables, as well as spared representations of all the properties of objects belonging to the other categories.

A selective (or disproportionate) deficit in accessing objects' visual properties other than colour, namely objects' shape properties, either at the structural or semantic level of processing, also seems unlikely to explain RS's disproportionate impairment for fruit and vegetables. There was no evidence for an impairment at the structural processing level: RS performed within the normal range in two object decision tasks, he showed similar scores in accessing semantic knowledge from a picture and from a word (as evidenced in the word and picture description task), and he could accurately retrieve the colour associated with fruit and vegetables from a picture—a task presumably requiring accurate access to a structural description.

As regards the semantic level of processing, RS's performance in the attribute verification task indicated that he was impaired at retrieving visual—that is, colour and shape—knowledge for fruit and vegetables from a spoken input. There was no evidence, however, for an impairment at retrieving shape knowledge for animals nor for manufactured objects. Such a pattern is inconsistent with the hypothesis of a selective damage to a shape knowledge store, which should impair shape knowledge for all categories of items to a certain extent. One must add that, under the knowledge-specific account, a deficit in retrieving the shape attributes of objects should result in equal if not greater difficulty in identifying animals than fruit and vegetables, because shape knowledge is assumed to be *relatively* more diagnostic for animals than for fruit and vegetables. In fact, the reverse pattern was found in the present case.

The most parsimonious account for RS's pattern of performance across all tasks is that RS's semantic deficit impaired all kinds of semantic properties associated with fruit and vegetables (with the exception of colour properties) while relatively sparing all kinds of semantic properties associated with the other categories of objects. Hence, RS's pattern of performance can be taken as evidence in support of a topographical category-like organisation of semantic knowledge within the brain. Our data are, however, silent on the issue of knowing which organising principle would have led to such a topographical organisation of knowledge, i.e., the strength of association among semantic properties (cf. the OUCH model, Caramazza et al., 1990), the prevailing object properties that were pertinently associated in experience (cf. Damasio, 1990; Tranel et al., 1997), or evolutionary pressure (cf. the domain-specific knowledge hypothesis, Caramazza & Shelton, 1998). RS's apparent association of deficits for fruit and vegetables and manufactured food items seems to be compatible with the three proposals. Within the framework of the OUCH model, it can be argued that manufactured food items share some properties in common with fruit and vegetables (e.g., gustatory properties and functional and associative properties related to eating) and are hence represented through partly overlapping property clusters within the semantic space. Consistent with Damasio and his collaborators' proposal, it could be argued that the properties that are pertinently associated in experience for food items and fruit and vegetables are quite similar (e.g., similar modalities of transactions). Finally, within the framework of the domain-specific knowledge hypothesis, it might be that the specialised neural systems dedicated to processing plant life, which evolved at the time of our hunter-gatherer ancestors, now also process objects that appeared later in the development of the human environment—especially if these objects, as might be the case for food items, share with the original domain (i.e., plant life) similar perceptual cues for accurate identification and similar types of behavioural responses.

## REFERENCES


Albanese, E., Capitani, E., Barbarotto, R., & Laiacona, M. (2000). Semantic category dissociations, familiarity and gender. *Cortex*, *36*, 733–746.

Bachy-Langedoc, N. (1988). *Batterie d'examen des troubles en dénomination*. Bruxelles: Editest.

Capitani, E., Laiacona, M., & Barbarotto, R. (1999). Gender affects word retrieval of certain categories in semantic fluency tasks. *Cortex*, *35*, 273–278.

Cappa, S. F., Frugoni, M., Pasquali, P., Perani, D., & Zorat, F. (1998). Category-specific naming impairment for artefacts: A new case. *Neurocase*, *4*, 391–397.

Caramazza, A. (1998). The interpretation of semantic category-specific deficits: What do they reveal about the organisation of conceptual knowledge in the brain? *Neurocase*, *4*, 265–272.

Caramazza, A., Hillis, A. E., Rapp, B. C., & Romani, C. (1990). The multiple semantics hypothesis: multiple confusions? *Cognitive Neuropsychology*, *7*, 161–189.

Caramazza, A., & Shelton, R. S. (1998). Domain-specific knowledge systems in the brain: The animate-inanimate distinction. *Journal of Cognitive Neuroscience*, *10*, 1–34.

Content, A., Mousty, P., & Radeau, M. (1990). Brulex. Une base de données lexicales informatisée pour le français écrit et parlé. *L'Année psychologique*, *90*, 551–566.

Damasio, A. R. (1990). Category-related recognition defects as a clue to the neural substrates of knowledge. *Trends in Neurosciences*, *13*, 95–98.

Davidoff, J. (1991). *Cognition through colour*. Cambridge, MA: MIT Press.

Della Sala, S., Kinnear, P., Spinnler, H., & Stangalino, C. (2000). Color-to-figure matching in Alzheimer's disease. *Archives of Clinical Neuropsychology*, *15*, 571–585.

de Partz, M.-P., Bilocq, V., De Wilde, V., Seron, X., & Pillon, A. (2001). *LEXIS. Tests pour le diagnostic des troubles lexicaux chez le patient aphasique*. Marseille, France: Solal.

De Renzi, E., & Lucchelli, F. (1994). Are semantic systems separately represented in the brain? The case of living categories impairment. *Cortex*, *30*, 3–25.

Devlin, J. T., Gonnerman, L. M., Andersen, E. S., & Seidenberg, M. S. (1998). Category-specific semantic deficits in focal and widespread brain damage: A computational account. *Journal of Cognitive Neuroscience*, *10*, 77–94.

Farah, M. J., & McClelland, J. L. (1991). A computational model of semantic memory impairment: Modality specificity and emergent category specificity. *Journal of Experimental Psychology: General*, *120*, 339–357.

Farah, M. J., & Wallace, M. A. (1992). Semantically bounded anomia: Implications for the neural implementation of naming. *Neuropsychologia*, *30*, 609–621.

Forde, E. M. E., Francis, D., Riddoch, M. J., Rumiati, R., & Humphreys, G. W. (1997). On the links between visual knowledge and naming: A single case study of a patient with a category-specific impairment for living things. *Cognitive Neuropsychology*, *14*, 403–458.

Forde, E. M. E., & Humphreys, G. W. (1999). Category-specific recognition impairments: A review of important case studies and influential theories. *Aphasiology*, *13*, 169–193.

Gaffan, D., & Heywood, A. (1993). A spurious category-specific visual agnosia for living things in normal human and nonhuman primates. *Journal of Cognitive Neuroscience*, *5*, 118–128.

Gaillard, M. J., Auzou, P., Miret, N., Ozsancak, C., & Hannequin, D. (1998). Trouble de la dénomination pour les objets manufacturés dans un cas d'encéphalite herpétique. *Revue Neurologique*, *154*, 683–689.

Gainotti, G., & Silveri, M. C. (1996). Cognitive and anatomical locus of lesion in a patient with a category-specific semantic impairment for living beings. *Cognitive Neuropsychology*, *13*, 357–389.

Garrard, P., Lambon Ralph, M. A., Watson, P. C., Powis, J., Patterson, K., & Hodges, J. R. (2001). Longitudinal profiles of semantic impairment for living and nonliving concepts in dementia of Alzheimer's type. *Journal of Cognitive Neuroscience*, *13*, 892–909.

Garrard, P., Patterson, K., Watson, P. C., & Hodges, J. R. (1998). Category specific semantic loss in dementia of Alzheimer's type: Functional–anatomical correlations from cross-sectional analyses. *Brain*, *121*, 633–646.

Hart, J., Berndt, R. S., & Caramazza, A. (1985). Category-specific naming deficit following cerebral infraction. *Nature*, *316*, 439–440.

Hart, J., & Gordon, B. (1992). Neural subsystems for object knowledge. *Nature*, *359*, 60–64.

Hillis, A. E., & Caramazza, A. (1991). Category-specific naming and comprehension impairment: A double dissociation. *Brain*, *114*, 2081–2094.

Humphreys, G. W., & Forde, E. M. E. (2001). Hierarchies, similarity and interactivity in object recognition: on the multiplicity of "category-specific" deficits in neuropsychological populations. *Behavioral and Brain Sciences*, *24*, 453–509.

Humphreys, G. W., Riddoch M. J., & Quinlan, P. T. (1988). Cascade processes in picture identification. *Cognitive Neuropsychology*, *5*, 67–103.

Ishihara, S. (1974). *Tests for color-blindness*. Tokyo: Kanehara Shup.

Laiacona, M., & Capitani, E. (2001). A case of prevailing deficit of nonliving categories or a case of prevailing sparing of living categories. *Cognitive Neuropsychology*, *18*, 39–70.

Laiacona, M., Capitani, E., & Barbarotto, R. (1997). Semantic category dissociations: A longitudinal study of two cases. *Cortex*, *33*, 441–461.

Lambon Ralph, M. A., Howard, D., Nightingale, G., & Ellis, A. W. (1998). Are living and non-living category-specific deficits causally linked to impaired perceptual or associative knowledge? Evidence from a category-specific double dissociation. *Neurocase*, *4*, 311–338.

Luzzatti, C., & Davidoff, J. (1994). Impaired retrieval of object-colour knowledge with preserved colour naming. *Neuropsychologia*, *32*, 933–950.

McKenna, P., & Parry, R. (1994). Category-specificity in the naming of natural and man-made objects: Normative data from adults and children. *Neuropsychological Rehabilitation*, *4*, 255–281.

McRae, K., & Cree, G. S. (2002). Factors underlying category-specific impairments. In E. M. E. Forde &

G. W. Humphreys (Eds.), *Category-specificity in brain and mind* (pp. 211–248). Hove, UK: Psychology Press.

Miceli, G., Fouch, E., Capasso, R., Shelton, J. R., Tomaiuolo, F., & Caramazza, A. (2001). The dissociation of color from form and function knowledge. *Nature Neuroscience, 4*, 662-667.

Moss, H. E., & Tyler, L. K. (2000). A progressive category-specific semantic deficit for non-living things. *Neuropsychologia, 38*, 60–82.

Moss, H. E., Tyler, L. K., & Devlin, J. T. (2002). The emergence of category-specific deficits in a distributed semantic system. In E. M. E. Forde & G. W. Humphreys (Eds.), *Category-specificity in brain and mind* (pp. 115–146). Hove, UK: Psychology Press.

Moss, H. E., Tyler, L. K., Durrant-Peatfield, M., & Bunn, E. M. (1998). "Two eyes of a see-through": Impaired and intact semantic knowledge in a case of selective deficit for living things. *Neurocase, 4*, 291–310.

Pietrini, V., Nertempi, P., Vaglia, A., Revello, M. G., Pinna, V., & Ferro-Milone, F. (1988). Recovery from herpes simplex encephalitis: Selective impairment of sepcific semantic categories with neuroradiological correlation. *Journal of Neurology, Neurosurgery and Psychiatry, 51*, 1284–1293.

Pillon, A., & Samson, D. (2001). On disentangling and weighting kinds of semantic knowledge. *Behavioral and Brain Sciences, 24*, 490.

Pillon, A., Samson, D., & Gilmont, V. (1995). *Batterie d'épreuves évaluant la reconnaissance, la compréhension et la production de verbes et substantifs concrets et abstraits.* Unpublished test.

Price, C. J., & Humphreys, G. W. (1989). The effects of surface detail on object categorization and naming. *Quarterly Journal of Experimental Psychology, 41A*, 797–828.

Riddoch, M. J., & Humphreys, G. W. (1993). *BORB: The Birmingham Object Recognition Battery.* Hove, UK: Lawrence Erlbaum Associates Ltd.

Sacchett, C., & Humphreys, G. W. (1992). Calling a squirrel a squirrel but a canoe a wigwam: A category-specific deficit for artefactual objects and body parts. *Cognitive Neuropscyhology, 9*, 73–86.

Samson, D., Pillon, A., & De Wilde, V. (1998). Impaired knowledge of visual and non-visual attributes in a patient with a semantic impairment for living entities: A case of a true category-specific deficit. *Neurocase, 4*, 273–290.

Shelton, J. R., Fouch, E., & Caramazza, A. (1998). The selective sparing of body part knowledge: A case study. *Neurocase, 4*, 339–351.

Silveri, M. C., & Gainotti, G. (1988). Interaction between vision and language in category-specific impairment. *Cognitive Neuropsychology, 5*, 677–709.

Silveri, M. C., Gainotti, G., Perani, D., Cappelletti, J. Y., Carbone, G., & Fazio, K. (1997). Naming deficit for non-living items: Neuropsychological and PET study. *Neuropsychologia, 35*, 359–367.

Snodgrass, J., & Vanderwart, M. (1980). A standardized set of 260 pictures: Norms for name agreement, familiarity, and visual complexity. *Journal of Experimental Psychology: Human Learning and Memory, 6*, 174–215.

Tranel, D., Damasio, H., & Damasio, A. R. (1997). A neural basis for the retrieval of conceptual knowledge. *Neuropsychologia, 35*, 1319–1327.

Tranel, D., Logan, C. G., Frank, R. J., & Damasio, A. R. (1997). Explaining category-related effects in the retrieval of conceptual and lexical knowledge for concrete entities: Operationalization and analysis of factors. *Neuropsychologia, 35*, 1329–1339.

Tyler, L. K., & Moss, H. E. (2001). Towards a distributed account of conceptual knowledge. *Trends in Cognitive Science, 5*, 244–252.

Tyler, L. K., Moss, H. E., Durrant-Peatfield, M., & Levy, J. (2000). Conceptual structure and the structure of categories: A distributed account of category-specific deficits. *Brain and Language, 75*, 195–231.

Warrington, E. K., & McCarthy, R. (1983). Category specific access dysphasia. *Brain, 106*, 859–878.

Warrington, E. K., & McCarthy, R. (1987). Categories of knowledge: Further fractionations and an attempted integration. *Brain, 110*, 1273–1296.

Warrington, E. K., & Shallice, T. (1984). Category specific semantic impairments. *Brain, 107*, 829–854.

COGNITIVE NEUROPSYCHOLOGY, 2003, 20 (3/4/5/6), 401–408

# GENETIC AND ENVIRONMENTAL INFLUENCES ON THE ORGANISATION OF SEMANTIC MEMORY IN THE BRAIN: IS "LIVING THINGS" AN INNATE CATEGORY?

Martha J. Farah and Carol Rabinowitz
*University of Pennsylvania, Philadelphia, USA*

The organisation of semantic memory into separately lesionable or imageable components must be determined by some combination of genetic and environmental factors. Little is known about the relative contributions of these two factors in establishing the functional architecture of semantic memory. By assessing the semantic memory impairment of an individual who sustained brain damage as a newborn, it is possible to place an upper bound on the contribution of post-natal experience. The present case study demonstrates a profound and enduring impairment in knowledge of "living things" following posterior cerebral artery infarctions at approximately 1 day of age. The design of the two experiments reported here allows us to characterise the subject's semantic memory impairment in terms of its scope and selectivity. The impairment affects both the naming of pictures of living things and the retrieval of verbal information about living things. It cannot be accounted for by differences in the difficulty of retrieving knowledge of living and nonliving things, as the living and nonliving items were equated for difficulty in each experiment. When visual and nonvisual information were queried separately for living and nonliving things, the impairment was manifest for both kinds of information about living things, but for neither kind of information about nonliving things. Because this impairment resulted from brain damage sustained too early for experience to have contributed to the organisation of semantic memory, this case study supports a genetic basis for the living–nonliving distinction in semantic memory.

Much of contemporary cognitive neuroscience is concerned with what has been called the "functional architecture" of cognition. What are the most meaningful large-scale groupings of the billions of neurons that underlie human intelligence, for the purposes of understanding such psychological processes as perception, memory, and language? In the field of semantic memory research, this issue has been central. Cognitive neuroscientists have considered a number of alternative subdivisions of semantic knowledge as it is implemented in the brain, including modality-specific components (e.g., Warrington & Shallice, 1984), attribute-specific components (e.g., Martin, 1998), and category-specific or meaning-specific components (e.g., Caramazza & Shelton, 1998). The vigorous testing and refinement of alternative hypotheses continues, as many of the articles in this Special Issue attest.

Requests for reprints should be addressed to Martha Farah, Center for Cognitive Neuroscience, University of Pennsylvania, 3815 Walnut Street, Philadelphia, PA 19104-6196, USA (Email: mfarah@psych.upenn.edu).

This research was supported by NIH grants R01-AG14082, R01-DA14129, and K02-AG0056 and by NSF grant 0226060. The authors thank Doctors Graham Quinn and Grant Liu for introducing us to Adam and sharing their insights on his neuro-ophthalmologic development, Sharon Thompson-Schill for insightful comments on an earlier draft of this article, and Adam and his mother for their time, effort, and cooperation.



http://www.tandf.co.uk/journals/pp/02643294.html DOI:10.1080/02643290244000293

A question that is considered less often in cognitive neuroscience is: Where do the components of the functional architecture come from? Are they innate or acquired through experience? The present study was designed to address this question in connection with the development of the separate components of semantic memory. The specific components under study have often been referred to as knowledge of "living things" and knowledge of "nonliving things." Disagreement exists over whether these labels are merely a convenient (if misleading) shorthand for some less obvious factor separating the impaired from preserved domains of knowledge, or whether the components truly correspond to semantic categories that are roughly equivalent to "living" and "nonliving." Although the results of our second experiment are relevant to this issue, the more general implications of the present case study do not depend on any particular hypothesis about the underlying distinctions. For simplicity, we will refer to the two components with the terms "living" and "nonliving."

Given that knowledge of living things is sufficiently segregated from knowledge of nonliving things in the brain that the two are doubly dissociable after brain damage (Hillis & Caramazza, 1991), what type of mechanism creates this segregation? The localisation of knowledge about living things could conceivably be innate. This alternative implies that the distinction between living and nonliving things, or some factor sufficient to distinguish between them, is explicitly encoded in the genome, along with a similarly explicit specification of the anatomical location for the knowledge of living things. As for any innate ability, some degree of experience would of course be necessary, for example there must eventually be exposure to information in order for a semantic memory system to function. However, according to the nativist account of the living–nonliving distinction, this information does not influence the organisation of semantic memory but is merely assimilated into an already-determined organisation. The special adaptive value of recognising and remembering animals and plants in the course of human evolution gives the innate alternative a degree of plausibility (Caramazza & Shelton, 1998).

At the other extreme, the specification of living things as a component of semantic memory, and its localisation, could emerge entirely as a result of postnatal experience. Principles of self-organisation have been shown to be capable of causing a segregation of the neural representations of even arbitrary categories in particular learning environments (Polk & Farah, 1995a, 1995b). According to this class of hypotheses, only the most minimal innate endowment, a general-purpose learning mechanism, would be needed in order to account for the segregation of knowledge of living and nonliving things. The organisation of semantic memory into components such as living and nonliving would then emerge from an interaction of this learning mechanism with properties of the environmental input, such as statistics of occurrence and cooccurrence of objects and features within objects. Between these two extremes lie mechanisms by which genes and environment both play a substantial role in distinguishing and localising knowledge of living things.

How can we study the determinants of the living–nonliving distinction and its implementation in distinct brain areas? An approach that allows us to put an upper limit on the contribution of the environment is to study a person whose semantic memory impairment followed perinatal brain damage. If the distinction between living and nonliving things, and the specific localisation for living things, are specified in the genome, then damage to that area prior to any relevant experience should result in an enduring category-specific knowledge impairment, comparable to those of adult onset. This contrasts with the alternatives of either no genetic preprogramming or genetic preprogramming of a default or "first choice" localisation which, if unavailable because of damage, is plastic enough to be shifted to a different brain region. Phrased in a different way, if it is possible to cause a lifelong selective impairment in knowledge of living things by brain damage occurring prior to experience with living and nonliving things, this implies that the designation of brain areas specialised for acquiring and/or representing knowledge of living things is accomplished prior to, and therefore independent of, experience. Here we describe a case with just such a history and outcome.

## EXPERIMENT 1

The goal of this experiment was to find out whether Adam has a truly selective impairment in knowledge of living things, when the confounding factors of visual complexity and familiarity are taken into account.

### Case description

Adam was 16 years old at the time of the testing reported here. Following a normal gestation and delivery, he developed Group B streptococcal meningitis at 1 day of age. Bilateral posterior cerebral artery infarction, common in such cases, was suspected on the basis of Adam's visual behaviour, and was confirmed by a CT scan at age 6 years showing bilateral occipital and occipitotemporal lesions. Adam's IQ tested at age 15 years was 101 (verbal) and 68 (performance). His residual neurological problems are primarily visual, and he has been able to attend a combination of mainstream and special education classes at his local public school. A previous published study of Adam's face and object recognition includes details of his neuro-ophthalmologic development (Farah, Rabinowitz, Quinn, & Liu, 2000), which in brief consist of bilateral homonymous visual field defects, mild object agnosia, and profound face agnosia.

### Materials and procedure

Pictures used by Funnell and Sheridan (1992) in their study of selective knowledge impairment were used. These were drawn from the Snodgrass and Vanderwart (1980) corpus, and consisted of 43 living and 42 nonliving items with equivalent average name frequency, familiarity, and complexity, according to Snodgrass and Vanderwart's ratings. An approximately 2" diameter copy of each picture was glued to a 3" × 5" picture card, and these were presented one at a time, in a random order, by placing them in front of Adam on the table at which he was seated. Adam was given about 4 seconds to name each item. This procedure was carried out twice in each testing session, for three testing sessions, giving a total of six naming attempts per picture. When uncertain he was encouraged, but not forced, to guess.

### Results and discussion

As noted in the Case Description, Adam is prosopagnosic and mildly object agnosic. Like other mild agnosics, he is sensitive to the visual quality of stimuli and finds line drawings more difficult than photographs or real objects (Farah, in press). His performance with the drawings of nonliving things was therefore impaired, with an average of 31.3 out of 42 drawings named, or 75%. When he misidentified objects, it was usually attributable to a visual confusion, for example, calling a cigar "a crayon" and a broom "a spatula." In contrast, Adam had significantly more difficulty with pictures of living things, naming just 17 out of 43 on average, or 40%. It is harder to classify these errors as visual versus semantic, given the high correlation between these dimensions of similarity for living things. In some cases the errors were clearly visual confusions, such as mistaking a cherry for "a Chinese yo-yo," whereas in other cases it was less clear, for example calling a mouse "a cat" and a monkey "an owl." The pattern of responses over repeated presentations of a picture was relatively consistent, with only 13 of the 85 pictures evoking inconsistent responses (8 living, 5 nonliving). Within the living things, errors were distributed over both animals and plants (including fruits and vegetables). A direct comparison between these two types of living things would fail to control for the difficulty factors that were matched between living and nonliving things. Nevertheless, for descriptive purposes, we can report that Adam made at least one naming error on 79% of the animals he was shown, and on 54% of the plants.

The difference between Adam's performance on the living and nonliving items was highly significant by $t$-test over the six sessions, $t(10) = 15.6$, $p <$ 001, despite the two picture sets' equivalence in average name frequency, complexity, and familiarity, and the equivalent levels of naming performance demonstrated by Funnell and Sheridan (1992) with these stimuli. This demonstrates that Adam has a relatively selective impairment in the knowledge of living things necessary for naming pictures.

## EXPERIMENT 2

The previous experiment tested only Adam's ability to recognise a visually presented stimulus. With these data we cannot tell whether his knowledge impairment is limited to knowledge required for visual recognition, or whether it constitutes a more general impairment of semantic knowledge. The present experiment answers this question by probing his knowledge of living and nonliving things verbally. It also contrasts the hypotheses of underlying modality-specific and category-specific organisation.

### Materials and procedure

Adam again participated, along with nine other neurologically normal children of the same age (four males and five females). The questionnaire of Farah, Hammond, Mehta, and Ratcliff (1989) was administered to Adam and the nine control subjects. The questionnaire has 4 questions about each of the 47 living and 48 nonliving items, for a total of 380 questions. These items were drawn from the work of Warrington and Shallice (1984), differing only in the exclusion of the living item "foxglove," a plant that was unfamiliar to the authors and to a number of colleagues whom they questioned. For each item two questions probe visual knowledge (e.g., "Does a guitar have a square-shaped opening?") and two probed nonvisual knowledge (e.g., "Is peacock served in French restaurants?") One question in each of the resulting pairs had a correct answer of "yes" and the other "no."

The questionnaire was printed on normal typing paper with a Y and an N next to each question. Subjects were tested individually, for two sessions each, with 190 questions administered in each session. Each question was read aloud by the experimenter while the subject also viewed it and had the opportunity to read it. The subject answered by circling the Y or the N.

### Results and discussion

As shown in Figure 1, the normal control subjects performed approximately the same in all four conditions: 82% and 83% for living-visual and living-nonvisual, and 79% and 84% for nonliving visual and nonliving nonvisual, respectively. From this we can conclude that normal children of Adam's age find the four different conditions of the questionnaire equally difficult, and that this equivalence is not attributable to floor or ceiling effects.

In contrast, Adam's performance in the different conditions ranged from being at chance to normal performance. As shown in Figure 1, he was at chance with both categories of question concerning living things, 40% and 45% for living visual and living nonvisual, questions, respectively. The significance of his impairment relative to the control subjects can be quantified by the $t$ value of his performance relative to the distribution of normal subjects' performance. For living visual questions, $t(8) = 5.38$ and for living nonvisual, $t(8) = 6.01$, $p < .001$ in both cases. Adam's performance on the two sets of nonliving questions could not be distinguished from that of the control subjects. He showed normal performance in answering nonliving visual questions, 78% correct (normal mean

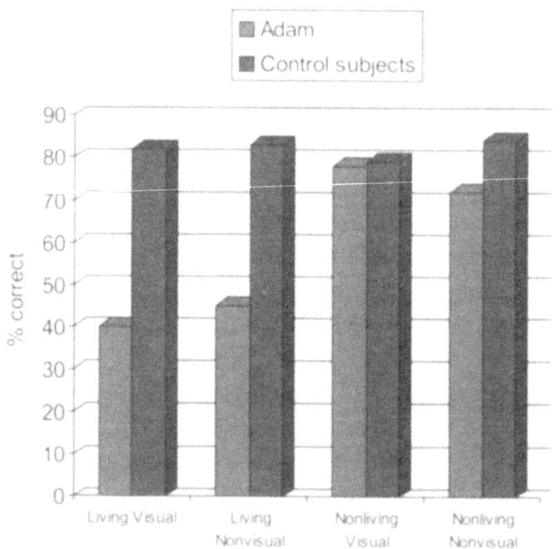


**Figure 1.** *Performance of Adam and nine age-matched control subjects on verbal questions concerning visual and nonvisual properties of living and nonliving things.*

79%, range 70–90%) and borderline performance in answering the nonliving nonvisual questions, 72% correct (normal mean 84%, range 73–92%). The $t$ values of his performance on these questions relative to normal control subjects was $t(8) = 0.16$, $p > .1$, and $t(8) = 1.96$, $.1 > p > .05$, for nonliving visual and nonliving nonvisual, respectively.

The most relevant comparison for testing the hypothesis that Adam has a selective impairment in knowledge of living things is between the size of Adam's performance disparity between the living and nonliving conditions and the size of that of the normal subjects. The tests so far reported consider each condition in isolation, and therefore fail to measure anything about the pattern of performance over conditions. If the normal subjects' means just reported reflect a mixture of some subjects with excellent performance in the living conditions and poor performance in the nonliving, and other subjects with the opposite pattern, then Adam would not differ from normal in any way other than his overall level of performance. To gauge the difference between Adam and the normal subjects in the size of his living–nonliving disparity, we computed the size of that disparity for each of the normal subjects and asked whether Adam's disparity differed significantly from this sample. It did, $t(8) = 50.6$, $p < .001$.

Two main conclusions emerge from these data. First, Adam's impaired performance with living things is not limited to naming pictures, as in the previous experiment, but extends to purely verbal tasks as well. The second conclusion concerns the nature of the underlying impairment, and whether or not it implies a category-specific organisation for normal semantic memory. From the earliest reports of "living things deficits" it has been noted that a category-specific organisation is only one possible organisation for semantic memory that could account for such deficits. Warrington and Shallice (1984) suggested that semantic memory could have a modality-specific organisation, with patients sustaining damage to components of semantic memory such as visual semantics (which represents knowledge of visual appearance). Given that visual knowledge predominates among the different forms of knowledge we have about living things, whereas it forms a smaller part of our knowledge of nonliving things (Farah & McClelland, 1991; Warrington & Shallice, 1984), damage to visual semantics could result in an apparently category-specific impairment in knowledge of living things.

The questionnaire used in this experiment was designed to address this issue, by independently varying the category (living/nonliving) and the modality (visual/nonvisual) of knowledge queried. In its previous use, with case LH, the outcome supported neither a simple category-specific hypothesis nor a modality-specific hypothesis (Farah et al., 1989). Rather, the patient's impairment was delineated by both category and modality, being most severe for visual knowledge of living things. Nonvisual knowledge of living things and visual knowledge of nonliving things were nonsignificantly depressed, and nonvisual knowledge of nonliving things was entirely normal. Farah and McClelland (1991) showed that this pattern would result from damage to the visual semantics component of a purely modality-specific system operating as a highly interactive associative network.

Adam's performance with the same questionnaire, relative to his control group, shows a very different pattern, one that is problematic for Farah and McClelland's (1991) hypothesis. His knowledge of living things, including nonvisual knowledge, is far from normal, whereas his knowledge of nonliving things is comparable to the control children's. Indeed, his performance on the nonliving-visual questions was unambiguously normal. This pattern is incompatible with a purely modality-specific system.

What about the visual attribute-specific account of Martin and colleagues (e.g., Martin, 1998)? They have proposed that a finer-grained distinction within the visual modality could form the basis of a categorical organisation for semantic memory. According to their account, form and motion information may be differentially involved in the representation of living things and tools, and these visual attributes may be responsible for the different brain regions implicated in knowledge of animals and tools across a variety of different tasks (Chao & Martin, 1999). Although the majority of the visual questions in the present questionnaire did concern some aspect of form, there was no systematic control over the types of visual or specifically of form information that was queried for living and nonliving things. Thus we cannot dismiss the possibility of a specific visual attribute-based distinction underlying Adam's semantic memory impairment. However, such an explanation would need to invoke the additional assumption that Adam's visual form areas were necessary for acquiring nonvisual knowledge of living things. Note that the cross-modal effects of visual semantic damage in the Farah and McClelland (1991) model result from the nonvisual components of the network having come to rely on collateral input from the visual components because those visual components were available during learning. The assumption that visual form information is required for the acquisition of nonvisual knowledge about living things is not, therefore, independently motivated by computational considerations. Although it is still a possibility, the most straightforward interpretation of these results is that Adam lacks a semantically defined component of semantic memory, dedicated to representing knowledge about living things.

## GENERAL DISCUSSION

The present case study is relevant to two issues in the cognitive neuroscience of semantic memory. The first issue concerns the components of the functional architecture of semantic memory, specifically, whether there are truly semantic category-specific components. The second issue concerns the development of the functional architecture of semantic memory, specifically, whether one of its major divisions is innate or whether it emerges through experience.

### Components of semantic memory: Living and nonliving things?

Adam has a relatively selective and severe impairment in his knowledge of living things, whether assessed by a visual recognition task or a verbal questionnaire. Although it is possible that some factor other than living versus nonliving is the true underlying distinction around which semantic memory is organised, the data from Adam rule out the most obvious candidates. It is not the case that the difference in difficulty between living and nonliving items can account for Adam's performance. His naming of the pictures in Funnell and Sheridan's (1992) stimulus set demonstrates that his selective impairment at naming nonliving things is not attributable to any of the measures of overall difficulty that these researchers had controlled for, specifically name frequency, familiarity, and visual complexity. Despite a mild degree of visual agnosia affecting his picture naming in general, the discrepancy in his performance on living and nonliving pictures in the Funnell and Sheridan set was wide and highly significant. Furthermore, his performance relative to age-matched control subjects on a verbal questionnaire ruled out a differential difficulty account with a completely different set of materials. The absence of ceiling effects in the normal subjects' data allowed us to verify that the living and nonliving questions were equivalent in difficulty, and although Adam performed like a control subject on the nonliving items, he performed at chance on the living items.

This same questionnaire allows us to test an alternative account in terms of modality-specific semantic systems. Adam's semantic memory impairment cannot be explained as an impairment of visual semantic memory, given that his ability to retrieve visual semantic knowledge of nonliving things appears intact. On 80 questions testing visual knowledge of nonliving things his performance was almost identical to the mean of the control subjects. This pattern of performance is inconsistent with an underlying visual semantic memory impairment. It is also inconsistent with an impairment in the acquisition of visual knowledge, even with the assumption that knowledge of any modality is initially reliant on visual learning. Adam's normal visual knowledge of nonliving things rules out a visual learning impairment. Instead, the present results suggest that the organisation revealed by Adam's impairment is either a genuinely semantic distinction between living and nonliving things, or a distinction closely related to this semantic distinction.

How can the present result be reconciled with a previous finding, using the same questionnaire, of both modality-specific and category-specific influences on semantic memory performance (Farah et al., 1989)? The subject of the earlier study was LH, an individual who, like Adam, had prosopagnosia, mild object agnosia, and poor semantic memory for living things. When compared to age- and education-matched control subjects, LH was significantly impaired only on visual questions about living things. He also showed a nonsignificant trend toward poor performance on visual questions about nonliving things and nonvisual questions about living things. This pattern is consistent with Farah and McClelland's modality-specific neural network model of semantic memory.

We suggest that another property of neural networks is relevant to understanding the discrepancy between the results of Adam and LH. That property is the need for multiple layers of neuronal units for mapping between different representational domains. Mapping between perceptual and semantic representations, for example, is best achieved in incremental transformations of the representations through one or more intermediate layers of units, rather than in a single step implemented in direct connections between perceptual and semantic units. Multilayer, or "deep" networks allow more complex mappings than are possible with two-layer perceptron-like networks in which inputs and outputs are associated through a single set of weighted connections (O'Reilly & Munakata, 2000, Ch. 3).

Associating knowledge of appearance with knowledge of other semantic information is a relatively complex mapping. In spatial terms, it involves transforming the similarity space of perceptual representations, in which a ball and an orange are similar, to the similarity space of semantic representations, in which an orange and a banana are similar. In this case the role of the intermediate layers is to represent partial transformations of the similarity space, for example increasing the distance between some similarly shaped objects. Thus, when a deep network learns a mapping between two representational domains, by whatever learning algorithm, the intermediate layers instantiate hybrid representations of the two end-layer domains, with some aspects of the similarity structure of each.

The implication of this general property of neural networks for the cognitive neuroscience of semantic memory is that, in addition to "purely" perceptual, lexical, and semantic representations, we should also expect to find evidence of hybrid representations. Coltheart, Inglis, Cupples, Michie, Bates, and Budd (1998) have made a similar suggestion based on the empirical patterns of impairment in different patients, with some seeming to show a pure semantic impairment and others having both semantic and perceptual specificity to their impairment. Thus a priori computational considerations and empirical observation are both consistent with this idea. LH's disproportionate impairment in visual knowledge of living things could be explained in terms of a functional lesion earlier in the chain of transformations from vision to semantics than Adam's.

## Components of semantic memory: Nature or nurture?

Although Adam is not the first subject to demonstrate an apparently category-specific impairment in semantic memory (see, e.g., Caramazza & Shelton, 1998), he is the first subject with a semantic memory impairment of any kind that has been present since birth. This aspect of Adam's history offers a unique insight into the determinants of the functional architecture of semantic memory. Specifically, it indicates a strong genetic contribution to the architectural distinction demonstrated by Adam's selective impairment, which, as best we can tell, is the distinction between living and nonliving things. Let us examine the reasoning behind this conclusion more explicitly.

Whatever tissue was destroyed when Adam was a newborn had different relations to semantic memory for living and nonliving things. Specifically, it was essential for acquiring semantic memory about living things and not essential for semantic memory about nonliving things. If the distinction between living and nonliving things were not fixed at birth, how then would localised perinatal brain damage have been able to prevent the acquisition of knowledge about living things while allowing the acquisition of knowledge about nonliving things? Conversely, phrased in terms of Adam's surviving brain tissue, despite its adequacy for acquiring semantic memory about nonliving things, it could not take over the function of semantic memory for living things. This implies that prior to any experience with living and nonliving things, we are destined to represent our knowledge of living and nonliving things with distinct neural substrates. This in turn implies that the distinction between living and nonliving things, and the anatomical localisation of knowledge of living things, are specified in the human genome.

## REFERENCES


Caramazza, A., & Shelton, J. R. (1998). Domain specific knowledge systems in the brain: The animate-inanimate distinction. *Journal of Cognitive Neuroscience, 10,* 1–34.

Chao, L. L., & Martin, A. (1999). Cortical representation of perception, naming, and knowledge of color. *Journal of Cognitive Neuroscience, 11,* 25–35.

Coltheart, M., Inglis, L., Cupples, L., Michie, P., Bates, A., & Budd, B. (1998). A semantic subsystem specific to the storage of information about visual attributes of animate and inanimate objects. *Neurocase, 4,* 353–370.

Farah, M. J. (in press). *Visual agnosia* (2nd ed.). Cambridge, MA: MIT Press.

Farah, M. J., Hammond, K. H., Mehta, Z., & Ratcliff, G. (1989). Category-specificity and modality-specificity in semantic memory. *Neuropsychologia, 27,* 193–200.

Farah, M. J., & McClelland, J. L. (1991). A computational model of semantic memory impairment: Modality-specificity and emergent category-specificity. *Journal of Experimental Psychology: General, 120,* 339–357.

Farah, M. J., Rabinowitz, C., Quinn, G., & Liu, G. (2000). Early commitment of the neural substrates of face recognition. *Cognitive Neuropsychology, 17,* 117–123.

Funnell, E., & Sheridan, J. (1992). Categories of knowledge? Unfamiliar aspects of living and non-living things. *Cognitive Neuropsychology, 9,* 135–154.

Hillis, A., & Caramazza, A. (1991). Category-specific naming and comprehension impairment: A double dissociation. *Brain, 114,* 2081–2094.

Martin, A. (1998). The organization of semantic knowledge and the origin of words in the brain. In N. G. Jablonski & L. C. Aiello (Eds.), *The origins and diversification of language memoirs of the California academy of sciences, Vol. 24* (pp. 69–88). San Francisco: California Academy of Sciences.

O'Reilly, R. C., & Munakata, Y. (2000). *Computational explorations in cognitive neuroscience.* Cambridge, MA: MIT Press.

Polk, T. A., & Farah, M. J. (1995a). Late experience alters vision. *Nature, 376,* 648–649.

Polk, T. A., & Farah, M. J. (1995b). Brain localization for arbitrary stimulus categories: A simple account based on Hebbian learning. *Proceedings of the National Academy of Sciences, 92,* 12370–12373.

Snodgrass, J. G., & Vanderwart, M. (1980). A standardized set of 260 pictures: Norms for name agreement, image agreement, familiarity, and visual complexity. *Journal of Experimental Psychology: Human Learning and Memory, 6,* 174–215.

Warrington, E. K., & Shallice, T. (1984). Category specific semantic impairments. *Brain, 107,* 829–854.

COGNITIVE NEUROPSYCHOLOGY, 2003, 20 (3/4/5/6), 409–432

# NEURAL CORRELATES OF CONCEPTUAL KNOWLEDGE FOR ACTIONS

Daniel Tranel, David Kemmerer, and Ralph Adolphs
*University of Iowa College of Medicine, Iowa City, USA*

Hanna Damasio and Antonio R. Damasio
*University of Iowa College of Medicine, Iowa City, and The Salk Institute for Biological Studies, La Jolla, USA*

The neural correlates of conceptual knowledge for actions are not well understood. To begin to address this knowledge gap, we tested the hypothesis that the retrieval of conceptual knowledge for actions depends on neural systems located in higher-order association cortices of left premotor/prefrontal, parietal, and posterior middle temporal regions. The investigation used the lesion method and involved 90 subjects with damage to various regions of the left or right hemisphere. The experimental tasks measured retrieval of knowledge for actions, in a nonverbal format: Subjects evaluated attributes of pictured actions, and compared and matched pictures of actions. In support of our hypothesis, we found that the regions of highest lesion overlap in subjects with impaired retrieval of conceptual knowledge for actions were in the left premotor/prefrontal sector, the left parietal region, and in the white matter underneath the left posterior middle temporal region. These sites are partially distinct from those identified previously as being important for the retrieval of words for actions. We propose that a key function of the sites is to operate as two-way intermediaries between perception and concept retrieval, to promote the retrieval of the multidimensional aspects of knowledge that are necessary and sufficient for the mental representation of a concept of a given action.

## INTRODUCTION

Within the past few decades, a considerable amount of research has explored the neural correlates of retrieval of conceptual (semantic)[1] knowledge for concrete entities such as animals, fruits/vegetables, tools, and persons (Arguin, Bub, & Dudek, 1996; Cappa, Perani, Schnur, Tettamanti, & Fazio, 1998; Caramazza & Shelton, 1998; Chao, Haxby, & Martin, 1999; A. R. Damasio, Damasio, Tranel, & Brandt, 1990; H. Damasio, Tranel, Grabowski, Adolphs, & Damasio, in press; Gainotti & Silveri, 1996; Gerlach, Law, Gade, & Paulson, 1999; Hart & Gordon, 1992; Hillis & Caramazza, 1991; Laiacona, Barbarotto, & Capitani, 1993; Martin, Wiggs, Ungerleider, & Haxby, 1996; Perani, Schnur, Tettamanti, Gorno-Tempini, Cappa, & Fazio, 1999; Sartori, Job, Miozza, Zaco, & Marchiori, 1993; Tranel, Damasio, & Damasio, 1997a; Warrington &

[1] Many authors have used the term "semantics" or "semantic memory" to designate conceptual knowledge. We prefer the term "conceptual knowledge," because it avoids the connotation of "verbal" that is frequently associated with "semantic," and also other potential unintended implications attached to older usage of "semantic memory" (e.g., Tulving, 1972).

Requests for reprints should be addressed to Daniel Tranel, PhD, Department of Neurology, University of Iowa Hospitals and Clinics, 200 Hawkins Drive, Iowa City, Iowa 52242, USA (Email: daniel-tranel@uiowa.com).

This study was supported in part by a grant from the National Institute for Neurological Diseases and Stroke (Program Project Grant NS 19632). We thank Ken Manzel and Denise Krutzfeldt for expert technical help.



http://www.tandf.co.uk/journals/pp/02643294.html
DOI:10.1080/02643290244000248

McCarthy, 1994; Warrington & Shallice, 1984; for reviews, see Caramazza, 1998, 2000; Forde & Humphreys, 1999; Humphreys & Forde, 2001; Saffran & Schwartz, 1994; Saffran & Sholl, 1999). Comparatively less work has addressed the neural underpinnings for the retrieval of conceptual knowledge for actions, although interest in this topic is gradually increasing (e.g., Chatterjee, Southwood, & Basilico, 1999; Grézes & Decety, 2001; Kable, Lease-Spellmeyer, & Chatterjee, 2002; Martin, Ungerleider, & Haxby, 2000; see also the recent Special Issues of *Cognitive Neuropsychology*, Vol. 15, 1998, and *Brain and Cognition*, Vol. 44, 2000, that focused on the cognitive neuroscience of actions). The current article reports a new investigation of the neural structures that mediate the retrieval of conceptual knowledge for actions.

## Representational components of action concepts

At the outset, it is important to explain what we mean by the designation "conceptual knowledge for actions." Our characterisation of action concepts is based on a theoretical framework regarding the cognitive and neural architecture of knowledge representation that has been elaborated in detail elsewhere (A. R. Damasio, 1989; A. R. Damasio & Damasio, 1994; H. Damasio et al., in press; Tranel, Adolphs, Damasio, & Damasio, 2001; Tranel et al., 1997a; for similar approaches, see Barsalou, 1999; Humphreys & Forde, 2001; Pulvermüller, 1999), and that we sketch briefly in the Discussion section. In general, we propose that action concepts embody knowledge about the behaviours of entities, especially animate entities such as people and animals, but also inanimate entities such as tools and vehicles (cf. Chatterjee, 2001; Klatzky, Pellegrino, McCloskey, & Doherty, 1989; Klatzky, Pellegrino, McCloskey, & Leiderman, 1993). These concepts not only contribute to the planning and programming of specific kinds of movement, but they also mediate recognition of the movements performed by other entities (Binkofski, Buccino, Posse, Seitz, Rizzolatti, & Freund, 1999a; Binkofski, Buccino, Stephan, Rizzolatti, Seitz, & Freund, 1999b; Di Pellegrino, Fadiga, Fogassi, Gallese, & Rizzolatti, 1992; Fadiga, Fogassi, Gallese, & Rizzolatti, 2000; Grafton, Arbib, Fadiga, & Rizzolatti, 1996; Iacoboni, Woods, Brass, Bekkering, Mazziotta, & Rizzolatti, 1999). Very little is known about the internal structure of action concepts; however, we suggest that the most important representational components or dimensions for these concepts include the following.

One of the most basic components is causal organisation (this component is akin to the older notion of transitive versus intransitive movements, e.g., Delay, 1935). Some physical actions involve purely body-internal behaviour, such as smiling, waving, or running, whereas others involve bringing about a particular kind of change in the state and/or location of another entity, either through direct contact—e.g., lifting a cup, crumpling a piece of paper—or by means of a tool—e.g., pounding a nail with a hammer, slicing a cucumber with a knife. Another representational dimension involves which body parts are typically used to execute certain actions—e.g., eyes, mouth, arms, hands, trunk, legs, feet. Closely related to this is the specific manner in which actions are executed. Thus, different hand configurations are used for punching, poking, and slapping (an early suggestion along these lines was put forth by Katz, 1925); different spatial trajectories are associated with bouncing a ball, rolling a ball, and throwing a ball; and different forms of locomotion are involved in walking, skipping, and running. Yet another component of action concepts involves temporal distribution. Some actions take place during a very short period of time and have an inherent endpoint, such as sneezing or hitting something; others usually have a more extended temporal contour and are not defined in terms of a necessary endpoint, such as singing or reading; still others are iterative in quality, such as beating a drum with a stick. An additional component that is very important for many action concepts involves the intention or purpose of the agent. For instance, the goal of chasing something is to catch it; the goal of washing something is to make it clean. Furthermore, actions vary with respect to the emotional valence typically associated with them. For example, some are inherently pleasurable whereas others are not; some lead to positive effects in other entities whereas others lead to negative effects; and so on.

## Action concepts and language

We turn here to a brief discussion of the distinction between conceptual knowledge and lexical knowledge, with regard to actions. At first glance, the distinction might seem to go without saying, but in fact, it is rather complex (and more so in regard to actions than in regard to concrete entities); moreover, the distinction is frequently ignored in the empirical literature (for some discussions of this issue, see Friston, Price, Fletcher, Moore, Frackowiak, & Dolan, 1996; Gainotti, Silveri, Daniele, & Giustolisi, 1995; Tranel & Damasio, 1999). Thus, a few words regarding this issue are warranted.

It is important to make two distinctions regarding the relation between action concepts and language. First, when an action concept is activated, it is often the case that a pool of phonological and/or orthographic forms of more or less appropriate words, especially verbs, is also activated. However, we believe that these two processes are separate, and that the retrieval of an action concept does not necessarily require the concomitant retrieval of a word-form. Tip-of-the-tongue phenomena in normal subjects (e.g., R. Brown & McNeill, 1966; Burke, MacKay, Worthley, & Wade, 1991; Maril, Wagner, & Schacter, 2001), and severe chronic anomia in aphasic subjects (e.g., Goodglass & Wingfield, 1997) demonstrate clearly that one can have an action concept in mind, and yet be incapable of activating and/or retrieving the desired word-form (see also Berndt, Mitchum, Haendiges, & Sandson, 1997; Kemmerer, Tranel, & Barrash, 2001; Tranel et al., 2001). In addition, there is evidence that young children develop many basic action concepts before they acquire the corresponding verbs (Nelson, 1986, 1996; Tomasello, 1992). Furthermore, it is likely that other animals, such as nonhuman primates, have a repertoire of action concepts despite not having conventional linguistic signs for them. In short, it is crucial to distinguish between conceptual knowledge retrieval (recognition) on the one hand, and word-form retrieval (naming) on the other, and we (H. Damasio, Grabowski, Tranel, Hichwa, & Damasio, 1996; H. Damasio et al., in press; Tranel et al., 2001; Tranel & Damasio, 1999; Tranel, Damasio, & Damasio, 1997b, 1998) and others (Caramazza & Shelton, 1998; Gainotti et al., 1995; Humphreys & Forde, 2001; Indefrey & Levelt, 2000; Levelt et al., 1999; Pulvermüller, 1999) have discussed this issue at some length previously.[2] A cross-linguistic study by Gennari, Sloman, Malt, and Fitch (2002) has also demonstrated that linguistic and nonlinguistic performances in regard to motion events are dissociable.

The second distinction that we would like to make is that the action concepts that people use for behavioural planning, perceptual categorisation, and inferential reasoning may not be fully identical to the meanings of verbs; instead, the meanings of verbs may be partially autonomous mental representations that "package" action concepts in language-specific ways (Levinson, 1997; Pinker, 1989; Talmy, 2000; Van Valin & LaPolla, 1997; Wienold, 1995). The strongest evidence for this view comes from research on cross-linguistic differences in verb meaning. Take, for example, a Native American language called Atsugewi. In order to compare the different ways in which English and Atsugewi encode actions, consider a situation in which a man spits out a grape seed onto a napkin. It may seem straightforward or even inevitable from the perspective of English speakers that the entire event would most naturally be expressed linguistically such that the verb *spit* specifies the particular manner of caused motion, the compound noun *grape seed* specifies the kind of entity that is caused to move, and the prepositional phrase *onto the napkin* specifies the endpoint of the motion. However, in Atsugewi the event is expressed very differently. There is a verb which means "for a small spherical object to move or be located," an instrumental prefix which means "from the mouth acting egressively

[2] Another important source of evidence for the separation of conceptual and lexical knowledge comes from patients with modality-specific naming defects (e.g., Caramazza & Hillis, 1991).

on an entity," and a directional suffix which means "onto a two-dimensional surface" (Talmy, 2000). Although these two ways of linguistically encoding the same objective event are quite different, presumably speakers of English and Atsugewi do not differ significantly in their nonlinguistic conceptualisation of spitting actions. Thus, we would suggest that it is only when a speaker decides to talk about a given event that it is necessary to engage in a form of "thinking for speaking" that requires mapping a nonlinguistic action concept onto the appropriate language-specific verb meaning (cf. Slobin, 1996).

The distinction between action concepts and verb meanings has been explored in recent research on language development in children (e.g., Bowerman & Choi, 2001; P. Brown, 2001; De Leon, 2001), but it is only beginning to be addressed in the field of cognitive neuroscience (cf. Chainay & Humphreys, 2002; Gennari et al., 2002; Kemmerer, 2000; Kemmerer & Wright, 2002). In the current study, we are concerned with nonlinguistic action concepts, not the language-specific meanings of verbs, but as noted earlier, this separation is challenging, and we have tried to be as clear as possible in regard to what our study does and does not allow us to conclude on this issue.

## The current study

It was noted above that very little is known about the neural basis of conceptual knowledge for actions. Overall, the gist of the available evidence points to structures in the left premotor/prefrontal, left parietal, and left posterior middle temporal (a region related to motion processing, known as MT) regions as being important for different aspects of action knowledge (Beauchamp, Lee, Haxby, & Martin, 2002; Chatterjee, 2001; Grézes & Decety, 2001; Jeannerod, 1994, 1997; Kable et al., 2002; see Discussion for a detailed review of this and related evidence). Accordingly, we formulated the following hypothesis: *The retrieval of conceptual knowledge for actions depends on neural systems located in higher-order association cortices of left premotor/prefrontal, parietal, and MT regions.* In the study reported here, we tested this hypothesis using the lesion approach in a large group of subjects. The specific prediction was that lesions in the target regions specified in the hypothesis would be associated with impaired retrieval of conceptual knowledge for actions.

It was also of interest to investigate how the neural systems for action concepts compared with those that have been identified previously as being important for various categories of concrete entities. To address this, we also measured retrieval of conceptual knowledge for the categories of *persons* and *tools* in the brain-damaged subjects. Previous findings have suggested that person knowledge is associated with right-hemisphere structures including the anterior and inferior temporal and occipito-temporal regions (e.g., Behrmann & Moscovitch, 2001; A. R. Damasio et al., 1990; Kanwisher & Moscovitch, 2000; Tranel, Damasio, & Damasio, 1995, 1997a), whereas tool knowledge is associated with the left occipital-temporal-parietal junction, in the vicinity of MT (e.g., Chao et al., 1999; Chao & Martin, 2000; Martin et al., 2000; Perani et al., 1995; Tranel et al., 1997a). Thus, we expected that the neural systems for action knowledge and person knowledge would differ, and accordingly, we predicted that subjects with impaired retrieval of action knowledge would not demonstrate impaired retrieval of person knowledge. By contrast, we expected that the systems for action knowledge and tool knowledge might be partially overlapping and, accordingly, we predicted that at least some subjects with impaired retrieval of action knowledge would also demonstrate impaired retrieval of tool knowledge.

# METHOD

## Subjects

Ninety subjects with circumscribed unilateral left ($n = 65$) or right ($n = 25$) hemisphere brain damage were selected from the Patient Registry of the University of Iowa's Division of Cognitive Neuroscience. All gave informed consent in accordance with the Human Subjects Committee of the University of Iowa. The subjects included 55 men and 35 women.

The distribution of lesions allowed us to probe most of the left hemisphere and a substantial portion of the right hemisphere (not all regions were sampled with equal density). Lesions were caused by either cerebrovascular disease (*n* = 72), temporal lobectomy (*n* = 16), or herpes simplex encephalitis (*n* = 2). To be eligible for the study, subjects had to have lesions that could be analysed with our MAP-3 technique (see below), and they had to have left-hemisphere language dominance (as determined from neurological, WADA, and neuropsychological testing). Handedness, measured with the Geschwind-Oldfield Questionnaire, which has a scale ranging from full right-handedness (+100) to full left-handedness (−100), was distributed as follows: 84 subjects were fully right-handed (+90 or greater); 3 were primarily right-handed (+70, +60, +30); 2 were fully left-handed (−90, −100); and 1 was primarily left-handed (−60).

All subjects had been extensively characterised neuropsychologically and neuroanatomically, according to standard protocols (H. Damasio & Frank, 1992; Frank, Damasio, & Grabowski, 1997; Tranel, 1996). All subjects had normal intelligence (as measured by the WAIS-R/WAIS-III), and had no difficulty attending to or perceiving visual stimuli, as determined by detailed neuropsychological assessment. The subjects had at least 8 years of formal schooling; for the sample as a whole, the average level of education was 13.0 years (*SD* = 2.6). The subjects ranged in age from 20 to 83 (*M* = 51.4, *SD* = 15.7). Some of the subjects with left-hemisphere lesions were recovered aphasics. However, none of the subjects had residual aphasia of such a degree as to preclude their comprehension of the experimental tasks (and verbal responses were not called for in this study). Given the nature of the experimental tasks (see below), this was a crucial consideration: We took care to exclude subjects who could not comprehend the tasks, and who had any difficulty understanding the content of the queries used in the tasks (4 subjects were excluded on this basis, prior to forming the group of 90 noted above; the determination of exclusion was made by a clinical neuropsychologist who was not involved in the planning or execution of the current study). The subjects were studied in the chronic phase, at least 3 months post-lesion onset. All data, including standard neuropsychological measures, neuroanatomical data, and the experimental tasks, were obtained in the chronic epoch (more than 3 months post-lesion onset), and they were obtained contemporaneously. The average time post-lesion onset was 5.6 years (*SD* = 4.0).

## Stimuli and procedures

### *Conceptual knowledge for actions*

The choice of tasks for measuring action knowledge is a challenging issue. The primary consideration in this regard was that the tasks be amenable to nonverbal problem solving, at least in principle—in other words, we wanted to avoid tasks that necessitate verbal mediation in order to be solved. The idea here is that the tasks should require subjects to conjure up knowledge about actions, without necessarily requiring the subjects to conjure up the associated words (e.g., verbs) that are often used to denote such actions (cf. Gennari et al., 2002). (A similar approach has been adopted by other investigators facing the same challenge—for example, see Kable et al., 2002, who used a Pyramids and Palm Trees type of task to prompt action concept retrieval). Two tasks were available that satisfied our criteria: the Picture Attribute Test and the Picture Comparison Test. Both tests were developed and standardised in our laboratory, and both were explicitly designed to measure retrieval of conceptual knowledge for actions, without requiring verbal mediation (Fiez & Tranel, 1997).[3] The tests also were developed to probe the various representational components of action concepts outlined earlier, although it is beyond the scope of the current study to investigate these different components in detail.

The Picture Attribute Test comprises 72 items, presented as colour photographs. Of these, 48 are single pictures of ongoing actions, and 24 are

[3] The original tests described in Fiez and Tranel (1997) had a few more items than were used in the current study. Some items were dropped from both tests due to unreliable performances in normal control subjects.

picture pairs depicting causative events, such that the first picture shows an initial state and the second shows a final result state. For each of the 72 items, the subject viewed two pictures (or two picture pairs), and was asked to choose the picture (or picture pair) that best met certain criteria. Across different items, the subject was asked to apply the following criteria: (1) Which action would make the loudest noise? (2) Which action would be most physically tiring? (3) Which action would take the longest time to complete? (4) Which action would require a specified kind of movement (e.g., moving hands closer together, moving hands up/down, moving hands in a circle)? (5) Which action would be most enjoyable/harmful/helpful? (6) Which change of state was accomplished using a specified tool or utensil (e.g., knife, hammer)? (7) Which change of state was most permanent? (8) Which change of state best represented an improvement to the object? An example of an item from the Picture Attribute Test is shown in Figure 1a (a complete list of all the items in the test is provided in Appendix C in Kemmerer et al., 2001). With respect to processing considerations, the Picture Attribute Test requires visual processing of the pictorial stimuli and retrieval of the appropriate action concepts. The main task of answering the attribute questions calls on the following types of additional operations: decomposing the internal structure of each action concept, identifying the attribute at issue, determining its value, comparing the values for the different concepts, and making a decision about which one fulfils the target criterion. For some of the items, it may also be necessary to imagine the specific kinds of dynamic motion patterns that the actions involve.

The Picture Comparison Test has 24 items, each of which consists of three individual photographs of ongoing actions. The subject is requested to select one picture from among the three that shows an action that is different from the other two ("odd one out"). An example of an item from the Picture Comparison Test is shown in Figure 1b (a complete list of all the items on this test is provided in Appendix E in Kemmerer et al., 2001). Although this test has much in common with the Picture Attribute Test, it also has some unique processing requirements. Most importantly, the subject is not given the relevant attributes for comparison, but must instead carry out the computational operations necessary to identify them. Also, the Picture Attribute and Picture Comparison tests vary with respect to the details of how action concepts must be cognitively manipulated (see Kemmerer et al., 2001). Despite such differences, however, it is important to emphasise that both tests require the activation and processing of conceptual knowledge for actions. We sought to improve the reliability of our measurement of action concepts by using both tests; however, it was not within the scope of this study to analyse the tests at a greater level of detail (e.g., different types of items), although we have provided some preliminary data on this issue in a previous publication (Kemmerer et al., 2001).

It is possible that during performance of these tests, normal subjects name (at least covertly) some of the actions, if only because using language is a natural, reflexive thing to do and may facilitate performance. It is also possible that some of the items in the tests reflect certain idiosyncratic ways in which English packages action concepts as verb meanings. However, it is likely that successful performance on the tests does not absolutely require or depend on retrieving either the phonological forms or the language-specific semantic structures of verbs (cf. Gennari et al., 2002). The tasks can be accomplished accurately *without* accessing these forms, and for this reason, we consider the tasks to be relatively pure measures of at least some aspects of action concept retrieval. Also, we have provided some empirical support for our contention that these two tasks have processing requirements that differ from those typically involved in action *naming* tests. Specifically, in the study reported in Kemmerer et al. (2001), we found in a principal components factor analysis that the Picture Attribute Test and the Picture Comparison Test loaded on factors that were quite distinct from those on which an action naming test, and other tests involving explicit verbal processing, loaded. In a similar vein, it should be noted that the issue of verb-form retrieval for the purpose of action naming was the subject of a previous investigation, and the reader is

**Which action would make the loudest sound?**

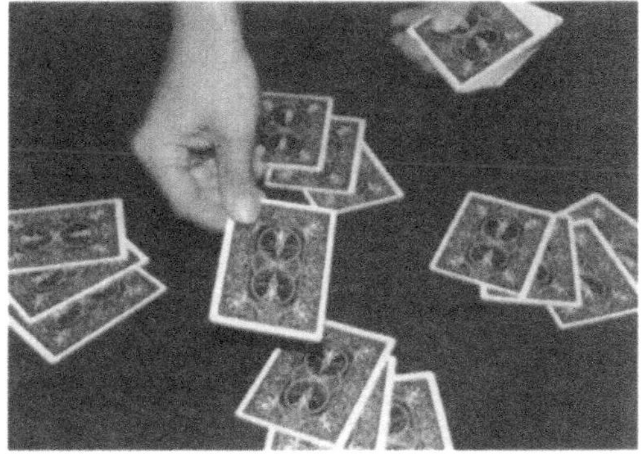

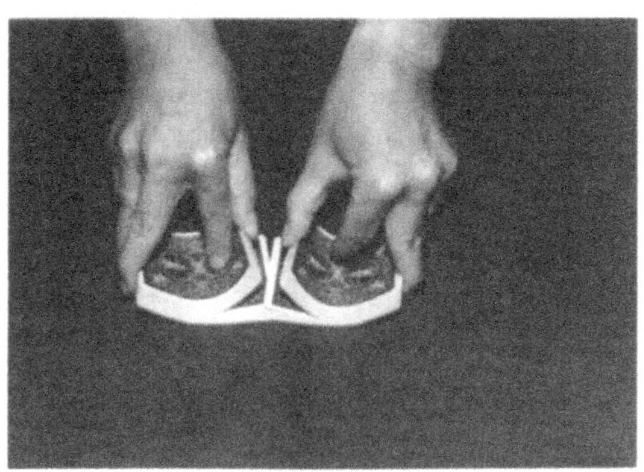

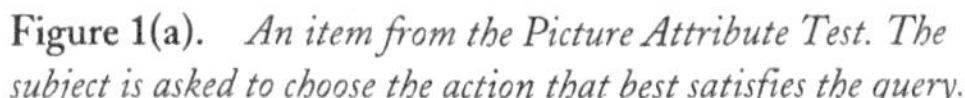

Figure 1(a). *An item from the Picture Attribute Test. The subject is asked to choose the action that best satisfies the query.*

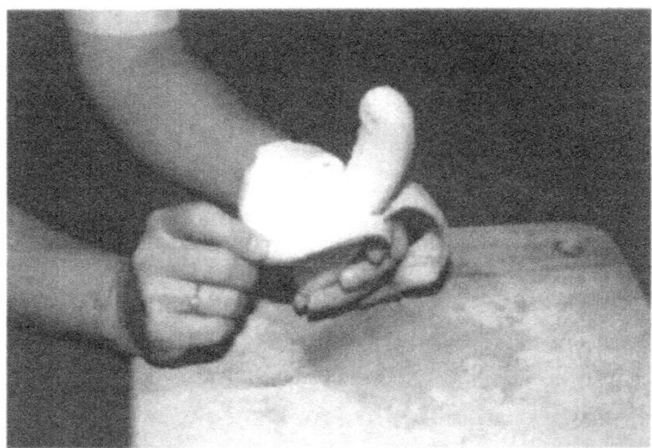

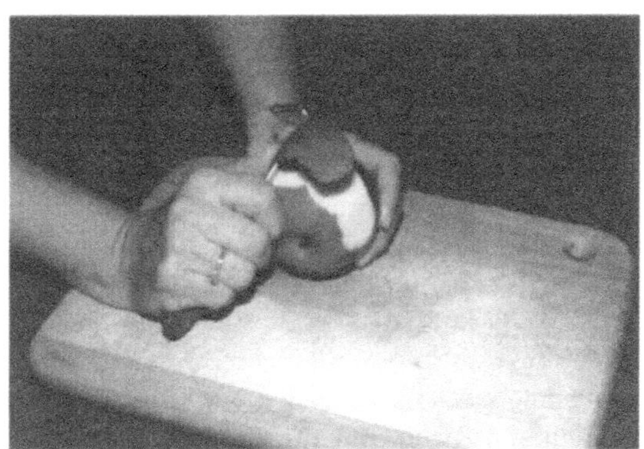

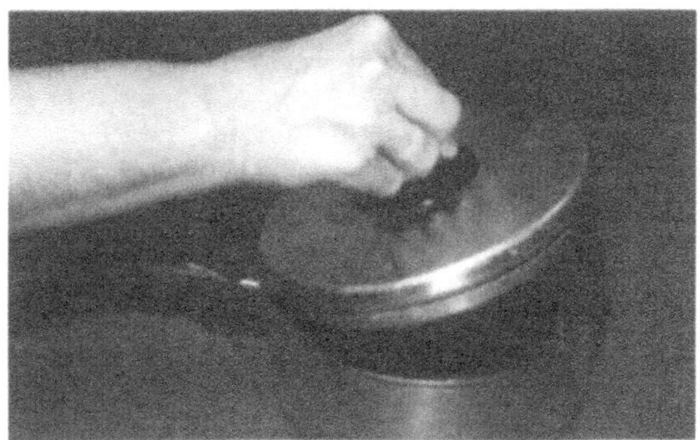

Figure 1(b). *An item from the Picture Comparison Test. The subject is asked to choose the action that "doesn't belong" with the other two.*

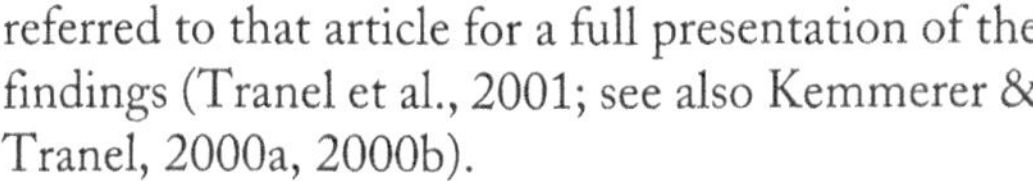

referred to that article for a full presentation of the findings (Tranel et al., 2001; see also Kemmerer & Tranel, 2000a, 2000b).

*Conceptual knowledge for persons and tools*

Measurement of conceptual knowledge for the concrete object categories of persons and tools was conducted using previously established methods (H. Damasio et al., in press; Tranel et al., 1997a). Briefly, these entailed the following. Subjects were presented pictures of famous faces ($n$ = 133) or tools ($n$ = 104), and asked to identify them. Accurate naming responses were accepted as correct identification. If naming was inaccurate or absent, subjects were prompted to generate specific, detailed descriptions of the stimuli. These were rated by experimenters to determine whether they conveyed sufficient information about the entity to support the scoring of the response as a correct identification, i.e., as adequate retrieval of conceptual knowledge.

We have discussed elsewhere the strengths and weaknesses of our method for measuring conceptual knowledge in the foregoing manner (H.

Damasio et al., in press). To briefly summarise, for items not named correctly, the subjects' responses were presented to two raters who were asked to determine who/what the stimulus was from the description alone, without having independent access to either the stimulus or its name. Recognition responses that either or both raters were able to use to generate the correct name of the entity were scored as correct. We appreciate that this procedure does not provide a direct probe of the full extent of the conceptual knowledge that a subject may possess for an entity; however, we do believe the procedure is actually quite demanding of conceptual knowledge, because for a naïve rater to be able to use a subject's definition in order to reach the name of an entity, the definition has to be fairly specific and detailed. By allowing subjects an open-ended opportunity to generate whatever information they can about the entities they cannot name (as opposed to asking specific questions about various properties of entities), we provide a situation that encourages subjects to substitute detailed descriptions for naming failures. Again, it is our contention that this procedure places fairly stringent demands on the subject's ability to access conceptual knowledge, even if it does not exhaust every conceivable means of measuring the status of such knowledge.

## Data quantification

*Neuropsychological data: Conceptual knowledge tests*
For each subject, performances on the Picture Attribute Test and the Picture Comparison Test were calculated as percentage correct (number of items answered correctly, divided by the number of items on the test, multiplied by 100). Scoring of items was based on the normative data from Fiez and Tranel (1997). Scoring is straightforward: For all items on both tests, there is a single correct answer, so subjects' answers are either right or wrong.

The following method, which we have used previously in a similar context (see Tranel et al., 2001), was used to determine a cut-off score for each test—i.e., a level above which subjects' scores were considered unimpaired, and below which subjects' scores were considered impaired. For each test, data from the 90 brain-damaged subjects were plotted according to percentage correct scores. To explore whether these scores were drawn from one or from more than one Gaussian normal distributions, we obtained quantile–quantile plots (actual data vs. the scores that would be expected if the data were normally distributed "N-scores"), as follows. Typically, the *i*th N-score for a sample of size N is obtained from the mean of the sampling distribution of the *i*th order statistic in a sample of N values drawn from a standard normal distribution. (In order to increase resistance to skewness, we conducted the analysis using the medians of the sampling distributions, rather than the means.) The *i*th median order statistic of a sample size N was approximated by the function: InvGaussian([i − 1/3]/[N + 1/3]), where InvGaussian is the inverse Gaussian (or normal) cumulative distribution function. We used a dynamic least-squares regression of actual scores versus N-scores to isolate those scores that were most likely to belong to the same distribution. Beginning at each extreme of the score range (the lowest score and the highest score), we calculated the least-squares fit continuously as additional scores were added, until a maximum was reached. At this point, a cut-off score was set. Both tests were subjected to this analysis, so that cut-off scores were set for both tests. For each test, scores below the cut-off were designated as impaired, and scores above the cut-off were designated as unimpaired.

For the persons and tools categories, the number of correctly named plus correctly identified items was divided by the number of items in the category, and multiplied by 100, to yield a percentage correct score. For each subject, the persons and tools scores were compared to previously established normative data (H. Damasio et al., in press; Tranel et al., 1997a) to determine whether the scores were unimpaired or impaired. Here, we present these data for a subset of the subjects (namely, those who had impaired action knowledge) in order to test the predictions outlined at the end of the Introduction (the reader is referred to Tranel et al., 1997a, for a complete presentation of these findings).

*Neuroanatomical data*

The neuroanatomical analysis was based on magnetic resonance (MR) data obtained in a 1.5 Tesla scanner with an SPg sequence of thin (1.5 mm) and contiguous $T_1$ weighted coronal cuts, and reconstructed in three dimensions using Brainvox (H. Damasio, 2000; H. Damasio & Frank, 1992; Frank et al., 1997). (In a few subjects in whom an MR could not be obtained, the analysis was based on computerised axial tomography—CT—data.) The final anatomical description of the lesion overlap and of its placement relative to neuroanatomical landmarks was performed with Brainvox, using the MAP-3 technique. All lesions in this set were transposed and manually warped into a normal 3-D reconstructed brain, so as to permit the determination of the maximal overlap of lesions relative to subjects grouped by neuropsychological defect according to the method specified above.

A detailed description of MAP-3 is provided in H. Damasio (2000); in brief, it entails: (1) a normal 3-D reconstructed brain is resliced so as to match the slices of the MR/CT of the subject and create a correspondence between each of the subject's MR/CT slices and the slices of the normal brain; (2) the contour of the lesion on each slice is then transposed onto the matched slices of the normal brain, taking into consideration the distance from the edge of the lesion to appropriate anatomical landmarks; (3) for each lesion, the collection of contours constitutes an "object" that can be co-rendered with the normal brain. The objects in any given group can intersect in space, and thus yield a maximal overlap relative to both surface damage and depth extension. We can then calculate the number of subjects contributing to this overlap.

## Data analysis

To analyse the data in regard to our hypothesis, we grouped the subjects according to their performances on the Picture Attribute Test and Picture Comparison Test, and analysed the neuroanatomical results. We utilised a lesion analysis approach that we have used previously with comparable datasets (Adolphs, Damasio, Tranel, Cooper, & Damasio, 2000; H. Damasio et al., in press; Tranel et al., 2001). Specifically, we contrasted the group of subjects who fell in the "impaired" partition of the distributions of scores for the Picture Attribute Test and the Picture Comparison Test ($n = 26$; see Results, below), with the group of subjects who fell in the "unimpaired" partition of the distributions ($n = 64$). Subjects were classified as impaired if they met the criterion for impairment (i.e., scores below the cut-off) on either or both of the action concept tests; to be classified as unimpaired, subjects had to have scores above the cut-off on *both* of the action concept tests. A MAP-3 lesion overlap was calculated for each group (impaired, unimpaired), and then the two MAP-3 overlaps were contrasted by subtracting one from the other. Thus, neuropsychological performance (action recognition) served as the independent variable, and lesion overlap (according to MAP-3) served as the dependent variable. Also, in order to confirm statistically the reliability of the findings, we used parametric techniques to compare neuropsychological performances of groups of subjects (see below).

The lesion subtraction proceeded arithmetically for each brain voxel (see Adolphs et al., 2000, for additional details about this method). We took the number of subjects with unimpaired action concept scores (as defined above) who had lesions at a given voxel, and subtracted this from the total number of subjects with impaired action concept scores who had lesions at that same voxel. Thus, the subtraction yields a difference in the number of lesions at each voxel, reflecting the proportion of subjects with impaired scores, compared with the proportion of subjects with unimpaired scores, who had damage at that voxel. This arithmetic subtraction of subject numbers was applied to all voxels in the brain.

The standard we used for defining a region of voxels as "significant" was a difference in the overlap subtraction of five subjects or more (H. Damasio et al., in press). That is, if subtracting the unimpaired subjects from the impaired subjects yielded a difference of five subjects or more for a particular region of voxels, that region was considered to be involved crucially in the experimental test performance (retrieving action concepts). The use of this five-subject threshold is based on extensive

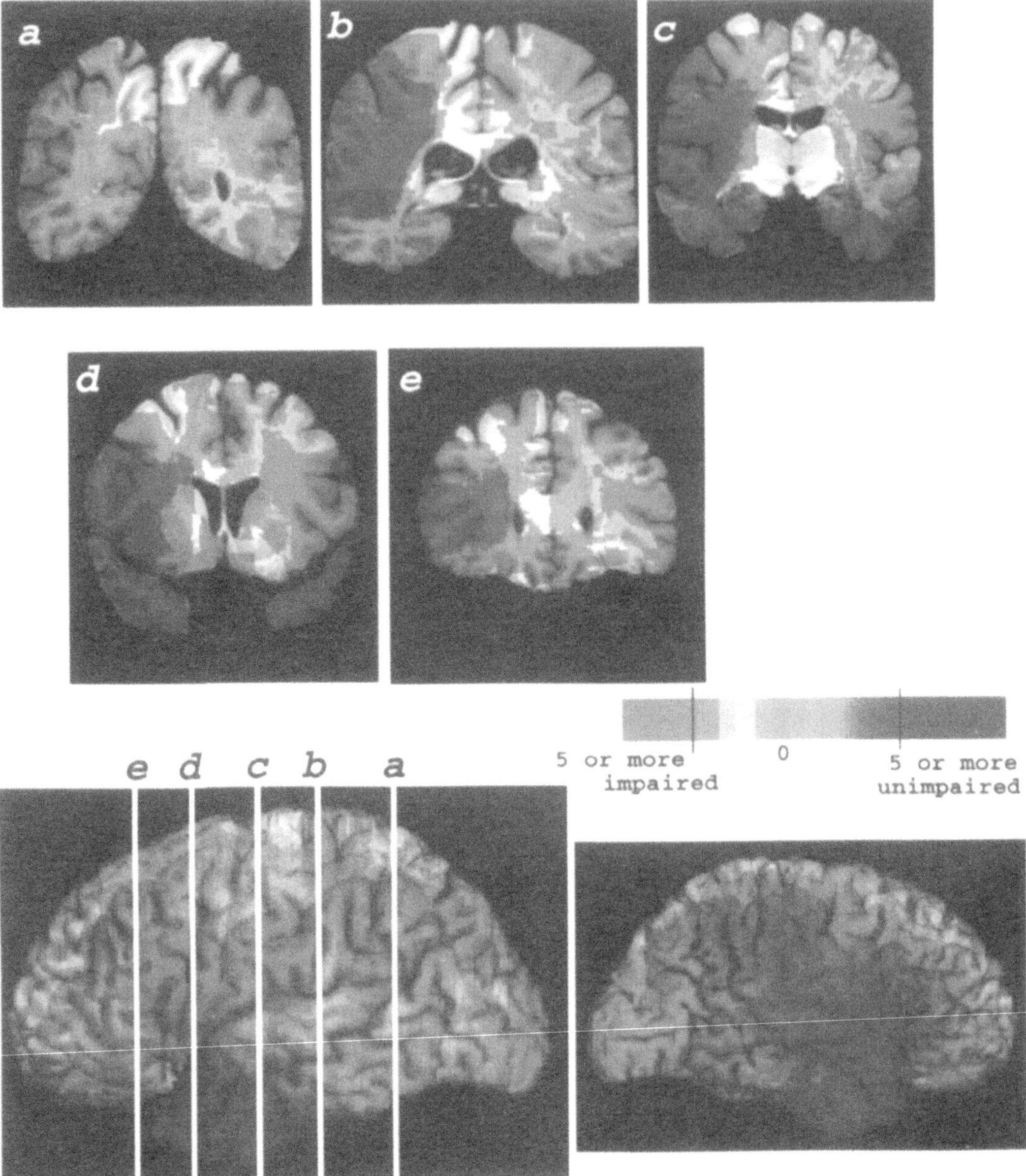


**Figure 2.** *The subtraction of lesion overlaps for 64 unimpaired subjects from the lesion overlaps for 26 impaired subjects, derived from MAP-3 (see text for methods). The colour bar indicates the number of lesions in the overlap difference. The white lines denote the planes of coronal sections depicted in the upper two rows of the figure (sections a–e). The subtraction image shows that the highest area of lesion overlap specific to the impaired subjects is in the left hemisphere (lower left), in the left frontal operculum, underlying white matter, and anterior sector of the insula (sections c, d, e). Significant areas of lesion overlap are also evident in the left parietal region (section b) and in the white matter underneath left MT (section a). No region of significant lesion overlap associated with impaired action recognition was identified in the right hemisphere (lower right); by contrast, the highest densities of lesion overlaps in the right hemisphere were associated with unimpaired action recognition performance.*

prior investigations in our laboratory, which have determined that this is a valid criterion for identifying, with a high degree of specificity and sensitivity, brain regions that are important for experimental task performance (see H. Damasio, in press, for a detailed presentation of this information). The overlap subtraction results were color coded, and the volumes were depicted on lateral and coronal brain views (see Figure 2).

**Table 1.** *Action concept retrieval; average percentage correct (and standard deviation)*

| | *Test* | |
|---|---|---|
| *Group* | *Picture attribute* | *Picture comparison* |
| Impaired ($n$ = 26) | 84.1 (7.3) | 57.8 (17.1) |
| Unimpaired ($n$ = 64) | 93.8 (3.4) | 87.5 (8.1) |
| $t$-test result[a] | $t$ = 8.59* | $t$ = 11.13* |
| Fiez/Tranel Ss[b] ($n$ = 56) | 91.7 (4.8) | 83.6 (8.3) |
| Cut-off scores[c] | <85 <68 | |

[a]The $t$-tests compared the two brain-damaged groups—impaired vs. unimpaired subjects—on each test.
[b]Slight modifications of the tests were implemented by Kemmerer et al. (2001), and the means and *SD*s shown here are derived from the modified versions of the tests. See Kemmerer et al. (2001) for details.
[c]Derived from analysis of entire distribution of scores; see text for details.
*$p$ < .0001.

## RESULTS

### Action knowledge

As noted, 26 subjects met the criterion for impairment on one or both of the action concept tests. The specific breakdown was as follows: 9 subjects were impaired on both the Picture Attribute Test and the Picture Comparison Test; 6 subjects were impaired on just the Picture Attribute Test; and 11 subjects were impaired on just the Picture Comparison Test. (Since we are concerned primarily with the action knowledge that both of the tests probe, and not with differences in processing requirements that distinguish the two tests, we will not explore further the behavioural dissociation between the tests that emerged for some of the subjects. Instead, we will concentrate on the entire group of 26 subjects who failed either one or both of the tests. In the same vein, we do not address here potential differences between various subtypes of items on the tests.) Taking this group as a whole, the average score on the Picture Attribute Test was 84.1 (*SD* = 7.3) and the average score on the Picture Comparison Test was 57.8 (*SD* = 17.1). These values are well below those for the normal control subjects reported by Fiez and Tranel (1997), and those for the unimpaired brain-damaged subjects in the current study (Table 1). Statistical comparisons of the impaired and unimpaired brain-damaged groups (Bonferroni corrected one-tailed $t$-tests) were highly significant for both tests ($p$s < .0001). Also, it is important to note that the performances of brain-damaged subjects classified as unimpaired in the current study were comparable to those of normal controls reported in Fiez and Tranel (1997).

Figure 2 shows the results of the MAP-3 overlap analysis. As noted earlier, the two group MAP-3 overlaps were contrasted by subtracting the MAP-3 overlap for the 64 unimpaired subjects from the MAP-3 overlap for the 26 impaired subjects. This subtraction revealed a maximal overlap difference encompassing the left premotor/prefrontal region (cortex and white matter), the left parietal region (cortex and white matter), and the white matter underlying the left MT region. Using the five-subject criterion defined earlier, the regions meeting this threshold for significant overlap are denoted by red in Figure 2. It can be seen that the most substantial overlap region is comprised by the left frontal operculum and its attendant white matter. The involvement of the white matter extends all the way to the edge of the lateral ventricle, and there is also involvement of the anterior insular cortex and white matter. The left parietal region is involved to a lesser extent, with some overlap in both the cortex and underlying white matter. There is also an area of significant overlap in the white matter underneath left MT.

In follow-up analyses, we calculated lesion overlaps for the three subgroups of subjects who were impaired on both the Picture Attribute Test and the Picture Comparison Test ($n = 9$), or on only the Picture Attribute Test ($n = 6$), or on only the Picture Comparison Test ($n = 11$). For all three subgroups, the results were similar to the subtraction overlap depicted in Figure 2, with the highest overlap in the left frontal operculum and in the white matter underneath this region, and other areas of greatest overlap in the left parietal region and in the white matter underneath MT. We did not observe notable discrepancies between the lesion overlaps for the nine subjects with impairments on both tests, versus the groups that were impaired on only one or the other of the tests.

One issue that can be raised in this context is the extent to which lesion volumes may differ systematically in the impaired versus unimpaired groups of subjects. We have addressed this question conceptually in previous publications (e.g., Adolphs et al., 2000), and have pointed out that the MAP-3 subtraction technique makes it highly unlikely that the regions identified in the subtraction (as being associated with a particular neuropsychological defect) would be an artifact of the impaired subjects having larger lesion volumes than the unimpaired subjects. To illustrate the point in the current study, we present results for three representative subjects (Figure 3). The subject in the upper left panel of Figure 3 has a small lesion located strategically in the left MT region (especially in underlying white matter, as shown in the coronal section), and this subject was impaired on *both* the Picture Attribute Test (78% correct) and the Picture Comparison Test (21% correct). The subject in the upper right panel of Figure 3 has a relatively large lesion in the left frontal operculum, involving cortex and underlying white matter, and this subject was impaired on the Picture Comparison Test (50% correct) but not on the Picture Attribute Test (93% correct). The subject in the bottom panel of Figure 3 has a large lesion in the anterior temporal region, and this subject was *normal* on both the Picture Attribute Test (96% correct) and the Picture Comparison Test (79% correct).

## Person and tool knowledge

Another objective of the study was to explore how the neural systems for action concepts compared to those that are important for various categories of concrete entities. As reviewed earlier, there is evidence that knowledge for persons is associated with right anterior/inferior temporal and occipitotemporal structures, whereas knowledge for tools is associated with structures in and near left MT. Accordingly, we had predicted that subjects with impaired retrieval of action knowledge would not demonstrate impaired retrieval of person knowledge, and by contrast, that some subjects with impaired retrieval of action knowledge would demonstrate impaired retrieval of tool knowledge. To test this, we calculated conceptual knowledge scores for the categories of persons and tools for all of the 26 subjects who had impaired action knowledge. The results were as follows (Table 2): For the persons category, the overall performance of the 26 subjects was nearly identical (actually slightly superior) to those that were reported previously for brain-damaged and normal control subjects (Tranel et al., 1997a). Taking the 26 subjects individually, only one met the conventional *2-SD* cutoff for impairment in the persons category, and this subject happened to be the one exceptional case that had a right occipital-temporal lesion (all of the other 25 subjects in this group had left-hemisphere lesions). Turning to the tools category, the overall performance of the 26 subjects was about 5 percentage points below the previously reported values for brain-damaged and normal control groups (statisti-

**Table 2.** *Person and tool concept retrieval; average percentage correct (and standard deviation)*

| | *Category* | |
|---|---|---|
| *Group* | *Persons* | *Tools* |
| Subjects with impaired action concepts ($n = 26$) | 79.2 (11.3) | 91.4 (7.8) |
| Brain-damaged unimpaired subjects (Tranel et al., 1997a) | 77.7 (8.0) | 96.1 (3.2) |
| Normal control subjects (Tranel et al., 1997a) | 75.7 (6.7) | 96.2 (3.3) |

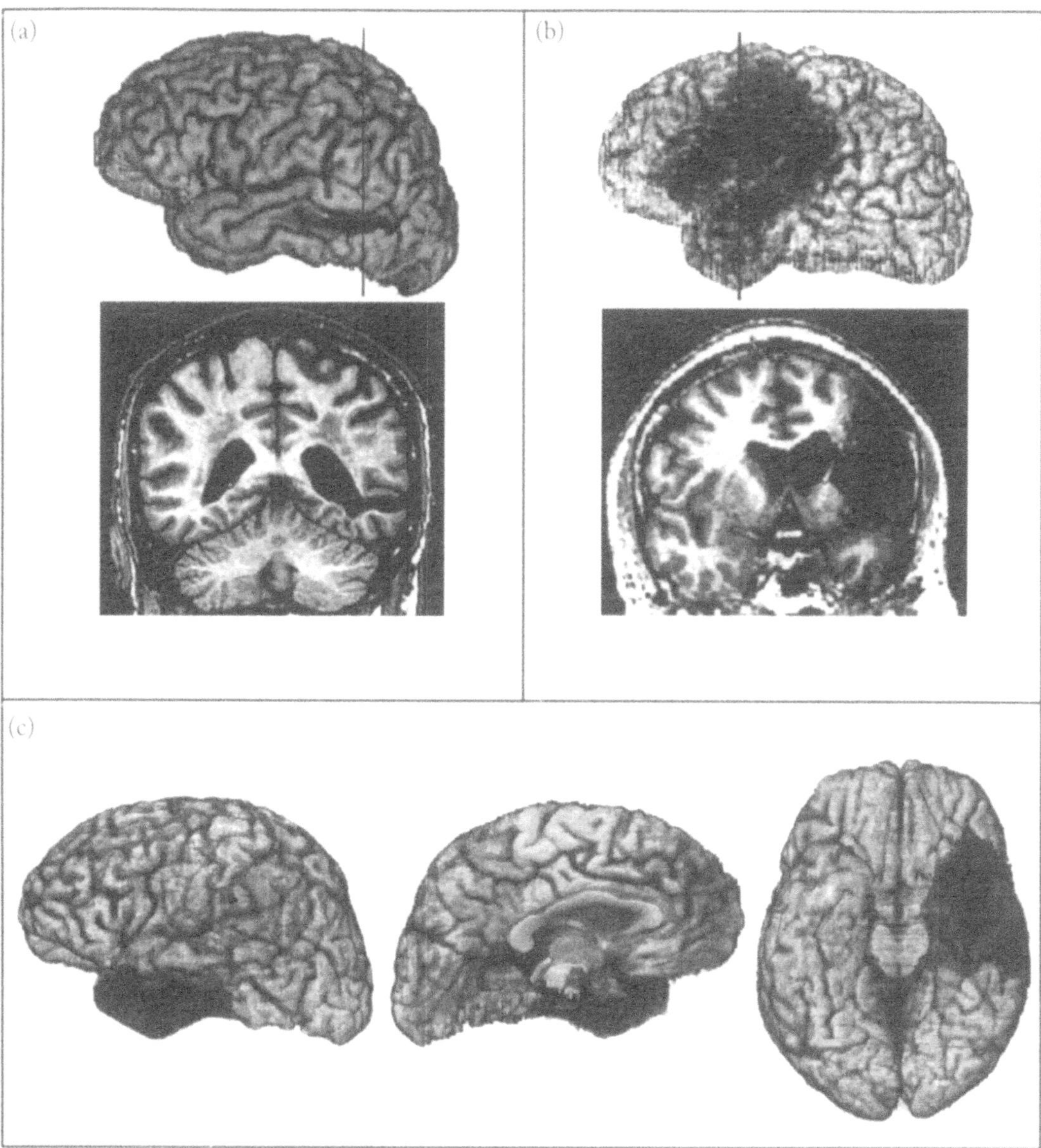


**Figure 3.** *Depiction of lesions in three representative subjects, based on MR data and our 3-dimensional reconstruction technique. (a) Upper left panel: This subject has a small left MT lesion, shown on the lateral view and in the coronal section taken at the level indicated by the vertical line. The subject has a severe defect in action recognition, and failed both experimental tasks. (b) Upper right panel: This subject has a relatively large left frontal opercular lesion, shown on the lateral view and in the coronal section taken at the level indicated by the vertical line. The subject has a defect in action recognition, and failed one (but not both) of the experimental tasks. (c) Lower panel: This subject has a relatively large left anterior temporal lesion, shown in lateral, mesial, and inferior views. The subject had normal action recognition, and performed normally on both experimental tasks.*

cal analyses were not applied to the data in Table 2, since most of the data were analysed and reported in Tranel et al., 1997a). Thus, at a group level there is evidence that subjects with impaired action concepts had somewhat poorer performance in tool recognition. And at an individual level, we found that 6 of the 26 subjects had impaired tool concepts, according to a *2-SD* cut-off classification.

Naturally, it was of interest to explore the lesion profiles of the six subjects who had impaired tool concepts in addition to impaired action concepts. Based on a simple lesion overlap analysis, we found that the highest area of overlap in this group was in the left MT region (four subjects). This is consistent with findings reported previously (Tranel et al., 1997a), and suggests that there is partial overlap in the neural systems important for action concepts and those important for tool concepts. We should also note that the four subjects with dual impairments in action concepts and tool concepts were a subset of those reported in the MT component of the lesion overlap depicted in Figure 2, which provides further evidence consistent with the idea that action knowledge and tool knowledge share a common neural substrate, to some extent.

## DISCUSSION

The findings from this study provide support for our hypothesis—specifically, in subjects with impaired retrieval of conceptual knowledge for actions, we found significant lesion overlap in the left premotor/prefrontal region, in the left parietal region, and in the white matter underneath left MT. The specificity of these findings is supported by the lesion overlap subtraction, which indicates that there is a significant over-representation of impaired subjects with lesions in these regions, as compared to unimpaired subjects. We turn now to situating the current results in the context of the relevant literature. Each of the identified sectors—the premotor/prefrontal region, the parietal region, and the MT region—is reviewed in turn.

### Premotor/prefrontal region

The premotor/prefrontal cortices, which are targets of parietal projections, appear related to the retrieval of specific visuomotor aspects of action concepts. In the ventral premotor cortex of the macaque monkey, area F5 contains two types of neurons—canonical neurons and mirror neurons (Fadiga et al., 2000; Rizzolatti & Fadiga, 1998). The first type responds to the mere visual presentation of prehensile objects, and the second type fires during the production of certain kinds of object-directed hand actions (e.g., holding, tearing, poking) as well as when the animal observes other individuals performing the same actions. Similarly, functional neuroimaging studies have found activation in the homologous region of the human premotor cortex when subjects view and name pictures of tools (Chao & Martin, 2000; H. Damasio et al., in press; Grabowski, Damasio, & Damasio, 1998; Grafton, Arbib, Fadiga, & Rizzolatti, 1997; Martin et al., 1996), and also when subjects execute, observe, or imagine various hand actions (Binkofski et al., 1999a, 1999b; Decety et al., 1994; Gerardin et al., 2000; Grafton, Arbib, Fadiga, & Rizzolatti, 1996; Iacoboni et al., 1999; Lotze et al., 1999; Moll, De Oliveira-Souza, Passman, Cunha, Souza-Lima, & Andreiuolo, 2000). In addition, damage to the premotor/prefrontal cortices sometimes leads to so-called "action disorganisation syndrome," which involves a disruption of the hierarchical and temporal structure of complex action sequences such as "making a pot of coffee" or "wrapping a present" (Humphreys & Forde, 1998; M. F. Schwartz, Montgomery, Fitzpatrick-DeSalme, Ochipa, Coslett, & Mayer, 1995; Schwartz, Reed, Montgomery, Palmer, & Mayer, 1991; Sirigu, Zalla, Pillon, Dubois, Grafman, & Agid, 1996b; West & Alain, 2000). (We did not assess this syndrome in connection with the current study, and the complexities of this issue are well beyond the scope of the current context—see, for example, Zanini, Rumiati, & Shallice, 2002.)

## Parietal region

Sectors of the parietal lobe contribute to the transformation of visual, auditory, and somatosensory input into a format that is appropriate for planning bodily movements, especially reaching and grasping movements within peripersonal space (Farne & Ladavas, 2000; Graziano, Cooke, & Taylor, 2000; Pisella et al., 2000; for review, see Jeannerod, Arbib, Rizzolatti, & Sakata, 1995). Single-cell recording studies in nonhuman primates have demonstrated that neurons in area 7b fire immediately prior to or during reaching and grasping movements (Andersen, 1995); and that neurons in area AIP (anterior intraparietal sulcus; see Binkofski et al., 1998, for a definition of this region in humans) are sensitive to the three-dimensional properties of objects (e.g., shape, size, orientation) that are relevant to determining how the hand and fingers should be configured to interact with various objects (Sakata, Taira, Murata, & Mine, 1995). Lesion and functional imaging studies in human subjects have provided some additional, consistent evidence. For example, damage to posterior parietal cortices, especially on the left, can produce impairments in object-directed actions, such as inaccurate preshaping of the hand during the approach phase (Perenin & Vighetto, 1988). Lesions in this region have also been reported to disrupt conceptual knowledge regarding the precise manner in which tools should be manipulated (Buxbaum, Veramonti, & Schwartz, 2000). In addition, parietal damage can impair temporal aspects of action concepts. Sirigu, Dumanel, Cohen, Pillon, Dubois, and Agid (1996a) found that lesions to the parietal cortex (especially on the left) produced impairments in the ability to predict, through mental imagery, the time necessary to perform differentiated finger movements and visually guided pointing gestures. Similarly, in functional imaging studies, the parietal region has been associated with perception of actions (Buccino et al., 2001; Decety et al., 1997; for review, see Goodale & Humphrey, 1998) and, more specifically, with the perception of scripts of goal-directed hand actions (Bonda, Petrides, Ostry, & Evans, 1996). This region has also been shown to be activated during conditions in which subjects either execute or imagine hand movements (Gerardin et al., 2000), as well as when subjects view and name pictures of tools that are typically manipulated in certain ways (Chao & Martin, 2000).

Furthermore, there is a classic literature regarding apraxia that has some bearing on the role of the parietal lobe in retrieving knowledge for actions (Critchley, 1953; Geschwind, 1975; Geschwind & Damasio, 1985; Heilman & Rothi, 1993; Liepmann, 1920; also see Sunderland & Sluman, 2000). In particular, the condition known as "ideational apraxia" is relevant—this condition has been defined as a loss of the ideas or concepts behind skilled movements, and traditionally it was associated with lesions in the left parieto-occipital junction (De Renzi, 1989; Heilman & Rothi, 1993; Kirshner, 1991). Relatively "pure" cases of ideational apraxia are exceedingly rare, and the most convincing examples actually come from patients with degenerative conditions (e.g., Ochipa, Rothi, & Heilman, 1992; R. L. Schwartz et al., 2000). Also, the neuroanatomical correlates of ideational apraxia have been repeatedly questioned, and it is even difficult to find a consensus on how to define the disorder (Kirshner, 1991; Tranel & Damasio, 1996). Nonetheless, evidence from this literature is consistent with the notion that cortices in the left occipital-parietal junction support the retrieval of conceptual knowledge for actions (Leiguarda & Marsden, 2000; Rothi, Raade, & Heilman, 1994). Our current findings are broadly compatible with this conclusion, although we did not specifically test our subjects for ideational apraxia.

## Posterior middle temporal (MT) region

There is a growing body of evidence suggesting that the region known as MT, a motion-related area in the posterior middle temporal region (Tootell et al., 1995; Watson et al., 1993; Zeki, Watson, Lueck, Friston, Kennard, & Frackowiak, 1991; for a review regarding this region in humans, see Dumoulin et al., 2000), may play a role in retrieving knowledge about the typical motion patterns of entities. Functional imaging studies have shown activation in and near this area in tasks in which subjects must generate verbs associated with visually presented nouns or objects (Fiez, Raichle, Balota, Tallal, & Petersen, 1996; Martin, Haxby, Lalonde, Wiggs, & Ungerleider, 1995; Warburton et al., 1996; Wise, Chollet, Hader, Friston, Hoffner, & Frackowiak, 1991; for review, see Martin et al., 2000). A recent PET study found MT activation (as well as activation in the left premotor cortex) during action recognition and naming (H. Damasio, Grabowski, Tranel, Ponto, Hichwa, & Damasio, 2001). In addition, it has been shown (in fMRI studies) that this region is activated when subjects view static images of implied motion (Kourtzi & Kanwisher, 2000; Senior et al., 2000; also see David & Senior, 2000). This is especially relevant to the results of the present study, because some of the stimuli in the two action concept tests portray actions whose recognition probably requires retrieval of implied dynamic motion patterns. Finally, it is worth noting that left MT was the site of maximal lesion overlap identified in our study of brain-damaged subjects with tool recognition defects (Tranel et al., 1997a). This was in the vicinity of the region identified by Martin et al. (1996) as activated by tool naming in a PET study. The association with tools may be to the fact that tools usually have characteristic patterns of movement, and tool processing may thus engage MT in a manner comparable to that seen for processing some action concepts.

There is also a recent functional imaging study that bears directly on our study. Kable et al. (2002) used fMRI to investigate the neural basis of what the investigators termed "action event knowledge." Subjects were presented tasks that were purported to require access to conceptual knowledge for actions, with minimal demands on lexical retrieval processes—specifically, subjects had to match pictures of actions, using a format derived from the Pyramids and Palm Trees task (cf. Howard & Patterson, 1992). This was compared to matching pictures of objects. A second group of subjects performed the same tasks, but with words (verbs and nouns) instead of pictures. The investigators found that the action matching tasks produced differential activation in the MT/MST region,[4] bilaterally; that is, there was more activation in MT/MST when subjects were performing the action matching task, compared to the object matching task. The MT/MST action-related activation was primarily left-sided for the word condition, whereas it was more bilateral for the picture condition. The investigators did not find greater activity during action matching in either the prefrontal or parietal regions, although this may have been due to the possibility that the object matching task engaged some of the same areas (especially the left frontal operculum) that would be engaged by the action matching task, thereby cancelling out the action-related activation. That is, in normal subjects, matching pictures of concrete entities is likely to evoke the names of those entities, reflexively. This would be expected to activate left frontal operculum, a finding that would be even more likely in the case of the word matching task. In fact, the authors reported that the action matching tasks, when compared to the baseline (as opposed to the object tasks), did produce activation in the left prefrontal and left inferior parietal regions. (We note that in the current study, we did not have a sufficient number of subjects with lesions in the right MT/MST region to address this interesting issue.)

## Action concepts and concrete entity concepts

Returning to the current study, another objective was to explore how the neural systems important for action concepts compare to those that are important for concepts of categories of concrete

[4] MT refers to posterior middle temporal, as noted; MST is middle superior temporal gyrus. The authors used a definition of these regions which follows that set forth by Kourtzi and Kanwisher (2000) and Tootell et al. (1995).

entities, such as persons and tools. In the case of persons, it appears that the systems are distinct. In previous work, we found that conceptual knowledge for persons was associated with structures in right hemisphere, including the anterior and inferior temporal region and the occipitotemporal region (H. Damasio et al., in press; Tranel et al., 1995, 1997a). In the current study, we found that only 1 of 26 subjects with impaired action concepts had impaired knowledge for persons. This subject was the only one of the 26 that had a right-hemisphere lesion (in the occipital-temporal region). By contrast, in the case of neural systems presumed to support conceptual knowledge for tools, there appears to be partial overlap with systems that support conceptual knowledge for actions—specifically, in the vicinity of MT. Our previous work has shown that lesions in this region impair conceptual knowledge for tools (H. Damasio et al., in press; Tranel et al., 1997a). In the current study, six subjects with impaired action concepts (four of whom had left MT lesions) had impaired tool knowledge. As alluded to earlier, this makes sense when one considers that characteristic motion is a defining feature of tools.

## Action concepts and action names

It is also worth considering how the current findings compare to the findings regarding action *naming* that were reported recently (Tranel et al., 2001). In that study, we found that lesions related to impaired action naming overlapped maximally in the left frontal operculum. A detailed comparison of the results from the two studies is beyond the scope of the current discussion, but on initial scrutiny, there appears to be some commonality in the findings. Specifically, both studies identified a region that includes the left frontal operculum, underlying white matter, and anterior insula.[5] The regions that stand out as being at least partially different in the current study are the left parietal and left MT regions; neither of these was strongly associated with action naming in the Tranel et al. study, whereas both were identified in the current study as being associated with action concepts. On balance, the results point to some overlap in the neural systems that subserve conceptual knowledge for actions, and those that subserve lexical knowledge for actions—specifically, in the left frontal operculum; however, the overlap does not appear to be complete. Further investigation of this issue is warranted.

## Concluding comment

We propose that the action concept retrieval tasks used in the experiments reported here depend for their execution on *intermediary* (or *mediational*) regions, which consist of collections of "convergence zones," articulated in systems (A. R. Damasio, 1989; A. R. Damasio & Damasio, 1994). To illustrate our interpretation, consider an example: when a stimulus depicting a particular action is shown to a subject and the visual properties of the stimulus are processed, a particular intermediary region becomes active and promotes the explicit sensorimotor representation of knowledge pertaining to the action, which occurs in the appropriate early sensory cortices and motor structures. The evocation of some part of the potentially large number of such images, over a brief lapse of time and in varied sensorimotor cortices, constitutes the conceptual evocation for the action.

In this framework, when we evoke the concept of an action, we activate collections of sensory and motor patterns in cerebral cortices appropriate to represent pertinent features of the concept (e.g., motion, sound, effort, speed). The patterns are generated from dispositions contained in convergence zones, and generate either mental images or actions or preparations for action. We assume that on different occasions, somewhat different combinations of features may be retrieved with different

[5] In fact, a number of subjects were common to both studies, and some of these had impairments in both action recognition and action naming. The typical lesion correlate in these subjects was left frontal opercular damage, and in these cases, the naming impairment tended to be disproportionately severe, relative to the recognition impairment (see Tranel et al., 2001, pp. 663–664, for further details regarding this comparison).

degrees of automaticity, depending on the circumstances in which concept retrieval occurs and on autobiographical factors. We also assume that the anatomical placement of convergence zones is suited for the most efficient interaction with the cortical regions that contain the relevant dispositions, and with the cortices where the dispositions ultimately generate images or drive actions. In the case of action stimuli, this placement is preferentially aimed at left MT, parietal, and frontal opercular sectors, and as reviewed above, this makes sense in light of considerable convergent evidence regarding the processing of action-related knowledge.

In our view, the basic neuroanatomical design of convergence zones is available in higher-order cortices prior to individual experience, and then is shaped by individual learning. The process of learning selects the micro-regions and the input-output projections that optimally perform particular tasks, under particular circumstances. The constraints of the brain's anatomical design mean that in most individuals, convergence zones involved in certain classes of tasks—e.g., retrieving knowledge about actions—are likely to be found in the same large-scale region of the brain, e.g., MT, frontal operculum. But this does not mean that at micro-scale level, convergence zones would be found in anatomically equal sites across individuals—on the contrary, we expect that the same task will be performable with the help of different convergence zones in the very same individual (depending on particulars of task demands, stimuli, etc.), and that the same task will require the engagement of somewhat different convergence zones across comparable individuals. Overall, then, the large-scale neuroanatomical sector in which certain convergence zones will be engaged by a task should be quite comparable, under similar experimental circumstances, but the micro-scale neuroanatomical sector may not be. The process of anatomical selection of convergence zones—both during learning and during subsequent operation—is probability-driven, flexible, and individualised. Thus, it should not be expected that nearly equal lesions will be associated with precisely the same neuropsychological defects; and likewise, it should not be expected that in functional imaging experiments, the same tasks activate or deactivate sites with precisely the same coordinates. At the macro-scale, though, the spatial placement of convergence zones is expected to be comparable across individuals.

## REFERENCES


Adolphs, R., Damasio, H., Tranel, D., Cooper, G., & Damasio, A. R. (2000). A role for somatosensory cortices in the visual recognition of emotion as revealed by three-dimensional lesion mapping. *Journal of Neuroscience, 20*, 2683–2690.

Andersen, R. (1995). Encoding of intention and spatial location in the posterior parietal cortex. *Cerebral Cortex, 5*, 457–469.

Arguin, M., Bub, D., & Dudek, G. (1996). Shape integration for visual object recognition and its implication in category-specific visual agnosia. *Visual Cognition, 3*, 221–275.

Barsalou, L. W. (1999). Perceptual symbol systems. *Behavioral and Brain Sciences, 22*, 577–609.

Beauchamp, M. S., Lee, K. E., Haxby, J. V., & Martin, A. (2002). Parallel visual motion processing streams for manipulable objects and human movements. *Neuron, 34*, 149–159.

Behrmann, M., & Moscovitch, M. (2001). Face recognition: Evidence from intact and impaired performance. In F. Boller & J. Grafman (Eds.), *Handbook of neuropsychology, Vol. 4* (2nd ed., pp. 181–205). Amsterdam: Elsevier Science.

Berndt, R. S., Mitchum, C. C., Haendiges, A. N., & Sandson, J. (1997). Verb retrieval in aphasia. I. Characterizing single word impairments. *Brain and Language, 56*, 68–106.

Binkofski, F., Buccino, G., Posse, S., Seitz, R. J., Rizzolatti, G., & Freund, H.-J. (1999a). A fronto-parietal circuit for object manipulation in man: evidence from an fMRI-study. *European Journal of Neuroscience, 11*, 3276–3286.

Binkofski, F., Buccino, G., Stephan, K. M., Rizzolatti, G., Seitz, R. J., & Freund, H.-J. (1999b). A parieto-premotor network for object manipulation: Evidence from neuroimaging. *Experimental Brain Research, 128*, 210–213.

Binkofski, F., Dohle, C., Posse, S., Stephan, K. M., Hefter, H., Seitz, R. J., & Freund, H.-J. (1998). Human anterior intraparietal area subserves prehension: A combined lesion and functional MRI activation study. *Neurology, 50*, 1253–1259.

Bonda, E., Petrides, M., Ostry, D., & Evans, A. (1996). Specific involvement of human parietal systems and the amygdala in the perception of biological motion. *Journal of Neuroscience, 16*, 3737–3744.

Bowerman, M., & Choi, S. (2001). Shaping meanings for language: Universal and language-specific in the acquisition of spatial semantic categories. In M. Bowerman & S. Levinson (Eds.), *Language acquisition and conceptual development* (pp. 475–511). Cambridge, MA: MIT Press.

Brown, P. (2001). Learning to talk about motion UP and DOWN in Tzeltal: Is there a language–specific bias for verb learning? In M. Bowerman & S. Levinson (Eds.), *Language acquisition and conceptual development* (pp. 512–543). Cambridge, MA: MIT Press.

Brown, R., & McNeill, D. (1966). The "tip of the tongue" phenomenon. *Journal of Verbal Learning and Verbal Behavior, 5*, 325–337.

Buccino, G., Binkofski, F., Fink, G. R., Fadiga, L., Fogassi, L., Gallese, V., Seitz, R. J., Zilles, K., Rizzolatti, G., & Freund, H. J. (2001). Action observation activates premotor and parietal areas in a somatotopic manner: An fMRI study. *European Journal of Neurology, 13*, 400–404.

Burke, D. M., MacKay, D. G., Worthley, J. S., & Wade, E. (1991). On the tip of the tongue: What causes word finding failures in young and older adults? *Journal of Memory and Language, 30*, 542–579.

Buxbaum, L. J., Veramonti, T., & Schwartz, M. F. (2000). Function and manipulation tool knowledge in apraxia: Knowing "what for" but not "how." *Neurocase, 6*, 83–97.

Cappa, S. F., Perani, D., Schnur, T., Tettamanti, M., & Fazio, F. (1998). The effects of semantic category and knowledge type on lexical-semantic access: a PET study. *Neuroimage, 8*, 350–359.

Caramazza, A. (1998). The interpretation of semantic category-specific deficits: What do they tell us about the organisation of conceptual knowledge in the brain? *Neurocase, 4*, 265–272.

Caramazza, A. (2000). The organization of conceptual knowledge in the brain. In M. S. Gazzaniga (Ed.), *The new cognitive neurosciences* (2nd ed., pp. 1037–1046). Cambridge, MA: The MIT Press.

Carammaza, A., & Hillis, A. (1991). Lexical organization of nouns and verbs in the brain. *Nature, 349*, 788–790.

Caramazza, A., & Shelton, J. R. (1998). Domain-specific knowledge systems in the brain: The animate-inanimate distinction. *Journal of Cognitive Neuroscience, 10*, 1–34.

Chainay, H., & Humphreys, G. W. (2002). Neuropsychological evidence for a convergent route model for action. *Cognitive Neuropsychology, 19*, 67–93.

Chao, L. L., Haxby, J. V., & Martin, A. (1999). Attribute-based neural substrates in temporal cortex for perceiving and knowing about objects. *Nature Neuroscience, 2*, 913–919.

Chao, L. L., & Martin, A. (2000). Representation of manipulable man-made objects in the dorsal stream. *NeuroImage, 12*, 478–484.

Chatterjee, A. (2001). Language and space: Some interactions. *Trends in Cognitive Sciences, 5*, 55–61.

Chatterjee, A., Southwood, M.H., & Basilico, D. (1999). Verbs, events and spatial representations. *Neuropsychologia, 37*, 395–402.

Critchley, M. (1953). *The parietal lobes*. London: Edward Arnold.

Damasio, A. R. (1989). Time–locked multiregional retroactivation: A systems-level proposal for the neural substrates of recall and recognition. *Cognition, 33*, 25–62.

Damasio, A. R., & Damasio, H. (1994). Cortical systems for retrieval of concrete knowledge: The convergence zone framework. In C. Koch (Ed.), *Large-scale neuronal theories of the brain* (pp. 61–74). Cambridge, MA: MIT Press.

Damasio, A. R., Damasio, H., Tranel, D., & Brandt, J. P. (1990). The neural regionalization of knowledge access: Preliminary evidence. *Quantitative Biology, 55*, 1039–1047.

Damasio, H. (2000). The lesion method in cognitive neuroscience. In F. Boller & J. Grafman (Eds.), *Handbook of neuropsychology, Vol. 1* (2nd ed., pp. 77–102). New York: Elsevier.

Damasio, H., & Frank, R. (1992). Three-dimensional in vivo mapping of brain lesions in humans. *Archives of Neurology, 49*, 137–143.

Damasio, H., Grabowski, T. J., Tranel, D., Hichwa, R., & Damasio, A. R. (1996). A neural basis for lexical retrieval. *Nature, 380*, 499–505.

Damasio, H., Grabowski, T. J., Tranel, D., Ponto, L. L. B., Hichwa, R. D., & Damasio, A. R. (2001). Neural correlates of naming actions and of naming spatial relations. *NeuroImage, 13*, 1053–1064.

Damasio, H., Tranel, D., Grabowski, T. J., Adolphs, R., & Damasio, A. R. (in press). Neural systems behind word and concept retrieval. *Cognition.*

David, A. S., & Senior, C. (2000). Implicit motion and the brain. *Trends in Cognitive Sciences, 4*, 293–295.

Decety, J., Grézes, J., Costes, N., Perani, D., Jeannerod, M., Procyk, E., Grassi, F., & Fazio, F. (1997). Brain activity during observation of actions. Influence of action content and subject's strategy. *Brain, 120*, 1763–1777.

Decety, J., Perani, D., Jeannerod, M., Bettinardi, V., Tadary, B., Woods, R., Mazziotta, J. C., & Fazio, F. (1994). Mapping motor representations with positron emission tomography. *Nature, 371*, 600–602.

Delay, J.-P. L. (1935). *Les astéréognosies: Pathologie du toucher*. Paris: Masson.

De Leon, L. (2001). Finding the richest path: Language and cognition in the acquisition of verticality in Tzotzil (Mayan). In M. Bowerman & S. Levinson (Eds.), *Language acquisition and conceptual development* (pp. 544–565). Cambridge, MA: MIT Press.

De Renzi, E. (1989). Apraxia. In F. Boller & J. Grafman (Eds.), *Handbook of neuropsychology, Vol. 2* (pp. 245–263). New York: Elsevier.

Di Pellegrino, G., Fadiga, L., Fogassi, L., Gallese, V., & Rizzolatti, G. (1992). Understanding motor events: A neurophysiological study. *Experimental Brain , 91*, 176–180.

Dumoulin, S. O., Bittar, R. G., Kabani, N. J., Baker, C. L., Le Goualher, G., Pike, G. B., & Evans, A. C. (2000). A new anatomical landmark for reliable identification of human area V5/MT: A quantitative analysis of sulcal patterning. *Cerebral Cortex, 10*, 454–463.

Fadiga, L., Fogassi, L., Gallese, V., & Rizzolatti, G. (2000). Visuomotor neurons: Ambiguity of the discharge or "motor" perception? *International Journal of Psychophysiology, 35*, 165–177.

Farne, A., & Ladavas, E. (2000). Dynamic size-change of hand peripersonal space following tool use. *NeuroReport, 11*, 1645–1649.

Fiez, J. A., Raichle, M. E., Balota, D. A., Tallal, P., & Petersen, S. (1996). PET activation of posterior temporal regions during auditory word presentation and verb generation. *Cerebral Cortex, 6*, 1–10.

Fiez, J. A., & Tranel, D. (1997). Standardized stimuli and procedures for investigating the retrieval of lexical and conceptual knowledge for actions. *Memory and Cognition, 25*, 543–569.

Forde, E. M. E., & Humphreys, G. W. (1999). Category-specific recognition impairments: A review of important case studies and influential theories. *Aphasiology, 13*, 169–193.

Frank, R. J., Damasio, H., & Grabowski, T. J. (1997). Brainvox: An interactive, multimodal, visualization and analysis system for neuroanatomical imaging. *NeuroImage, 5*, 13–30.

Friston, K. J., Price, C. J., Fletcher, P., Moore, C., Frackowiak, R. S. J., & Dolan, R. J. (1996). The trouble with cognitive subtraction. *NeuroImage, 4*, 97–104.

Gainotti, G., & Silveri, M. C. (1996). Cognitive and anatomical locus of lesion in a patient with a category-specific semantic impairment for living beings. *Cognitive Neuropsychology, 13*, 357–389.

Gainotti, G., Silveri, M. C., Daniele, A., & Giustolisi, L. (1995). Neuroanatomical correlates of category–specific semantic disorders: A critical survey. *Memory, 3*, 247–264.

Gennari, S. P., Sloman, S. A., Malt, B. C., & Fitch, W. T. (2002). Motion events in language and cognition. *Cognition, 83*, 49–79.

Gerardin, E., Sirigu, A., Lehéricy, S., Poline, J.-B., Gaymard, B., Marsault, C., Agid, Y., & Le Bihan, D. (2000). Partially overlapping neural networks for real and imagined hand movements. *Cerebral Cortex, 10*, 1093–1104.

Gerlach, C., Law, I., Gade, A., & Paulson, O. B. (1999). Perceptual differentiation and category effects in normal object recognition: A PET study. *Brain, 122*, 2159–2170.

Geschwind, N. (1975). The apraxias: Neural mechanisms of disorders of learned movement. *American Scientist, 63*, 188–195.

Geschwind, N., & Damasio, A. R. (1985). Apraxia. In J. A. M. Frederiks (Ed.), *Handbook of clinical neurology* (pp. 423–432). Amsterdam: Elsevier.

Goodale, M. A., & Humphrey, G. K. (1998). The objects of action and perception. *Cognition, 67*, 181–207.

Goodglass, H., & Wingfield, A. (1997). Word-finding deficits in aphasia: Brain–behavior relations and clinical symptomatology. In H. Goodglass & A. Wingfield (Eds.), *Anomia: Neuroanatomical and cognitive correlates* (pp. 3–27). New York: Academic Press.

Grabowski, T. J., Damasio, H., & Damasio, A. R. (1998). Premotor and prefrontal correlates of category-related lexical retrieval. *NeuroImage, 7*, 232–243.

Grafton, S. T., Arbib, M. A., Fadiga, L., & Rizzolatti, G. (1996). Localization of grasp representations in humans by PET: 2. Observation compared with imagination. *Experimental Brain Research, 112*, 103–111.

Grafton, S. T., Fadiga, L., Arbib, M. A., & Rizzolatti, G. (1997). Premotor cortex activation during observation and naming of familiar tools. *Neuroimage, 6*, 231–236.

Graziano, M. S. A., Cooke, D. F., & Taylor, C. S. R. (2000). Coding the location of the arm by sight. *Science, 290*, 1782–1786.

Grézes, J., & Decety, J. (2001). Functional anatomy of execution, mental simulation, observation, and verb generation of actions: A meta-analysis. *Human Brain Mapping, 12*, 1–19.

Hart, J., & Gordon, B. (1992). Neural subsystems for object knowledge. *Nature, 359*, 60–64.

Heilman, K. M., & Rothi, L. J. (1993). Apraxia. In K. M. Heilman & E. Valenstein (Eds.), *Clinical neuropsychology* (3rd ed., pp. 141–163). New York: Oxford University Press.

Hillis, A. E., & Caramazza, A. (1991). Category-specific naming and comprehension impairment: A double dissociation. *Brain, 114*, 2081-2094.

Howard, D., & Patterson, K. (1992). *Pyramids and Palm Trees: A test of semantic access from pictures and words.* Bury St. Edmunds, UK: Thames Valley Test Company.

Humphreys, G. W., & Forde, E. M. E. (1998). Disordered action schema and action disorganisation syndrome. *Cognitive Neuropsychology, 15*, 771–811.

Humphreys, G. W., & Forde, E. M. E. (2001). Hierarchies, similarity, and interactivity in object recognition: "Category-specific" neuropsychological deficits. *Behavioural Brain Sciences, 24*, 453–509.

Iacoboni, M., Woods, R. P., Brass, M., Bekkering, H., Mazziotta, J. C., & Rizzolatti, G. (1999). Cortical mechanisms of human imitation. *Science, 286*, 2526–2528.

Indefrey, P., & Levelt, W. J. M. (2000). The neural correlates of language production. In M. S. Gazzaniga (Ed.), *The new cognitive neurosciences* (2nd ed., pp. 845–865). Cambridge, MA: The MIT Press.

Jackendoff, R. (1990). *Semantic structures.* Boston: MIT Press.

Jeannerod, M. (1994). The representing brain: Neural correlates of motor intention and imagery. *Behavioral Brain Sciences, 17*, 187–245.

Jeannerod, M. (1997). *The cognitive neuroscience of action.* Cambridge, MA: Blackwell.

Jeannerod, M., Arbib, M. A., Rizzolatti, G., & Sakata, H. (1995). Grasping objects: The cortical mechanisms of visuomotor transformation. *Trends in Neurosciences, 18*, 314–320.

Kable, J. W., Lease-Spellmeyer, J., & Chatterjee, A. (2002). Neural substrates of action event knowledge. *Journal of Cognitive Neuroscience, 14*, 795–805.

Kanwisher, N., & Moscovitch, M. (2000). The cognitive neuroscience of face processing: An introduction. *Cognitive Neuropsychology, 17*, 112.

Katz, D. (1925). Der Aufbau der Tastwelt. *Zeitschrift Psychol Physio Sinnesorg, 2*, 1–270.

Kemmerer, D. (2000). Grammatically relevant and grammatically irrelevant features of verb meaning can be independently impaired. *Aphasiology, 14*, 997–1020.

Kemmerer, D., & Tranel, D. (2000a). Verb retrieval in brain-damaged subjects: I. Analysis of stimulus, lexical, and conceptual factors. *Brain and Language, 73*, 347–392.

Kemmerer, D., & Tranel, D. (2000b). Verb retrieval in brain-damaged subjects: II. Analysis of errors. *Brain and Language, 73*, 393–420.

Kemmerer, D., Tranel, D., & Barrash, J. (2001). Patterns of dissociation in the processing of verb meanings in brain-damaged subjects. *Language and Cognitive Processes, 16*, 1–34.

Kemmerer, D., & Wright, S. K. (2002). Selective impairment of knowledge underlying *un-* prefixation: Further evidence for the autonomy of grammatical semantics. *Journal of Neurolinguistics, 15*, 403–432.

Kirshner, H.S. (1991). The apraxias. In W. G. Bradley, R. B. Daroff, G. M. Fenichel, & C. D. Marsden (Eds.), *Neurology in clinical practice, Vol. 1* (pp. 117–122). Boston: Butterworth-Heinemann.

Klatzky, R. L., Pellegrino, J. W., McCloskey, B. P., & Doherty, S. (1989). Can you squeeze a tomato? The role of motor representations in semantic sensibility judgments. *Journal of Memory and Language, 28*, 56–77.

Klatzky, R. L., Pellegrino, J., McCloskey, B. P., & Lederman, S. (1993). Cognitive representations of functional interactions with objects. *Memory and Cognition, 21*, 294–303.

Kourtzi, Z., & Kanwisher, N. (2000). Activation in human MT/MST by static images with implied motion. *Journal of Cognitive Neuroscience, 12*, 48–55.

Laiacona, M., Barbarotto, R., & Capitani, E. (1993). Perceptual and associative knowledge in category specific impairment of semantic memory: A study of two cases. *Cortex, 29*, 727–740.

Leiguarda, R. C., & Marsden, C. D. (2000). Limb apraxias: Higher-order disorders of sensorimotor integration. *Brain*, *123*, 860–879.

Levelt, W. J. M., Roelofs, A., & Meyer, A. S. (1999). A theory of lexical access in speech production. *Behavioural and Brain Sciences*, *22*, 1-75.

Levinson, S. C. (1997). From outer space to inner space: Linguistic categories and nonlinguistic thinking. In J. Nuyts & E. Pederson (Eds.), *Language and conceptualization* (pp. 13–45). Cambridge: Cambridge University Press.

Liepmann, H. (1920). *Apraxie: Brusch's Ergebnisse der Gesamten Medizin* (pp. 518–543). Berlin: Urban & Schwarzenberg.

Lotze, M., Montoya, P., Erb, M., Hulsmann, E., Flor, H., Klose, U., Birbaumer, N., & Grodd, W. (1999). Activation of cortical and cerebellar motor areas during executed and imagined hand movements: An fMRI study. *Journal of Cognitive Neuroscience*, *11*, 491–501.

Maril, A., Wagner, A. D., & Schacter, D. L. (2001). On the tip of the tongue: An event-related fMRI study of semantic retrieval failure and cognitive conflict. *Neuron*, *31*, 653–660.

Martin, A., Haxby, J. V., Lalonde, F. M., Wiggs, C. L., & Ungerleider, L. G. (1995). Discrete cortical regions associated with knowledge of color and knowledge of action. *Science*, *270*, 102–105.

Martin, A., Ungerleider, L. G., & Haxby, J. V. (2000). Category specificity and the brain: The sensory/motor model of semantic representations of objects. In M. S. Gazzaniga (Ed.), *The new cognitive neurosciences* (2nd ed., pp. 1023–1036). Cambridge, MA: The MIT Press.

Martin, A., Wiggs, C. L., Ungerleider, L. G., & Haxby, J. V. (1996). Neural correlates of category-specific knowledge. *Nature*, *379*, 649–652.

Moll, J., De Oliveira-Souza, R., Passman, L. J., Cunha, F. C., Souza-Lima, F., & Andreiuolo, P. A. (2000). Functional MRI correlates of real and imagined tool–use pantomimes. *Neurology*, *54*, 1331–1336.

Nelson, K. (1986). *Event knowledge*. Hillsdale, NJ: Lawrence Erlbaum Associates Inc.

Nelson, K. (1996). *Language in cognitive development*. Cambridge: Cambridge University Press.

Ochipa, C., Rothi, L. J. G., & Heilman, K. M. (1992). Conceptual apraxia in Alzheimer's disease. *Brain*, *115*, 1061–1071.

Perani, D., Cappa, S. F., Bettinardi, V., Bressi, S., Gorno-Tempini, M., Matarrese, M., & Fazio, F. (1995). Different neural systems for the recognition of animals and man-made tools. *NeuroReport*, *6*, 1637–1641.

Perani, D., Schnur, T., Tettamanti, M., Gorno-Tempini, M., Cappa, S. F., & Fazio, F. (1999). Word and picture matching: A PET study of semantic category effects. *Neuropsychologia*, *37*, 293–306.

Perenin, M. T., & Vighetto, A. (1988). Optic ataxia: A specific disruption in visuomotor mechanisms. *Brain*, *111*, 643–674.

Pinker, S. (1989). *Learnability and cognition: The acquisition of argument structure*. Cambridge, MA: MIT Press.

Pisella, L., Grea, H., Tilikete, C., Vighetto, A., Desmurget, M., Rode, G., Boisson, D., & Rossetti, Y. (2000). An "automatic pilot" for the hand in human posterior parietal cortex: Toward reinterpreting optic ataxia. *Nature Neuroscience*, *3*, 729-736.

Pulvermüller, F. (1999). Words in the brain's language. *Behavioral and Brain Sciences*, *22*, 253–336.

Rizzolatti, G., & Fadiga, L. (1998). Grasping objects and grasping meanings: The dual role of monkey rostroventral premotor cortex (area F5). *Novart FDN Symposium*, *218*, 81–103.

Rothi, L. J. G., Raade, A. S., & Heilman, K. M. (1994). Localization of lesions in limb and buccofacial apraxia. In A. Kertesz (Ed.), *Localization and neuroimaging in neuropsychology* (pp. 407–427). New York: Academic Press.

Saffran, E. M., & Schwartz, M. F. (1994). Of cabbages and things: Semantic memory from a neuropsychological perspective—A tutorial review. *Attention and Performance*, *15*, 507–536.

Saffran, E. M., & Sholl, A. (1999). Clues to the functional and neural architecture of word meaning. In C. M. Brown & P. Hagoort (Eds.), *The neurocognition of language* (pp. 241–272). New York: Oxford University Press.

Sakata, H., Taira, M., Murata, A., & Mine, S. (1995). Neural mechanisms of visual guidance of hand action in the parietal cortex of the monkey. *Cerebral Cortex*, *5*, 429–438.

Sartori, G., Job, R., Miozzo, M., Zago, S., & Marchiori, G. (1993). Category-specific form-knowledge deficit in a patient with herpes simplex virus encephalitis. *Journal of Clinical and Experimental Neuropsychology*, *15*, 280–299.

Schwartz, M. F., Montgomery, M. W., Fitzpatrick-DeSalme, E. J., Ochipa, C., Coslett, H. B., & Mayer,

N. H. (1995). Analysis of a disorder of everyday action. *Cognitive Neuropsychology, 12*, 863–892.

Schwartz, M. F., Reed, E. S., Montgomery, M., Palmer, C., & Mayer, N. H. (1991). The quantitative description of action disorganisation after brain damage: A case study. *Cognitive Neuropsychology, 8*, 381–414.

Schwartz, R. L., Adair, J. C., Raymer, A. M., Williamson, D. J. G., Crosson, B., Rothi, L. J. G., Nadeau, S. E., & Heilman, K. M. (2000). Conceptual apraxia in probable Alzheimer's disease as demonstrated by the Florida Action Recall Test. *Journal of the International Neuropsychological Society, 6*, 265–270.

Senior, C., Barnes, J., Giampietro, V., Simmons, A., Bullmore, E. T., Brammer, M., & Davis, A. S. (2000). The functional neuroanatomy of implicit-motion perception or "representational momentum." *Current Biology, 10*, 16–22.

Sirigu, A., Duhamel, J.-R., Cohen, L., Pillon, B., Dubois, B., & Agid, Y. (1996a). The mental representation of hand movements after parietal cortex damage. *Science, 273*, 1564–1568.

Sirigu, A., Zalla, T., Pillon, B., Dubois, B., Grafman, J., & Agid, Y. (1996b). Encoding of sequence and boundaries of script following prefrontal lesions. *Cortex, 32*, 297–310.

Slobin, D. I. (1996). From "thought and language" to "thinking for speaking." In J. J. Gumperz & S. C. Levinson (Eds.), *Rethinking linguistic relativity* (pp. 70–96). Cambridge: Cambridge University Press.

Sunderland, A., & Sluman, S.-M. (2000). Ideomotor apraxia, visuomotor control and the explicit representation of posture. *Neuropsychologia, 38*, 923–934.

Talmy, L. (2000). *Towards a cognitive semantics*. Cambridge, MA: MIT Press.

Thompson-Schill, S. L., Swick, D., Farah, M. J., D'Esposito, M., Kan, I. P., & Knight, R. T. (1998). Verb generation in patients with focal frontal lesions: A neuropsychological test of neuroimaging findings. *Proceedings of the National Academy of Sciences, 95*, 15855–15860.

Tomasello, M. (1992). *First verbs*. Cambridge: Cambridge University Press.

Tootell, R. B. H., Reppas, J. B., Kwong, K. K., Malach, R., Born, R. T., Brady, T. J., Rosen, B. R., & Belliveau, J. W. (1995). Functional analysis of human MT and related visual cortical areas using functional magnetic resonance imaging. *Journal of Neuroscience, 15*, 3215–3230.

Tranel, D. (1996). The Iowa-Benton school of neuropsychological assessment. In I. Grant & K. M. Adams (Eds.), *Neuropsychological assessment of neuropsychiatric disorders* (2nd ed., pp. 81–101). New York: Oxford University Press.

Tranel, D., Adolphs, R., Damasio, H., & Damasio, A. R. (2001). A neural basis for the retrieval of words for actions. *Cognitive Neuropsychology, 18*, 655–670.

Tranel, D., & Damasio, A. R. (1996). The agnosias and apraxias. In W. G. Bradley, R. B. Daroff, G. M. Fenichel, & C. D. Marsden (Eds.), *Neurology in clinical practice* (2nd ed., pp. 119–129). Stoneham, MA: Butterworth Publishers.

Tranel, D., & Damasio, A. R. (1999). The neurobiology of knowledge retrieval. *Behavioral and Brain Sciences, 22*, 303.

Tranel, D., Damasio, H., & Damasio, A. R. (1995). Double dissociation between overt and covert face recognition. *Journal of Cognitive Neuroscience, 7*, 425–432.

Tranel, D., Damasio, H., & Damasio, A. R. (1997a). A neural basis for the retrieval of conceptual knowledge. *Neuropsychologia, 35*, 1319–1327.

Tranel, D., Damasio, H., & Damasio, A. R. (1997b). On the neurology of naming. In H. Goodglass & A. Wingfield (Eds.), *Anomia: Neuroanatomical and cognitive correlates* (pp. 65–90). New York: Academic Press.

Tranel, D., Damasio, H., & Damasio, A. R. (1998). The neural basis of lexical retrieval. In R. W. Parks, D. S. Levine, & D. L. Long (Eds.), *Fundamentals of neural network modeling: Neuropsychology and cognitive neuroscience* (pp. 271–296). Cambridge, MA: MIT Press.

Tulving, E. (1972). Episodic and semantic memory. In E. Tulving & W. Donaldson (Eds.), *Organization of memory* (pp. 381–403). New York: Academic Press.

Van Valin, R., & LaPolla, R. (1997). *Syntax*. Cambridge, MA: Cambridge University Press.

Warburton, E., Wise, R. J. S., Price, C. J., Weiller, C., Hadar, U., Ramsay, S., & Frackowiak, R. S. J. (1996). Noun and verb retrieval by normal subjects: Studies with PET. *Brain, 119*, 159–179.

Warrington, E. K., & McCarthy, R. A. (1994). Multiple meaning systems in the brain: A case for visual semantics. *Neuropsychologia, 32*, 1465–1473.

Warrington, E. K., & Shallice, T. (1984). Category specific semantic impairments. *Brain, 107*, 829–853.

Watson, J. D. G., Myers, R., Frackowiak, R. S. J., Hajnal, J. V., Woods, R. P., Mazziota, J. C., Shipp, S., & Zeki, S. (1993). Area V5 of the human brain: Evidence from a combined study using positron emission tomography and magnetic resonance imaging. *Cerebral Cortex*, *3*, 79–94.

West, R., & Alain, C. (2000). Evidence for the transient nature of a neural system supporting goal-directed action. *Cerebral Cortex*, *10*, 748–752.

Wienold, G. (1995). Lexical and conceptual structures in expressions for movement and space: With reference to Japanese, Korean, Thai, and Indonesian as compared to English and German. In U. Egli, P. E. Pause, C. Schwartze, A. Stechow, & G. Wienold (Eds.), *Lexical knowledge in the organization of language* (pp. 301–340). Amsterdam: Benjamins.

Wise, R., Chollet, F., Hader, U., Friston, K., Hoffner, E., & Frackowiak, R. (1991). Distribution of cortical neural networks involved in word comprehension and word retrieval. *Brain*, *114*, 1803-1817.

Zanini, S., Rumiati, R. I., & Shallice, T. (2002). Action sequencing deficit following frontal lobe lesion. *Neurocase*, *8*, 88–99.

Zeki, S., Watson, J. D. G., Lueck, C. J., Friston, K. J., Kennard, C., & Frackowiak, R. S. J. (1991). A direct demonstration of functional specialisation in human visual cortex. *Journal of Neuroscience*, *11*, 641–649.

COGNITIVE NEUROPSYCHOLOGY, 2003, 20 (3/4/5/6), 433–450

# CONSTRAINING QUESTIONS ABOUT THE ORGANISATION AND REPRESENTATION OF CONCEPTUAL KNOWLEDGE

**Bradford Z. Mahon and Alfonso Caramazza**
*Harvard University, Cambridge, USA*

In this article we assume a domain-specific organisation of conceptual knowledge and consider two questions: How does this architecture constrain further assumptions that might be made regarding (1) the organisation of conceptual knowledge in the brain, and (2) the representation of conceptual knowledge in the brain? Data from category-specific semantic deficits, functional neuroimaging, and apraxia are recruited in attempt to clarify these questions. It is shown that the domain-specific hypothesis can account for the extant facts. Furthermore, we outline one possible theoretical framework that imposes empirical constraints on proposals that might be advanced in response to the two questions raised above.

## INTRODUCTION

The patterns of differential impairment/sparing of cognitive function subsequent to brain damage can provide strong constraints on theories of the organisation and representation of cognitive systems in the brain. As the articles in this Special Issue of *Cognitive Neuropsychology* attest, the phenomenon of category-specific semantic[1] deficit is a compelling case in point. One well-iterated demonstration of the types of constraints imposed on theories of cognitive organisation is provided by recent evaluations of a widely received explanation of category-specific semantic deficits: the sensory/functional theory (e.g., Warrington & McCarthy, 1983, 1987, 1994; Warrington & Shallice, 1984). This theory assumes that category-specific semantic deficits emerge as a result of damage to a type or modality of information (e.g., visual/perceptual vs. functional/associative) upon which successful recognition/naming of objects from the impaired category differentially depends (i.e., living things vs. nonliving things, respectively). However, a nearly exhaustive review of the literature on category-specific deficits (Capitani, Laiacona, Mahon, & Caramazza, 2003-this issue) establishes the *fact* that the majority of patients with such impairments *do not* present with a disproportionate deficit for a type or modality of knowledge. From this fact it can be concluded that the cause of category-specific semantic deficits cannot be damage to a type or modality of information. This conclusion

[1] In this article we use the terms "semantic" and "conceptual" interchangeably.

Requests for reprints should be addressed to Alfonso Caramazza, Department of Psychology, William James Hall, Harvard University, 33 Kirkland Street, Cambridge, MA 02138, USA (Email: caram@wjh.harvard.edu).

Preparation of this manuscript was supported in part by NIH grant DC 04542 to Alfonso Caramazza. The authors are grateful to Laurel Buxbaum and Alex Martin for their comments on an earlier version of this manuscript. We would also like to thank Lauren Moo for her insights into the functional neuroimaging data that have been reviewed.



http://www.tandf.co.uk/journals/pp/02643294.html DOI:10.1080/02643290342000014

implies the rejection of the sensory/functional theory as a viable theoretical framework with which to explain the existence of category-specific semantic deficits (see also Caramazza & Shelton, 1998).

How, then, does one account for the facts of category-specific semantic deficits? Perhaps the most straightforward proposal is that the organisation of conceptual knowledge in the brain is subject to domain-specific principles (Caramazza & Shelton, 1998). In this article, we assume a domain-specific organisation of conceptual knowledge, and ask two questions: If we assume a domain-specific architecture, (1) what constraints are placed on further theoretical assumptions that might be made regarding the organisation of conceptual knowledge in the brain, and (2) what constraints are placed on assumptions about how conceptual knowledge is represented? Relevant neuropsychological and functional neuroimaging data, as well as alternative theoretical proposals, are recruited in an attempt to clarify these two questions.

## Clues from category-specific semantic deficits

The central assumption of the domain-specific hypothesis (Caramazza & Shelton, 1998) is that evolutionary pressures have resulted in specialised (and functionally dissociable) neural circuits dedicated to processing, perceptually and conceptually, different categories of objects. In this way, the domain-specific hypothesis provides a principled way of specifying what constitutes a conceptual category in the brain, since it is restricted to only those categories for which rapid and efficient identification could have had survival and reproductive advantages. Plausible candidates are the categories "animals," "plant life," "conspecifics," and possibly "tools."[2] The plausibility of the domain-specific hypothesis is established by the fact that the grain of category-specific deficits is as fine as the above-mentioned evolutionarily salient object domains (see, e.g., Crutch & Warrington, 2003-this issue; Samson & Pillon, 2003-this issue; for review see Capitani et al., 2003-this issue).

The domain-specific hypothesis generates several predictions: First, at a functional level, the prediction is made that there will not be a necessary association between a deficit for a type or modality of knowledge and a conceptual deficit for a specific category of objects. This prediction follows from the assumption that processes/information are not *functionally* organised within object domain. In line with this prediction,[3] the majority of cases that presented with a disproportionate deficit for living things also presented with *equivalent* impairments for visual/perceptual and functional/associative knowledge. For instance, cases EA (Barbarotto, Capitani, & Laiacona, 1996; Laiacona, Capitani, & Barbarotto, 1997), EW (Caramazza & Shelton, 1998), FM (Laiacona, Barbarotto, & Capitani, 1993), Jennifer (Samson, Pillon, & De Wilde, 1998), and SB (Sheridan & Humphreys, 1992) all had disproportionate semantic deficits for living things compared to nonliving things, but *equivalent* deficits to visual/perceptual and functional/associative knowledge of living things (for review, see Capitani et al., 2003-this issue).

A second prediction made by the domain-specific hypothesis is that there should be relatively poor recovery of lost function for impaired categories. This prediction receives striking support from a recent case study (Farah & Rabinowitz, 2003-this issue) of a patient, Adam, who suffered a bilateral posterior cerebral artery infarction at age 1 day. When tested at age 16 years, Adam was disproportionately impaired at naming pictures of living

[2] For discussion of the domain-specific hypothesis in developmental psychology and comparative work with nonhuman primates, see, e.g., Carey (2000); Carey and Markman (1999); Keil (1989); Santos and Caramazza (2002); Santos, Hauser, and Spelke (2002).

[3] Early reports seemed contrary to this prediction: Patients were reported with deficits for living things who were also disproportionately impaired for the visual attributes of objects compared to functional/associative attributes (Basso, Capitani, & Laiacona, 1988; Farah, Hammond, Mehta, & Ratcliff, 1989; Silveri & Gainotti, 1988). However, these studies have been criticised methodologically on the grounds that the tasks accessing visual and functional/associative knowledge were not matched for difficulty (see Caramazza & Shelton, 1998).

things (40% correct) compared to nonliving things (75% correct). Furthermore, Adam's deficit for living things affected all types of semantic information investigated: The patient was at chance for both visual/perceptual and functional/associative knowledge for living things (visual/perceptual = 40%; functional/associative = 45% correct), while performance was within the normal range for both types of knowledge for nonliving things (visual/perceptual = 78%, normal range = 70–90%; functional/associative = 72%, normal range = 73–92%).

A third prediction made by the domain-specific hypothesis follows from the assumption that relatively early (i.e., pre-semantic or perceptual) stages of object processing will be organised by domain. With respect to the visual modality, this hypothesis generates the prediction that the structural description system will be functionally organised by object domain. Perhaps the strongest evidence consistent with this prediction is provided by the performance of patient Michelangelo (Sartori, Coltheart, Miozzo, & Job, 1994; Sartori & Job, 1988; Sartori, Miozzo, & Job, 1993b). Michelangelo was disproportionately impaired for the category "living things" and was also disproportionately impaired on an object decision task for living things compared to nonliving things (see also, for example, patient EW, Caramazza & Shelton, 1998; Capitani et al., 2003-this issue, Table 3).

Another aspect of Michelangelo's profile of category-specific deficit for living things is that he was disproportionately impaired for visual/perceptual knowledge of living things compared to functional/associative knowledge (see also patient Giulietta: Sartori, Job, Miozzo, Zago, & Marchiori, 1993a). If we take these data to be a fact of category-specific deficits (but see Capitani et al., 2003-this issue), these data could suggest that object domain is not the only constraint on the organisation of conceptual knowledge in the brain. Specifically, one possibility would be to adopt the domain-specific hypothesis (in order to account for the data from category-specific semantic deficits) but *not* dispose of the modality-specific assumption.

To be clear: It is an established fact that the majority of patients who have presented with category-specific semantic deficits have not presented with a disproportionate impairment to a modality or type of knowledge. The conclusion that follows from this fact is that it cannot be assumed that the *cause* of category-specific semantic deficits is damage to a type (i.e., modality) of knowledge upon which successful recognition/naming differentially depends. However, this conclusion is silent with respect to the possibility that one organising constraint on the physical distribution of conceptual knowledge in the brain is modality or type of information. The conjunction of the domain-specific hypothesis with the modality-specific assumption would imply that, within for instance the visual modality, information would be organised by object domain.

The assumption that conceptual knowledge corresponding to visual/perceptual properties of objects is stored in a different area of the brain from knowledge about the functional/associative properties of objects must be distinguished from the claim that there are modality-specific semantic subsystems specialised for processing a specific type of information. In the context of the domain-specific hypothesis, there are two reasons why it would not be theoretically coherent to refer to the "system" that stores information about the visual properties of objects as a "modality-specific semantic subsystem." First, information internal to such a "system" would be functionally organised (and thus functionally dissociable) by object domain. Second, information across these "modality-specific semantic subsystems" would be functionally unitary within any given object domain. In other words, we would no longer have functionally defined modality-specific semantic subsystems, but rather neuroanatomically defined modality-specific semantic subsystems. In order to avoid confusion, we will refer to the "systems" that represent/process conceptual knowledge of a given type (e.g., visual/perceptual vs. functional/associative) as modality-specific semantic *stores* (for further discussion of these issues, see Caramazza, Hillis, Rapp, & Romani, 1990; and Mahon & Caramazza, in press).

Modality-specific semantic stores must be further distinguished from modality-specific input/output representations. For instance, with respect to visual knowledge, we will adopt as a working assumption a distinction between the modality-specific semantic store that represents/processes conceptual knowledge about the visual properties of objects and the structural description system. Representations contained in the structural description system are pre-semantic, and thus provide one route for *accessing* information contained in the visual modality-specific semantic store. Assuming the validity of this distinction for discussion amounts to a strong (and by no means uncontroversial) claim about the independence of conceptual knowledge from modality-specific input/output representations. We will return to an evaluation of this distinction in our Conclusion in light of the empirical evidence to be discussed below.

Distinguishing between modality-specific semantic stores and modality-specific input/output representations requires some specification of why information in a modality-specific semantic store is modality-specific. In other words: What is *visual* about "visual" semantic knowledge? At least three (nonmutually exclusive) possibilities could be envisioned. First, it could be argued that what makes "visual" semantic information *visual* is that it is stored in a visual *format*. Second, it could be argued that what makes this information *visual* is that it is *about* the visual properties of objects. Third, it could be that what is *visual* about "visual" knowledge is that it was *learned* or *acquired* through the visual modality. These are questions for future research (see Caramazza et al., 1990, for extended discussion). Our present interest is not in arguing *for* the architecture just described, but rather is of the form: *If* we were to assume such an organisation, then what further expectations might we have regarding the neuroanatomical organisation and representation of conceptual knowledge?

In the next section, we approach the question of whether conceptual knowledge is organised by object domain within the visual modality from the perspective of functional neuroimaging.

## Clues from functional neuroimaging

If we assume that conceptual knowledge is organised by domain-specific constraints within neuroanatomically defined modalities, then the strongest prediction that can be made is that there will be spatial segregation of processes/information by semantic category *within* modality. We limit our discussion to functional neuroimaging studies that have investigated category-specific patterns of activation in inferior and lateral temporal areas, as these neural areas correspond to (at least part of) the "visual modality."

A number of investigators have observed differential activation in the ventral object processing stream for different categories of objects. For instance, Chao, Haxby, and Martin (1999a) reported activation in the medial aspect of the fusiform gyri bilaterally across viewing, naming, and matching tasks involving pictures of "tools," as well as for a task in which subjects were reading the names of "tool" stimuli. In the same study, activation was reported in the lateral aspect of the fusiform gyri for the same tasks conducted over "animal" stimuli. A similar pattern of results has been found when contrasting the activation produced by "face" stimuli and "house" stimuli: Compared to houses, faces activated more lateral regions of the fusiform gyrus (e.g., Haxby, Ungerleider, Clark, Schouten, Hoffman, & Martin, 1999; Kanwisher, McDermott, & Chun, 1997; McCarthy, Puce, Gore, & Allison, 1997), whereas the reverse comparison (houses–faces) yielded disproportionate activation in more medial regions of the fusiform gyrus (Aguirre, Zarahn, & D'Esposito, 1998) as well as in parahippocampal cortex (Epstein & Kanwisher, 1998). To sum up, differential and spatially dissociable (although overlapping) foci of activation have been found for each of the categories "animals," "tools," "houses," and "faces" (Chao et al., 1999a; Chao, Martin, & Haxby, 1999b; see Martin & Chao, 2001).[4]

Similar patterns have been observed in lateral temporal cortex. Items corresponding to "living

[4] Not all investigators have observed category-specific effects with functional neuroimaging. For instance, Devlin et al., (2002) did not find reliable category-specific foci of activation for the categories "animals," "fruit," "tools," and "vehicles."

things" differentially activated the superior temporal sulcus (faces: Chao et al., 1999a, 1999b; Haxby et al., 1999; Hoffman & Haxby, 2000; Kanwisher et al., 1997; animals: Chao et al., 1999a, 1999b). In contrast, activation associated with identifying pictures of tools activated more inferior regions centred on the left middle temporal gyrus (e.g., Chao et al., 1999a; Martin, Wiggs, Ungerleider, & Haxby, 1996). Furthermore, lateral temporal cortex seems to be specialised for processing object-associated motion. In a recent study, Beauchamp, Lee, Haxby, and Martin (2002) found that the superior temporal sulci and gyri responded differentially to biological motion (right » left) while the middle temporal gyri and inferior temporal sulci responded differentially to tool associated-motion (left » right) (see also Senior et al., 2000, for related findings; see Beauchamp et al., 2002, for review and discussion).

Taken together, these data would seem to provide strong prima facie support for the hypothesis that conceptual knowledge is organised by object domain within inferior and lateral temporal areas. However, a reductio counterargument that has been raised against a domain-specific interpretation of these data is based on the observation (Ishai, Ungerleider, Martin, Schouten, & Haxby, 1999) that "chair" stimuli activated an area in inferior temporal cortex lateral to that elicited by faces. In other words: Why would the category "chairs" elicit a discrete area of activation, since this category clearly does not constitute an evolutionarily significant object domain? In the context of this argument, Martin and Chao (2001, p. 196) propose that these data are consistent with the notion that conceptual representations are distributed over features: "A feature-based model can accommodate the observation that an arbitrary category such as chairs elicited a pattern of neural activity distinct from other object categories (i.e., faces and houses). Clearly, it would be difficult, as well as unwise, to argue that there is a 'chair area' in the brain." The premise upon which this argument is based is that a feature-based model *could* accommodate the results reported by Ishai and colleagues (1999). But wouldn't a feature-based model face the same dilemma that the domain-specific hypothesis purportedly faces? In other words, if conceptual knowledge is organised by the features that define objects, so that the conceptual representations of objects that share features are stored in adjacent neural areas, then why would "chair" stimuli activate an area next to an area that has previously shown disproportionate activation for "animal" stimuli? What features are shared between the conceptual representations of exemplars from the categories "chairs" and "animals?" Is the claim that animals and chairs share the feature "legs?" Would this still be the claim if the word referring to the feature [+LEG$_{[animal]}$] was not homonymous with the feature [+LEG$_{[chair]}$]? What about the feature [+ARM$_{[human]}$] and [+ARM$_{[chair]}$]: Are these the same feature too because the word referring to each is the same?

Data from a recent functional neuroimaging study (Martin & Weisberg, 2003) lends some support to the argument that the patterns of differential activation by object category in inferior and lateral temporal areas are driven by domain-specific processes, and not object-specific features. The authors compared the activation produced when subjects viewed the *same physical stimuli* (e.g., coloured triangles) depicting either social or mechanical motion. When these two conditions were compared, activation associated with social motion (e.g., scaring, sharing etc.) was observed in the lateral fusiform gyrus and superior temporal sulcus, while activation associated with mechanical motion (e.g., bowling, conveyor belt, etc.) was observed in the medial aspect of the fusiform gyrus and the left middle temporal gyrus.[5] These data indicate that seemingly category-specific patterns of activation can be invoked by stimuli that must be *interpreted* (at a relatively abstract level) as pertaining to one or another semantic domain. Crucially, this level of interpretation must be more abstract than the level at which the physical properties of stimuli are represented, since the stimuli in the mechanical and social conditions were physically identical.

[5] Activation associated with social motion was also found in the amygdala and ventromedial prefrontal cortex (Martin & Weisberg, 2003-this issue; see also Castelli, Frith, Happé, & Frith, 2002; Castelli, Happé, Frith, & Frith, 2000).

## Interim summary and directions

To this point, we have been discussing issues concerning the organisation of conceptual knowledge from two perspectives: category-specific semantic deficits (for review, see Capitani et al., 2003-this issue) and the patterns of differential activation observed for stimuli from different semantic categories in functional neuroimaging (see Joseph, 2001; Martin & Chao, 2001; Price & Friston, 2002; Thompson-Schill, 2002, for recent reviews). Both methods provide evidence in line with the basic expectations that follow from the assumption that conceptual knowledge is organised by the domains of "animals," "fruit/vegetables," "conspecifics," and possibly "tools." Furthermore, the data from category-specific semantic deficits lend tentative support to the possibility that there are two orthogonal constraints on the organisation of conceptual knowledge: domain and modality. This architecture receives independent support from the functional neuroimaging data that have been reviewed. For instance, differential effects of object category have been observed in inferior temporal cortex, which is specialised for processing visual information. A domain-specific interpretation of these differential effects of semantic category in inferior temporal regions is consistent with either of two possibilities regarding the nature of the information stored in these regions. First, it could be that these data reflect the activation of modality-specific visual structural descriptions of objects (see Whatmough, Chertkow, Murtha, & Hanratty, 2002, for discussion). In this case, these data would be consistent with the view that even at relatively low (i.e., pre-semantic) levels of representation, processes/information are organised by object domain. Second, these data could reflect semantic processing of the visual properties of objects. If this were the case, these data would be consistent with the proposal that conceptual knowledge is organised by object domain within neuroanatomically defined modality-specific semantic stores.[6]

A domain-specific interpretation of category-specific patterns of activation in functional neuroimaging is by no means the received view. In fact, the received view assumes that differential effects of object category reflect the activation of object-specific features, but that these features are not explicitly organised by object domain (e.g., Bookheimer, 2002; Gerlach, Law, Gade, & Paulson, 2000; Ishai et al., 2000; Kraut, Moo, Segal, & Hart, 2002; Martin & Chao, 2001; Moore & Price, 1999; Mummery, Patterson, Hodges, & Price, 1998; Perani et al., 1995; Thompson-Schill, 2002; but see, e.g., Kanwisher, 2000). The primary empirical motivation for this proposal is the observation that the same brain regions are activated by objects from different categories (e.g., Martin & Chao, 2001). For instance, in inferior temporal cortex, the areas of activation observed for animals, tools, houses, and faces were differential and not selective.[7]

There may be methodological limitations regarding this inference: Many functional neuroimaging studies first identify regions of interest (ROIs) that are activated by objects from all of the categories being investigated. For instance, Chao et al. (1999a) first identified "... brain regions that responded to visually presented objects ..." (p. 918) and then looked within those areas for differential effects of object category, in this case "animals" vs. "tools" and "houses" vs. "faces." This methodological approach is biased against the possibility of observing patterns of activation that are "selective," and it is perhaps, then, not surprising that there is substantial overlap between the

[6] It is a separate question as two *why* inferior temporal areas are activated: Are they activated by object-specific properties or is activation in these regions driven (in part) by higher-level processes organised by domain-specific constraints (e.g., see above discussion of Martin & Weisberg, 2003-this issue)?

[7] The assumption that conceptual knowledge is represented as features or conceptual primitives is not in itself contrary to the domain-specific hypothesis: This hypothesis is aimed at articulating the organization of information at the level of domain, and is thus silent with respect to whether or not concepts are assumed to decompose into conceptual primitives or features (for further discussion, see Mahon & Caramazza, in press).

activation produced by objects from different categories. For discussion we will set this methodological concern aside (for further discussion, see Joseph, 2001).

The most articulated version of the proposal that conceptual knowledge is represented in the brain in terms of the features that define objects is the sensory/motor theory of Martin, Chao, and colleagues (e.g., Martin & Chao, 2001; Martin, Ungerleider, & Haxby, 2000). There are two important differences between the sensory/motor theory and the sensory/functional theory. First, whereas the sensory/functional theory assumes that conceptual knowledge and *modality-specific representations* are functionally and physically dissociable, the sensory/motor theory assumes that *conceptual knowledge is distributed over* modality-specific representations. The second way in which the two theories diverge is that, whereas the sensory/functional theory assumes that functional/associative information is crucial for recognising/naming tools, the sensory/motor theory assumes that information about how tools are physically manipulated is required in order recognise/name tools. We can thus evaluate our working assumption that a distinction is required between conceptual information and modality-specific input/output representations by considering whether or not the sensory/motor theory can account for the extant facts. Specifically, we can evaluate the assumption that conceptual knowledge is distributed over modality-specific representations by asking whether this is a plausible assumption for the category "tools." In the next section we briefly outline the functional neuroimaging data that have been marshalled in support of the sensory/motor theory. Empirical predictions are generated from the assumption that conceptual knowledge of tools is distributed over modality-specific representations and these predictions are evaluated with neuropsychological data. We argue that the sensory/motor theory is not tenable in light of the reviewed data. We conclude by considering the implications of the data reviewed in this article for the two questions with which we began.

## The sensory/motor theory

### *Over what is conceptual knowledge of tools distributed?*

The distinguishing assumption of the sensory/motor theory is that conceptual knowledge of manipulable artifacts and information about the correct motor movements associated with their use are distributed over the same features.[8] For instance, Martin et al. (2000; p. 1028) write: "...[T]he position proposed here is that the information about object function *needed* to support tool recognition and naming is information about the patterns of visual motion and patterns of motor movements associated with the actual use of the object [emphasis added]." If information regarding the correct use of a tool, or the visual motions associated with its use, is *needed* to identify the object, then how is such information accessed? None of this information is transparent in the visual presentation of the object. In other words, a plausible processing story is required of how the information about object use *specific* to the object being recognised is accessed, *given that the object has not yet been recognised.* One possibility is that there are systematic mappings from the structural description system to information encoding the ways in which objects are manipulated (for proposals in line with this, but which also assume a unitary-amodal semantic system, see Caramazza et al., 1990; Plaut, 2002; Riddoch, Humphreys, Coltheart, & Funnell, 1988).

The sensory/motor theory has been motivated by two well-established results in the functional neuroimaging literature: It has been found that (for instance, naming) tasks performed over tool stimuli (compared to animal stimuli) differentially activated (1) the left middle temporal gyrus (e.g.,

[8] Note the similarity between the sensory/motor theory of object recognition and the motor theory of speech perception (e.g., Liberman, Cooper, Shankweiler, & Studdert-Kennedy, 1967): Both theories assume that information required for production (i.e., motor engrams for using tools or producing speech sounds) must be retrieved in the course of successful recognition (of tools or speech sounds, respectively).

Chao et al., 1999a; Martin et al., 1996; Moore & Price, 1999; Mummery et al., 1998; Perani, Schnur, Tettamanti, Gorno-Tempini, Cappa, & Fazio, 1999), and (2) left premotor cortex (e.g., Chao & Martin, 2000; Chao, Weisberg, & Martin, 2002; Grabowski, Damasio, & Damasio, 1998; Martin et al., 1996). Relevant to these findings is the observation that the area activated in the left middle temporal gyrus is at most 8 mm away from an area assumed to store information about object movement (e.g., Corbetta, Miezin, Dobmeyer, Shulman, & Petersen, 1990; see also Beauchamp et al., 2002). Likewise, Martin and colleagues interpret the differential activation observed in left premotor cortex in the context of the observation that this area is activated when subjects are asked to imagine grasping objects, but not to actually do so (Decety et al., 1994).

Because the sensory/motor theory assumes that conceptual knowledge is distributed over modality-specific representations, this proposal is a species of a broader theoretical view which holds that conceptual knowledge does not constitute (physically) distinct information from modality-specific input/output representations.[9] The question is: Does the sensory/motor theory make empirically tractable predictions?

In order to generate empirical predictions from the sensory/motor theory we will interpret this theory in its strongest form. The reason for this is straightforward: It is not clear in what ways the theory might be "weakened" while remaining empirically distinguishable from other theoretical alternatives. For instance, a weaker version of the theory might propose to combine a unitary-amodal account of semantic memory with the assumption that different types of knowledge are differentially important for different categories of objects and/or tasks. This was the route taken by Plaut (2002). The author presented a model of optic aphasia in which a central semantic store received input from two modalities, vision and touch, and made two types of output projections: action naming and object naming. This architecture was implemented in a distributed connectionist model, in which there was a topographic learning bias favouring short connections between semantic representations and modality-specific representations. When focal areas of semantic space were lesioned, the model demonstrated what Plaut referred to as a *graded degree of modality-specific functional specialisation within semantics*. However, the theory and the implemented model are indistinguishable from an amodal account of semantic memory in which there is a privileged relationship between the semantic representations of a certain class of objects and the information contained in a certain type of modality-specific input or output representation (for discussion, see Caramazza et al., 1990).[10]

Assuming the sensory/motor theory in its strongest form, it is important to be clear about what is meant by "information about the visual motion and patterns of motor movements associated with the actual use of the object." We reason as follows: Since modality-specific input/output representations and conceptual knowledge are distributed over the *same* features, this information *must* be modality-specific. Following conventions of the literature regarding modality-specific representations encoding information about how to manipulate objects, we refer to such representations as "sensorimotor representations" (these can also be referred to as visual/kinaesthetic representations). Two straightforward empirical predictions follow from the basic assumptions of the sensory/motor theory. *Prediction 1:* A deficit for conceptual knowledge of manipulable artefacts will be associated with damage to modality-specific input/output representations (i.e., sensorimotor knowledge); and *Prediction 2:* Damage to sensorimotor representations will *necessarily* be associated with a deficit for conceptual knowledge of manipulable artefacts. Note that the structure of these predictions, and the empirical arguments to be developed below, exactly

9 For instance, Allport (1985) sums up this position as follows: "The essential idea is that the *same* neural elements that are involved in coding the sensory attributes of a (possibly unknown) object presented to eye or ear also make up the elements of the auto-associated activity patterns that represent familiar object-concepts in 'semantic memory'" (p. 53).

10 We thank Laurel Buxbaum (personal communication) for raising this issue.

parallel recent evaluations of the sensory/functional theory (e.g., see Capitani et al., 2003-this issue; Caramazza & Shelton, 1998).

*Empirical evaluation of Prediction 1*
A deficit for conceptual knowledge of manipulable artefacts will be associated with damage to modality-specific input/output representations (i.e., sensorimotor knowledge).

Consider the performance of patients FB (Sirigu, Duhamel, & Poncet, 1991) and DM (Buxbaum, Schwartz, & Carew, 1997), who could indicate the correct use associated with an object despite being impaired for semantic knowledge of manipulable objects. For example, when FB was asked to verbally provide both function information (what an object is used for) and manipulation information (how an object is used) in response to a safety pin (presented visually), he responded: "You open on one side, stick something on it, close it, and it stays in. I can tell you how it works, but I don't see its exact use. I don't think I have seen one like this before, it is not a very common object (Sirigu et al., 1991, p. 2555). It seems, from this example, that the patient has knowledge of *how* a safety pin is used, but no knowledge of what it might be *used for*.

Similarly, patient DM presented with impaired conceptual knowledge of objects but relatively intact ability to use objects. For instance, on a function matching test, the patient was asked to match two pictures out of three that are used for similar purposes (e.g., given pictures of a can opener, a hand mixer, and an electric mixer, the latter two would be the correct choice). The unrelated foil on this task was always visually similar to one of the two target items, and on many trials, all three items were associated (e.g., in the above example, all of the items are found in a kitchen). DM's performance was impaired on this task (61%; 22/36) compared to normal control subjects (94%; 34/36; range: 29–36/36). In contrast, DM's performance was flawless on a task in which real objects were presented in both the visual and tactile modalities and the patient was asked to demonstrate the correct use associated with the object. Crucially, DM's performance was also very good (91%; 10/11) at demonstrating the correct use associated with objects when they were presented only in the visual modality (and the patient was not allowed to touch them). This last result indicates that visual information alone was sufficient to support relatively unimpaired performance on a task requiring objects to be used, but the same information (provided in pictures) was not sufficient to support performance on a function matching task.

The performance of patients FB and DM indicates that (1) there is a dissociation between function knowledge (what an object is for) and manipulation knowledge (how an object is used); and (2) it is possible to observe, within the same patient, a *semantic* impairment for tools without an associated impairment in *using* tools. These data would seem to indicate that it can't be the case that conceptual knowledge of tools is distributed over the same features as knowledge of how tools are used, since these patients could access knowledge of how tools are used but were impaired at accessing conceptual knowledge about tools. However, the strength of this conclusion is mitigated by the alternative hypothesis that patients such as FB and DM are succeeding on object use tests through general mechanical problem-solving abilities and not through accessing stored representations of the correct gestures associated with objects (e.g., Goldenberg & Hagmann, 1998; Hodges, Bozeat, Lambon Ralph, Patterson, & Spatt, 2000; Hodges, Spatt, & Patterson, 1999).

In the case of FB, support for this alternative hypothesis is provided by the fact that on an object decision task, the patient accepted nonobjects that were not functionally anomalous as real objects, suggesting that the patient was not accessing stored representations but was making judgements based on the extraction of object properties. Furthermore, neither FB nor DM were tested on a novel tool use task, which is generally regarded as informative of a patient's ability to infer the function of a tool from its physical structure. Finally, it could also be noted that neither FB nor DM had lesions extending into the parietal lobes, and that parietal lobe lesions have been associated with impairments in novel tools selection tasks (Goldenberg & Hagmann, 1998).

The possibility that FB and DM are succeeding on object use tests through general mechanical problem-solving skills raises an important theoretical question: On the assumption that part of the conceptual representation of a tool includes knowledge of how to use that tool, a distinction is required between the semantic system *storing* such information and the semantic system *reading* this information from sensorimotor engrams (see, e.g., Sirigu et al., 1991; and Buxbaum, Veramonti, & Schwartz, 2000, for discussion). That is, how might we distinguish between the semantic system storing the information that a hammer is used by swinging the hand in an arc from the semantic system retrieving this information by reading a modality-specific sensorimotor engram? It is the burden of those theories for which knowledge of the ways in which objects are manipulated figures critically in the conceptual representations of those objects to give a principled account of how these two possibilities might be empirically distinguished.

*Empirical evaluation of Prediction 2*

Damage to sensorimotor representations will *necessarily* be associated with a deficit for conceptual knowledge of manipulable artefacts.

We turn now to the second, and *determining* prediction made by the sensory/motor theory: There *cannot* be patients who are impaired at using tools but can nevertheless access intact semantic information about tools and/or recognise/name tools. If there were to be a patient whose performance was contrary to this prediction, then we could conclude that it is not the case that conceptual knowledge of artefacts is distributed over the same features that constitute sensorimotor knowledge. In fact, there are a number of such patients reported in the literature (Buxbaum et al., 2000; Hodges et al., 1999; Montomura & Yamadori, 1994; Ochipa, Rothi, & Heilman, 1989; Rumiati, Zanini, Vorano, & Shallice, 2001). For instance, Ochipa and colleagues reported the performance of a patient who was relatively unimpaired at naming tools (17/20 correct) as well as pointing them out to name (19/20). However, he was severely impaired at (1) pointing to a correct tool when given its function (7/20); (2) verbally describing the function of a visually presented tool (3/20); (3) verbally identifying a tool described by its function (3/10); (4) pantomiming the use of a tool to a verbal command (0/20); and (5) demonstrating tool use when holding a tool (2/20). Crucially, the same 20 tools were used for all tasks with this patient, and yet he was able to name and identify tools but was not able to use them or identify them based on their function (see Figure 1).

The patient reported by Ochipa and colleagues (1989) was also impaired at imitating symbolic gestures (4/20); symbolic gestures are learned manual movements, such as making the "peace sign" or the "hitch-hiking fist." Based on this deficit for symbolic gestures, it might be argued that the patient had an uninteresting production deficit that did not compromise sensorimotor representations. However, the patient reported by Montomura and Yamadori (1994) was unimpaired at making symbolic gestures to command, imitating symbolic gestures, pantomiming tool use to command, and pantomiming tool use to imitation, indicating that the inability of the patient to use the same tools correctly cannot be dismissed in terms of a motor deficit. This patient was impaired at imitating and pantomiming to command "meaningless" gestures (i.e., manual gestures that do not have a conventional meaning). This pattern of performance suggests damage to a mechanism for directly converting observed hand movements to motor commands, without accessing stored representations of what those movements mean; see Rothi, Ochipa, and Heilman (1991) and Cubelli, Marchetti, Boscolo, and Della Sala (2000) for discussion.

The performance of the patient reported by Ochipa and colleagues (1989) seems to indicate

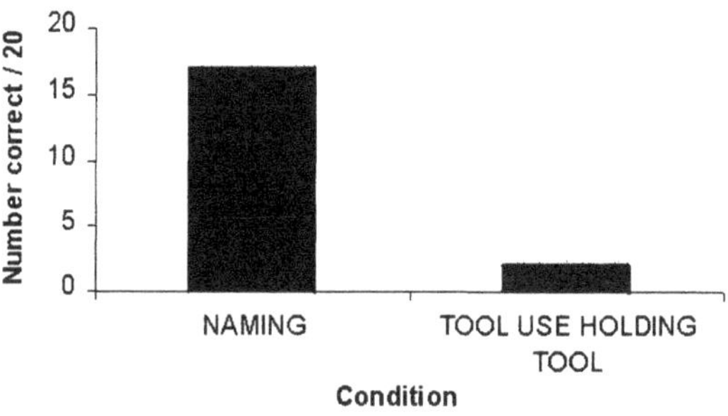


Figure 1. *Dissociation of tool use from tool naming (Ochipa et al., 1989).*

that the ability to recognise/name objects does not require that either functional knowledge (what an object is used for) or manipulation knowledge (how an object is used) must be intact and/or accessible. However, it might be argued that it has not been demonstrated that the patient reported by Ochipa and colleagues had damage to stored knowledge of how tools are used. Specifically, it might be argued that this patient was impaired at producing the correct actions associated with a tool, but the patient was nevertheless able to access stored knowledge of the movements associated with objects in order to succeed at naming tasks; this position entails the hypothesis that the damage in Ochipa and colleagues' patient was to the *connections* between sensorimotor engrams and the production system. A similar position has been advanced by Buxbaum et al. (2000) to distinguish between what the authors term "central" and "peripheral" apraxics: Central apraxics can neither recognise nor produce gestures, while peripheral apraxics are only impaired at producing the correct gesture associated with an object. It is assumed that central apraxics have damage to sensorimotor representations, while peripheral apraxics have damage to the connections between sensorimotor representations and the production system. The question is: Are there any central apraxics (i.e., patients with impairments in both recognising and producing gestures) who can nevertheless access intact semantic information about objects?

*Further empirical evaluation of Prediction 2*

Damage to sensorimotor representations will *necessarily* be associated with a deficit for conceptual knowledge of manipulable artefacts.

Patient WC (Buxbaum et al., 2000) presented with an impairment for knowledge of how objects are manipulated but perfect performance on a number of tasks requiring access to conceptual knowledge of objects. For instance, WC was impaired at choosing the correct object out of four to match an observed gesture, indicating an impairment in recognising gestures (80%; control mean 97%). WC was also impaired in using actual objects presented in the visual and tactile modalities, indicating an impairment in producing the correct gestures associated with an object (73%; control mean 99%). The combination of a deficit in both gesture production and recognition indicates that there is damage to stored sensorimotor representations of the correct gestures associated with objects (Buxbaum et al., 2000). Perhaps even more convincing that the impairment in WC was to the knowledge (per se) of how to manipulate objects is the patient's contrasting performance on picture matching tasks requiring objects to be matched based on either their function or their manner of manipulation. In this task, the patient is presented with three pictures and must choose the two that are most similar. In the manipulation condition, all three items on a given trial differ in terms of their function, while two of the three are similar in their manner of manipulation (for instance, given pictures of a piano, typewriter, and stove, the correct response would be to choose piano and typewriter). For this manipulation condition, WC was severely impaired (50%; control mean 96%). Contrastively, for the function condition, all three items on a given trial differ in their manner of manipulation, and the patient must pick the two pictures out of three that have similar functions (i.e., given radio, record player, and telephone, the correct response would be to select radio and record player). WC was at ceiling (100%) on this task. WC was also administered semantic probe questions testing his knowledge of specific conceptual properties of tools. For instance, given a picture of, for instance, a knife, the patient might be asked: "Is it used for tightening or for cutting?" WC was at ceiling (100% correct) for answering semantic probe questions about tools.

*Refuting the sensory/motor theory*

A final aspect of WC's profile should be noted: WC presented with severe anomia. This aspect of the patient's performance seems to indicate, at least at first glance, that an impairment to knowledge of how to use objects is associated with a naming deficit. However, we know from the performance of the patient reported by Ochipa and colleagues (see Figure 1) that this association of impairments is not necessary. Regardless, even setting aside Ochipa and colleagues' patient, the association of anomia and an impairment for using tools is not relevant to an evaluation of the assumption that conceptual knowledge of tools is distributed over modality-specific sensorimotor representations.[11] It is this assumption that is under evaluation.

Patient WC was at ceiling on several tasks requiring access to conceptual knowledge of tools and at the same time disproportionately impaired for knowledge of how to use tools. On the assumption that WC had damage to sensorimotor representations that store information about the ways in which objects are used, it would not be possible, given the assumptions of the sensory/motor theory, to account for the ceiling performance of this patient on several tasks requiring access to conceptual knowledge.[12] Furthermore, recall that the sensory/motor theory also appealed to knowledge of the visual movements associated with using tools: The performance of WC speaks to this assumption as well, as the patient was impaired at recognising the correct gestures associated with the use of tools. The performance of patient WC refutes the hypothesis that conceptual knowledge of manipulable objects is distributed over the same modality-specific representations that are active when such objects are being used. Given that this is the central (and distinguishing) assumption of the sensory/motor theory, the theory as a whole can be provisionally rejected.[13] Our conclusion is *not* that conceptual knowledge of artefacts does not include knowledge of the ways in which artifacts are used. Rather, we have been arguing against the claim, in the terms in which it has been proposed, that conceptual knowledge of artefacts is distributed over modality-specific sensorimotor representations.

One possible counterargument to our conclusion is the following: It might be argued by a sensory/motor theorist that while WC had damage to sensorimotor representations, this damage was not so extensive as to cause a deficit for the conceptual knowledge that is distributed over these representations. There is an empirical argument against this: If there were patients with disproportionate conceptual deficits for artefacts compared to other categories of objects, then we could infer (based on the sensory/motor theory) that these patients must also have presented with disproportionate deficits for the type of conceptual knowledge that is hypothesised to be distributed over sensorimotor representations. Specifically, the prediction is the same as is made by the original formulation of the sensory/functional theory: Patients with disproportionate deficits for artefacts will also have disproportionate deficits for functional/associative knowledge compared to visual/perceptual knowledge. Contrary to this prediction is the performance of patients PL (Laiacona & Capitani, 2001), CN98 (Gaillard, Auzou, Miret, Ozsancak, & Hannequin, 1998), and ES (Moss & Tyler, 1997, 2000). These patients presented with disproportionate deficits for artifacts, but *equivalent* impairments for perceptual and functional/associative knowledge of artifacts. Furthermore, the structural description system was spared in patient PL, indicating that the impairment to visual/perceptual knowledge of nonliving things was not an artefact of having damage to the structural descriptions of those objects. Even more striking is the performance of patient IW (Lambon Ralph, Howard, Nightingale, & Ellis, 1998) who presented with a

[11] Data is not reported on WC's naming performance by semantic category. However, on a triplet matching task, the patient was presented with three words, and had to choose the two that were most semantically similar (e.g., given hammer, mallet, and saw, the correct answer would be hammer and mallet). Contrary to what would be predicted by the sensory/motor theory, WC's performance on this test was actually slightly *better* for tool triplets (94%) than for animal triplets (83%).

[12] Another task administered to WC investigated whether he could choose the correct object corresponding to a given tool. For instance, when presented with a hammer, WC had to choose between a nail and screw as the correct object to use with a hammer. WC was just below ceiling on this task (96%); however, when WC was asked to demonstrate the use of the *same* tools on the *same* objects that the patient had just selected, the patient was severely impaired (58%). For instance, on the trial with a hammer and nail, after selecting the nail, WC grasped the hammer at the wrong end and pounded the nail with the hammer's handle.

[13] The "other half" of the theory concerns living things. The assumption here is the same made by the sensory/functional theory: The ability to recognise living things differentially depends on visual/perceptual information. (But see Capitani et al., 2003-this issue; Humphreys & Forde, 2001; Mahon & Caramazza, 2001.)

disproportionate (albeit small) impairment for nonliving things compared to living things (33% and 42% respectively). In direct contrast to what would be expected based on the assumption that functional/associative knowledge is needed to support correct recognition/naming of artefacts, this patient was disproportionately impaired for visual/perceptual knowledge compared to functional/associative knowledge for both living and nonliving things. At this point, it seems the only option left for a sensory/motor theorist is to assume that visual/perceptual knowledge is what is crucial for recognising/naming artifacts, and that it is *this* knowledge that is distributed over sensorimotor engrams. However, at this point, the theory cannot explain the cause of category-specific deficits, since both living things and artefacts would be hypothesised to depend on visual/perceptual knowledge.

One way in which the sensory/motor theory might be modified in an attempt to account for the neuropsychological evidence that has been reviewed would be to drop the assumption that conceptual knowledge of manipulable artefacts is distributed over the same representations that are active when such objects are being used. In other words, it could be that sensorimotor knowledge is functionally (and physically) dissociable from conceptual knowledge, but that sensorimotor information is nevertheless required in order to perform correctly on naming and recognition tasks. Note that the revised sensory/motor theory *must* assume that knowledge of the ways in which objects are used is required, or at least differentially important, for recognising tools; if the theory does not assume sensorimotor knowledge is (at least) differentially important for recognising/naming tools, then it would not have provided an explanatory account of the cause of category-specific semantic deficits.

However, even on the basis of the neuropsychological evidence that has already been reviewed, it is clear that revising the sensory/motor theory in this way will not be sufficient to save it. For instance, if knowledge of the ways in which objects are manipulated is required (or differentially important) in order to recognize/name objects, then one cannot account for the performance of the patient reported by Ochipa and colleagues (1989). Recall that this patient was relatively unimpaired at naming tools (17/20 correct) but was severely impaired at demonstrating the use of the same tools (2/20) (see Figure 1).

Another version of the sensory/motor theory stresses the contexts in which different types of information are recruited:

> Consistent with the notion of 'privileged access' to various kinds of stored information (e.g., sensorimotor versus verbal/propositional) according to the modality of the task (e.g., action versus verbal), it may be that on naturalistic action tasks, manipulation nodes for objects are the most strongly and rapidly activated, whereas on verbal tasks concerned with man-made objects, function nodes receive greater and/or more rapid activation. The hypothesized privileged role of manipulation knowledge in naturalistic action may explain why JD [reported in Buxbaum et al., 2000] and WC are unable to use their relatively intact function knowledge to prevent object misuse errors in naturalistic action (Buxbaum et al., 2000, p. 94).

It is not clear what work the notion of "privileged access" could be doing, unless the proposal is that there is an amodal semantic system. In other words, if the semantic system is assumed to be modality-specific, then there would be no need for the assumption of a *privileged* relationship between a certain type of semantic information and a certain type of modality-specific input/output representation, since the semantic representations themselves would *already be* modality-specific. However, if an amodal semantic system is assumed, then this is not a "weaker" version of the sensory/motor theory, but rather an amodal account of the organisation of semantic knowledge that stresses the importance of different types of semantic information as a function of task demands (see, e.g., Caramazza et al., 1990, and above discussion of Plaut, 2002).[14]

In this section we have critically evaluated two assumptions: First, we have shown that the assumption that conceptual knowledge of manipulable artefacts is distributed over modality-specific sensorimotor representations is contrary to the performance of patient WC. Second, we have shown that the (weaker) assumption that in order to name/recognise tools, information about their use

[14] We are grateful to Laurel Buxbaum (personal communication) for bringing these issues to our attention.

must be accessible, is contrary to the performance of patients such as the one reported by Ochipa and colleagues (1989). In the next section we consider how the data reviewed in this article constrain questions about the organisation and representation of conceptual knowledge.

## CONCLUSION

The structure of the argument that has been developed against the sensory/motor theory is not new: Arguments of the same structure have been articulated against the basic assumptions of the sensory/functional theory by a number of authors. For example, some sensory/functional theorists have proposed that the specific type of visual/perceptual information required in order to recognise fruit/vegetables consists of knowledge of their colour (e.g., Humphreys & Forde, 2001). If we interpret this claim literally and in its strongest form, the prediction is made that a deficit for knowledge of object colour must be associated with a disproportionate deficit for fruit/vegetables. Notice that any weaker interpretation of the proposal renders it unable to account for a category-specific deficit for fruit/vegetables. Evidence contrary to this proposal has been reported by Miceli, Fouch, Capasso, Shelton, Tomaiuolo, and Caramazza (2001): Patient IOC presented with intact colour perception but impaired knowledge of the colours associated with objects. IOC did not present with a disproportionate deficit for fruit/vegetables compared to other semantic categories. These data indicate that the existence of category-specific deficits for fruit/vegetables cannot be explained in terms of an impairment to knowledge of object colour. Similarly with respect to the sensory/motor theory: Patient WC was impaired for both producing and recognising the correct movements associated with the actual use of objects, but was unimpaired for conceptual knowledge of objects across a wide range of tests. This indicates that it cannot be the case that conceptual knowledge of tools is distributed over sensorimotor representations.

The argument that has been developed against the sensory/motor theory with respect to the category of tools is thus a species of a broader and more general argument that has been articulated against the sensory/functional theory. The fact that the majority of well-studied patients with category-specific deficits have presented with equivalent impairments to both visual/perceptual and functional/associative knowledge of items from the impaired category (Capitani et al., 2003-this issue) demonstrates the inadequacy of the sensory/functional theory to explain the existence of category-specific deficits. In this article we have suggested that the simplest solution is to assume that the broadest constraint on the organisation of conceptual knowledge is object domain. Furthermore, as discussed above, adopting the domain-specific hypothesis does not entail rejecting the assumption that conceptual knowledge is organised in the brain into modality-specific stores. If the domain-specific hypothesis is conjoined with the modality-specific store assumption, the prediction is made that that there will be segregation of information corresponding to different categories of objects within neuroanatomically defined modalities. Functional neuroimaging data consistent with this prediction were reviewed: A number of investigators have observed that living things and nonliving things produced differential and spatially dissociable peaks of activation in inferior and lateral temporal cortex.

The critical issue in regard to these functional neuroimaging data concerns the nature of the information that is activated in a seemingly category-specific pattern. For instance, does the activation in fusiform regions reflect the activation of modality-specific representations (i.e., visual/structural descriptions) or rather *conceptual* knowledge about the visual properties of objects? The same question must be addressed prior to an interpretation of the observation that tool stimuli differentially activated left premotor cortex. Does this finding reflect the activation of conceptual knowledge of tools or rather of modality-specific sensorimotor representations? Either possibility is consistent with a domain-specific interpretation, since this hypothesis assumes that both pre-conceptual and conceptual levels of representation/processing will be organised by domain-specific constraints. Thus, there is currently at best equivocal evidence from neuropsychology (e.g., patient Michelangelo) and functional neuroimaging that *conceptual* knowledge is organised in the brain into modality-specific semantic stores.

However, *if* one assumes that conceptual information is organised by object domain within neuroanatomically defined modalities, then it must also be assumed that conceptual information within a given domain is not functionally dissociable across modalities. But then the following question arises: Why did WC not present with a general conceptual deficit? In other words, if WC had a deficit for *conceptual* knowledge of how objects are used, *and* it is assumed that conceptual knowledge cannot be functionally dissociated across modalities, then this case presents a paradox. A straight-forward solution is to assume that the functional locus of damage in this patient is to the system that stores sensorimotor engrams. In other words, we might draw an analogy between the functional impairment in patient WC and the functional impairment in patients with damage to the visual/structural description system. However, this interpretation of the impairment in patient WC presupposes a positive answer to the question: Must we distinguish between modality-specific input/output representations and conceptual knowledge?

## REFERENCES

Aguirre, G. K., Zarahn, E., & D'Esposito, M. (1998). An area within human ventral cortex sensitive to "building" stimuli: Evidence and implications. *Neuron, 21*, 373–383.

Allport, D. A. (1985). Distributed memory, modular subsystems and dysphasia. In S. K. Newman & R. Epstein (Eds.), *Current perspectives in dysphasia*. New York: Churchill Livingstone.

Barbarotto, R., Capitani, E., & Laiacona, M. (1996). Naming deficit in herpes simplex isingencephalitis. *Acta Neurologica Scandinavica, 93*, 272–280.

Basso, A., Capitani, E., & Laiacona, M. (1988). Progressive language impairment without dementia: A case study with isolated category-specific semantic defect. *Journal of Neurology, Neurosurgery, and Psychiatry, 51*, 1201–1207

Beauchamp, M. S., Lee, K. E., Haxby, J. V., & Martin, A. (2002). Parallel visual motion processing streams for manipulable objects and human movements. *Neuron, 34*, 149–159.

Bookheimer, S. (2002). Functional MRI of language: New approaches to understanding the cortical organisation of semantic processing. *Annual Review of Neuroscience, 25*, 151–88

Buxbaum, L. J., Schwartz, M. F., & Carew, T. G. (1997). The role of semantic memory in object use. *Cognitive Neuropsychology, 14*, 219–254.

Buxbaum, L. J., Veramonti, T., Schwartz, M. F. (2000). Function and manipulation tool knowledge in apraxia: Knowing "what for" but not "how." *Neurocase, 6*, 83–97.

Capitani, E., Laiacona, M., Mahon, B., & Caramazza, A. (2003). What are the facts of category-specific deficits? A critical review of the clinical evidence. *Cognitive Neuropsychology, 20*, 213–261.

Caramazza, A., Hillis, A. E., Rapp, B. C., & Romani, C. (1990). The multiple semantics hypothesis: Multiple confusions? *Cognitive Neuropsychology, 7*, 161–189.

Caramazza, A., & Shelton, J. R. (1998). Domain specific knowledge systems in the brain: The animate–inanimate distinction. *Journal of Cognitive Neuroscience, 10*, 1–34.

Carey, S. (2000). The origins of concepts. *Journal of Cognition and Development, 1*, 37–41.

Carey, S., & Markman, E. M. (1999). Cognitive development. In B. Martin & D. E. Rumelhart (Eds), *Cognitive science. Handbook of perception and cognition* (2nd ed., pp. 201–254). San Diego, CA: Academic Press.

Castelli, F., Frith, C., Happé, F., & Frith, U. (2002). Autism, Asperger syndrome and brain mechanisms for the attribution of mental states to animated shapes. *Brain, 125*, 1839–1849.

Castelli, F., Happé, F., Frith, U., & Frith, C. (2000). Movement and mind: A functional imaging study of perception and interpretation of complex intentional movement patterns. *NeuroImage, 12*, 314–325.

Chao, L. L., Haxby, J. V., & Martin, A. (1999a). Attribute-based neural substrates in posterior temporal cortex for perceiving and knowing about objects. *Nature Neuroscience, 2*, 913–919.

Chao, L. L., & Martin, A. (2000). Representation of manipulable man-made objects in the dorsal stream. *NeuroImage, 12*, 478–84

Chao, L. L., Martin, A., & Haxby, J. V. (1999b). Are face-responsive regions selective only for faces? *NeuroReport, 10,* 2945–50

Chao, L. L., Weisberg, J., & Martin, A. (2002). Experience-dependent modulation of category-related cortical activity. *Cerebral Cortex, 12,* 545–551.

Corbetta, M., Miezin, F. M., Dobmeyer, S., Shulman, G. L., & Petersen, S. E. (1990). Attentional modulation of neural processing of shape, color, and velocity in humans. *Science, 248,* 1556–1559

Crutch, S. J., & Warrington, E. K. (2003). The selective impairment of fruit and vegetable knowledge: A multiple processing channels account of fine-grain category specificity. *Cognitive Neuropsychology, 20,* 355–372.

Cubelli, R., Marchetti, C., Boscolo, G., & Della Sala, S. (2000). Cognition in action: Testing a model of limb apraxia. *Brain and Cognition, 44,* 144–165.

Decety, J., Perani, D., Jeannerod, M., Bettinardi, V., Tadary, B., Woods, R., Mazziotta, J. C., & Fazio, F. (1994). Mapping motor representations with positron emission tomography. *Nature, 371,* 600–602.

Devlin, J. T., Russell, R. P., Davis, M. H., Price, C. J., Moss, H. E., Fadili, M. J., & Tyler, L. K. (2002). Is there an anatomical basis for category-specificity? Semantic memory studies in PET and fMRI. *Neuropsychologia, 40,* 54–75.

Epstein, R., & Kanwisher, N. (1998). A cortical representation of the local visual environment. *Nature, 392,* 598–601

Farah, M. J., Hammond, K. M., Mehta, Z., & Ratcliff, G. (1989). Category-specificity and modality-specificity in semantic memory. *Neuropsychologia, 27,* 193–200.

Farah, M. J., & Rabinowitz, C. (2003). Genetic and environmental influences on the organisation of semantic memory in the brain: Is "living things" an innate category? *Cognitive Neuropsychology, 20,* 401–408.

Farah, M. J., & Wallace, M. A. (1992). Semantically bounded anomia: Implication for the neural implementation of naming. *Neuropsychologia, 30,* 609–621.

Gaillard, M. J., Auzou, P., Miret, M., Ozsancak, C., & Hannequin, D. (1998). Trouble de la dénomination pour les objets manufacturés dans un cas d'encéphalite herpétique. *Révue Neurologique, 154,* 683–689.

Gerlach, C., Law, I., Gade, A., & Paulson, O. B. (2000). Categorization and category-effects in normal object recognition: A PET study. *Neuropsychologia, 38,* 1693–1703.

Goldenberg, G., & Hagmann, S. (1998). Tool use and mechanical problem solving in apraxia. *Neuropsychologia, 36,* 581–589.

Gonnerman, L., Andersen, E. S., Devlin, J. T., Kempler, D., & Seidenberg, M. (1997). Double dissociation of semantic categories in Alzheimer's disease. *Brain and Language, 57,* 254–279.

Grabowski, T. J., Damasio, H., & Damasio, A. R. (1998). Premotor and prefrontal correlates of category-related lexical retrieval. *NeuroImage, 7,* 232–243.

Haxby, J. V., Ungerleider, L. G., Clark, V. P., Schouten, J. L., Hoffman, E. A., & Martin, A. (1999). The effect of face inversion on activity in human neural systems for face and object perception. *Neuron, 22,* 189–199

Hodges, J. R., Bozeat, S., Lambon Ralph, M., Patterson, K., & Spatt, J. (2000). The role of conceptual knowledge in object use. Evidence from semantic dementia. *Brain, 123,* 1913–1925.

Hodges, J. R., Spatt, J., & Patterson, K. (1999). "What" and "how": Evidence for the dissociation of object knowledge and mechanical problem-solving skills in the human brain. *Proceedings of the National Academy of Science, USA, 96,* 9444–9448.

Hoffman, E. A., & Haxby, J. V. (2000). Distinct representations of eye gaze and identity in the distributed human neural system for face perception. *Nature Neuroscience, 3,* 80–84.

Humphreys, G. W., & Forde, E. M. E. (2001). Hierarchies, similarity, and interactivity in object recognition: "Category-specific" neuropsychological deficits. *Behavioral and Brain Sciences, 24,* 453–509.

Ishai, A., Ungerleider, L. G., Martin, A., Schouten, J. L., & Haxby, J. V. (1999). Distributed representation of objects in the human ventral visual pathway. *Proceedings of the National Academy of Science, USA, 96,* 9379–9384

Joseph, J. E. (2001). Functional neuroimaging studies of category specificity in object recognition: A critical review and meta-analysis. *Cognitive, Affective and Behavioral Neuroscience, 1,* 119–136.

Kanwisher, N. (2000). Domain specificity in face perception. *Nature, 3,* 759–763.

Kanwisher, N., McDermott, J., & Chun, M. M. (1997). The fusiform face area: A module in human extrastriate cortex specialized for face perception. *Journal of Neuroscience, 17,* 4302–4311.

Keil, F. C. (1989). *Concepts, kinds, and cognitive development.* Cambridge, MA: MIT Press.

Kraut, M. A., Moo, L. R., Segal, J. B., & Hart, J. Jr. (2002). Neural activation during an explicit categorisation task: Category- or feature-specific effects? *Cognitive Brain Research*, *13*, 213–220.

Laiacona, M., Barbarotto, R., & Capitani, E. (1993). Perceptual and associative knowledge in category specific impairment of semantic memory: A study of two cases. *Cortex*, *29*, 727–740.

Laiacona, M., & Capitani, E. (2001). A case of prevailing deficit for nonliving categories or a case of prevailing sparing of living categories? *Cognitive Neuropsychology*, *18*, 39–70

Laiacona, M., Capitani, E., & Barbarotto, R. (1997). Semantic category dissociations: A longitudinal study of two cases. *Cortex*, *33*, 441–461.

Lambon Ralph, M. A., Howard, D., Nightingale, G., & Ellis, A. W. (1998). Are living and non-living category-specific deficits causally linked to impaired perceptual or associative knowledge? Evidence from a category-specific double dissociation. *Neurocase*, *4*, 311–338.

Liberman, A. M., Cooper, F. S., Shankweiler, D. P., & Studdert-Kennedy, M. (1967). Perception of the speech code. *Psychological Review*, *74*, 431–461.

Mahon, B., & Caramazza, A. (2001). The sensory/functional assumption or the data: Which do we keep? *Behavioral and Brain Sciences*, *24*, 488–489.

Mahon, B., & Caramazza, A. (in press). The organization of conceptual knowledge in the brain: Living kinds and artifacts. In E. Margolis & S. Laurence (Eds.), *Creations of the mind: Essays on artefacts and their representation*. Oxford: Oxford University Press.

Martin, A., & Chao, L. L. (2001). Semantic memory and the brain: Structure and processes. *Current Opinion in Neurobiology*, *11*, 194–201.

Martin, A., Ungerleider, L. G., & Haxby, J. V. (2000). Category specificity and the brain: The sensory/motor model of semantic representations of objects. In M. S. Gazzaniga (Ed.), *Higher cognitive functions: The new cognitive neurosciences* (pp. 1023–1036). Cambridge, MA: The MIT Press.

Martin, A., & Weisberg, J. (2003). Neural foundations for understanding social and mechanical concepts. *Cognitive Neuropsychology*, *20*, 575–587.

Martin, A., Wiggs, C. L., Ungerleider, L. G., & Haxby, J. V. (1996). Neural correlates of category-specific knowledge. *Nature*, *379*, 649–652.

McCarthy, C., Puce, A., Gore, J. C., & Allison, T., (1997). Face-specific processing in the human fusiform gyrus. *Journal of Cognitive Neuroscience*, *9*, 605–610.

Miceli, G., Fouch, E., Capasso, R., Shelton, J. R., Tomaiuolo, F., & Caramazza, A. (2001). The dissociation of color from form and function knowledge. *Nature Neuroscience*, *4*, 662–667.

Montomura, N., & Yamadori, A. (1994). A case of ideational apraxia with impairment of object use and preservation of object pantomime. *Cortex*, *30*, 167–170.

Moore, C. J., & Price, C. J. (1999). A functional neuroimaging study of the variables that generate category-specific object processing differences. *Brain*, *122*, 943–962

Moss, H. E., & Tyler, L. K. (1997). A category-specific semantic deficit for nonliving things in a case of progressive aphasia. *Brain and Language*, *60*, 55–58.

Moss, H. E., & Tyler, L. K. (2000). A progressive category-specific semantic deficit for non-living things. *Neuropsychologia*, *38*, 60–82.

Mummery, C. J., Patterson, K., Hodges, J. R., & Price, C. J. (1998). Functional neuroanatomy of the semantic system: Divisible by what? *Journal of Cognitive Neuroscience*, *10*, 766–777

Ochipa, C., Rothi, L. J. G., & Heilman, K. M., (1989). Ideational apraxia: A deficit in tool selection and use. *Annals of Neurology*, *25*, 190–193.

Perani, D., Cappa, S. F., Bettinardi, V., Bressi, S., Gorno-Tempini, M., Matarrese, M., & Fazio, F. (1995). Different neural systems for the recognition of animals and man-made tools. *NeuroReport*, *6*, 1637–1641.

Perani, D., Schnur, T., Tettamanti, M., Gorno-Tempini, M., Cappa, S. F., & Fazio, F. (1999). Word and picture matching: A PET study of semantic category effects. *Neuropsychologia*, *37*, 293–306.

Plaut, D. C. (2002). Graded modality-specific specialisation in semantics: A computational account of optic aphasia. *Cognitive Neuropsychology*, *19*, 603–639.

Price, C. J., & Friston, K. J. (2002). Functional imaging studies of category specificity. In E. M. E. Forde & G. W. Humphreys (Eds.), *Category-specificity in the brain and mind*. Hove, UK: Psychology Press.

Riddoch, M. J., Humphreys, G. W., Coltheart, M., & Funnell, E., (1988). Semantic systems or system? Neuropsychological evidence re-examined. *Cognitive Neuropsychology*, *5*, 3–25.

Rothi, L. J. G., Ochipa, C., & Heilman, K. M (1991). A cognitive neuropsychological model of limb praxis. *Cognitive Neuropsychology*, *8*, 443–458.

Rumiati, R. I, Zanini, S., Vorano, L., & Shallice, T. (2001). A form of ideational apraxia as a selective deficit of contention scheduling. *Cognitive Neuropsychology, 18*, 617–642.

Samson, D., & Pillon, A. (2003). A case of impaired knowledge for fruit and vegetables. *Cognitive Neuropsychology, 20*, 373–400.

Samson, D., Pillon, A., & De Wilde, V. (1998). Impaired knowledge of visual and nonvisual attributes in a patient with a semantic impairment for living entities: A case of a true category-specific deficit. *Neurocase, 4*, 273–290

Santos, L. R., & Caramazza, A. (2002). The domain-specific hypothesis: A developmental and comparative perspective on category-specific deficits. In E. M. E. Forde & G. W. Humphreys (Eds.), *Category-specificity in the brain and mind* (pp. 1–24). Hove, UK: Psychology Press.

Santos, L. R., Hauser, M. D., & Spelke, E. S. (2002). Domain-specific knowledge in human children and non-human primates: Artifacts and foods. In M. Bekoff, C. Allen, & G. M. Burghardt (Eds.), *The cognitive animal: Empirical and theoretical perspectives on animal cognition* (pp. 205–216). Cambridge, MA: MIT Press.

Sartori, G., Coltheart, M., Miozzo, M., & Job, R. (1994). Category specificity and informational specificity in neuropsychological impairment of semantic memory. In C. A. Umiltà & M. Moscovitch (Eds.), *Attention and performance XV* (pp. 537–550). Cambridge, MA: MIT Press.

Sartori, G., & Job, R. (1988). The oyster with four legs: A neuropsychological study on the interaction between vision and semantic information. *Cognitive Neuropsychology, 5*, 105–132.

Sartori, G., Job, R., Miozzo, M., Zago, S., & Marchiori, G. (1993a). Category-specific form-knowledge deficit in a patient with herpes simplex virus encephalitis. *Journal of Clinical and Experimental Neuropsychology, 15*, 280–299.

Sartori, G., Miozzo, M., & Job, R. (1993b). Category-specific naming impairments? Yes. *Quarterly Journal of Experimental Psychology, 46A*, 489–504.

Senior, C., Barnes, J., Giampietro, V., Simmons, A., Bullmore, E. T., Brammer, M., & David, A. S. (2000). The functional neuroanatomy of implicit-motion perception or representational momentum. *Current Biology, 10*, 16–22.

Sheridan, J., & Humphreys, G. W. (1993). A verbal-semantic category-specific recognition impairment. *Cognitive Neuropsychology, 10*, 143–184.

Silveri, M. C., & Gainotti, G. (1988). Interaction between vision and language in category-specific semantic impairment. *Cognitive Neuropsychology, 5*, 677–709.

Sirigu, A., Duhamel, J., & Poncet, M. (1991). The role of sensorimotor experience in object recognition. *Brain, 114*, 2555–2573.

Thompson-Schill, S. L. (2002). Neuroimaging studies of semantic memory: Inferring "how" from "where." *Neuropsychologia, 40*, 280–292.

Warrington, E. K., & McCarthy, R. (1983). Category specific access dysphasia. *Brain, 106*, 859–878.

Warrington, E. K., & McCarthy, R. (1987). Categories of knowledge: Further fractionations and an attempted integration. *Brain, 110*, 1273–1296.

Warrington, E. K., & McCarthy, R. A. (1994). Multiple meaning systems in the brain: A case for visual semantics. *Neuropsychologia, 32*, 1465–1473.

Warrington, E. K., & Shallice, T. (1984). Category-specific semantic impairment. *Brain, 107*, 829–854.

Whatmough, C., Chertkow, H., Murtha, S., & Hanratty, K. (2002). Dissociable brain regions process object meaning and object structure during picture naming. *Neuropsychologia, 40*, 174–186.

COGNITIVE NEUROPSYCHOLOGY, 2003, 20 (3/4/5/6), 451–486

# THE SIMILARITY-IN-TOPOGRAPHY PRINCIPLE: RECONCILING THEORIES OF CONCEPTUAL DEFICITS

W. Kyle Simmons and Lawrence W. Barsalou
*Emory University, Atlanta, USA*

Three theories currently compete to explain the conceptual deficits that result from brain damage: sensory-functional theory, domain-specific theory, and conceptual structure theory. We argue that all three theories capture important aspects of conceptual deficits, and offer different insights into their origins. Conceptual topography theory (CTT) integrates these insights, beginning with A. R. Damasio's (1989) convergence zone theory and elaborating it with the similarity-in-topography (SIT) principle. According to CTT, feature maps in sensory-motor systems represent the features of a category's exemplars. A hierarchical system of convergence zones then conjoins these features to form both property and category representations. According to the SIT principle, the proximity of two conjunctive neurons in a convergence zone increases with the similarity of the features they conjoin. As a result, conjunctive neurons become topographically organised into local regions that represent properties and categories. Depending on the level and location of a lesion in this system, a wide variety of deficits is possible. Consistent with the literature, these deficits range from the loss of a single category to the loss of multiple categories that share sensory-motor properties.

## INTRODUCTION

Following certain insults to the brain, an individual may lose knowledge of some categories while retaining knowledge of others. Over the past 25 years, many clinical cases have been reported that demonstrate various patterns of category-specific deficits. Most commonly, patients lose knowledge of living things; in particular, animals. Less commonly, patients lose knowledge of nonliving things, such as manipulable artefacts. In some cases, patients lose a single category, such as living things. In others, they lose multiple categories, such as living things and musical instruments.[1]

In describing these deficits, researchers have used a variety of terms, sometimes referring to them as agnosias, and sometimes as *semantic deficits*. Whereas agnosia implies that a deficit reflects damage to a particular sensory-motor modality, semantic deficit implies damage to a higher-order conceptual representation. As will be seen, it is not always clear whether the loss of category knowledge

[1] "Category" will refer to a set of exemplars in the world, and "concept" will refer to a cognitive representation of the category in the brain.

Requests for reprints should be addressed to Lawrence W. Barsalou, Department of Psychology, Emory University, Atlanta, GA 30322, USA (Email: barsalou@emory.edu).

We are grateful to Alex Martin and Alfonso Caramazza for the opportunity to write this article. We are also grateful to Aron Barbey, Sergio Chaigneau, George Cree, Glyn Humphreys, Jay McClelland, and Ken McRae for helpful comments on earlier drafts. This work was supported by National Science Foundation Grants SBR-9905024 and BCS-0212134 to Lawrence W. Barsalou.



http://www.tandf.co.uk/journals/pp/02643294.html
DOI:10.1080/02643290342000032

reflects damage to sensory-motor modalities or to conceptual structures. Furthermore, particular theories tend to favour one term over the other, based on their particular assumptions about the conceptual system. To avoid terminology that favours one position, we adopt the term *conceptual deficit*, and use it inclusively in referring to deficits of both types. When known, the specific origins of a deficit should be clear from the surrounding text.

In this article, we develop a new account of conceptual deficits—conceptual topography theory (CTT)—that draws on A. R. Damasio's (1989) theory of *convergence zones*. To increase the explanatory power of convergence zone theory, we add the *similarity-in-topography (SIT) principle*. We then show that this revised theory is at least roughly compatible with the main theories of conceptual deficits in the literature. In particular, this theory predicts the particular findings that each theory explains most naturally, plus those that each theory alone cannot.

## Theories of conceptual deficits

Three accounts of conceptual deficits currently dominate the literature: sensory-functional theory, domain-specific theory, and conceptual structure theory. We address each in turn.

*Sensory-functional theory.* The first attempt to explain conceptual deficits was the sensory-functional theory proposed by Warrington and her colleagues (e.g., Warrington & McCarthy, 1987; Warrington & Shallice, 1984), and later implemented computationally by Farah and McClelland (1991). Other formulations of this view include Humphreys and Forde's (2001) HIT theory, McRae and Cree's (2002) property profile theory, and Damasio's (1989) convergence zone theory.[2] Sensory-functional theory assumes that knowledge of a specific category is located near the sensory-motor areas of the brain that process its instances. Thus knowledge of living things is stored near sensory areas (especially vision), because sensory mechanisms dominate the processing of these categories. Conversely, knowledge of manipulable artefacts is stored near motor and somatosensory areas, because mechanisms involved in the functional use of artifacts dominate processing. Given the proximity of category knowledge to sensory-motor mechanisms, damage to a sensory-motor system may produce deficits in the specific categories that rely on them. Thus, a deficit for living things may arise from damage to brain regions that process sensory information, whereas a deficit for manipulable artefacts may arise from damage to regions that implement functional action.[3]

An important prediction from sensory-functional theory is that conceptual deficits should often include multiple categories. Because conceptual deficits arise from damage to a particular sensory-motor system, any category that relies on that system for processing its instances may suffer. Because a given sensory-motor system almost always serves multiple categories, more than one category should suffer if the system is damaged. Clearly other factors are relevant, such as how strongly one property type is correlated with other property types, and how dominant a given modality is for processing a category (e.g., Farah & McClelland, 1991). Regardless, sensory-functional theory generally predicts that multiple categories should show deficits when a given sensory-motor system is damaged. When sensory areas are damaged, multiple categories whose processing relies heavily on sensory analysis should suffer. When motor areas are damaged, multiple categories whose processing relies heavily on motor execution should suffer.

[2] Readers may find it confusing that an elaborated version of A. R. Damasio's (1989) convergence zone theory integrates all three theories, while being an instance of sensory-functional theories. In its original form, convergence zone theory is closest to sensory-functional theories because of the central roles that sensory-motor areas play in representation. Adding the SIT principle, however, changes the theory's character such that it exhibits central properties of domain-specific and conceptual structure theories as well.

[3] A major issue in the sensory-functional literature concerns the specific nature of functional information. McRae and Cree (2002) address this issue extensively. Barsalou, Sloman, and Chaigneau (in press) provide a detailed theory of the conceptual content that underlies function.

*Domain-specific theory.* According to the domain-specific theory, knowledge of a category is not distributed across the sensory-motor systems that process its instances. Instead knowledge of a category is stored in a circumscribed brain system that solely represents the category downstream from sensory-motor processing (e.g., Caramazza, 1998; Caramazza & Shelton, 1998; also see Capitani, Laiacona, Mahon, & Caramazza, 2003-this issue). According to this view, evolutionary contingencies led to at least three dissociable brain systems that represent animals, plants, and conspecifics, respectively. One further representational system of a more generic variety represents knowledge about categories having less evolutionary significance, such as artefacts.

Most importantly, the domain-specific theory predicts that conceptual deficits should typically affect a single category. When damage to the evolutionary system for a category occurs, a deficit in processing that category should follow, but not a deficit for others. In contrast to the sensory-functional theory, deficits should typically not occur for different categories that share the same type of core information. Instead deficits should be observed for individual types of categories.

*Conceptual structure theory.* According to this final view, all categories are represented in a single conceptual system (e.g., Caramazza, Hillis, Rapp, & Romani, 1990; Tyler & Moss, 2001; Tyler, Moss, Durrant-Peatfield, & Levy, 2000).[4] Prior to developing the domain-specific theory, Caramazza and his colleagues proposed the organized unitary content hypothesis (OUCH), which Tyler, Moss, and colleagues developed further into the conceptual structure theory. Similar to OUCH, the conceptual structure theory proposes that knowledge of objects is represented in a single semantic space. Within this continuous semantic space, the structure of categories arises from: (1) property correlations, (2) distinctive properties, and (3) interactions between property correlations and distinctive properties. Together, property correlations and property distinctiveness create a similarity metric within semantic space, such that the information for a particular category tends to lump together in a specific subregion. If the instances of a category share many correlated properties, its instances lump tightly in semantic space, whereas a category with diverse instances is distributed more broadly. Furthermore, as a category's distinctive properties increase, so does its distance to other categories.

The conceptual structure account proposes that three factors determine how susceptible a category is to brain injury. First, a category is more robust when its instances share many correlated properties. For example, different instances of mammals, such as dog, horse, and lion, share many properties, such as *four legs*, *fur*, and *bear live young*. If one property in a correlation is compromised, other properties in its correlational structure can help retrieve it, or stand in for it.

The second factor that increases a category's robustness is its number of distinctive properties. Categories become lost when their distinctive properties no longer distinguish them from similar categories. The more distinctive properties a category has, the more damage is necessary to make it indistinguishable.

Finally, a category's robustness increases as its distinctive properties increasingly correlate with other properties, thereby protecting distinguishing information from damage. In artefacts, distinctive structural properties are often correlated with corresponding functions, thereby increasing their robustness. For example, *curved prong* for corkscrew distinguishes it from other artefacts and is uniquely correlated with its function—opening wine bottles. In natural kinds, distinctive properties are often not uniquely correlated. For example, *stripes* distinguish zebra from related categories but are not uniquely correlated with other zebra properties (e.g., *hooves*), which occur for other categories

[4] Correlated and distinctive properties are also central to McRae and Cree's (2002) account of category deficits (also see Cree & McRae, in press). However, they attempt to explain the importance of these factors within an elaborated version of sensory-functional theory, rather than within a single semantic space.

(e.g., horse, mule). Thus, correlated and distinctive properties work together to represent categories, with the weak points of statistical structure being most prone to damage.

*Reconciling conflicting theories.* Three different theories purport to account for the same data. Sensory-functional theory proposes that the conceptual system is organised around different types of sensory-motor information. Domain-specific theory argues that the conceptual system is organised into separate processing systems for evolutionarily significant categories. Conceptual structure theory holds that the conceptual system is organised by statistical relationships between categories and their properties.

A typical assumption in such debates is that one theory is correct and the others false. The spirited discussion on conceptual deficits often appears to proceed on this assumption. Significantly, however, the history of science is replete with rapprochements between competing theories. Theories viewed as conflicting and mutually exclusive often turn out to each capture important elements of truth and to even be compatible. In the early and mid-nineteenth century, British physicists argued heatedly over whether light was a particle or a wave. As we now know, both were correct (Chen, 1995). A major debate over the mechanisms of biological respiration similarly ended in rapprochement (Bechtel & Richardson, 1993). Closer to home, early research on the localisation of vision in the brain hotly debated whether vision resides in the occipital vs. parietal lobes. As became clear, both views were correct (Bechtel & McCauley, 1999; McCauley & Bechtel, 2001).

We believe that such a resolution may exist for theories of conceptual deficits. Although these theories may appear mutually exclusive at first blush, each captures important aspects of the conceptual system. Given this system's complexity, much room exists for different theories to capture different elements of truth about it.

*Convergence zone (CZ) theory.* An existing sensory-functional theory offers a preliminary basis for synthesising the three theories of conceptual deficits: Damasio's convergence zone (CZ) theory (A. R. Damasio, 1989; A. R. Damasio & Damasio, 1994). As argued in the next section, additional principles must be added to CZ theory to accomplish this synthesis. Here we review the theory's basic components: (1) modality-specific representations in sensory-motor areas, and (2) the binding of modality-specific information in convergence zones.

CZ theory begins with a widespread assumption about sensory-motor processing. When an entity is perceived, it activates feature detectors in the relevant sensory-motor areas (from hereon, we will refer to systems of these detectors as *feature maps*). During visual processing of a cat, for example, some neurons respond to line orientations, vertices, and planar surfaces. Others fire for colour, orientation, and direction of movement. The overall pattern of activation across this hierarchically organised distributed system represents the entity in visual perception (Palmer, 1999; Zeki, 1993). Similar patterns of activation in feature maps on other modalities represent how the entity might sound and feel, and also the actions performed on it. A similar account can be given for introspective states that arise while interacting with an entity. For example, patterns of activation in the amygdala represent emotional states produced in response to perceived entities. A tremendous amount of neuroscience research has addressed the structure of these feature maps across modalities and the states that arise in them.

The second core component of CZ theory concerns storage of the states that arise in feature maps. When a pattern in a feature map becomes active, neurons in an association area bind the pattern's features for later use (from hereon, we will refer to neurons in association areas as *conjunctive neurons*). Damasio refers to these association areas as "convergence zones" and assumes that they exist at multiple hierarchical levels, ranging from posterior to anterior in the brain. Most locally, CZs near a particular modality capture patterns of activation within it. Thus association areas near visual processing areas capture patterns of activation there, whereas association areas near motor processing areas capture patterns of activation there. Further downstream, higher-level association areas in more anterior areas, such as the temporal and frontal lobes, conjoin patterns of activation *across* modalities. We will say more about the localisation of these areas later.

In a given CZ, conjunctive neurons link active neurons in feature maps together. According to A. R. Damasio (1989, p. 129), neurons notice "combinatorial arrangements" of neurons active in a feature map, and establish associative relationships between them. On viewing a chair, for example, a subset of the conjunctive neurons in a visual CZ captures the active features across the hierarchically organised feature maps in vision. On sitting in the chair, a subset of the conjunctive neurons in a motor CZ captures the active features that executed the movement. At a higher level, a subset of the neurons in a cross-modal CZ correlates the visual form of the chair with the action taken on it. As will become clear, we assume that higher-level conjunctive neurons conjoin lower-level conjunctive neurons. Rather than conjoining feature map neurons directly, cross-modal conjunctions conjoin earlier conjunctions, thereby conjoining states in feature maps indirectly. Thus the conjunctive neurons that link visual and motor properties do so indirectly by linking modality-specific conjunctive neurons in the visual and motor systems.

This architecture of feature maps and convergence zones has the following functional implication: Once conjunctive neurons in a CZ capture an active pattern in a feature map, these neurons can later reactivate the pattern in the absence of bottom-up sensory stimulation (A. R. Damasio, 1989). In recollecting a perceived object, conjunctive neurons in CZs re-enact the sensory-motor states active while encoding it. Similarly, when representing a concept, conjunctive neurons in CZs reactivate the sensory-motor states characteristic of its instances. A given re-enactment is never complete, and biases may affect its reactivation, but at least some semblance of the original state occurs. This basic idea of re-enactment is essentially the same as neural accounts of mental imagery (e.g., Farah, 2000; Grezes & Decety, 2001; Jeannerod, 1995; Kosslyn, 1994). The one difference might be that imagery typically creates more complete and vivid re-enactments than those in memory, conceptualisation, and comprehension (Barsalou, 1999, in press-b).

Barsalou (1999, in press-a) takes the basic CZ architecture and shows how a fully functional conceptual system can be built upon it. Within this architecture, it is possible to implement categorical inference, the type-token distinction, argument binding, recursion, productivity, propositions, and abstract concepts. Because these phenomena are largely unrelated to the issue of how conceptual deficits originate, however, we do not pursue them here. Instead our interest is in how an elaborated CZ architecture synthesises the sensory-functional, domain-specific, and conceptual structure theories, thereby providing a unified account of conceptual deficits.

*Distributed representations in CZ theory.* As is evident, the representation of a concept in CZ theory is distributed across many brain areas that serve a variety of processes. On the one hand, a concept's representation resides in subsets of conjunctive neurons across multiple association areas. On the other hand, these conjunctive neurons re-enact sensory-motor states in feature maps, often in several modalities at once. Thus the representation of a concept may span the brain from frontal and temporal association areas to a variety of sensory-motor feature maps.

An important issue concerns the roles that parts of a distributed representation play in conceptual tasks. A. R. Damasio (1989, p. 46) proposes that conjunctive neurons in CZs play no representational roles. Instead they only constitute a means of reactivating previously active patterns in feature maps. Consider the representation of chairs. According to Damasio, the conjunctive neurons that conjoin the visual features of chairs cannot function as a stand-alone representation of this category. Instead these neurons only serve to reactivate chair features in visual feature maps, which then constitute a conceptual representation of chairs.

We agree that conjunctive neurons play the important role of reactivating patterns in feature maps during imagery, conceptual processing, and other cognitive tasks (Barsalou, 1999).

Reactivating features provides a powerful means of representing and processing categories. Unlike Damasio, however, we believe that patterns of conjunctive neurons in CZs can also function as stand-alone representations, in particular, during automatised feed-forward processes such as categorisation. During the categorisation of familiar objects (e.g., chairs), active feature detectors feed activation into the conjunctive neurons that integrate chair features. These conjunctive neurons then feed activation to response systems, such as the system that vocally produces a category name (e.g., "chair"). In this chain of feed-forward processing, the pattern of active conjunctive neurons functions as a representation sufficient to produce a correct response—reactivating a feature map pattern is not necessary. Nevertheless, research has shown that the visual system may be reactivated when categorisations are difficult (e.g., Humphreys & Forde, 2001; Kosslyn, Alpert, Thompson, Chabris, Rauch, & Anderson, 1994; Kosslyn, Thompson, & Alpert, 1997). Under demanding conditions, re-entrant activation produces visual representations that guide further feature extraction.

An open question is whether patterns of conjunctive neurons can function as stand-alone representations in other tasks that require the construction, manipulation, and evaluation of conceptual representations. For example, can people construct novel conceptual combinations using patterns of conjunctive neurons alone, or must they reactivate feature maps and then perform conceptual combination on these simulations? Similarly, can people perform language comprehension by simply manipulating patterns of conjunctive neurons, or are simulations in feature maps required (cf. Glenberg & Kaschak, 2002; Spivey, Tyler, Richardson, & Young, 2000; Stanfield & Zwaan, 2001; Zwaan, Stanfield, & Yaxley, 2002)?

We conjecture that conjunctive neurons only function as stand-alone representations when they feed forward automatically to responses under highly routinised conditions, such as categorisation and word association. When nonautomatised strategic processing must be performed to construct, manipulate, or evaluate a conceptual representation, simulations in feature maps are necessary. We increasingly believe that the componential symbolic operations that underlie complex conceptual processing can only be performed on simulations, not on stand-alone patterns of conjunctive neurons (cf. Kan, Barsalou, Solomon, Minor, & Thompson-Schill, 2003-this issue).

*Distributed representations in other theories.* Distributed representations are certainly not unique to CZ theory. Many theories, especially those grounded in connectionism, assume that knowledge is distributed across multiple systems. In sensory-functional theories, for example, a concept's representation resides in different knowledge stores for visual vs. functional properties.

In most other theories, however, conceptual content does not exist in feature maps—content exists only in other systems that *recode* patterns of feature map activation. In sensory-functional theories, for example, a sensory store is assumed to contain conceptual content that has presumably been recoded from the original sensory systems. Similarly, a functional store is assumed to contain conceptual content that has been recoded from the motor system. Typically, pools of hidden units in these theories recode sensory-motor properties into new representations, which then function as stand-alone representations.

Consider Humphreys and Forde's (2001) HIT theory. In their distributed architecture, knowledge stores exist for properties on different modalities (e.g., see their Figure 3 on p. 474). Importantly, however, "descriptions" of these properties represent them in conceptual knowledge—not simulations of them in sensory-motor systems. Furthermore, Forde and Humphreys' re-entrant activation is primarily a way to support difficult categorisation—it does not function as a simulation mechanism for representing imagery and knowledge in general. Thus a key difference between our approach and others is that simulations of content in feature maps represent categories, not re-descriptions of that content into amodal description languages.

Furthermore, nothing like our similarity-in-topography (SIT) principle (described later) exists in other current theories. Applying this principle to

A. R. Damasio's (1989) convergence zone theory produces a novel architecture that can be mapped to neural systems in ways that other theories have not. Additionally, this architecture makes novel predictions about conceptual deficits.[5]

Knowledge stores in the domain-specific and conceptual structure theories appear to have a similar status. In the domain-specific theory, stores outside sensory-motor systems recode the sensory-motor content of specific categories. In the conceptual structure theory, descriptions stored outside sensory-motor systems represent this content in a continuous semantic space. Furthermore, nothing like the SIT principle organises conceptual content in these theories.

*Overview.* In the first of the remaining sections, we supplement A. R. Damasio's (1989) CZ theory with the SIT principle, along with its corollary, the variable dispersion principle. These principles allow CZ theory to explain critical findings on conceptual deficits, and also to synthesise the sensory-functional, domain-specific, and conceptual structure theories. Within this framework, the second remaining section presents the conceptual topography theory (CTT). In the third remaining section, we bring neuroscience evidence to bear on CTT's neuroanatomical predictions. In the fourth section, we list critical findings in the lesion literature that any model of conceptual deficits must explain. In the final section, we show that CTT's architecture naturally predicts these findings.

## TWO SUPPLEMENTARY PRINCIPLES FOR CONVERGENCE ZONE THEORY

On its own, A. R. Damasio's (1989) CZ theory is not sufficient to explain what is known about conceptual deficits; nor is it sufficient to synthesise the sensory-functional, domain-specific, and conceptual structure theories. At least, two additional principles are necessary: (1) *the similarity-in-topography (SIT) principle*, and its corollary, (2) *the variable dispersion principle.*

### The similarity-in-topography (SIT) principle

We offer the SIT principle in the spirit of a conjecture that rests on modest empirical support but that clearly requires further examination and evidence. Perhaps the strongest current source of evidence is the SIT principle's ability to explain conceptual deficits, as the final section illustrates. Modest independent evidence, however, comes from the electrophysiological and neuroimaging literatures, as will be seen. Clearly much additional evidence is necessary before accepting this principle. Nevertheless we propose it here, first, because it seems like a conjecture worth pursuing, and second, because of its ability to explain conceptual deficits and to integrate theories.

The SIT principle concerns the organisation of the conjunctive neurons in CZs. Essentially the SIT principle claims that categorical structure in the world becomes instantiated in the topography of the brain's association areas. Specifically, the SIT principle states that:

> The spatial proximity of two neurons in a CZ reflects the similarity of the features they conjoin. As two sets of conjoined features become more similar, the conjunctive neurons that link them lie closer together in the CZ's spatial topography.

Consider the faces of a human, a monkey, and an elephant, and their representation in Figure 1. While viewing a given face, large numbers of neurons distributed throughout visual feature maps

[5] At the very end of their article, Humphreys and Forde (2001, p. 475) introduce something along the lines of our SIT principle, which they then dismiss as not being needed in the formulation of HIT that dominates their account of the literature. We originally and independently arrived at this principle earlier after reviewing the literature on conceptual deficits during a 1999 graduate seminar and seeing its potential for explaining the literature. This current article continues our application of A. R. Damasio's (1989) convergence zone theory to perceptual symbol systems (Barsalou, 1999), and shows how adding the SIT principle explains conceptual deficits within this framework.

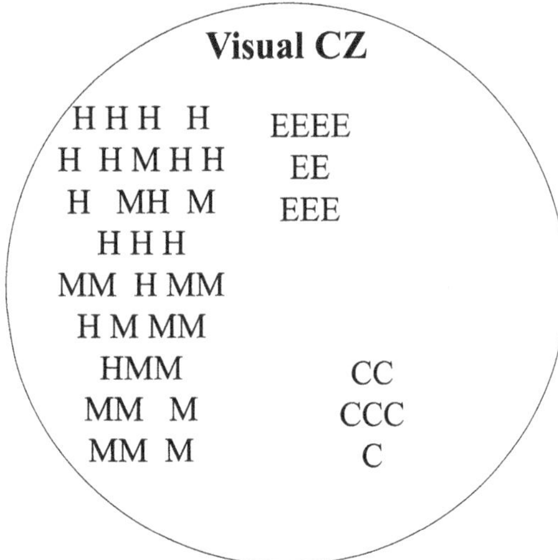


**Figure 1.** *Illustration of localised conjunctive neurons in a visual CZ for the features of a human (H), a monkey (M), an elephant (E), and a chair (C).*

become active to represent its features. Subsequently, neurons in a visual CZ conjoin these features by associating the respective feature map neurons. Of interest is the spatial proximity of the conjunctive neurons for the three faces. According to the SIT principle, the populations of conjunctive neurons for the human and monkey faces lie closer together on average in the visual CZ than does the population for the elephant face. Furthermore, the conjunctive neurons that represent all three faces lie closer together than the conjunctive neurons that represent some completely different type of object, such as a chair. In general, the topographic proximity of two conjunctive neurons reflects the similarity of the features they link.

The SIT principle has an important connection to the conceptual structure theory. As described earlier, this theory proposes that semantic space is "lumpy." Where clusters or "lumps" of correlated properties arise in the space, categories typically exist. Thus, one region of semantic space contains the correlated properties for mammals, whereas another contains those for plants. The SIT principle reproduces these lumps in the spatial topography of CZs. Whereas one population of neurons in the visual CZ tends to capture conjunctions of visual properties for animals, another population—perhaps partially overlapping—tends to capture conjunctions of visual properties typical of plants. Via the SIT principle, lumpiness at the conceptual level manifests itself physically at the topographical level of the CZ.[6]

Although statistical structure is central for both conceptual structure theory and the SIT principle, the actual implementation of this structure varies in the two approaches. Whereas the SIT principle realises statistical structure topographically in the brain's association areas, conceptual structure theories do not. Consequently, the two theories make somewhat different predictions about how statistical structure produces conceptual deficits, as we will see later.

*Problems in specifying conjunctive similarity.* To what feature combinations are conjunctive neurons tuned? How do conjunctive neurons acquire their tunings? We do not have space to address these issues in detail but briefly note their potential implications for our account.

In principle, any given feature could co-occur with any other feature. In the daunting face of this possibility, theorists often argue that biases must constrain the feature combinations that organisms anticipate (e.g., Murphy, 2002; Murphy & Medin, 1985). Perhaps some tunings evolve to anticipate feature combinations that are evolutionarily significant, such as those for animals. Similarly, other conjunctive neurons may be predisposed to link the feature correlations that pair words with their meanings, emotional expressions with emotional feelings, motor actions with visual outcomes, etc. The well-known fact that some associations are learned more easily than others is consistent with this proposal (e.g., Garcia & Koelling, 1966). By no

[6] As Barsalou (1983, 1985, 1991) shows, many categories do not share correlated properties (e.g., ad hoc categories). Because the lesion literature has not addressed these categories, we do not address them here. We assume, however, that other mechanisms beyond those in conceptual topography theory are necessary to account for ad hoc categories and other abstract concepts (see Barsalou, 1999, for accounts within the framework of perceptual symbol systems).

means do we imply that this categorical knowledge is "innate" or genetically encoded! To the contrary, we merely suggest that some tunings evolve that *anticipate* useful knowledge—category knowledge is not represented genetically. Only after actual experience utilises these conjunctive neurons does category knowledge develop epigenetically (cf. Elman, Bates, Johnson, Karmiloff-Smith, & Plunkett, 1996).

Clearly, though, people learn many categories that have little or no evolutionarily significance. Thus additional principles must determine the tunings of the conjunctive neurons that link the features of these categories. One possibility is that some tunings develop through learning. As new categories are encountered, free contiguous conjunctive neurons are recruited and tuned in the process. Another possibility is that constraints from higher-level knowledge establish tunings (cf. Murphy & Medin, 1985). For example, the belief that an organism's internal organs control its external behaviour might tune conjunctive neurons to these particular correlations.

*Topography as a general organising principle.* Substantial evidence exists for topographic organisation in feature maps, ranging from the visual system to the motor, somatosensory, and auditory systems. In these areas, feature maps are often laid out according to the physical structure of the world. Such organisation in feature maps does not concern us here—our interest is in the topographic organisation of association areas. Nevertheless, it is intriguing to consider the possibility that topographic organisation underlies both. If so, this would suggest that topographical mapping constitutes a fundamental principle of brain organisation at multiple levels.

## The variable dispersion principle

We do *not* assume that the conjunctive neurons for a category reside in a neatly circumscribed topographical region that only contains conjunctive neurons for that category and no other. To the contrary, we assume that the conjunctive neurons for a category are dispersed in clumps, with clumps for other categories falling between. Furthermore, a given clump may contain conjunctive neurons used by more than one category. As described later, both electrophysiological and fMRI evidence support these conclusions. Figure 2 summarises them. Unlike Panel A, the conjunctive neurons for a category are typically *not* contiguous in a CZ. Panel B illustrates instead how noncontiguous clusters of conjunctive neurons represent a category.

The variable dispersion principle applies to these noncontiguous clusters of conjunctive neurons, stating that:

> In a CZ, the proximity of the noncontiguous clusters for a category reflects the similarity of its instances. As the instances of a category decrease in similarity, its noncontiguous clusters of conjunctive neurons become increasingly dispersed in the CZ's spatial topography.

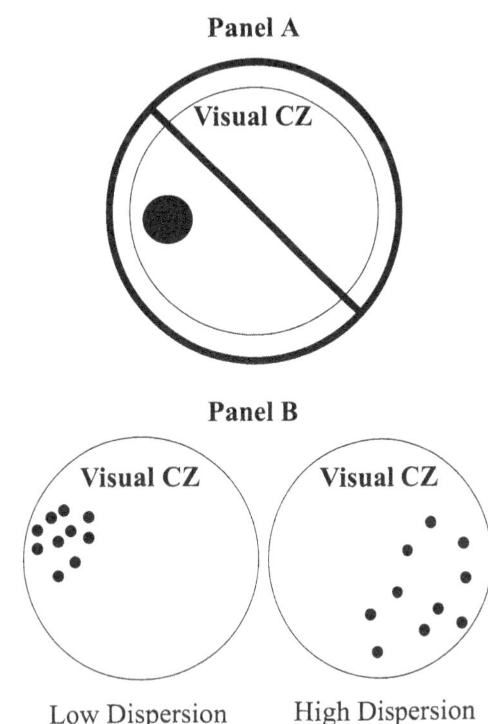


**Figure 2.** *Illustration of the variable dispersion principle. Panel A illustrates that the conjunctive neurons for a category are typically not contiguous in a CZ. Panel B illustrates how noncontiguous clusters of conjunctive neurons represent a category, with low dispersion for a category on the left, and high dispersion for a category on the right.*

Panel B in Figure 2 illustrates the variable dispersion principle, showing both low and high dispersion profiles for categories having similar vs. dissimilar instances respectively (e.g., mammals vs. artefacts).

The variable dispersion principle follows naturally from the SIT principle: Because similarity is instantiated in topography, the clusters of conjunctive neurons that represent a category lie closer together as within-category similarity increases. As will become clear later, this has significant implications for conceptual deficits. To the extent that the clusters for a category are tightly localised, a lesion can more easily disrupt the category. When a category's clusters are distributed more broadly, a single lesion is less likely to compromise them all.

## CONCEPTUAL TOPOGRAPHY THEORY (CTT)

CTT develops a specific formulation of A. R. Damasio's (1989) CZ theory, coupling it with the SIT and variable dispersion principles. We begin with a general overview of CTT, and then turn to its specific components.

### Overview

As Figure 3 illustrates, CTT contains the same configuration of four sub-systems on each of the six sensory-motor modalities, and also for emotion. Specifically, each modality contains *feature maps analytic CZs, holistic CZs*, and *modality CZs*. Although these four subsystems are only shown for the visual system, an analogous set is assumed to exist for each other modality. As Figure 3 further illustrates, cross-modal CZs integrate the modality-specific CZs. Together, all of these subsystems implement a core component of the human conceptual system.[7]

CTT further assumes that the lexicon is closely coupled with the conceptual system. Figure 3 does not illustrate a separate lexicon, however, because CTT assumes that the same modality-specific systems and cross-modal CZs that implement the conceptual system also implement the lexicon (as described later). The remainder of this section describes CTT's specific sub systems in greater detail.

### Feature maps

Each modality is assumed to contain feature maps that code the content of modality-specific states. Thus feature maps code colour, line orientation, pitch, physical pressure at bodily locations, and so forth. It almost goes without saying that the perception of an object produces a tremendous amount of activity across multiple feature maps. Furthermore, because a category's instances vary, their feature map representations vary as well. As will become clear later, variability across a category's instances has implications for how the CTT model operates, and for how it explains conceptual deficits.

### Analytic CZs

Thus far we have failed to address an important issue regarding CZs: Exactly what properties does a CZ capture for a category instance? A simple-minded possibility is that a CZ stores a complete image of them all. As Barsalou (1999) discusses, however, there is little evidence for complete images of this sort, and there are substantial theoretical problems as well (also see Hochberg, 1998; Wolfe, 2000).

Another much more likely possibility is that a CZ selectively stores information about *properties* of an entity, guided by selective attention. Barsalou (1999, in press-a) suggests that selective attention identifies informative subregions of a perceived entity and stores their content as perceptual symbols. Once selective attention focuses on a configuration of features in a particular subregion, the features become bound together in an analytic CZ (cf. Treisman & Gelade, 1980). As a result of being

[7] As mentioned earlier, a variety of additional components are necessary to handle intuitive theories, ad hoc categories, abstract concepts, and so forth.

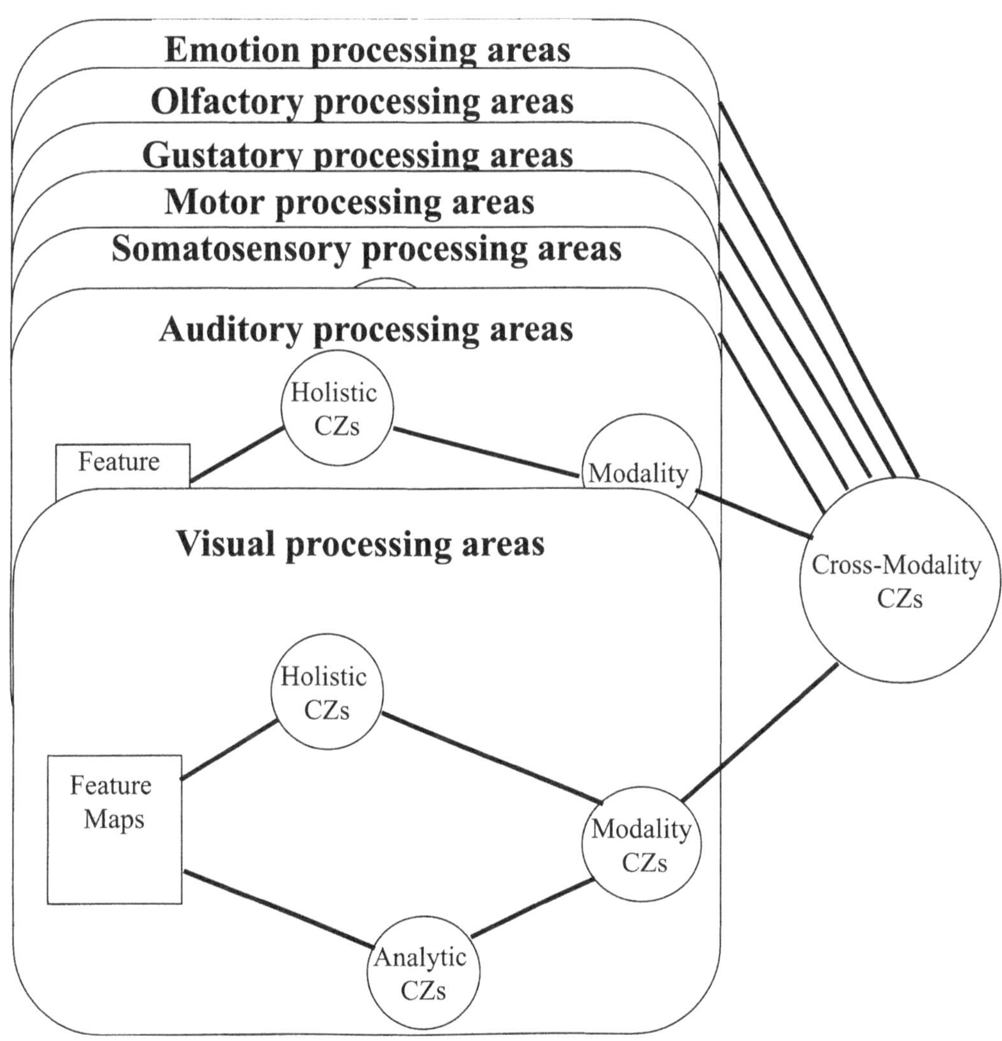


**Figure 3.** *The architecture of conceptual topography theory. The same configuration of four subsystems occurs in each of the six sensory-motor modalities and also for emotion, with cross-modality CZs integrating information across modalities.*

bound together, the features form an analytic property, which can then be used for a variety of conceptual tasks, such as categorisation and inference.

Consider *wheel* for car. On perceiving a car, the edges of a wheel are represented in visual feature maps. If selective attention focuses on this region of the perceived car, conjunctive neurons in an analytic CZ capture the features in this region. Later, on reactivating these conjunctive neurons, the visual representation of this particular wheel is partially re-enacted. As the perceived wheels of subsequent cars similarly receive attentional processing, they activate overlapping conjunctive neurons in the analytic CZ, thereby linking the visual features across different wheels to each other. The result is what Barsalou (1999) and Solomon and Barsalou (2001) refer to as a *property simulator*, namely, a system that can simulate the various forms a property takes in different categories. As the simulator for wheel develops, it produces simulations of different wheels in different objects, such as cars, bicycles, and skates. Furthermore, on perceiving a new car, processing its wheels might activate the simulator for wheel, which in turn might contribute to categorising the object as a car, given that the analytic property and the category are positively correlated.

As a result of such learning, knowledge of analytic properties develops. For car, such properties might include *wheels*, *doors*, *windshields*, *engines*, *exhaust fumes*, *steer*, and so forth. It is essential to note that analytic properties are not the same as features in feature maps—indeed, we use *feature* for one, and *property* for the other. Whereas the features in feature maps are sensory, supporting the construction of perceptions, analytic properties are conceptual, supporting the representation of cognitive-level categories. Whereas the features in feature maps are largely processed independently of attention, analytic properties typically result from applying attention to perception, thereby allowing conjunctive neurons to integrate the attended features. The results of this process are the "high-level" properties that constitute conceptual knowledge.

We assume that analytic properties arise on every modality, such as *loud* in audition, *pungent* in olfaction, and *sad* in emotion. Analytic properties need not have names. In many cases, feature configurations may become fused into unnamed analytic properties, such as the diagnostic properties that determined the categorisation of Martian rocks in Schyns and Murphy (1994). Many tastes and smells similarly appear unnamed. In general, any configuration of features that attention can select is a potential candidate for an analytic property (Schyns, Goldstone, & Thibaut, 1998). Sometimes these configurations have names and some times they do not. What is common across all analytic properties is that they play roles in the processing of concepts.

*Property organisation according to the SIT principle.* In CTT, the conjunctive neurons in analytic CZs are organised according to the SIT principle. Notably, the SIT principle does not generally organise analytic properties by category. Instead, it generally organises them by *property type*. As the SIT principle states, two conjunctive neurons are spatially close to the extent that they conjoin similar information. At the level of analytic properties, this similarity manifests itself in how similar two sets of conjoined features are. Because two different shapes are more similar than a shape and a colour, the conjunctive neurons for the two shapes should lie closer together than the conjunctive neurons for the shape and the colour. Figure 4 illustrates this state of affairs. As can be seen, regions of conjunctive neurons develop that represent shape, colour, movement, and other property types.

Notably, strong organisation by category should *not* be apparent in analytic CZs. For example, the properties of animals should not be tightly clustered. Because animals have diverse types of visual properties, these properties should be distributed widely throughout analytic CZs in vision. Following the SIT principle, the large differences between property types should cause them to be dispersed broadly, rather than being adjacent. Furthermore the visual properties for animals should be heavily mixed with those for other categories that have similar property types. To the extent that multiple categories share shape, colour, texture, and movement, their properties should reside in highly similar regions, such that the categories are not distinguished topographically.

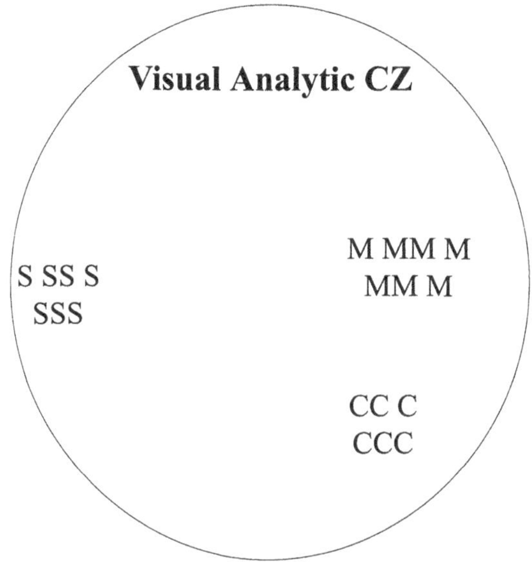


**Figure 4.** *Illustration of the conjunctive neurons in a visual analytic CZ that capture properties for colour (C), shape (S), and movement (M).*

Nevertheless, limited potential for category-specific topographic organisation exists in analytic CZs. Imagine that a category has a relatively unique type of property that no other category has, and that this property type is central to the category's identity. Following the SIT principle, the conjunctive neurons that capture these properties should be set off topographically from the conjunctive neurons that capture other property types. Furthermore, if the area holding these conjunctive neurons were lesioned, this category, and only this category, might show a deficit. In general, though, deficits at this level are unlikely to eliminate specific categories selectively, given that so many categories usually depend on a given property type. We pursue this issue later when we describe CTT's account of classic conceptual deficits.

## Holistic CZs

Much research indicates that global and configural properties are extracted during the holistic processing of perceived entities. For example, the extraction of low spatial frequency information establishes the rough shape of an object and the location of its major and minor axes, in contrast to the extraction of high spatial frequency information that yields classic analytic properties (e.g., De Valois & De Valois, 1988; Morrison & Schyns, 2001). Similarly, holistic processing captures the configural relations between multiple analytic properties, such as the configuration of the eyes, nose, and mouth in a face (e.g., Macrae & Lewis, 2002). In general, holistic properties are relatively large, being distributed across much or even most of a perceived entity.

Research suggests that holistic processing often finishes before analytic processing (e.g., Breitmeyer & Ganz, 1976, 1977; Navon, 1977). Other research suggests that holistic processing dominates early category learning, with analytic processing refining subsequent learning (Kemler Neslon, 1989). Such differences between holistic and analytic processing suggest that different neural systems underlie them.

Analogous to analytic CZs, we assume that holistic CZs contain conjunctive neurons that capture activation patterns in feature maps for holistic properties. Following the SIT principle, we assume that two conjunctive neurons are topographically close to the extent that the holistic properties they link are similar. Thus one region of a holistic CZ in vision might capture overall shape information, another might capture information about major axes, and another might capture configural relations between analytic parts. As a result, holistic information about a category may be distributed across holistic CZs, rather than being localised spatially, analogous to the distribution of analytic properties across analytic CZs (Figure 4).

Holistic CZs may also play important roles in expertise. Recent evidence suggests that the acquisition of configural information underlies various forms of visual expertise, ranging from face perception, to greeble perception, to bird watching (e.g., Gauthier, Tarr, Anderson, Skudlarski, & Gore, 1999; Johnson & Mervis, 1997; Rackover, 2002). In some cases, this configural information allows experts to shift the basic level of categorisation down to the subordinate level. We assume that holistic CZs capture the relevant configural properties. Of interest, though, is whether the configural properties that underlie expertise are processed before analytic properties, like nonexpert holistic properties, or whether they are processed afterwards. Current theories of skill learning suggest that the storage of exemplars underlies expert performance, and that these exemplars are learned *after* the initial formation of rules during analytic processing (Logan, 1988). This suggests that different kinds of holistic properties may be extracted early vs. late during perception, with those extracted later being relevant to expertise. Regardless, we assume that these properties are organised around the SIT principle in holistic CZs.

## Modality CZs

As the conceptual structure theory emphasises, the members of taxonomic categories tend to share correlated properties. As a result, the distributed pattern of activity for a category in analytic CZs provides a rich brew of statistical information just waiting to be extracted by higher-level systems. This is the task of modality CZs.

During perception, conjunctive neurons in modality CZs capture statistical regularities across the distributed activity in analytic and holistic CZs. Modality CZs neither process features (the job of feature maps), nor do they conjoin features into conceptual properties (the job of analytic and holistic CZs). Instead modality CZs capture correlations between various analytic and holistic properties. Because such property correlations are central to category structure, modality CZs are essentially category learners—they form category representations. At this point, however, modality CZs are only learning a category in *one* modality. Whereas modality CZs for vision capture the visual properties of a category, modality CZs for motor movement capture its action properties. As Figure 3 shows, modality CZs exist for each modality. As discussed in the next section, cross-modal CZs integrate the category's properties across modalities.

Within a modality CZ, conjunctive neurons are tuned to particular conjunctions of properties within the respective modality. Thus, a conjunctive neuron in the modality CZ for vision might capture the co-occurring presence of *red*, *round*, and *smooth*. Following the SIT principle, conjunctive neurons should be near each other to the extent that they capture similar conjunctions of properties. Conversely, conjunctive neurons that capture completely different sets of conjunctive properties should be far apart. To make this clearer, consider the categories of dogs, cats, and shoes. As different dogs are perceived, similar but somewhat different properties will be linked for them in analytic and holistic CZs. Because the property conjunctions for different dogs tend to be similar, conjunctive neurons in the modality CZ that are topographically close will capture them, as Panel A of Figure 5 illustrates. Next consider cats. Because different cats have similar analytic and holistic properties, conjunctive neurons that are spatially close in modality CZs will capture them. As Figure 5a illustrates, however, the greater similarity within dogs and within cats than between them results in some separation between their conjunctive neurons in modality CZs. Finally, consider shoes. Again, conjunctive neurons will

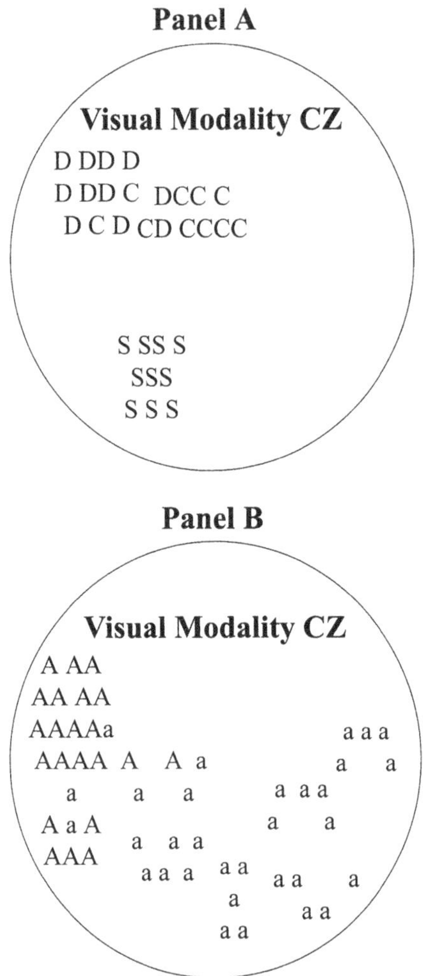


**Figure 5.** *Panel A illustrates the conjunctive neurons in a visual modality CZ that capture property correlations for dogs (D), cats (C), and shoes (S). Panel B illustrates the differential dispersion of the conjunctive neurons in a visual modality CZ for animals (A) vs. artefacts (a).*

cluster for the category in modality CZs. Because shoes differ more from dogs and cats than dogs and cats differ from each other, the conjunctive neurons for shoes lie relatively far from those for dogs and cats. As this example illustrates, modality CZs topographically capture the statistical "lumps" of conceptual information important in conceptual structure theory.

Another important property of modality CZs follows from the variable dispersion principle, which states that the dispersion of conjunctive neurons for a category reflects the similarity of the category's instances. Panel B of Figure 5 illustrates this principle in modality CZs. First consider conjunctive neurons in visual modality CZs for animals. Because different animals share many visual properties, the conjunctive neurons that capture their property conjunctions should lie near each other. Conversely, consider the conjunctive neurons for artefacts. Because different artefacts have more diverse visual properties, the conjunctive neurons that capture their property conjunctions should be more dispersed. As discussed later, these differences in dispersion play important roles in explaining various conceptual deficits.

## Cross-modal CZs

Whereas modality CZs conjoin properties within modalities, cross-modal CZs conjoin properties between modalities. Within a modality, the modality CZ creates a category representation but only on that modality. In contrast, cross-modal CZs create the complete representation of a category across modalities. Cross-modal CZs operate according to the same principles as modality CZs, except that the conjunctive neurons in cross-modal CZs link the conjunctive neurons in modality CZs, which in turn link conjunctive neurons in analytic and holistic CZs.

One might think that cross-modal integration of this sort is impossible: Because information on different modalities is represented in different formats (e.g., visual, auditory, olfactory, motor), they could not possibly be recoded into a common format. This is not a problem for CTT's cross-modal CZs, because conjunctive neurons in cross-modal CZs simply note the simultaneous firings of conjunctive neurons in modality CZs—they do not care about the format of the information ultimately represented in feature maps. Recoding into a common format is not necessary.

*Complex property profiles.* As we saw earlier, the sensory-functional theory divides conceptual properties into two types—sensory and functional—and proposes that conceptual deficits result from the loss of one property type or the other. In recent work, McRae and Cree (2002) showed that this simple division of property information is not adequate to explain the patterns of conceptual deficits in the literature (also see Cree & McRae, in press). However, a more detailed analysis of property types, based on a coding scheme developed by Wu and Barsalou (2003), does explain these deficits. Specifically, McRae and Cree coded categories for the extent to which they included external components, internal components, external surface features, internal surface features, materials, functions, and entity behaviours. McRae and Cree then computed how similar different categories are in possessing these different property types. For example, artefacts and foods are similar in both having *functions.* Most importantly, how categories cluster based on sharing these property types predicts the clusters of categories lost in category deficits.

This result bears on the organisation of conjunctive neurons in cross-modal CZs. To the extent that two categories are similar on one or more of McRae and Cree's seven property types, the closer their conjunctive neurons lie in cross-modal CZs, following the SIT principle. The closer two categories are, the easier it is for a localised brain lesion to compromise both.

One further implication of McRae and Cree's analysis concerns the relation of cross-modal CZs to modality CZs: It would be incorrect to presume that the topographic organisation of cross-modal CZs mirrors the topographic organisation of modality CZs. When two categories have similar properties on a specific modality, but different properties across modalities, their conjunctive neurons should be closer in modality CZs than in cross-modal CZs. For example, live animals and stuffed animals look similar visually, thereby causing their conjunctive neurons in visual modality CZs to lie close. However, because these categories differ substantially in auditory and olfactory properties, their conjunctive neurons in cross-modal CZs lie farther apart. As this example illustrates, the SIT principle interacts with complex property profiles to determine the proximity of conjunctive neurons at each level of analysis.

## The lexicon

Thus far we have discussed the organisation of the human conceptual system. Clearly, though, words are tied closely to the use of concepts in humans. Although we believe that the lexicon plays a central role in conceptual processing, we do not show it as a separate system in Figure 3. This reflects our belief that the lexicon is distributed throughout the same brain systems as the conceptual system. Perhaps the main difference is that the lexicon's primary presence is in the left hemisphere, whereas the conceptual system is bilateral (e.g., Gainotti, Silveri, Daniele, & Giustolisi, 1995; Lambon Ralph, McClelland, Patterson, Galton, & Hodges, 2001).

At the level of feature maps, the perception of words in vision, audition, and touch is represented in the respective modalities. Maps that represent the acoustic features of phonemes in the auditory system detect spoken words; line and vertex feature maps in the visual system detect written words; analogous feature maps in the somatosensory system detect Braille. Clearly these feature maps may play roles in the processing of nonlinguistic stimuli as well. For spoken language, however, certain auditory feature maps may be relatively specialised for linguistic processing.

At the level of analytic and holistic CZs, localised areas may develop for linguistic stimuli in the respective modalities. Following the SIT principle, the conjunctive neurons that link analytic and holistic features for words may be relatively localised, because the conjunctions of features that constitute phonemes and letters are relatively unique. For example, the conjunction of a bilabial stop and voicing that specifies /b/ may be relatively unlike most other auditory properties.

At the level of modality CZs, the conjunctive neurons that integrate phonemes and letters into words may be relatively localised. Again, following the SIT principle, the uniqueness of these conjunctions may distinguish them. In auditory CZs, spoken words may be relatively distinct from other auditory stimuli, with analogous distinctions existing for written language and Braille. As a result, the conjunctive areas representing words may be separate topographically from the conjunctive areas representing concepts, creating the appearance that lexical and conceptual knowledge are processed in separate systems.

Finally, at the level of cross-modal CZs, subsets of conjunctive neurons link different forms of the same word across modalities. Thus, conjunctive neurons link the spoken and written forms of "chair" in the auditory and visual modalities, respectively, thereby providing a higher-order lexical entry of sorts. On this view, a "lexical item" is simply a population of conjunctive neurons that point to other conjunctive neurons that ultimately organise the respective features in feature maps.

As this account illustrates, the lexicon is distributed throughout the same brain systems that represent conceptual knowledge (except not as bilaterally). Because of the SIT principle, however, the representations of words are somewhat localised within these systems. The unique perceptual features of words isolate them, especially in the topographies of higher-order CZs.

Finally additional cross-modal CZs integrate conjunctive neurons for words with conjunctive neurons for concepts. Following the SIT principle, conjunctive neurons in these CZs are topographically close to the extent that the words and concepts they conjoin are similar. Specifically, the spatial proximity of two conjunctive neurons should be a function of two factors: (1) the similarity of the words they link in terms of their phonological and orthographic properties, and (2) the similarity of the concepts they link in terms of their analytic and holistic properties. An intriguing issue is whether word organisation or conceptual organisation dominates topographical clustering in these CZs, or whether clustering is an equal function of both.

# NEURAL LOCALISATION OF CTT COMPONENTS

The previous section outlined a functional architecture for representing knowledge. As Table 1 illustrates, various anatomical predictions follow from this architecture. The current section reviews neuroscience evidence for these predictions. A later section analogously presents predictions for

**Table 1.** *Neuroanatomical predictions from conceptual topography theory (CTT)*

| *CTT component* | *Neuroanatomical predictions* |
|---|---|
| Feature maps | 1. Early topographic regions in sensory-motor processing streams detect and represent features that are utilised, not only in perception and action, but also in conceptual processing. |
| Analytic CZs | 2. Just downstream from feature maps, modality-specific association areas conjoin conjunctions of features into analytic conceptual properties. |
| | 3. Analytic CZs are organised topographically by property, not by category. |
| Holistic CZs | 4. Also just downstream from feature maps, modality-specific association areas conjoin conjunctions of features into holistic conceptual properties. |
| | 5. Holistic CZs are organised topographically by property, not by category. |
| Modality CZs | 6. Modality CZs near the end of the processing stream on a sensory-motor modality conjoin analytic and holistic properties only on that modality. |
| | 7. Modality CZs are organised topographically by category. The organisation of conjunctive neurons by similarity produces a rough categorical topography implicitly (there are no category-specific CZs). |
| Cross-modal CZs | 8. Cross-modal CZs reside in brain regions having projections to multiple modality CZs, thereby supporting the integration of category properties across modalities. |
| | 9. Modality CZs are organised topographically by category, again implicitly. |
| | 10. Some cross-modal CZs may be specialised for conjoining properties across modalities for evolutionarily important categories, such as emotions, words, etc. |

conceptual deficits and reviews the clinical evidence for them.

## Feature maps

Feature maps are some of the most well-understood systems in the brain. Each modality contains hierarchically organised regions of neurons that capture specific features. Perhaps the most studied system is the macaque visual cortex. Starting in primary visual cortex, V1, and moving into areas V2, V3, V4, MT, and TEO, columns of neurons tuned to specific features process the visual stream (Tanaka, 1997a). Neurons in area MT, for example, extract movement direction, whereas neurons in V4 extract colour. Analysis in these regions occurs largely in parallel, with each area typically having projections to the others (Kandel, 1991).

Similar feature systems reside in other modalities besides vision. In somatosensory cortex, columns of neurons along the post-central gyrus are arranged somatotopically to detect physical stimulation at specific bodily locations (Dodd & Kelly, 1991). In the motor system, neurons along the pre-central gyrus are analogously arranged to generate movements in specific muscle groups (Ghez, 1991). In the auditory system, columns of neurons along the superior temporal gyrus are ordered tonotopically, from the lowest frequencies at the anterior end of primary auditory cortex, to the highest frequencies at the posterior end (Schreiner, Read, & Sutter, 2000).

*The distribution of feature maps.* An open question is how far feature maps are distributed down the processing stream. Some evidence suggest that the borders between visual feature maps and adjacent CZs are graded, not discrete. For example, Tanaka (1997a) reports that the percentage of neurons responsive to moderately complex feature conjunctions increases gradually as one moves from V4 to TEO to TE. Thus feature detectors and the conjunctive neurons that integrate them appear mixed together in transitional regions. Findings from the visual imagery literature can be interpreted as telling a similar story. In some studies, imagery activates primary sensory-motor areas, whereas in other studies it just activates secondary ones (e.g., Thompson & Kosslyn, 2000). In both cases, human subjects appear to experience imagery, which suggests that feature maps are distributed from primary to secondary visual areas.

Regardless of how far feature maps are distributed down processing streams, their task is to analyse complex sensory signals and extract the information to which they are tuned. Activation of specific neurons constitutes a signal that a particular feature is present in the input stream.

## Analytic CZs

As described earlier, conjunctive neurons in analytic CZs link patterns of active feature detectors to represent analytic conceptual properties. According to the SIT principle, conjunctive neurons that link similar features lie near each other topographically in analytic CZs.

If this account is correct, two neuroanatomical predictions follow. First, neurons that conjoin features into higher-level conjunctions should lie just downstream from feature maps in the processing stream for a modality. Second, the proximity of conjunctive neurons in analytic CZs should follow the SIT principle. The evidence reviewed in this section offers preliminary evidence for both predictions.

*Evidence from area TE in the macaque.* Much evidence for the existence and placement of analytic CZs comes from work on the macaque visual system. According to Tanaka (1997a, 1997c), neurons along the occipital-temporal juncture, and also in the ventral and inferior temporal cortex, capture relatively complex feature conjunctions in earlier areas that contain feature maps (e.g., V1, V2, V4, TEO). Using a combination of single-unit recording and optical imaging techniques, Tanaka and his colleagues have focused on area TE in the inferior temporal cortex, mapping its functional and topographic organisation (e.g., Fujita, Tanaka, Ito, & Cheng, 1992; Kobatake & Tanaka, 1994; Tanaka, 1996, 1997b, 1997c; Wang, Tanaka, & Tanifuji, 1996). Consistent with CTT, these researchers show that TE has significant projections back to virtually all earlier visual processing areas (TEO, V4, V2, V1), with TE's cells tuned selectively to the presence of specific feature arrangements (Tanaka, 1997a).[8]

Conjunctive neurons in TE are organised into columns that stretch nearly the depth of the cortex, from layers two to six. Consistent with the SIT principle, these columns appear to be organised around the similarity of feature conjunctions. Fujita et al. (1992) inserted electrodes vertically into TE columns, isolated single neurons, and then recorded spike activity to three-dimensional objects. When a cell was particularly responsive to an object, the researchers produced a digital image of the object and used a computer to systematically pare down its features. Images were simplified until the minimum feature combination that maximally activated the neuron was identified, thereby isolating the feature combination for which the cell was tuned selectively. For example, a neuron that initially responded to an upside-down water bottle with a straw hanging out of the lid was eventually found to respond selectively to a vertically aligned ellipse with a small, thin line protruding from the bottom (for more on this technique see Tanaka, 1997a). Within a TE column, Fujita et al. found that all of its neurons responded to similar feature conjunctions. In further research using optical imaging, Wang et al. (1996) found that adjacent columns responded to related, but not identical, feature conjunctions.

Based on these findings, Tanaka (1997c, p. 524) speculated that "one function of the inferotemporal columns may be to augment feature variations around selected center points in the feature space; they may also facilitate computations among these variations. One or two principle components of the variations are mapped along the cortical surface." Such organisation follows directly from the SIT principle: Because two different orientations of a feature configuration are so similar, the conjunctive neurons that capture their respective features lie close to one another.

Although Tanaka and his colleagues report evidence consistent with the SIT principle, they note an important limitation. The sheer size of the feature space that must be laid out across a two-dimensional cortical surface means that the global organisation of TE cannot be a smooth function of similarity. Instead discontinuities should arise

[8] TE neurons are not the earliest cells that respond to co-occurring features—some cells in V4 respond in this way—but the proportion of such cells is significantly greater in TE (Kobatake & Tanaka, 1994).

where adjacent columns conjoin feature conjunctions that vary considerably. Nevertheless, two findings clearly support the SIT principle, first, the finding that neurons within a column represent a common conjunction, and second, that adjacent columns sometimes code similar conjunctions. Although it is physically impossible for an entire analytic CZ to reflect similarity, similarity still has considerable influence on the CZ's topography. We assume that such discontinuities are likely to arise in CZs at all levels of abstraction.

*Distributed representation in analytic CZs.* As we just saw, similar properties are often located near one another topographically. As described earlier, an implication of this organisation is that the representation of a particular category should be distributed widely over analytic CZs. The category's representation should not be localised at this level, because the SIT principle organises conjunctive neurons by property type—not by category. Because a given category typically has many types of properties, its representation in analytic CZs is distributed broadly. Because the members of a category tend to share properties, however, a shared set of distributed regions develops to represent these properties. Findings from two recent studies support this prediction.

Thomas, Van Hulle, and Vogels (2001) recorded from neurons distributed across macaque inferior temporal cortex (IT) during a simple categorisation task (e.g., whether a pictured object was a tree or something else). Using a Kohonen self-organising map to model the information-bearing properties of IT neurons, Thomas et al. found that, as a whole, these neurons contained sufficient information to distinguish the categories from one another.

Thomas et al. report two further findings in support of the conclusion that IT neurons code the analytic properties of categories. First, Thomas et al. observed some neurons that only responded to a single category, versus other neurons that responded to both categories, but to one more than to the other. These latter neurons, which were distributed throughout the recording region, played the most important role in categorisation. The authors concluded that these "broadly tuned feature detecting (almost certainly complex features) neurons" were central to the visual categorisation task (p. 198).

Thomas et al. further found that none of the recorded neurons responded to all of a category's exemplars. This finding is consistent with the idea that different exemplars of a category have somewhat different properties, linked by somewhat different sets of conjunctive neurons. Although all of these neurons may be useful in predicting category membership, none represents a property true of every exemplar, given that no such properties exist. Furthermore, the finding that some neurons responded to multiple categories is consistent with the fact that some properties occur in many categories, not just one.

Together, these findings support the conclusion that IT neurons capture the informational structure of visual categories at the level of conceptual properties. Consistent with CTT, a widely distributed set of conjunctive neurons in IT appears to represent the properties of a category, with some properties being unique for particular categories, and other properties being shared.

A second line of work further supports these conclusions. Using fMRI, Haxby et al. (2001) imaged the ventral temporal lobe in humans as they viewed pictures of cats, faces, houses, chairs, scissors, shoes, bottles, and nonsense patterns. Similar to Thomas et al., Haxby et al. found that a unique pattern of widely distributed activity predicted membership in each category. By observing a given pattern of brain activation, it was possible to predict the category viewed with 67% to 100% accuracy.

The structure of these activation patterns conforms to both Thomas et al.'s findings and to CTT's proposals about analytic CZs. First, the activation pattern that predicted each category contained topographically distributed regions of active neurons. This is again consistent with CTT's proposal that the multiple properties representing a category are distributed widely throughout analytic CZs. Within each activation pattern, one region was always more active than any of the others, namely, the *local maximum*. Interestingly, when the local maxima were excluded from analyses, the remaining active areas still predicted the category viewed. Thus multiple distributed regions represent a category's informational structure, not just one (i.e., the local maximum). Enough distinguishing information exists in the remaining properties to perform categorisation.

Haxby et al. further found that the activation patterns for different categories often overlapped, suggesting that a shared subregion represented a property common to multiple categories. Similar to Thomas et al.'s findings, these brain areas appear to capture a category's informational structure. Because categories often overlap in their properties, the brain regions that represent properties overlap as well.

Haxby et al. make an additional claim that is relevant to later sections on conceptual deficits: A lesion to the ventral temporal lobe could not produce a deficit in one and only one category. Because any given subregion responded to multiple categories, no well-placed lesion could knock out a single one. Haxby and colleagues conclude that "ventral temporal cortex has a topographically organized representation of attributes of form that underlie face and object recognition" (Haxby, Gobbini, Furey, Ishai, Schowten, & Pietriui, 2001, p. 2425). At this time, it is not known which particular properties these regions represent. Nevertheless, these regions do appear to represent category properties, given that they differentially predict category membership (if these regions were used to process all categories, they wouldn't be diagnostic). Regardless, these results are consistent with CTT's predictions about analytic CZs: Property information is distributed widely throughout these CZs, and multiple categories typically share properties.

*Localised property representations in occipital-temporal cortex.* In neuroimaging studies, Martin and his colleagues have extensively assessed the neural localisation of property representations (for reviews, see Martin, 2001; Martin & Chao, 2001; Martin, Ungerleider, & Haxby, 2000). In particular, these researchers have identified the brain regions that process object colour, form, and motion, for both animals and tools. Their findings indicate that brain regions just downstream from early vision areas capture these object properties. Furthermore, these properties appear organized according to the SIT principle, with similar properties lying nearer to each other than dissimilar properties.

For object colour, areas just anterior to V4 represent colour properties. For object form, areas in ventral occipito-temporal cortex represent *form* properties. For object motion, areas in the lateral temporal cortex represent *motion* properties. The localised representations of these three property types conform to the SIT principle's prediction that property types should cluster separately in analytic CZs. Different property types reside in different neural areas.

The representations of these property types for animals vs. tools offers even stronger support for the SIT principle. Form properties for animals reside right next to form properties for tools (lateral fusiform vs. medial fusiform gyrus, respectively). As the SIT principle predicts, form properties for animals and tools lie closer to each other than to colour and motion properties. The same relationship holds for motion properties. Motion properties for animals reside in superior temporal sulcus, whereas motion properties for tools reside just adjacently in middle temporal gyrus. Both of these areas are just anterior to area MT that underlies visual motion perception.

The overall layout of properties in occipital-temporal cortex provides evidence that the SIT principle organises analytic CZs. Not only are property types localised separately, the spatial proximity of property types reflects their conceptual similarity. The same property type for animals and tools (e.g., form) resides in different but adjacent areas, which lie closer together than two different property types for the same category (e.g., form and motion for animals).

## Holistic CZs

We only address the possible location of holistic CZs in the visual system, but assume that similar CZs exist for other modalities. It is not clear where the feature maps for holistic processing in vision end, and where the CZs for capturing holistic properties begin. We suspect that holistic feature maps reside in early visual processing areas. For example, Zhou, Friedman, and Von der Heydt (2000) report that cells in V2 and V4 (and to a lesser extent in V1) code invariant boundaries of objects. In contrast, holistic CZs probably lie further along the visual processing stream. For example, Kanwisher and her colleagues report that the lateral occipital complex (LOC) and fusiform gyrus are important for processing configurations of object parts (Kanwisher, Woods, Iacoboni, & Mazziotta, 1997; Kourtzi & Kanwisher, 2001). Other research similarly localises configural processing in both the LOC (Hasson, Hendler, Ben Bashat, & Malach, 2001) and the fusiform gyrus (Gauthier et al., 1999). Currently we know of no evidence that the SIT principle organises these areas, although we predict that it does, just as we saw for the Martin studies in analytic CZs. Analogous to property CZs, conjunctive neurons in holistic CZs should be organised by the type of holistic property they encode. In addition, distributed regions of conjunctive neurons should capture the holistic property structures of different categories, with the same conjunctive neurons often representing holistic information across multiple categories.

## Modality CZs

As we have seen, analytic and holistic CZs extract property information about categories. Furthermore, the topography of these CZs appears to reflect informational structure. Because properties vary across exemplars, no single conjunctive area becomes essential for a given category. Because multiple categories often share properties, a given conjunctive area is active for multiple categories. Thus analytic and holistic CZs contain the requisite information for a later processing stage that captures categories, not just their properties. In this spirit, Thomas et al. (2001, p. 190) state, "only one additional layer of processing is required to extract the categories from a population of IT neurons." In CTT, modality CZs and cross-modal CZs extract these category-level representations. We discuss the neural localisation of modality CZs in this section, and the localisation of cross-modal CZs in the next.

As described earlier, CTT proposes that conjunctive neurons in modality CZs link the conjunctions of analytic and holistic properties for a category exemplar in a given modality (where these properties are represented by earlier conjunctive neurons that link features in feature maps). Furthermore, the SIT principle specifies that the topographical proximity of conjunctive neurons in modality CZs generally increases with the similarity of the property conjunctions they link.

Importantly, these neurons are *not* tuned to categories. Instead these neurons are tuned to specific conjunctions of properties that may happen to occur for a category's exemplars, but not necessarily so. *There are no category-specific CZs.* Nevertheless, to the extent that a category's exemplars share many properties, the conjunctive neurons in modality CZs that link them should cluster together topographically. As a result, an imprecise category-specific region may emerge for the category within the CZ. Although individual conjunctive neurons do not represent categories, larger groups of them may, although conjunctive neurons for other categories may be somewhat interspersed, following the variable dispersion principle. In the terms of conceptual structure theory, lumpy conceptual space becomes represented in lumpy neural space.

In the visual system, the modality CZ should be located at the end of the ventral pathway, most likely in the anterior inferior temporal cortex, or in parts of the perirhinal and/or entorhinal cortices. Staining and lesion studies indicate that these locations receive significant projections from the IT cortex (Tanaka, 1997a, 1997c), and that they also have projections to and from other polymodal brain areas, which will be important in the next section for cross-modal CZs (e.g., Murray & Richmond, 2001).

Perhaps the most compelling evidence for modality CZs in these visual areas comes from Kreiman, Koch, and Fried (2000a, 2000b). In these studies, single neuron responses to visual stimuli were recorded from electrodes implanted in the medial temporal lobes of human epilepsy patients. In Kreiman et al. (2000a), the stimuli were complex images of objects drawn from various categories: animals, foods, manipulable objects, cars, famous faces, emotional faces, spatial layouts, and complex patterns. Neurons in the entorhinal cortex, amygdala, and hippocampus exhibited category-specific changes in firing rates. Some responded selectively to all animal pictures in the stimulus set. Others responded selectively to all face pictures. Category-selective neurons were observed for every category presented.[9]

Kreiman et al. (2000b) replicated these findings and observed firing rate changes in category-specific neurons, not only during picture presentation, but also for mental imagery of previously viewed pictures. Interestingly, many of the same neurons were active during both the perception and imagery conditions, a finding that coincides nicely with CTT's assumption that perceptual and conceptual processing share neural mechanisms (Barsalou, 1999).

These findings support CTT's prediction that conjunctive neurons in modality CZs capture regularities in the properties for specific categories. At this time, we know of no direct evidence that the SIT principle organises these conjunctive neurons, although we predict that the more similar two categories are, the closer their conjunctive neurons should lie in modality CZs. The later section on conceptual deficits provides indirect support for such organisation.

## Cross-modal CZs

As we just saw, CTT assumes that modality CZs integrate the properties of a category on a single modality. At that level, multiple representations of the category exist on all the modalities for which it has properties. What remains is to integrate information for the category across modalities. Cross-modal CZs play this role.

*Perirhinal cortex.* To accomplish cross-modal integration, cross-modal CZs must be located in brain areas that are highly connected to lower-order convergence zones for the various modalities. One region with such connections is the hippocampus. However, because patients with near total loss of the hippocampus often maintain conceptual knowledge (e.g., Mishkin, Vargha-Khadem, & Gadian, 1998), this structure is an unlikely candidate for the respective cross-modal CZs. The perirhinal cortex is a more likely possibility. Accumulating evidence indicates that perirhinal cortex is important for (1) integrating information about objects across sensory modalities, and (2) establishing associative relations between different concepts (e.g., Murray & Richmond, 2001). For example, lesion studies with monkeys demonstrate that perirhinal cortex is required for learning arbitrary associations between visual objects and the taste/smell of particular foods (Parker & Gaffan, 1998). Furthermore, monkeys with perirhinal lesions are impaired at visually identifying foods that taste good. Together these results suggest that perirhinal cortex integrates visual and gustatory information, implicating this area as a cross-modal CZ.

Perirhinal lesions similarly impair the ability to link an object's auditory and tactile properties with its visual and gustatory properties (e.g., Goulet & Murray, 2001; Higuchi & Miyashita, 1996; Holdstock, Gutnikov, Gaffan, & Mayes, 2000; Murray, Gaffan, & Mishkin, 1993; Parker & Gaffan, 1998). Based on these accumulating findings, Murray and Richmond (2001, p. 191) conclude that the perirhinal cortex "is an essential part of a system for storing fact-like information about objects . . . [and that] this 'object knowledge' system appears to be analogous to a semantic memory system in humans."

In this spirit, many models of conceptual deficits in humans propose "encyclopaedic knowledge" stores that are tantamount to associative, fact-like representation systems. In CTT, cross-modal CZs such as the perirhinal cortex implement this type of knowledge via associations between multiple concepts across modalities. Thus the knowledge

[9] Such neurons should not be confused with the infamous grandmother cell. As should be clear in the text, we assume that *populations* of conjunctive neurons integrate category features—not just a single conjunctive neuron. Also a given conjunctive neuron is likely to participate in the representation of *multiple* categories—not just one.

that a beaver builds a dam may be mediated by conjunctive neurons in the perirhinal cortex that link concepts for beavers, build, dam, trees, river, etc. Notably, however, cross-modal CZs do not literally contain this conceptual content, as is typically the case in current theories that employ knowledge stores. Instead conjunctive neurons in these CZs point to a hierarchy of lower-order conjunctive neurons that eventually activate features in feature maps. Ultimately the representation of a fact is a complex simulation of its content involving multiple concepts on multiple modalities.

*Cross-modal CZs in emotion.* Recent research suggests that specific areas organise emotion representations across modalities. For example, Anderson and Phelps (2000) suggested that somatosensory areas in the right hemisphere integrate "functionally distinct affective maps at different levels of organization" (also see Adolphs, Damasio, Tranel, Cooper, & Damasio, 2000). In particular, these CZs appear to integrate facial and bodily information for particular emotions.

Following A. R. Damasio's (1994) somatic marker theory, various researchers have similarly found that orbito-frontal cortex integrates emotional and conceptual information (e.g., Davidson, 2000; Davidson, Jackson, & Kalin, 2000). Specifically, conjunctive neurons in orbitofrontal cortex link a category's properties with associated emotional states (somatic markers). When a new category instance is encountered, the category's properties become active, which then activate its somatic markers, via conjunctive neurons in orbitofrontal cortex. The average of the activated somatic markers then provides a plausible emotional response to the new instance.

Besides providing evidence for cross-modal CZs, this work on emotion suggests an important constraint on them: Cross-modal CZs may often be tailored to conjoin particular sets of modalities that serve an important role in the cognitive system. For example, because different sources of information about emotion must be integrated, cross-modal CZs may develop in right somatosensory cortex for this purpose. Similarly, because conceptual and emotional information must be integrated, cross-modal CZs may develop in orbito-frontal cortex. Such cases suggest that some cross-modal CZs develop to integrate specific sources of modality-specific information that serve some purpose.

*Cross-modal CZs in language.* Similar sorts of cross-modal CZs appear tailored to language. Based on lesion studies, Tranel and his colleagues found that left prefrontal and premotor regions underlie the retrieval of words for actions, whereas left anterior and inferior temporal regions underlie the retrieval of words for concrete objects (Tranel, Adolphs, Damasio, & Damasio, 2001; Tranel, Damasio, & Damasio, 1998). In these studies, lesion patients had to name actions or concrete objects, thereby requiring them to link conceptual representations of categories with the respective words. When patients had lesions in left prefrontal and premotor regions, they could not make these mappings for action words; when they had lesions in left anterior and inferior temporal regions, they could not make these mappings for object words. These findings suggest that the respective brain areas constitute cross-modal CZs that link concepts and words.

### Summary

Findings in the neuroscience literature support predictions of the CTT architecture. We hasten to add, however, that this evidence is open to alternative interpretations. Furthermore, we are the first to agree that much more evidence is necessary before embracing CTT with high confidence. Although we find the existing evidence encouraging, much further research is clearly needed. The evidence that initially motivated CTT—conceptual deficits—is the topic of the next two sections.

## CONCEPTUAL DEFICITS

We next describe six findings for conceptual deficits that we believe any account must explain. In the subsequent section, we systematically step through CTT, addressing how damage to its various components produces these findings.

## Finding #1: Multiple-category deficits that reflect property profiles

In many cases, patients who suffer a conceptual deficit lose more than one category. In their review, McRae and Cree (2002) list seven common forms that multiple-category deficits take: (1) Multiple categories that constitute creatures, (2) multiple categories that constitute nonliving things, (3) fruits and vegetables, (4) fruits and vegetables with either creatures or nonliving things, (5) foods with living things, (6) musical instruments with living things, (7) gemstones with living things.

The standard goal of sensory-functional theories has been to explain these patterns (e.g., Farah & McClelland, 1991; Humphreys & Forde, 2001; Warrington & Shallice, 1984). As McRae and Cree note, however, the standard forms of sensory-functional theory cannot explain all seven (also see Caramazza & Shelton, 1998). Standard theories typically distinguish only between sensory and functional properties, which provide too few parameters for explaining all seven patterns. McRae and Cree's contribution is to extend the number of critical property types significantly, with each pattern resulting from loss to one or more property types.

This set of findings offers two important constraints on theories of conceptual deficits. First, a conceptual deficit can include multiple categories, not just one. Second, when multiple categories are lost, they reflect damage to specific property types that the lost categories share.

## Finding #2: Single-category deficits

At the opposite end of the deficit continuum lie single-category deficits. Rather than losing multiple categories, some individuals lose just one (Capitani, Laiacona, Mahon, & Caramazza, 2003-this issue; Caramazza & Shelton, 1998; Hart & Gordon, 1992). Furthermore, some of these patients lose the ability to process the category across all the sensory modalities tested—the deficit is not limited to a single modality. For example, EW demonstrated impaired recognition, naming, and knowledge comprehension for animals, whether tested in the visual or auditory/verbal modalities (Caramazza & Shelton, 1998). Her deficit cannot be attributed to low familiarity and frequency of animals, given careful control of these factors. In addition, perceptual deficits did not accompany her conceptual deficits, thereby implicating higher-order conceptual structures.

Other patients exhibit different single-category deficits. One patient reportedly lost knowledge of number (Cipolotti, Butterworth, & Denes, 1991); another lost knowledge of medical concepts (Crosson, Moberg, Boone, Rothi, & Raymer, 1997); yet another lost knowledge of musical notation (Cappelletti, Waley-Cohen, Butterworth, & Kopelman, 2000). Because of such cases, theories must account for single-category deficits as well as multiple ones.

## Finding #3: Deficits for nonliving things are infrequent

Relative to deficits for living things, deficits for nonliving things are relatively infrequent. Reports of the former are much more common than the latter, as reviewers of this literature often note (Caramazza & Shelton, 1998; Humphreys & Forde, 2001; Tyler et al., 2000).

## Finding #4: Deficits occur at the superordinate level, not at the basic level

Conceptual deficits are typically characterised by the loss of relatively large categories, such as superordinates, that reside toward the top of taxonomic hierarchies (Rosch, Mervis, Gray, Johnson, & Boyes-Braem, 1976). To our knowledge, there are no reported cases of conceptual deficits for basic or subordinate categories. For example, deficits occur for categories like musical instruments, jewels, artefacts, or animals, but not for individual categories like violins, diamonds, chairs, or dogs. The relatively broad loss of categorical knowledge may offer an important constraint on theories of conceptual deficits.

### Finding #5: Equal loss of functional and visual properties in some living things deficits

The sensory-functional theory asserts that knowledge of living things depends more on visual/sensory information than on functional information, whereas knowledge of nonliving things depends more on functional information. As a consequence, the sensory-functional theory predicts that living things deficits should be more associated with impairments in visual/sensory properties than with impairments in functional properties. The literature does not always support this prediction. Many researchers have reported patients with living things deficits whose knowledge of functional properties was just as impaired as their knowledge of visual/sensory properties (Capitani et al., 2003-this issue; Caramazza & Shelton, 1998; Funnell & De Mornay Davies, 1996; Laiacona, Barbarotto, & Capitani, 1993; Lambon Ralph, Howard, Nightingale, & Ellis, 1998; Samson, Pillon, & De Wilde, 1998). We believe that this finding offers another important constraint on theories of conceptual deficits.

### Finding #6: Loss of visual properties, but a greater deficit for artefacts than for living things

A related problem for sensory-functional theory is a patient with an artefacts deficit whose knowledge of visual properties was more impaired than her knowledge of functional properties (Lambon Ralph et al., 1998). If living things depend more on visual properties than nonliving things, this patient should have exhibited a deficit for living things, not for artefacts. Coltheart, Inglis, Cuples, Michie, Bates, and Budd (1998) report another patient who offers a similar challenge, namely, significant loss of visual property knowledge, but equivalent knowledge of living things and non-living things. Similar to Finding #5, the relationship of living things and nonliving things to visual and functional information is far from systematic, offering a further challenge for theories.

## EXPLAINING CONCEPTUAL DEFICITS WITH CTT

The CTT architecture makes natural predictions about the types of conceptual deficits that should be observed in the clinical literature. Three mechanisms underlie CTT's predictions:

1. The presence of modality-specific processing systems that begin with feature maps and proceed through holistic, analytic, and modality CZs.
2. The presence of cross-modal CZs that integrate properties for a category across all the relevant modalities.
3. The organisation of CZs according to the SIT principle, thereby organising analytic and holistic CZs topographically by property type, but organising modality and cross-modal CZs topographically by category.

Given this hierarchical, topographically organised architecture, diverse possibilities for localised lesions exist, along with correlated possibilities for conceptual deficits. Table 2 summarises CTT's predictions. The potential for diverse deficits is realised in the literature. Indeed, such diversity is one of CTT's primary predictions. No other current theory predicts the full range of deficits. In this next section, we step through CTT's systems, discuss the implications of lesions in each, and show how such lesions produce the six findings reviewed in the previous section.

### Damage to feature maps

Damage to feature maps can disrupt both perceptual and conceptual processing. When a feature map is damaged, perception in the modality is likely to be impaired. Such perceptual deficits are not uncommon. For example, damage to V4 in the occipital lobe often produces impaired colour perception (Kandel, 1991). Similarly, bilateral lesions of the superior temporal gyrus can produce cortical deafness (Coslett, Brashear, & Heilman, 1984).

According to CTT, one function of feature maps is to help represent knowledge during conceptual processing. Thus damage to feature maps should produce conceptual deficits, not just

**Table 2.** *Deficit predictions from conceptual topography theory (CTT)*

| *CTT component* | *Deficit prediction* |
|---|---|
| General prediction | 1. A wide variety of conceptual deficits should be observed, each reflecting the part of the CTT architecture damaged. Damage to feature maps, analytic CZs, holistic CZs, modality CZs, or cross-modal CZs should each produce a different deficit. All possible deficits could, in principle, be observed. |
| Feature maps | 2. A feature map lesion should not only compromise perception on the respective modality, it should also produce conceptual deficits across those categories that utilise these features conceptually (Finding #1).<br>3. Feature map damage should primarily impair performance on strategic conceptual tasks, not on automatic ones. |
| Analytic CZs | 4. Following a lesion to an analytic CZ, perception on the respective modality should remain relatively intact, while a conceptual deficit should arise for categories that rely on the analytic property damaged.<br>5. A lesion to an analytic CZ should typically disrupt multiple categories that utilise the damaged analytic property (Finding #1). Deficits for single categories should not be observed, unless the damaged analytic property is unique to a category (Finding #2). |
| Holistic CZs | 6. Following a lesion to a holistic CZ, low-level perception on the respective modality should remain relatively intact, while a conceptual deficit should arise for categories that rely on the holistic property damaged.<br>7. A lesion to a holistic CZ should typically disrupt multiple categories that utilise the damaged holistic property (Finding #1). Deficits for single categories should not be observed, unless the damaged holistic property is unique to a category (Finding #2). |
| Modality CZs | 8. When a lesion falls largely on the conjunctive neurons for one category in a modality CZ, a category-specific deficit may result (Finding #2), but only on that modality.<br>9. When a lesion falls on the conjunctive neurons for multiple categories in a modality CZ, multiple categories should be compromised (Finding #1).<br>10. A localised lesion should be more likely to eliminate the conjunctive neurons for a narrowly dispersed category on a modality than a broadly dispersed one (Finding #3).<br>11. Because basic level categories tend to share many properties with each other, damage to a modality CZ will usually compromise multiple basic level categories. As a result, conceptual deficits will occur mostly for superordinate categories, not for basic ones (Finding #4).<br>12. Contrary to the sensory-functional theory, a category can exhibit a deficit following damage to a secondary—not a primary—modality CZ (Finding #6) (e.g., an artefacts deficit following damage to a visual CZ, not to a motor CZ). |
| Cross-modal CZs | 13. When a lesion falls largely on the conjunctive neurons for one category in a cross-modal CZ, a category-specific deficit may result across all modalities for which the category has properties (Finding #2).<br>14. When a lesion falls on conjunctive neurons for multiple categories in a cross-modal CZ, multiple categories should be compromised (Finding #1).<br>15. A localised lesion should be more likely to eliminate the conjunctive neurons for a narrowly dispersed category on a modality than for a broadly dispersed one (Finding #3).<br>16. Because basic level categories tend to share many properties with each other, damage to a cross-modal CZ will usually compromise multiple basic level categories. As a result, conceptual deficits will occur mostly for superordinate categories, not for basic ones (Finding #4).<br>17. Contrary to the sensory-functional theory, a category can exhibit deficits for properties on both primary and secondary modalities, following a lesion to cross-modal CZs (Finding #5) (e.g., equal losses of functional and visual properties for nonliving things). |

perceptual ones. Indeed, classic agnosias offer such examples, where damage to a sensory system produces impairments in conceptual knowledge: For example, damage to colour processing areas produces deficits in colour knowledge (e.g., A. R. Damasio & Damasio, 1994; De Renzi & Spinnler, 1967).

If a particular modality is important for representing the properties of a concept, then damage to its feature maps should produce conceptual deficits on strategic tasks. Because animals depend heavily on visual properties, damage to visual feature maps should compromise knowledge of animals. Conversely, because tools depend heavily on motor properties, damage to motor maps should compromise knowledge of tools. As described earlier in the section on Distributed Representation in CZ Theory, the top-down reactivation of feature maps may only occur in conceptual tasks that require the strategic construction, manipulation, and evaluation of conceptual representations. Thus we only predict conceptual deficits on such tasks following feature map lesions. In routinised tasks, where automatised feed-forward pathways are sufficient for satisfactory task performance, we don't predict conceptual deficits in these patients.[10]

In general, damage to feature maps has the potential to produce multiple-category deficits, as described for Finding #1 in the previous section. Consistent with the sensory-functional theory, damage to a particular property type should have repercussions for any category whose instances rely on it. Because multiple categories typically use a given property type, multiple categories may often show deficits when it is damaged.

A potential problem for this account arises when patients lose perception on a modality but can still conceptualise properties on it. CTT explains such cases in several ways. First, loss of bottom-up pathways into feature maps may disable perception, while intact feature maps, along with intact top-down projections, still implement conceptualisation. Similarly, damage to feature maps may be incomplete, such that a partially intact feature map retains the capacity to support conceptual processing but not perception. Finally, it is unclear to what extent the intact conceptual performance of patients with damaged feature maps reflects their reliance on word associations to support seemingly conceptual processing (Kan et al., 2003-this issue; Solomon & Barsalou, 2003). Most, if not all, standard neuropsychological tests of conceptual knowledge are not designed to limit the degree to which patients can use word association strategies to perform tasks, thereby precluding assessments of knowledge.

## Damage to analytic CZs

Lesions in analytic CZs should impair conceptual knowledge, and possibly late perceptual processes, while leaving early sensation largely intact. In sensation, the bottom-up channels that activate feature maps remain unaffected, as do the feature maps themselves, while conjunctive neurons in an analytic CZ that combine features into conceptual properties are lost. As a result, activating the corresponding feature conjunctions is no longer possible. The content of the respective properties can no longer be retrieved, and the concepts that utilise them suffer.

As we saw earlier, the SIT principle organises analytic CZs by property type. Topographically, the conjunctive neurons that represent similar properties reside in the same region of an analytic CZ. In vision, conjunctive neurons for shape reside together, whereas conjunctive neurons for visual motion lie elsewhere. As a consequence of this organisation, localised lesions should tend to disrupt knowledge of specific property types, thereby producing multiple category deficits (i.e., Finding #1). Consistent with the sensory-functional theory, all categories that utilise a property type should be affected by its loss. Unlike damage to feature maps, however, perception should remain relatively unaffected. Many cases of conceptual deficits in the literature fit this pattern, namely, multiple category loss with no perceptual deficits.

The multiple category deficits that result from damage to an analytic CZ should exhibit certain patterns (Cree & McRae, in press; McRae & Cree, 2002). Given the wide variety of property types represented in analytic CZs, there should not just be one or two patterns, there should be many. From McRae and Cree's perspective, deficit patterns that initially appeared puzzling become straightforward. For example, fruits/vegetables and nonliving things may sometimes be lost together when the shared property type of function is lesioned.

[10] One problem in diagnosing such cases is that debilitating perceptual deficits often mask accompanying conceptual deficits, making the latter difficult to detect. Thus it would be useful to assess more thoroughly whether patients with feature map damage tend to have corresponding conceptual deficits.

Second, when multiple categories are lost, they should share properties on the damaged modality, but not necessarily on any other. Because damage is to a single modality, the categories lost should exhibit salient similarities only on it. As we will see later, when the categories lost are similar on multiple modalities, this implicates damage to cross-modal CZs instead.

Typically, loss to a particular property type should not produce a single-category deficit. However, if a property type is relatively unique for a category—no other categories share it—then damage to this area of an analytic CZ could compromise only that category (i.e., Finding #2). In general, though, because properties are generally shared across categories, single-category deficits should rarely arise this way. Instead they should typically arise after lesions to higher-order CZs that are organised by category, as we will see shortly.

## Damage to holistic CZs

Analogous to damage in an analytic CZ, damage to a holistic CZ should typically affect multiple categories that share the holistic property which is lost (i.e., Finding #1). In audition, for example, failure to apprehend the temporal envelope of a sound could reflect damage to a holistic CZ in the auditory system (Lorenzi, Wable, Moroni, Derobert, Frachet, & Belin, 2000). In vision, some patients with apperceptive visual agnosia may have suffered damage to a visual holistic CZ. Although these patients can typically perceive and recognise object parts, they cannot organise these parts into integrated perceptual wholes (e.g., Shelton, Bowers, Duara, & Heilman, 1994). When asked to copy a complex figure, these patients can occasionally draw and remember image fragments, but cannot organise them properly (e.g., Lezak, 1995). Such patterns suggest that feature maps and analytic CZs are intact, but that holistic CZs are not. Furthermore, the categories that pattern on such deficits should be similar on the same modality, but not necessarily on others.

## Damage to modality CZs

Whereas the SIT principle organises analytic and holistic CZs by property type, it organises modality CZs by category to a considerable extent. Because the proximity of conjunctive neurons reflects the similarity of the properties they conjoin, neurons that capture the correlated properties of a category tend to be localised topographically. Following the variable dispersion principle, however, the conjunctive neurons for a category are mixed with those for other categories that share similar property correlations. When high similarity exists between a category's exemplars (e.g., mammals), the dispersion of its conjunctive neurons is relatively low. Although these conjunctive neurons are somewhat dispersed, they nevertheless cluster within a relatively well-circumscribed region of the modality CZ. Conversely, when low similarity exists between a category's exemplars (e.g., artefacts), the dispersion of its conjunctive neurons is relatively high, covering a relatively broad region of the modality CZ (Figure 5b).

*Modality-specific single-category deficits.* When a lesion in a modality CZ falls squarely on the region containing the conjunctive neurons for a particular category, loss of category knowledge on that modality should result. Although other categories may have conjunctive neurons in the region, the bulk may lie elsewhere, thereby preserving them (e.g., Farah & McClelland, 1991). The result is a single-category deficit, but only on one modality, thereby making it a special case of Finding #2 (i.e., where a category is lost across all modalities).

Consider the patient Michelangelo, who exhibited impaired knowledge of visual properties for animals, relative to artefacts, but whose knowledge of functional/associative properties for animals appeared relatively intact (e.g., where they live, what they eat, how they sound, etc.; Sartori & Job, 1988). CTT explains this pattern as the result of localised damage to the visual modality CZ that integrates visual properties for animals. Because the conjunctive neurons that integrate functional/associative properties reside in different modality CZs, knowledge of these properties remained intact.

*Modality-specific multiple-category deficits.* Whenever a lesion fails to fall squarely on a categorical region in a modality CZ, multiple categories may be affected (i.e., Finding #1). Under such conditions, the categories affected should pattern according to the shared properties on the damaged modality (but again not on other modalities). Patterns of the sort addressed by McRae and Cree (2002) should arise. One prediction is that the lost categories may typically share multiple properties. Because conjunctive neurons at this level capture *correlations* of properties, a lesion should compromise the ability to represent complex *conjunctions* of properties, such that the multiple categories affected have multiple properties in common. In contrast, a lesion to an analytic or holistic CZ should be more likely just to disrupt a single property type, such that the multiple categories affected tend to be similar on one (or at least fewer) properties.

*The relative infrequency of artefact deficits.* The variable dispersion principle explains the relatively low probability that a localised lesion compromises artefacts (Finding #3). Consider Figure 5b. To the extent that the conjunctive neurons for a category are distributed broadly throughout a modality CZ, it should be difficult for a localised lesion to disrupt them completely. Because within-category similarity is relatively low for artefacts, its conjunctive neurons should be highly dispersed, thereby making it less susceptible to damage. Conversely, because animals has much higher within-category similarity, its conjunctive neurons should be more localised, and therefore more susceptible to damage.

A related implication is that certain concepts may be more susceptible to lesions in some modality CZs than in others. If a category has a narrow dispersion on one modality CZ but a broad dispersion on another, a deficit should be more likely after damage to the narrow dispersion than to the broad one. It follows that deficits for tools should be particularly associated with lesions in fronto-parietal areas that mediate action, whereas deficits for animals should be particularly associated with lesions in temporal areas that support vision (Gainotti et al., 1995; Tranel, Damasio, & Damasio, 1997). If the actions associated with tools are more similar than their visual properties, tool deficits should be more likely following lesions to motor areas than to visual areas. Conversely, if the visual properties for animals are more similar than their other properties, animal deficits should be most likely to follow lesions to visual areas.

*Deficits at high taxonomic levels.* The SIT and variable dispersion principles offer an explanation for why conceptual deficits cover superordinate categories, not basic level ones (i.e., Finding #4). Because the members of superordinate categories share many properties in a family resemblance structure (Rosch & Mervis, 1975), the conjunctive neurons that code them should all be mixed together topographically within a modality CZ. Thus a lesion that damages the conjunctive neurons for one basic level category is likely to damage the conjunctive neurons for other basic level categories that share its family resemblance features. The result is the loss of a superordinate category, or at least much of it. The relative sparing of a few exemplars that often occurs may reflect the sparing of conjunctive neurons for properties that represent a subset of the category's family resemblance structure.

*Simultaneous deficits in visual properties and nonliving things.* Damage to a modality CZ also explains Finding #6, in which patients with a deficit for visual properties also have a deficit for nonliving things. Again such findings constitute a problem for the sensory-functional theory, because it predicts that loss of visual properties should affect animals more than nonliving things. According to CTT, however, the large region in a visual modality CZ that integrates the visual properties of nonliving things has been damaged, while the relatively circumscribed region that integrates the visual properties of animals has been spared. Because the categories are topographically localised, such lesions are possible. Paradoxically, in this case, the tight clustering of animal properties in the visual modality CZ spares it.

## Damage to cross-modal CZs

As for modality CZs, CTT predicts that the conjunctive neurons in cross-modal CZs exhibit considerable topographic organisation by category. The difference is that the category knowledge linked in cross-modal CZs is multi-modal, whereas it is unimodal in modality CZs. Because of their similar organisation, however, many of the phenomena that arise in modality CZs also arise in their cross-modal counterparts.

*Single-category deficits.* When a lesion lands largely on the region of a cross-model CZ that integrates the multi-modal properties of a category, only that category may be lost (i.e., Finding #2). Unlike analogous lesions in modality CZs, such lesions in cross-modal CZs produce complete single-category deficits across modalities—the entire category is lost.

Forde, Francis, Riddoch, Rumiati, and Humphreys (1997) report a patient, SRB, with such a deficit. Following damage to an area stretching from his left medial temporal lobe to his occipital lobe, SRB exhibited impaired naming of living things, whether tested in the visual, gustatory, somatosensory, or auditory modality. SRB's loss of the category was apparently complete, consistent with a localised lesion in cross-modal CZs. Although SRB could have suffered individual damage on each of these modalities, it is more parsimonious to assume that he suffered damage to a single system that integrated information across them. The primary location of SRB's lesion—the inferior medial temporal lobe—is consistent with this conclusion. As described earlier, this area is widely implicated in cross-modal integration.

*Findings #1, #3, and #4.* Analogous to lesions in modality CZs, lesions in cross-modal CZs can produce a variety of important deficits noted in the literature. If a lesion does not fall squarely on a region that links a category but falls on a region that links multiple categories, a multiple category deficit should occur (i.e., Finding #1). Again the categories lost should tend to be similar on multiple properties, not just on one, because the conjunctive neurons in these CZs link conjunctions of properties. Furthermore, the similarities on which multiple deficits pattern should typically be multi-modal, not unimodal. Because conjunctive neurons in cross-modal CZs capture statistical regularities across modalities, conjunctive neurons lying together should link similar conjunctions of properties on different modalities.

Notably, categories that pattern together in a modality CZ may not necessarily pattern together in a cross-modal CZ. As described earlier, two categories may have similar properties on one modality but very different properties on another. Thus the same category may be lost with different other categories depending on whether the lesion falls in a modality or cross-modal CZ.

Because the variable dispersion principle applies to cross-modal CZs, categories having low within-category similarity at this level should be distributed more broadly than categories having high within-category similarity. As a result, a localised lesion should be less likely to completely disrupt all the conjunctive neurons for highly dispersed categories, such as artefacts (i.e., Finding #3).

Finally, deficits in cross-modal CZs should again primarily disrupt high-level categories, such as superordinates, rather than low-level categories, such as those at the basic level (i.e., Finding #4). Because the conjunctive neurons for different basic level categories are highly intermixed topographically, a localised deficit never disrupts just one—instead the larger superordinate is typically affected.

*Equal loss of visual and functional properties for living things.* Patients with a lesion that falls on conjunctive neurons for living things in a cross-modal CZ could exhibit equal loss of visual and functional properties (i.e., Finding #5). Again this pattern is difficult to reconcile with the sensory-functional theory, given its prediction that visual properties should suffer more than functional properties in a living things deficit. Nevertheless, this deficit is consistent with localised damage in cross-modal CZs. According to CTT, the conjunctive neurons for animals in these CZs conjoin properties across modalities. Two types of properties likely to be conjoined are those for visual recognition and function. Most importantly, a lesion to the conjunctive neurons that conjoin these properties would not only produce a deficit for animals, it would also produce roughly equivalent deficits in the retrieval of visual and functional properties for this category.

## CONCLUSIONS

Rather than being mutually exclusive, competing theories of conceptual deficits complement each other in important ways, all contributing important insights. The sensory-functional theory stresses the modality-specific representation of knowledge. The domain-specific theory stresses the circumscribed representation of individual categories. The conceptual structure theory stresses the statistical relationships that hold for properties within and between categories.

CTT integrates these insights into a single theory. Feature maps, analytic CZs, holistic CZs, and modality CZs capture the importance of modality-specific representations. The SIT principle maps the statistical structure of property information into the topographical organisation of CZs. In modality CZs and cross-modal CZs, this organisation produces representations of individual categories that are relatively circumscribed. Lesioning this distributed system produces a variety of deficits that correspond to many reported in the literature, ranging from single category deficits to multiple category deficits organised around various patterns of similarity.

A concern might be that such a theory is too complex and powerful. The conceptual system, however, is far from a simple structure, and conceptual deficits exhibit tremendous variability (Coltheart et al., 1998). CTT's ability to produce a diverse array of deficits does justice to the complexity of the phenomena. Indeed, CTT predicts that conceptual deficits should take a variety of specific forms, which they do.

Perhaps CTT's most unique contribution is the SIT principle. Although topographic organisation is well established for feature maps, its role in CZs is much less clear. Nevertheless, modest independent evidence exists for this principle in the neuroimaging and electrophysiological literatures, as we saw earlier. Perhaps the strongest evidence, though, is the SIT principle's ability to explain the wide variety of conceptual deficits. By assuming topographical organisation, we were able explain these deficits within a single framework, organised around one principle. Clearly additional direct evidence for the SIT principle is needed. Future assessments of the relation between conceptual similarity and topography within CZs are critical to assessing CTT. We would be most grateful to hear from readers who know of findings that bear on this issue.

Surprisingly little direct evidence for A. R. Damasio's (1989) convergence zone hypothesis exists as well. To what extent do conjunctive neurons in association areas reactivate feature configurations in feature maps? Again further research is essential to answering this critical question. Clearly much evidence across many literatures indicates that high-level conceptualisations re-enact sensory-motor processing. Nevertheless, little if any direct evidence exists that this re-enactment is the result of conjunctive neurons reactivating assemblies of feature detectors. Even if our assumptions about re-enactment and the SIT principle turn out to be false, the research required to rule them out may lead to the discovery of important new mechanisms. Electrophysiological studies of the relations between associative and feature neurons may be particularly informative on this issue.

Conversely, CTT fits well with a variety of new findings in the literature that implicate the modality-specific representation of knowledge. Such evidence has not just been reported in the lesion and neuroimaging literatures on concepts, but also in the neuroimaging literatures on imagery (Farah, 2001; Grezes & Decety, 2001; Jeannerod, 1995; Kosslyn, 1994) and episodic memory (Nyberg, Habib, McIntosh, & Tulving, 2000; Wheeler, Petersen, & Buckner, 2000). The behavioural literatures similarly report increasing evidence that modality-specific representations underlie concepts (Barsalou, 1999, in press-b), memory (Glenberg, 1997), and language comprehension (Glenberg, 1997; Glenberg & Kaschak, 2002; Spivey et al., 2000; Stanfield & Zwaan, 2001; Zwaan et al., 2002). Thus there is reason to believe that CTT's basic assumptions are on the right track, although much further assessment is required.

Finally, we are intrigued by the potential importance of topography throughout the brain. The topographical organisation of feature maps is well known, but the topographical organisation of CZs is not. On reflection, it is not so surprising that evolution capitalised on such a simple principle to organise the brain at multiple levels. McClelland (personal communication, 2002) suggests that related representations in the brain need to influence each other frequently, and that being topographically close minimises the use of long-distance connections. For example, the facilitory relations that produce thematic priming benefit from close connections, as do the inhibitory relations that allow one category to suppress close competitors during object recognition. In general, understanding why topographical organisation exists at multiple brain levels may lead to insights about the brain's evolution and function.

## REFERENCES


Adolphs, R., Damasio, H., Tranel, D., Cooper, G., & Damasio, A. R. (2000). A role for somatosensory cortices in the visual recognition of emotion as revealed by three-dimensional lesion mapping. *Journal of Neuroscience, 20*, 2683–2690.

Anderson, A. K., & Phelps, E. A. (2000). Perceiving emotion: There's more than meets the eye. *Current Biology, 10*, R551–R554.

Barsalou, L. W. (1983). Ad hoc categories. *Memory and Cognition, 11*, 211–227.

Barsalou, L. W. (1985). Ideals, central tendency, and frequency of instantiation as determinants of graded structure in categories. *Journal of Experimental Psychology: Learning, Memory, and Cognition, 11*, 629–654.

Barsalou, L. W. (1991). Deriving categories to achieve goals. In G. H. Bower (Ed.), *The psychology of learning and motivation: Advances in research and theory, Vol. 27* (pp. 1–64). San Diego, CA: Academic Press.

Barsalou, L. W. (1999). Perceptual symbol systems. *Behavioral and Brain Sciences, 22*, 577–660.

Barsalou, L. W. (in press-a). Abstraction as dynamic construal in perceptual symbol systems. In L. Gershkoff-Stowe & D. Rakison (Eds.), *Building object categories. Carnegie Symposium Series*. Mahwah, NJ: Lawrence Erlbaum Associates, Inc.

Barsalou, L. W. (in press-b). Situated simulation in the human conceptual system. *Language and Cognitive Processes.*

Barsalou, L. W., Sloman, S. A., & Chaigneau, S. E. (in press). The HIPE theory of function. In L. Carlson & E. van der Zee (Eds.), *Representing functional features for language and space: Insights from perception, categorization and development*. Oxford: Oxford University Press.

Bechtel, W., & McCauley, R. N. (1999). *Heuristic identity theory (or back to the future): The mind-body problem against the background of research strategies in cognitive neuroscience*. Paper presented at the Twenty-First Meeting of the Cognitive Science Society. Mahwah, New Jersey, USA.

Bechtel, W., & Richardson, R. C. (1993). *Discovering complexity: Decomposition and localization as strategies in scientific research*. Princeton, NJ: Princeton University Press.

Breitmeyer, B. G., & Ganz, L. (1976). Implications of sustained and transient channels for theories of visual-pattern masking, saccadic suppression, and information-processing. *Psychological Review, 83*, 1–36.

Breitmeyer, B. G., & Ganz, L. (1977). Temporal studies with flashed gratings: Inferences about human transient and sustained channels. *Vision Research, 17*, 861–865.

Capitani, E., Laiacona, M., Mahon, B., & Caramazza, A. (2003). What are the facts of semantic category-specific deficits? A critical review of the clinical evidence. *Cognitive Neuropsychology, 20*, 213–261.

Cappelletti, M., Waley-Cohen, H., Butterworth, B., & Kopelman, M. (2000). A selective loss of the ability to read and to write music. *Neurocase, 6*, 321–331.

Caramazza, A., Hillis, A. E., Rapp, B. C., & Romani, C. (1990). The multiple semantics hypothesis: Multiple confusions? *Cognitive Neuropsychology, 7*, 161–189.

Caramazza, A., & Shelton, J. R. (1998). Domain-specific knowledge systems in the brain: The animate–inanimate distinction. *Journal of Cognitive Neuroscience, 10*, 1–34.

Chen, X. (1995). Taxonomic changes and the particle-wave debate in early 19th-century Britain. *Studies in History and Philosophy of Science, 26*, 251–271.

Cipolotti, L., Butterworth, B., & Denes, G. (1991). A specific deficit for numbers in a case of dense acalculia. *Brain, 114*, 2619–2637.

Coltheart, M., Inglis, L., Cupples, L., Michie, P., Bates, A., & Budd, B. (1998). A semantic subsystem of visual attributes. *Neurocase, 4*, 353–370.

Coslett, H. B., Brashear, H. R., & Heilman, K. M. (1984). Pure word deafness after bilateral primary auditory-cortex infarcts. *Neurology, 34*, 347–352.

Cree, G. S., & McRae, K. (in press). Analyzing the factors underlying the structure and computation of the meaning of chipmunk, cherry, chisel, cheese, and cello (and many other such concrete nouns). *Journal of Experimental Psychology: General.*

Crosson, B., Moberg, P. J., Boone, J. R., Rothi, L. J., & Raymer, A. (1997). Category-specific naming deficit for medical terms after dominant thalamic/capsular hemorrhage. *Brain and Language, 60*, 407–442.

Damasio, A. R. (1989). Time-locked multiregional retroactivation: A systems-level proposal for the neural substrates of recall and recognition. *Cognition, 33*, 25–62.

Damasio, A. R. (1994). *Descartes' error: Emotion, reason, and the human brain.* New York: Grosset/Putnam.

Damasio, A. R., & Damasio, H. (1994). Cortical systems for retrieval of concrete knowledge: The convergence zone framework. In C. Koch & J. L. Davis (Eds.), *Large-scale neuronal theories of the brain. Computational neuroscience* (pp. 61–74). Cambridge, MA: The MIT Press.

Damasio, H., Grabowski, T. J., Tranel, D., Hichwa, R. D., & Damasio, A. R. (1996). A neural basis for lexical retrieval. *Nature, 380*, 499–505.

Davidson, R. J. (2000). Cognitive neuroscience needs affective neuroscience (and vice versa). *Brain and Cognition, 42*, 89–92.

Davidson, R. J., Jackson, D. C., & Kalin, N. H. (2000). Emotion, plasticity, context, and regulation: Perspectives from affective neuroscience. *Psychological Bulletin, 126*, 890–906.

De Valois, R., & De Valois, K. (1988). *Spatial vision.* New York: Oxford University Press.

De Renzi, E., & Spinnler, H. (1967). Impaired performance on color tasks in patients with hemispheric damage. *Cortex, 3*, 194–217.

Dodd, J., & Kelly, J. P. (1991). Trigeminal system. In E. R. Kandel, J. H. Schwartz, & T. M. Jessell (Eds.), *Principles of neural science* (3rd ed., pp. 701–710). New York: Elsevier.

Elman, J. L., Bates, E. A., Johnson, M. H., Karmiloff-Smith, A., & Plunkett, K. (1996). *Rethinking innateness: A connectionist perspective on development.* Cambridge, MA: MIT Press.

Farah, M. J. (2000). The neural bases of mental imagery. In M. S. Gazzaniga (Ed.), *The new cognitive neurosciences* (pp. 965–974). Cambridge, MA: MIT Press.

Farah, M. J. (2001). Consciousness. In B. Rapp (Ed.), *The handbook of cognitive neuropsychology: What deficits reveal about the human mind* (pp. 159–182). Philadelphia, PA: Psychology Press.

Farah, M. J., & McClelland, J. L. (1991). A computational model of semantic memory impairment: Modality specificity and emergent category specificity. *Journal of Experimental Psychology: General, 120*, 339–357.

Forde, E. M. E., Francis, D., Riddoch, M. J., Rumiati, R. I., & Humphreys, G. W. (1997). On the links between visual knowledge and naming: A single case study of a patient with a category-specific impairment for living things. *Cognitive Neuropsychology, 14*, 403–458.

Fujita, I., Tanaka, K., Ito, M., & Cheng, K. (1992). Columns for visual features of objects in monkey inferotemporal cortex. *Nature, 360*, 343–346.

Funnell, E., & De Mornay Davies, P. (1996). JBR: A reassessment of concept familiarity and a category-specific disorder for living things. *Neurocase, 2*, 461–474.

Gainotti, G., Silveri, M. C., Daniele, A., & Giustolisi, L. (1995). Neuroanatomical correlates of category-specific semantic disorders: A critical survey. *Memory, 3*, 247–264.

Garcia, J., & Koelling, R. (1966). Relation of cue to consequence in avoidance learning. *Psychonomic Science, 4*, 123–124.

Gauthier, I., Tarr, M. J., Anderson, A. W., Skudlarski, P., & Gore, J. C. (1999). Activation of the middle fusiform "face area" increases with expertise in recognizing novel objects. *Nature Neuroscience, 2*, 568–573.

Ghez, C. (1991). Voluntary movement. In E. R. Kandel, J. H. Schwartz, & T. M. Jessell (Eds.), *Principles of neural science* (3rd ed., pp. 609–625). New York: Elsevier.

Glenberg, A. M. (1997). What memory is for. *Behavioral and Brain Sciences, 20*, 1–18.

Glenberg, A. M., & Kaschak, M. P. (2002). Grounding language in action. *Psychonomic Bulletin & Review, 9*, 558–565.

Gonnerman, L. M., Andersen, E. S., Devlin, J. T., Kempler, D., & Seidenberg, M. S. (1997). Double dissociation of semantic categories in Alzheimer's disease. *Brain and Language, 57*, 254–279.

Goulet, S., & Murray, E. A. (2001). Neural substrates of crossmodal association memory in monkeys: The amygdala versus the anterior rhinal cortex. *Behavioral Neuroscience, 115,* 271–284.

Grezes, J., & Decety, J. (2001). Functional anatomy of execution, mental simulation, observation, and verb generation of actions: A meta-analysis. *Human Brain Mapping, 12,* 1–19.

Hart, J., & Gordon, B. (1992). Neural subsystems for object knowledge. *Nature, 359,* 60–64.

Hasson, U., Hendler, T., Ben Bashat, D., & Malach, R. (2001). Vase or face? A neural correlate of shape-selective grouping processes in the human brain. *Journal of Cognitive Neuroscience, 13,* 744–753.

Haxby, J. V., Gobbini, M. I., Furey, M. L., Ishai, A., Schouten, J. L., & Pietrini, P. (2001). Distributed and overlapping representations of faces and objects in ventral temporal cortex. *Science, 293,* 2425–2430.

Higuchi, S., & Miyashita, Y. (1996). Formation of mnemonic neuronal responses to visual paired associates in inferotemporal cortex is impaired by perirhinal and entorhinal lesions. *Proceedings of the National Academy of Sciences of the United States of America, 93,* 739–743.

Hillis, A. E., & Caramazza, A. (1991). Category-specific naming and comprehension impairment: A double dissociation. *Brain, 114,* 2081–2094.

Hochberg, J. (1998) Gestalt theory and its legacy: Organization in eye and brain, in attention and mental representation. In J. Hochberg (Ed.), *Perception and cognition at century's end: Handbook of perception and cognition* (2nd ed., pp. 253–306). San Diego, CA: Academic Press.

Holdstock, J. S., Gutnikov, S. A., Gaffan, D., & Mayes, A. R. (2000). Perceptual and mnemonic matching-to-sample in humans: Contributions of the hippocampus, perirhinal and other medial temporal lobe cortices. *Cortex, 36,* 301–322.

Humphreys, G. W., & Forde, E. M. E. (2001). Hierarchies, similarity, and interactivity in object recognition: "Category-specific" neuropsychological deficits. *Behavioral and Brain Sciences, 24,* 453–509.

Jeannerod, M. (1995). Mental-imagery in the motor context. *Neuropsychologia, 33,* 1419–1432.

Johnson, K. E., & Mervis, C. B. (1997). Effects of varying levels of expertise on the basic level of categorization. *Journal of Experimental Psychology: General, 126,* 248–277.

Kan, I. P., Barsalou, L. W., Solomon, K. O., Minor, J. K., & Thompson-Schill, S. L. (2003). Role of mental imagery in a property verification task: fMRI evidence for perceptual representations of conceptual knowledge. *Cognitive Neuropsychology, 20,* 525–540.

Kandel, E. R. (1991). Perception of motion, depth, and form. In E. R. Kandel, J. H. Schwartz, & T. M. Jessell (Eds.), *Principles of neural science* (3rd ed., pp. 440–466). New York: Elsevier.

Kanwisher, N., Woods, R. P., Iacoboni, M., & Mazziotta, J. C. (1997). A locus in human extrastriate cortex for visual shape analysis. *Journal of Cognitive Neuroscience, 9,* 133–142.

Kemler Nelson, D. G. (1989). The nature and occurrence of holistic processing. In B. E. Shepp & S. Ballesteros (Eds.), *Object perception: Structure and process* (pp. 357–386). Hillsdale, NJ: Lawrence Erlbaum Associates, Inc.

Kobatake, E., & Tanaka, K. (1994). Neuronal selectivities to complex object features in the ventral visual pathway of the Macaque cerebral cortex. *Journal of Neurophysiology, 71,* 856–867.

Kosslyn, S. M. (1994). *Image and brain: The resolution of the imagery debate.* Cambridge, MA: The MIT Press.

Kosslyn, S. M., Alpert, N. M., Thompson, W. L., Chabris, C. F., Rauch, S. L., & Anderson, A. K. (1994). Identifying objects seen from different viewpoints: A PET investigation. *Brain, 117,* 1055–1071.

Kosslyn, S. M., Thompson, W. L., & Alpert, N. M. (1997). Neural systems shared by visual imagery and visual perception: A positron emission tomography study. *NeuroImage, 6,* 320–334.

Kourtzi, Z., & Kanwisher, N. (2001). Representation of perceived object shape by the human lateral occipital complex. *Science, 293,* 1506–1509.

Kreiman, G., Koch, C., & Fried, I. (2000a). Category-specific visual responses of single neurons in the human medial temporal lobe. *Nature Neuroscience, 3,* 946–953.

Kreiman, G., Koch, C., & Fried, I. (2000b). Imagery neurons in the human brain. *Nature, 408,* 357–361.

Laiacona, M., Barbarotto, R., & Capitani, E. (1993). Perceptual and associative knowledge in category-specific impairment of semantic memory: A study of two cases. *Cortex, 29,* 727–740.

Lambon Ralph, M., Howard, D., Nightingale, G., & Ellis, A. (1998). Are living and non-living category-specific deficits causally linked to impaired perceptual or associative knowledge? Evidence from a category-specific double dissociation. *Neurocase, 4,* 311–338.

Lambon Ralph, M. A., McClelland, J. L., Patterson, K., Galton, C. J., & Hodges, J. R. (2001). No right to speak? The relationship between object naming and semantic impairment: Neuropsychological evidence and a connectionist model. *Journal of Cognitive Neuroscience, 13*, 341–356.

Lezak, M. (1995). *Neuropsychological assessment* (4th ed.). Oxford: Oxford University Press.

Logan, G. D. (1988). Toward an instance theory of automatization. *Psychological Review, 95*, 492–527.

Lorenzi, C., Wable, J., Moroni, C., Derobert, C., Frachet, B., & Belin, C. (2000). Auditory temporal envelope processing in a patient with left- hemisphere damage. *Neurocase, 6*, 231–244.

Martin, A. (2001). Functional neuroimaging of semantic memory. In R. Cabeza & A. Kingstone (Eds.), *Handbook of functional neuroimaging of cognition* (pp. 153–186). Cambridge, MA: MIT Press.

Martin, A., & Chao, L. (2001). Semantic memory and the brain: structure and process. *Current Opinion in Neurobiology, 11*, 194–201.

Martin, A., Ungerleider, L. G., & Haxby, J. V. (2000). Category-specificity and the brain: The sensory-motor model of semantic representations of objects. In M. S. Gazzaniga (Ed.), *The new cognitive neurosciences* (2nd ed., pp. 1023–1036). Cambridge, MA: MIT Press.

McCauley, R. N., & Bechtel, W. (2001). Explanatory pluralism and heuristic identity theory. *Theory and Psychology, 11*, 736–760.

Macrae, C. N., & Lewis, H. L. (2002). Do I know you? Processing orientation and face recognition. *Psychological Science, 13*, 194–196.

McRae, K., & Cree, G. S. (2002). Factors underlying category-specific semantic deficits. In E. M. E. Forde & G. W. Humphreys (Eds.), *Category-specificity in mind and brain* (pp. 211–249). Hove, UK: Psychology Press.

Mishkin, M., Vargha-Khadem, F., & Gadian, D. G. (1998). Amnesia and the organization of the hippocampal system. *Hippocampus, 8*, 212–216.

Morrison, D. J., & Schyns, P. G. (2001). Usage of spatial scales for the categorization of faces, objects, and scenes. *Psychonomic Bulletin and Review, 8*, 454–469.

Murphy, G. L. (2002). *The big book of concepts*. Cambridge, MA: MIT Press.

Murphy, G. L., & Medin, D. L. (1985). The role of theories in conceptual coherence. *Psychological Review, 92*, 289–316.

Murray, E. A., & Bussey, T. J. (1999). Perceptual-mnemonic functions of the perirhinal cortex. *Trends in Cognitive Sciences, 3*, 142–151.

Murray, E. A., Gaffan, D., & Mishkin, M. (1993). Neural substrates of visual stimulus association in Rhesus monkeys. *Journal of Neuroscience, 13*, 4549–4561.

Murray, E. A., & Richmond, B. J. (2001). Role of perirhinal cortex in object perception, memory, and associations. *Current Opinion in Neurobiology, 11*, 188–193.

Navon, D. (1977). Forest before trees: The precedence of global features in visual processing. *Cognitive Psychology, 9*, 353–383.

Nyberg, L., Habib, R., McIntosh, A. R., & Tulving, E. (2000). Reactivation of encoding-related brain activity during memory retrieval. *Proceedings of the National Academy of Sciences of the United States of America, 97*, 11120–11124.

Palmer, S. E. (1999). *Vision science: Photons to phenomenology*. Cambridge, MA: MIT Press.

Parker, A., & Gaffan, D. (1998). Lesions of the primate rhinal cortex cause deficits in flavour: Visual associative memory. *Behavioural Brain Research, 93*, 99–105.

Rackover, S. S. (2002). Featural vs. configurational information in faces: A conceptual and empirical analysis. *British Journal of Psychology, 93*, 1–30.

Rosch, E., & Mervis, C. B. (1975). Family resemblances: Studies in the internal structure of categories. *Cognitive Psychology, 7*, 573–605.

Rosch, E., Mervis, C. B., Gray, W. D., Johnson, D. M., & Boyes-Braem, P. (1976). Basic objects in natural categories. *Cognitive Psychology, 8*, 382–439.

Samson, D., Pillon, A., & De Wilde, V. (1998). Impaired knowledge of visual and non-visual attributes in a patient with a semantic impairment for living entities: A case of a true category-specific deficit. *Neurocase, 4*, 273–290.

Sartori, G., & Job, R. (1988). The oyster with four legs: A neuropsychological study on the interaction of visual and semantic information. *Cognitive Neuropsychology, 5*, 105–132.

Schreiner, C. E., Read, H. L., & Sutter, M. L. (2000). Modular organisation of frequency integration in primary auditory cortex. *Annual Review of Neuroscience, 23*, 501–529.

Schyns, P. G., Goldstone, R. L., & Thibaut, J. P. (1998). The development of features in object concepts. *Behavioral and Brain Sciences, 21*, 1–54.

Schyns, P. G., & Murphy, G. L. (1994). The ontogeny of part representation in object concepts. In D. Medin (Ed.), *The psychology of learning and motivation* (Vol. 31, pp. 305–349). San Diego, CA: Academic Press.

Shelton, P. A., Bowers, D., Duara, R., & Heilman, K. M. (1994). Apperceptive visual agnosia: A case study. *Brain and Cognition*, *25*, 1–23.

Silveri, M. C., Gainotti, G., Perani, D., Cappelletti, J. Y., Carbone, G., & Fazio, F. (1997). Naming deficit for non-living items: Neuropsychological and PET study. *Neuropsychologia*, *35*, 359–367.

Solomon, K. O., & Barsalou, L. W. (2001). Representing properties locally. *Cognitive Psychology*, *43*, 129–169.

Solomon, K. O., & Barsalou, L. W. (2003). *Perceptual simulation in property verification.* Manuscript under review.

Spivey, M., Tyler, M., Richardson, D., & Young, E. (2000). Eye movements during comprehension of spoken scene descriptions. *Proceedings of the 22nd Annual Conference of the Cognitive Science Society* (pp. 487–492). Mahwah, NJ: Lawrence Erlbaum Associates Inc.

Stanfield, R. A., & Zwaan, R. A. (2001). The effect of implied orientation derived from verbal context on picture recognition. *Psychological Science*, *12*, 153–156.

Tanaka, K. (1996). Representation of visual features of objects in the inferotemporal cortex. *Neural Networks*, *9*, 1459–1475.

Tanaka, K. (1997a). Columnar organization in the inferotemporal cortex. In K. Rockland, J. Kaas, & A. Peters (Eds.), *Cerebral cortex* (pp. 469–498). New York: Plenum Press.

Tanaka, K. (1997b). Inferotemporal cortex and object recognition. In J. W. Donahoe & V. P. Dorsel (Eds.), *Neural-network models of cognition: Biobehavioral foundations* (Vol. 121, pp. 160–188). Amsterdam, The Netherlands: North-Holland/Elsevier Science Publishers.

Tanaka, K. (1997c). Mechanisms of visual object recognition: Monkey and human studies. *Current Opinion in Neurobiology*, *7*, 523–429.

Thomas, E., Van Hulle, M. M., & Vogels, R. (2001). Encoding of categories by noncategory-specific neurons in the inferior temporal cortex. *Journal of Cognitive Neuroscience*, *13*, 190–200.

Thompson, W. L., & Kosslyn, S. M. (2000) Neural systems activated during visual mental imagery. In A. W. Toga & J. Mazziotta (Eds.), *Brain mapping: The systems* (pp. 535–560). San Diego, CA: Academic Press.

Tranel, D., Adolphs, R., Damasio, H., & Damasio, A. R. (2001). A neural basis for the retrieval of words for actions. *Cognitive Neuropsychology*, *18*, 655–674.

Tranel, D., Damasio, H., & Damasio, A. R. (1997). A neural basis for the retrieval of conceptual knowledge. *Neuropsychologia*, *35*, 1319–1327.

Tranel, D., Damasio, H., & Damasio, A. R. (1998). The neural basis of lexical retrieval. In R. W. Parks & D. S. Levine (Eds.), *Fundamentals of neural network modeling: Neuropsychology and cognitive neuroscience* (pp. 271–296). Cambridge, MA: MIT Press.

Treisman, A. M., & Gelade, G. (1980). A feature integration theory of attention. *Cognitive Psychology*, *12*, 97–136.

Tyler, L. K., & Moss, H. E. (2001). Towards a distributed account of conceptual knowledge. *Trends in Cognitive Sciences*, *5*, 244–252.

Tyler, L. K., Moss, H. E., Durrant-Peatfield, M. R., & Levy, J. P. (2000). Conceptual structure and the structure of concepts: A distributed account of category-specific deficits. *Brain and Language*, *75*, 195–231.

Wang, G., Tanaka, K., & Tanifuji, M. (1996). Optical imaging of functional organization in the monkey inferotemporal cortex. *Science*, *272*, 1665–1668.

Warrington, E. K., & McCarthy, R. A. (1987). Categories of knowledge: Further fractionations and an attempted integration. *Brain*, *110*, 1273–1296.

Warrington, E. K., & McCarthy, R. A. (1994). Multiple meaning systems in the brain: A case for visual semantics. *Neuropsychologia*, *32*, 1465–1473.

Warrington, E. K., & Shallice, T. (1984). Category specific semantic impairments. *Brain*, *107*, 829–854.

Wheeler, M. E., Petersen, S. E., & Buckner, R. L. (2000). Memory's echo: Vivid remembering reactivates sensory-specific cortex. *Proceedings of the National Academy of Sciences of the United States of America*, *97*, 11125–11129.

Wolfe, J. (2000). Visual attention. In K. K. De Valois (Ed.), *Seeing* (2nd ed., pp. 335–386). San Diego, CA: Academic Press.

Wu, L., & Barsalou, L. W. (2003). *Perceptual simulation in property generation.* Manuscript submitted for publication.

Zeki, S. (1993). *A vision of the brain.* Cambridge, MA: Blackwell Scientific Publications.

Zhou, H., Friedman, H. S., & Von der Heydt, R. (2000). Coding of border ownership in monkey visual cortex. *Journal of Neuroscience*, *20*, 6594–6611.

Zwaan, R. A., Stanfield, R. A., & Yaxley, R. H. (2002). Do language comprehenders routinely represent the shapes of objects? *Psychological Science*, *13*, 168–171.

COGNITIVE NEUROPSYCHOLOGY, 2003, 20 (3/4/5/6), 487–506

# THREE PARIETAL CIRCUITS FOR NUMBER PROCESSING

**Stanislas Dehaene, Manuela Piazza, Philippe Pinel, and Laurent Cohen**
*INSERM-CEA, Service Hospitalier Frédéric Joliot, Orsay, France*

Did evolution endow the human brain with a predisposition to represent and acquire knowledge about numbers? Although the parietal lobe has been suggested as a potential substrate for a domain-specific representation of quantities, it is also engaged in verbal, spatial, and attentional functions that may contribute to calculation. To clarify the organisation of number-related processes in the parietal lobe, we examine the three-dimensional intersection of fMRI activations during various numerical tasks, and also review the corresponding neuropsychological evidence. On this basis, we propose a tentative tripartite organisation. The horizontal segment of the intraparietal sulcus (HIPS) appears as a plausible candidate for domain specificity: It is systematically activated whenever numbers are manipulated, independently of number notation, and with increasing activation as the task puts greater emphasis on quantity processing. Depending on task demands, we speculate that this core quantity system, analogous to an internal "number line," can be supplemented by two other circuits. A left angular gyrus area, in connection with other left-hemispheric perisylvian areas, supports the manipulation of numbers in verbal form. Finally, a bilateral posterior superior parietal system supports attentional orientation on the mental number line, just like on any other spatial dimension.

## INTRODUCTION

Did evolution endow the human brain with a predisposition to represent dedicated domains of knowledge? We have previously argued that the number domain provides a good candidate for such a biologically determined semantic domain (Dehaene, 1997; Dehaene, Dehaene-Lambertz, & Cohen, 1998a). Three criteria for domain specificity suggest that number and arithmetic are more than cultural inventions, and may have their ultimate roots in brain evolution. First, a capacity to attend to numerosity, and to manipulate it internally in elementary computations, is present in animals even in the absence of training (Hauser, Carey, & Hauser, 2000). Second, a similar capacity for elementary number processing is found early on in human development, prior to schooling or even to the development of language skills (Spelke & Dehaene, 1999; Xu & Spelke, 2000). This suggests that numerical development follows a distinct developmental trajectory based on mechanisms with a long prior evolutionary history.

Third, it has been suggested that number processing rests on a distinct neural circuitry, which can be reproducibly identified in different subjects with various neuroimaging, neuropsychological, and brain stimulation methods (Dehaene et al., 1998a). The present paper focuses on this last issue, taking into account the considerable progress that has recently been made in neuroimaging methods. The involvement of parietal cortex in number processing was initially discovered on the basis of lesion data (Gerstmann, 1940; Hécaen, Angelergues, &

Requests for reprints should be addressed to Stanislas Dehaene, INSERM Unit 562, Service Hospitalier Frédéric Joliot, CEA/DRM/DSV, 4 place du Général Leclerc, 91401 Orsay cedex, France (Email: dehaene@shfj.cea.fr).





http://www.tandf.co.uk/journals/pp/02643294.html DOI:10.1080/02643290244000239

Houillier, 1961; Henschen, 1919). Subsequently, a systematic activation of the parietal lobes during calculation, together with precentral and prefrontal cortices, was discovered (Roland & Friberg, 1985) and extensively replicated using positron emission tomography (PET) (Dehaene et al., 1996; Pesenti, Thioux, Seron, & De Volder, 2000; Zago, Pesenti, Mellet, Crivello, Mazoyer, & Tzourio-Mazoyer, 2001) and later fMRI (Burbaud, Camus, Guehl, Bioulac, Caille, & Allard, 1999; Rueckert et al., 1996). On this basis, some of us proposed that the parietal lobe contributes to the representation of numerical quantity on a mental "number line" (Dehaene & Cohen, 1995). Unfortunately, due to poor spatial resolution and limits on experimental designs, those studies did not permit a finer exploration of the regions involved in different kinds of numerical tasks. This has become critical, however, because recent behavioural studies have made it clear that mental arithmetic relies on a highly composite set of processes, many of which are probably not specific to the number domain. For instance, studies of language interference in normal subjects suggest that language-based processes play an important role in exact but not approximate calculation (Spelke & Tsivkin, 2001). Likewise, concurrent performance of a spatial task interferes with subtraction, but not multiplication, while concurrent performance of a language task interferes with multiplication, but not subtraction (Lee & Kang, 2002). Such behavioural dissociations suggest that the neural bases of calculation must be heterogeneous.

The triple-code model of number processing predicts that, depending on the task, three distinct systems of representation may be recruited: a quantity system (a nonverbal semantic representation of the size and distance relations between numbers, which may be category specific), a verbal system (where numerals are represented lexically, phonologically, and syntactically, much like any other type of word), and a visual system (in which numbers can be encoded as strings of Arabic numerals) (Dehaene, 1992; Dehaene & Cohen, 1995). We initially proposed that the parietal activations during number processing reflected solely the contribution of the quantity system. However, it is now clear that this hypothesis requires further elaboration. First, the left perisylvian language network clearly extends into the inferior parietal lobe. Second, the posterior superior parietal lobes are strongly engaged in visual attention processes that may contribute to the visual processing of numbers. It is thus crucial to distinguish, within the observed parietal lobe activations during number processing, which activation sites, if any, are associated with a semantic representation of numerical quantity and which correspond to nonspecific verbal or visual/attentional systems.

Fortunately, functional magnetic resonance imaging (fMRI) has recently allowed much finer-grained studies of the neuroanatomy of number processing, using paradigms adapted from cognitive psychology. The present review focuses entirely on the parietal lobe activations identified by those recent neuroimaging studies. We use three-dimensional visualisation software to investigate how the parietal activations reported by various studies relate to one another in cortical space. On this basis, we propose that three circuits coexist in the parietal lobe and capture most of the observed differences between arithmetic tasks: a bilateral intraparietal system associated with a core quantity system, a region of the left angular gyrus associated with verbal processing of numbers, and a posterior superior parietal system of spatial and nonspatial attention.

It should be emphasised that our description provides only a tentative model. Although it is based on a synthesis of the existing literature, this model remains speculative and will require further validation by direct experimentation. For each postulated circuit, we first examine the relevant neuroimaging literature, and then consider how those brain-imaging results impinge on our understanding of neuropsychological impairments of number processing. Our account predicts that depending on lesion localisation, three different categories of numerical impairments should be observed: genuine semantic impairments of the numerical domain following intraparietal lesions; impairments of verbal fact retrieval following lesions to the left perisylvian cortices, including the left angular gyrus; and impairments of spatial attention on the number line following lesions to the dorsal parietal attention system.

## THE BILATERAL HORIZONTAL SEGMENT OF THE INTRAPARIETAL SULCUS AND QUANTITY PROCESSING

### Neuroimaging evidence

The horizontal segment of the intraparietal sulcus (hereafter HIPS) is a major site of activation in neuroimaging studies of number processing. As shown in Figure 1a, this region lies at the intersection of the activations observed in many different number processing tasks (see Table 1). What seems to be common to those tasks is the requirement to access a semantic representation of the quantity that the numbers represent. We propose that a nonverbal representation of numerical quantity, perhaps analogous to a spatial map or "number line," is present in the HIPS of both hemispheres. This representation would underlie our intuition of what a given numerical size means, and of the proximity relations between numbers. In support of this view, several features of its responsiveness to experimental conditions are worth noting.

*Mental arithmetic.* The HIPS seems to be active whenever an arithmetic operation calls upon a quantitative representation of numbers. For example, it is more active when subjects calculate than when they merely have to read numerical symbols (Burbaud et al., 1999; Chochon, Cohen, Van de Moortele, & Dehaene, 1999; Pesenti et al., 2000), suggesting that it plays a role in the semantic manipulation of numbers. Its activation increases, at least in the right hemisphere, when subjects have to compute two addition or subtraction operations instead of one (Menon, Rivera, White, Glover, & Reiss, 2000). Furthermore, even within calculation, the HIPS is more active when subjects estimate the approximate result of an addition problem than when they compute its exact solution (Dehaene, Spelke, Stanescu, Pinel, & Tsivkin, 1999). Finally, it shows greater activation for subtraction than for multiplication (Chochon et al., 1999; Lee, 2000). Multiplication tables and small exact addition facts can be stored in rote verbal memory, and hence place minimal requirements on quantity manipulation. Contrariwise, although some subtraction problems may be stored in verbal memory, many are not learned by rote and therefore require genuine quantity manipulations. In another study, relative to five different visuospatial and phonological non-numerical tasks, subtraction was the only task that led to increased activation of the HIPS (Simon, Cohen, Mangin, Bihan, & Dehaene, 2002).

*Number comparison.* The HIPS is also active whenever a comparative operation that needs access to a numerical scale is called for. For instance, it is more active when comparing the magnitudes of two numbers than when simply reading them (Chochon et al., 1999). The systematic contribution of this region to number comparison processes is replicated in many paradigms using tomographic imaging (Le Clec'H et al., 2000; Pesenti et al., 2000; Pinel, Dehaene, Riviere, & LeBihan, 2001; Thioux, Pesenti, Costes, De Volder, & Seron, 2002) as well as scalp recordings of event-related potentials (Dehaene, 1996). Parietal activation in number comparison is often larger in the right than in the left hemisphere (Chochon et al., 1999; Dehaene, 1996; Pinel et al., 2001). This may point to a possible right-hemispheric advantage in comparison and in other tasks requiring an abstraction of numerical relations (Langdon & Warrington, 1997; Rosselli & Ardila, 1989). However, in comparison, the parietal activation, although it may be asymmetric, is always present in both hemispheres, compatible with the observation that numerical comparison is accessible to both hemispheres in split-brain patients (Cohen & Dehaene, 1996; Seymour, Reuter-Lorenz, & Gazzaniga, 1994).

*Specificity for the number domain.* Several studies have reported greater HIPS activation when processing numbers than when processing other categories of objects on non-numerical scales (such as comparing the ferocity of animals, the relative positions of body parts, or the orientation of two

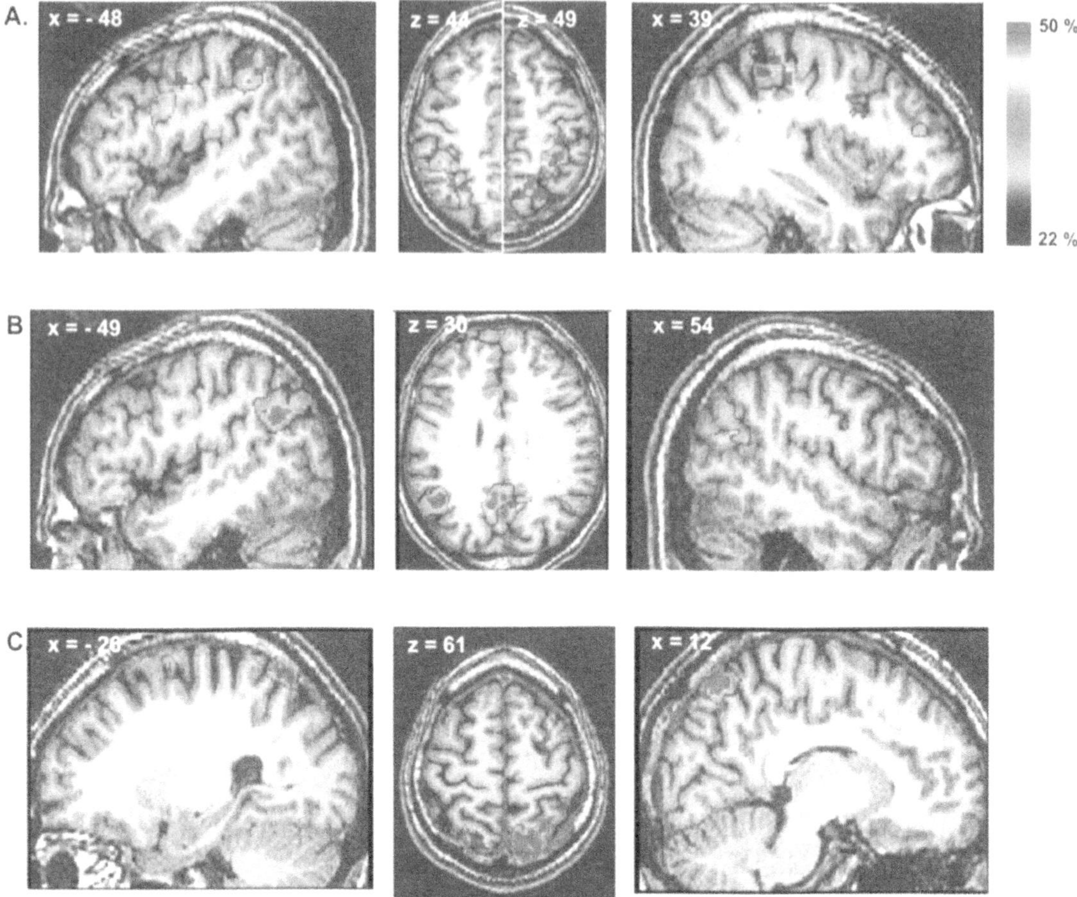


**Figure 1.** *Regions of overlapping activity for three groups of studies, superimposed on axial and sagittal slices of a normalised single-subject anatomical image. The overlap was calculated by averaging binarised contrast images indicating which voxels were significant for a given contrast (studies and contrasts are listed in Table 1). The colour scale indicates the percentage of studies showing activation in a given voxel. The same colour scale (from 22% to 50% of overlap) is applied to all images. Although no single voxel was shared by 100% of studies in a group, probably due to variability across groups of subjects, laboratories, and imaging methods, Table 1 revealed a high consistency of activations. (A) The horizontal segment of the intraparietal sulcus (HIPS) was activated bilaterally in a variety of contrasts sharing a component of numerical quantity manipulation. The barycentre of the region of maximum overlap (>50%) was at Talairach Coordinates (TC) 41, –42, 49 in the left hemisphere, and –48, –41, 43 in the right hemisphere. Activation overlap is also visible in the precentral gyrus. (B) The angular gyrus (AG) was activated with a strong left lateralisation (TC –48, –59, 30) in 5 studies of arithmetic tasks with a strong verbal component. Posterior cingulate as well as superior frontal regions also show some degrees of overlap. (C) The posterior superior parietal lobule (PSPL) was activated bilaterally in a few numerical tasks (left and right barycentres at TC –26, –69, 61 and 12, –69, 61; and see Table 1). To emphasise the nonspecificity of this region, the image shows the intersection of the overlap between four numerical tasks with an image of posterior parietal activity during a non-numerical visual attention shift task (Simon et al., 2002).*

**Table 1.** *Studies and contrasts used to isolate the three parietal regions in Figures 1 and 2*[a]

| | | *Coordinates of maxima* | | | | | |
|---|---|---|---|---|---|---|---|
| | | *Left* | | | *Right* | | |
| *Reference* | *Contrast* | *x* | *y* | *z* | *x* | *y* | *z* |
| | *Horizontal segment of intraparietal sulcus (HIPS)* | | | | | | |
| Chochon et al. (1999) | Comparison of one-digit numbers vs. letter naming | −45 | −42 | 39 | 39 | −42 | 42 |
| Chochon et al. (1999) | Subtraction of one-digit numbers from 11 vs. comparison | −42 | −48 | 48 | 39 | −42 | 42 |
| Dehaene et al. (1999) | Approximate vs. exact addition of one-digit numbers | −56 | −44 | 52 | 44 | −36 | 52 |
| Lee (2000) | Subtraction vs. multiplication of one-digit numbers | −31 | −52 | 49 | 28 | −54 | 52 |
| Naccache and Dehaene (2001) | Subliminal quantity priming across notations | −44 | −56 | 56 | 36 | −44 | 44 |
| Piazza et al. (2002[b]) | Numerosity estimation vs. physical matching | n.s. | | | 44 | −56 | 54 |
| Pinel et al. (2001) | Distance effect in comparison of two-digit numbers | −40 | −44 | 36 | 44 | −56 | 48 |
| Simon et al. (2002) | Subtraction of one-digit numbers from 11 vs. letter naming | −48 | −44 | 52 | 52 | −44 | 52 |
| Stanescu-Cosson et al. ( 2000) | Size effect in exact addition of one-digit numbers | −44 | −52 | 48 | | n.s. | |
| Mean | | −44 | −48 | 47 | 41 | −47 | 48 |
| *SD* | | 7 | 5 | 6 | 7 | 7 | 5 |
| | *Angular gyrus (AG)* | | | | | | |
| Chochon et al. (1999) | Multiplication vs. comparison of one-digit numbers | −30 | −69 | 39 | n.s. | | |
| Dehaene et al. (1999) | Exact vs. approximate addition of one-digit numbers | −44 | −72 | 36 | 40 | −76 | 20 |
| Lee (2000) | Multiplication vs. subtraction of one-digit numbers | −49 | −54 | 31 | n.s. | | |
| Simon et al. (2002) | Intersection of subtraction and phoneme detection tasks | −31 | −70 | 43 | n.s. | | |
| Stanescu-Cosson et al. (2000) | Inverse size effect in exact addition of one-digit numbers | −52 | −68 | 32 | n.s. | | |
| Mean | | −41 | −66 | 36 | | | |
| *SD* | | 9 | 6 | 4 | | | |
| | *Posterior superior parietal lobule (PSPL)* | | | | | | |
| Dehaene et al. (1999) | Approximate vs. exact addition of one-digit numbers | −32 | −68 | 56 | 20 | −60 | 60 |
| Lee (2000) | Subtraction vs. multiplication of one-digit numbers | −29 | −64 | 69 | 21 | −61 | 65 |
| Naccache and Dehaene (2001) | Subliminal quantity priming across notations | n.s. | | | 12 | −60 | 48 |
| Pinel et al. (2001) | Distance effect in comparison of two-digit numbers | −4 | −72 | 44 | 8 | −72 | 52 |
| Mean | | −22 | −68 | 56 | 15 | −63 | 56 |
| *SD* | | 15 | 4 | 12 | 6 | 6 | 8 |

[a]In each case, we report the coordinates of activation maxima, their mean, and their standard deviation (n.s. = not significant).
[b]In some studies, we report the coordinates of subpeaks not reported in the digital papers, which only reported a single global maximum for each cluster.

visually presented characters: Le Clec'H et al., 2000; Pesenti et al., 2000; Thioux et al., 2002). Event-related potentials have also revealed greater parietal activation for numbers than for other categories of words such as action verbs, names of animals, or names of famous persons (Dehaene, 1995). In this study, the first point in time in which category-specific semantic effects emerge during visual word processing was found to be 250–280 ms following stimulus onset.

One study directly tested the specificity of the HIPS for the numerical domain in multiple tasks (Thioux et al., 2002). Subjects were presented with number words and names of animals matched for length. The HIPS showed greater activation, bilaterally, to numbers than to animal names. This was true whether subjects were engaged in a comparison task (larger or smaller than 5; more or less ferocious than a dog), a categorisation task (odd or even; mammal or bird), or even a visual judgement of character shape. Thus, the HIPS shows category specificity independently of task context. Further research will be needed, however, to decide whether it is strictly specific for numbers or whether it extends to other categories that have a strong spatial or serial component (e.g., the alphabet, days, months, spatial prepositions, etc.).

*Parametric modulation.* Parametric studies have revealed that the activation of the HIPS is modulated by semantic parameters such as the absolute magnitude of the numbers and their value relative to a reference point. Thus, intraparietal activity is larger and lasts longer during operations with large numbers than with small numbers (Kiefer & Dehaene, 1997; Stanescu-Cosson, Pinel, Van de Moontele, Le Bihan, Cohen, & Delaene, 2000). It is also modulated by the numerical distance separating the numbers in a comparison task (Dehaene, 1996; Pinel et al., 2001). On the other hand, the activation of the HIPS is independent of the particular modality of input used to convey the numbers. Arabic numerals, spelled-out number words, and even nonsymbolic stimuli like sets of dots or tones can activate this region if subjects attend to the corresponding number (Le Clec'H et al., 2000; Piazza, Mechelli, Butterworth, & Price, 2002a; Piazza, Mechelli, Price, & Butterworth, 2002b; Pinel et al., 2001). In one study, subjects attended either to the numerosity or to the physical characteristics (colour, pitch) of series of auditory and visual events. The right HIPS was active whenever the subjects attended to number, regardless of the modality of the stimuli (Piazza et al., 2002b). In another study, the activation of the bilateral HIPS was found to correlate directly with the numerical distance between two numbers in a comparison task, and this effect was observed whether the numbers were presented as words or as digits (Pinel et al., 2001). Those parametric studies are all consistent with the hypothesis that the HIPS codes the abstract quantity meaning of numbers rather the numerical symbols themselves.

*Unconscious quantity processing.* Quantity processing and HIPS activation can be demonstrated even when the subject is not aware of having seen a number symbol (Dehaene et al., 1998b; Naccache & Dehaene, 2001). In this experiment, subjects were asked to compare target numbers to a fixed reference of 5. Unbeknownst to them, just prior to the target, another number, the prime, was briefly present in a subliminal manner. FMRI revealed that the left and right intraparietal regions were sensitive to the unconscious repetition of the same number. When the prime and target corresponded to the same quantity (possibly in two different notations, such as ONE and 1), less parietal activation was observed than when the prime and target corresponded to two distinct quantities (e.g., FOUR and 1). This result suggests that this region comprises distinct neural assemblies for different numerical quantities, so that more activation can be observed when two such neural assemblies are activated than when only one is. It also indicates that this region can contribute to number processing in a subliminal fashion.

Taken together, these data suggest that the HIPS is essential for the semantic representation of numbers as quantities. This representation may provide a foundation for our "numerical intuition," our immediate and often unconscious understanding of where a given quantity falls with respect to others, and whether or not it is appropriate to a given context (Dehaene, 1992, 1997; Dehaene & Marques, 2002).

## Neuropsychological evidence

Neuropsychological observations confirm the existence of a distinct semantic system for numerical quantities and its relation to the vicinity of the intraparietal sulcus. Several single-case studies indicate that numbers doubly dissociate from other categories of words at the semantic level. On the one hand, spared calculation and number comprehension abilities have been described in patients with grossly deteriorated semantic processing (Thioux, Pillon, Samson, De Partz, Noel, & Seron, 1998) or semantic dementia (Butterworth, Cappelletti, & Kopelman, 2001; Cappelletti, Butterworth, & Kopelman, 2001). In both cases, the lesions broadly affected the left temporo-frontal cortices while sparing the intraparietal regions. On the other hand, Cipolotti, Butterworth, and Denes (1991) reported a striking case of a patient with a small left parietal lesion and an almost complete deficit in all spheres of number processing, sparing only the numbers 1 through 4, in the context of otherwise largely preserved language and semantic functions. Although such a severe and isolated degradation of the number system has never been replicated, other cases confirm that the understanding of numbers and their relations can be specifically impaired in the context of preserved language and semantics (e.g., Dehaene & Cohen, 1997; Delazer & Benke, 1997).

In many cases, the deficit can be extremely incapacitating. Patients may fail to compute operations as simple as 2 + 2, 3 – 1, or 3 × 9. Several characteristics indicate that the deficit arises at an abstract, notation-independent level of processing. First, patients may remain fully able to comprehend and to produce numbers in all formats. Second, they show the same calculation difficulties whether the problem is presented to them visually or auditorily, and whether they have to respond verbally or in writing, or even merely have to decide whether a proposed operation is true or false. Thus, the calculation deficit is not due to an inability to identify the numbers or to produce the operation result. Third, the deficit often extends to tasks outside of calculation per se, such as comparison or bisection. For instance, patient MAR (Dehaene & Cohen, 1997) showed a mild impairment in deciding which of two numbers is the larger (16% errors), and was almost totally unable to decide what number falls in the middle of two others (bisection task: 77% errors). He easily performed analogous comparison and bisection tasks in non-numerical domains such as days of the week, months, or the alphabet (What is between Tuesday and Thursday? February and April? B and D?). This type of deficits seems best described as a category-specific impairment of the semantic representation and manipulation of numerical quantities (Dehaene & Cohen, 1997), rather than with the mere clinical label of "acalculia."

In such patients, calculation impairments often co-occur with other deficits, forming a cluster of deficits called Gerstmann's syndrome (Benton, 1992; Gerstmann, 1940), which comprises agraphia, finger agnosia, and left–right distinction difficulties (to which one may often add constructive apraxia). The lesions that cause acalculia of the Gerstmann's type are typically centred in the depth of the left intraparietal sulcus (Mayer, Martory, Pegna, Landis, Delavelle, & Annoni, 1999; Takayama, Sugishita, Akiguchi, & Kimura, 1994). This is compatible with the above brain-imaging results showing intraparietal activation during various numerical manipulation tasks independently of language. Results from a recent brain-imaging study (Simon et al., 2002) shed some light on why the various elements of Gerstmann's syndrome often co-occur following left intraparietal lesions. In this study, fMRI was used to compare, in the same subjects, the localisation of parietal activations during a number subtraction task with those observed during various tasks that also involve the parietal lobe, such as eye or attention movements, finger pointing, hand grasping, and a language task of phoneme detection. The results revealed a systematic topographical organisation of activations and their intersections. In particular, the intraparietal sulcus appears to contains a "four-corners" region in which four areas of activation are juxtaposed: calculation only, calculation and language, manual tasks only, and an area activated during the four visuospatial tasks (eye and attention movements, pointing, and grasping). The simultaneous lesion of those four areas would predictably result in joint impairments of calculation, word processing (possibly including agraphia), finger knowledge and movement, and high-level spatial reference (possibly including understanding of left–right coordinates). Such a joint lesion might be frequent because this cortical territory is jointly irrigated by a branch of the middle cerebral artery, the angular gyrus artery. Inter-individual variability in the boundaries between cortical territories as well as in the branching patterns of this artery would explain that the different elements of Gerstmann's syndrome can be dissociated (Benton, 1961, 1992). Note that this interpretation implies that, contrary to a frequent speculation, Gerstmann's syndrome does not result from a homogeneous impairment to a single representation that would somehow intermingle fingers, numbers, and space (Butterworth, 1999; Gerstmann, 1940; Mayer et al., 1999). Rather, the syndrome may represent a happenstance conjunction of distinct, but dissociable, deficits that frequently co-occur due to a common vascularisation, and that are only loosely connected at the functional level due to the overarching spatial and sensorimotor functions of the parietal lobe.

## THE LEFT ANGULAR GYRUS AND VERBAL NUMBER MANIPULATIONS

### Neuroimaging evidence

The left angular gyrus (hereafter AG) is also often activated in neuroimaging studies of number processing (see Figure 1b and Table 1). This region is left-lateralised and located posterior and inferior to the HIPS (see Figure 2 for their respective locations). A closer look at the types of numerical tasks that activate this region, detailed below, reveals that its functional properties are very different from the properties of the HIPS. The left AG does not seem to be concerned with quantity processing, but shows increasingly greater activation as the task puts greater requirement on verbal processing. We therefore propose that this region is part of the language system, and contributes to number processing only inasmuch as some arithmetic operations, such as multiplication, make particularly strong demands on a verbal coding of numbers.

In support of this hypothesis, the left AG is not merely involved in calculation, but in different types of language-mediated processes such as reading or verbal short-term memory tasks (for reviews, see Fiez & Petersen, 1998; Paulesu, Frith, & Frackowiak, 1993; Price, 1998). In Simon et al.'s (2002) fMRI study of six different tasks, the left angular gyrus was the only parietal site where there

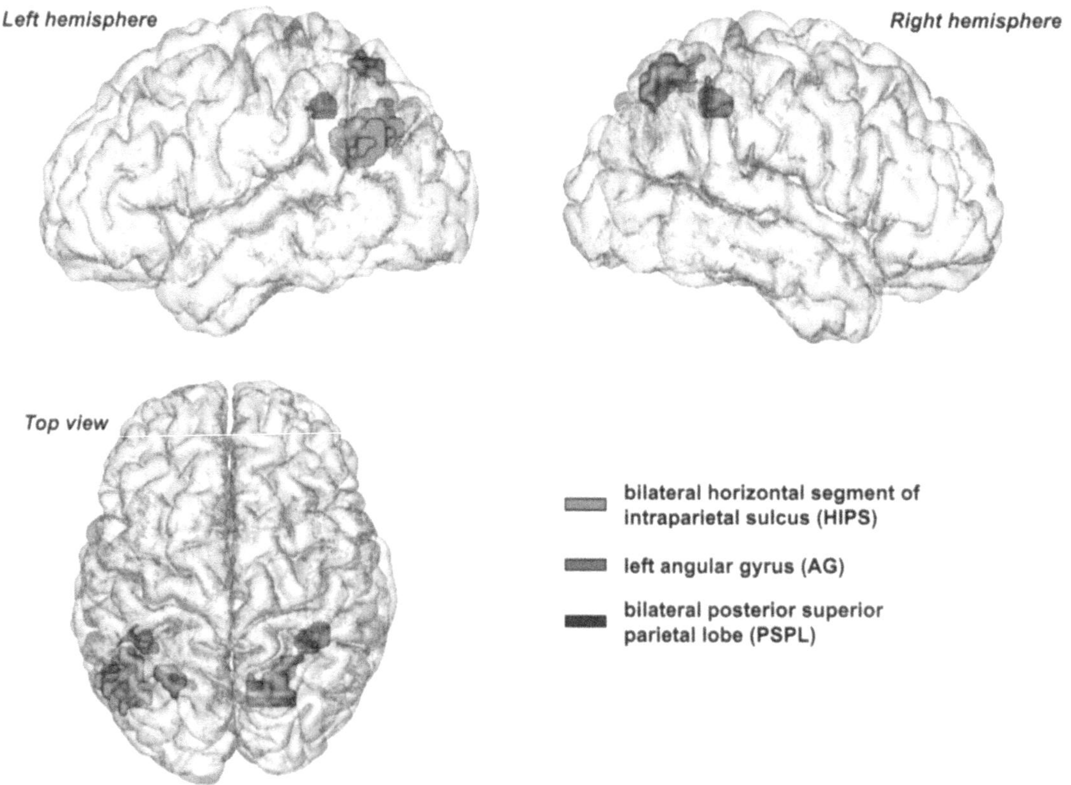


Figure 2. *Three-dimensional representation of the parietal regions of interest. For better visualisation, the clusters show all parietal voxels activated in at least 40% of studies in a given group.*

was overlapping activity for calculation and phoneme detection, but no activation during the other four visuospatial tasks. This clearly indicates that the left AG is not specific for calculation, but jointly recruited by language and calculation processes.

Even within calculation, several studies indicate a modulation of AG activation in direct proportion to the verbal requirements of the task. First, the AG is more active in exact calculation than in approximation (Dehaene et al., 1999). This fits with behavioural data indicating that exact arithmetic facts are stored in a language-specific format in bilinguals, while approximate knowledge is language-independent and shows the classical numerical distance effect associated with the nonverbal quantity system (Xu & Spelke, 2000). Second, within exact calculation, the left AG shows greater activation for operations that require access to a rote verbal memory of arithmetic facts, such as multiplication, than for operations that are not stored and require some form of quantity manipulation. For instance, the left AG shows increased activation for multiplication relative to both subtraction and number comparison (Chochon et al., 1999; Lee, 2000), for multiplication and division relative to a letter substitution control (Gruber, Indefrey, Steinmetz, & Kleinschmidt, 2001), and for multidigit mulplication relative to a digit-matching control (Fulbright, Molfese, Stevens, Skudlarski, Lacadie, & Gore, 2000).

Even within a given operation, such as single-digit addition, the left angular gyrus is more active for small problems with a sum below 10 than for large problems with a sum above 10 (Stanescu-Cosson, Pinel, Van de Moortele, Le Bihan, Cohen, & Dehaene, 2000). This probably reflects the fact that small addition facts, just like multiplication tables, are stored in rote verbal memory, while behavioural evidence indicates that larger addition problems are often solved by resorting to various semantic elaboration strategies (Dehaene & Cohen, 1995; Lefevre, 1996).

In summary, the contribution of the left angular gyrus in number processing may be related to the linguistic basis of arithmetical computations. Its contribution seems essential for the retrieval of facts stored in verbal memory, but not for other numerical tasks (like subtraction, number comparison, or complex calculation) that call for a genuinely quantitative representation of numbers and relate more to the intraparietal sulcus.

## Neuropsychological evidence: Dissociations between operations

The finding that the intraparietal sulcus and the angular gyrus exhibit functionally differentiated properties can shed light on the neuropsychology of acalculia. One of the most striking findings is the occurrence of sharp dissociations between arithmetic operations. It is not rare for a patient to be much more severely impaired in multiplication than in subtraction (Cohen & Dehaene, 2000; Dagenbach & McCloskey, 1992; Dehaene & Cohen, 1997; Lampl, Eshel, Gilad, & Sarova-Pinhas, 1994; Lee, 2000; Pesenti, Seron, & Van der Linden, 1994; Van Harskamp & Cipolotti, 2001), while other patients are much more impaired in subtraction than in multiplication (Dehaene & Cohen, 1997; Delazer & Benke, 1997; Van Harskamp & Cipolotti, 2001). Some have proposed that such dissociations reflect random impairments in a system with distinct stores of arithmetic facts for each operation (Dagenbach & McCloskey, 1992). Here, however, we would like to show that there is much more systematicity behind those observations. Our views suggest that dissociations between operations reflect a single, basic distinction between overlearned arithmetic facts such as the multiplication table, which are stored in rote verbal memory, and the genuine understanding of number meaning that underlies nontable operations such as subtraction (Dehaene & Cohen, 1997; Delazer & Benke, 1997; Hittmair-Delazer, Sailer, & Benke, 1995). According to this interpretation, multiplication requires the integrity of language-based representations of numbers, because multiplication facts are typically learned by rote verbal memorisation. Subtraction, on the other hand, is typically not learned by rote. Although the mechanisms by which simple subtraction problems are resolved are not yet understood, it is likely that some form of internal manipulation of nonverbal quantities on the internal number line is involved, as attested by the fact that very simple subtractions are accessible to preverbal infants (Wynn, 1992) and nonhuman primates (Hauser et al., 2000).

Support for this view comes from several lines of research. First, as noted earlier, imaging studies in normals confirm that distinct sites of activations underlie performance in simple multiplication and subtraction (Chochon et al., 1999; Cohen, Dehaene, Chochon, Lehéricy, & Naccache, 2000; Lee, 2000). Second, all patients in whom subtraction was more impaired than subtraction had left parietal lesions and/or atrophy, most often accompanied by Gerstmann's syndrome, compatible with an impairment to the left HIPS and to the semantic representation of numerical quantities (Dehaene & Cohen, 1997; Delazer & Benke, 1997; Van Harskamp & Cipolotti, 2001). Conversely, although this is not always thoroughly documented, patients in whom multiplication is more impaired than subtraction typically have associated aphasia (e.g., Cohen et al., 2000; Dehaene & Cohen, 1997). Furthermore, the lesions often spare the intraparietal cortex and can affect multiple regions known to be engaged in language processing, such as the left perisylvian cortices including the inferior parietal lobule (Cohen et al., 2000), the left parieto-temporal carrefour (Lampl et al., 1994), or the left basal ganglia (Dehaene & Cohen, 1997).

Multiplication impairments with spared subtraction have also been reported in two patients with reading deficits in whom the lesion affected access to the language system from visual symbols (Cohen & Dehaene, 2000; McNeil & Warrington, 1994). Amazingly, one of those patients was able to subtract better than she could read the same problems (Cohen & Dehaene, 2000). This confirms the relative independence of subtraction, but not multiplication, from the language system.

Perhaps the best evidence for a dissociation between quantity processing in the HIPS and verbal number processing in the left AG comes from two studies of the temporary calculation impairments caused by electrical brain stimulation. In one patient with strips of subdural electrodes arranged over the left parietal, superior temporal, and posterior frontal regions, a single electrode site was found whose stimulation systematically disrupted multiplication performance much more than addition performance (27% vs. 87% correct; subtraction was not tested; Whalen, McCloskey, Lesser, & Gordon, 1997). Although limited information is available on localisation, this electrode was located in the left inferior parietal region, apparently close to the angular gyrus. Interestingly, multiplication performance was worse when the responses were given orally (27% correct) than when they were typed with a key pad (64% correct), suggesting that stimulation also interfered with the verbal coding of numbers.

A second case presented a double dissociation between subtraction and multiplication (Duffau et al., 2002). Cortical stimulation was performed intra-operatively during the resection of a parieto-occipital glioma. Two neighbouring sites were found within the left parietal lobe. The first, located within the angular gyrus proper (approximate Talairach coordinates −50, −60, +30), disrupted multiplication but not subtraction when stimulated. The second, located more superiorily and anteriorily within the intraparietal sulcus (TC −45, −55, +40), disrupted subtraction but not multiplication. An intermediate location was also found where stimulation disrupted both operations. The reported coordinates, although imprecise given the distortions possibly induced by the glioma and the surgery, are completely compatible with the dissociated areas of activation observed in functional brain imaging (Chochon et al., 1999; Lee, 2000).

To close on the issue of dissociations between operations, we briefly consider the case of addition (see also Cohen & Dehaene, 2000). Addition is complex because it can be solved in at least two ways. It is similar to multiplication in that many people have memorised most of the basic addition table (single digit addition facts with a sum below 10). However, addition is also similar to subtraction in that simple addition problems can also be solved by quantity manipulation strategies, something that would be utterly impractical with multiplication. Thus, addition performance is hard to predict. Indeed, in our experience, it varies considerably across patients or even within patients, depending on the strategy that they adopt. The only clear prediction from our model is that addition performance cannot dissociate from *both* subtraction and multiplication together. That is to say, a patient cannot be impaired in addition, but not in subtraction nor in multiplication (since the latter would imply that both the verbal and the quantity circuits are intact); nor can a patient show preserved addition with impaired subtraction and multiplication (since the latter would imply that both systems are impaired).

If dissociations between operations followed a chance pattern, this prediction should be violated in about one third of cases. In fact, however, it is confirmed by essentially all patients to date (10 out of 11 patients: Cohen & Dehaene, 2000; Dagenbach & McCloskey, 1992; Dehaene & Cohen, 1997; Delazer & Benke, 1997; Lampl et al., 1994; Lee, 2000; Pesenti et al., 1994; Van Harskamp & Cipolotti, 2001). The only exception (patient FS, Van Harskamp & Cipolotti, 2001) is worth discussing. Overall, this patient was 96.3% correct (156/162) in single-digit subtraction and multiplication, but only 61.7% correct (100/162) in single-digit addition, thus superficially qualifying as a straightforward violation of our hypothesis. However, the pattern of errors in this patient was quite different from other cases of acalculia; 87% of his addition errors consisted of selecting the wrong operation (he almost always solved the corresponding multiplication problem, e.g., 3 + 3 = 9). This is very different from the other two patients reported in the same paper: patient DT, who was impaired in subtraction, made only 12.5% operation errors, and patient VP, who was impaired in multiplication, only 3.5%.

In a reanalysis, we excluded patient FS's operation errors and analysed only the remaining trials, in which he was presumably really attempting to add the operands. In this way, we can estimate patient FS's conditional success rate in addition, given that he is really trying to add. This success rate is 92.6% correct (100/108), a value which does not differ from the performance observed in the other two operations (96.3% correct). Thus, it can be argued that patient FS experiences little difficulty with arithmetic operations per se, but exhibits a selective deficit in choosing the appropriate operation. Exactly how subjects transform the task instructions and operation signs into the selection of an appropriate information-processing circuit is left largely unspecified in current models. Nevertheless, deficits affecting this task-setting level should be kept conceptually distinct from the genuine impairments in arithmetical computation itself.

In summary, a review of neuropsychological dissociations between arithmetic operations indicates that it is not necessary to postulate as many brain circuits as there are arithmetical operations (Dagenbach & McCloskey, 1992). Rather, most if not all cases so far can be accommodated by the postulated dissociation between a quantity circuit (supporting subtraction and other quantity-manipulation operations) and a verbal circuit (supporting multiplication and other rote memory-based operations).

## THE POSTERIOR SUPERIOR PARIETAL SYSTEM AND ATTENTIONAL PROCESSES

### Neuroimaging evidence

A third region, observed bilaterally in the posterior superior parietal lobule (hereafter PSPL), with a frequent mesial extension into the precuneus, is also active in several tasks requiring number manipulations. This region is posterior to the HIPS, and occupies a location superior and mesial to the AG in the superior parietal lobule (see Figure 1c and Figure 2). It is active during number comparison (Pesenti et al., 2000; Pinel et al., 2001), approximation (Dehaene et al., 1999), subtraction of two digits (Lee, 2000), and counting (Piazza et al., 2002a). It also appears to increase in activation when subjects carry out two operations instead of one (Menon et al., 2000). However, this region is clearly not specific to the number domain. Rather, it also plays a central role in a variety of visuospatial tasks including hand reaching, grasping, eye and/or attention orienting, mental rotation, and spatial working memory (Corbetta, Kincade, Ollinger, McAvoy, & Shulman, 2000; Culham & Kanwisher, 2001; Simon et al., 2002). For example, Wojciulik and Kanwisher (1999) have observed overlapping activations in this region in three tasks that all shared a component of attention-orienting. Similarly, Simon et al. (2002) observed that this region was activated during eye movement, attention movements, grasping, and pointing.

The contribution of this region to spatial attention and/or eye orienting probably explains its activation during counting, where subjects are sequentially attending to the enumerated objects. However, spatial attention does not seem to explain its activation during purely numerical operations of comparison, approximation, or subtraction. In all of those tasks, number-related activation in the PSPL was observed relative to a control that used the same spatial distribution of stimuli on screen, as well as a very similar motor response.

Obviously, any reconciliation of those sparse and disparate data set must remain tentative. The hypothesis that we would like to propose is that this region, in addition to being involved in attention orienting in space, can also contribute to attentional selection on other mental dimensions that are analogous to space, such as time (Coull & Nobre, 1998; Wojciulik & Kanwisher, 1999) or number. Psychological experiments indicate that the core semantic representation of numerical quantity can be likened to an internal "number line," a quasispatial representation on which numbers are organised by their proximity (Dehaene, Bossini, & Giraux, 1993; Moyer & Landauer, 1967). It is then conceivable that the same process of covert attention that operates to select locations in space can also be engaged when attending to specific quantities on the number line. Such number-based attention would be particularly needed in tasks that call for the selection of one amongst several quantities, for instance when deciding which of two quantities is the larger (Pesenti et al., 2000; Pinel et al., 2001), or which of two numbers approximately fits an addition problem (Dehaene et al., 1999).

## Neuropsychological evidence: Joint impairments of attention and number processing

Only a few neuropsychological and brain stimulation findings provide some support for our admittedly speculative theory. In a recent study using transcranial magnetic stimulation with normal subjects, Gobel, Walsh, and Rushworth (2001) first located left and right dorsal posterior parietal sites where stimulation interfered with performance in a visual serial search task. The coordinates of those regions correspond to those of the bilateral posterior parietal regions found active in neuroimaging studies of eye and attention orienting (Corbetta et al., 2000; Simon et al., 2002; Wojciulik & Kanwisher, 1999). They then tested the effect of magnetic stimulation at those locations on a two-digit number comparison task. On stimulated trials, comparison performance was significantly slower. Interestingly, the numerical distance effect itself was still present and relatively unchanged (although stimulation on the left tended to interfere more with numbers close to the reference, particularly those that were larger than the reference). This suggests that the stimulation did not directly interfere with a core representation of numerical quantity, but rather with the response decision process itself. At the very least, this experiment confirms that spatial attention orienting and numerical comparison both engage this parietal region, thus confirming previous brain-imaging evidence (Pinel et al., 2001).

Further support for a close interplay between the representations of space and numbers is provided by a study with unilateral neglect patients (Zorzi, Priftis, & Umiltà, 2002). It is a well-known, indeed almost a defining feature of those patients that they perform poorly in spatial bisection tests. When asked to locate the middle of a line segment, neglect patients with right parietal lesions tend to indicate a location further to the right, consistent with their failure to attend to the left side of space. Zorzi et al. tested their performance in a *numerical* bisection task, where they were asked to find the middle of two orally presented numbers. Strikingly, patients erred systematically, often selecting a number far larger than the correct answer (e.g., Q: What number falls in between 11 and 19? A: 17). This suggests that spatial attention can be oriented on the left-to-right oriented number line, and that this attention-orienting process contributes to the resolution of simple arithmetic problems such as the bisection test. Interestingly, these patients were said not to be acalculic and did not show any deficit in other numerical tasks such as simple arithmetic fact retrieval. Indeed, Vuilleumier and Rafal (1999) demonstrated, on a different group of patients with neglect, that a posterior parietal lesion does not impair the mere quantification of small number of items. Neglect patients were able to estimate numerosity with sets of up to four objects even when some of enumerated items fell in the neglected field. Again, this suggests that attentional and numerical systems are dissociable. However, Zorzi et al.'s finding of "representational neglect" on the numerical continuum indicates that spatial attention processes do contribute to some numerical tasks.

## DEVELOPMENTAL DYSCALCULIA AND THE ONTOGENY OF NUMBER REPRESENTATIONS

Whether or not our functional characterisation of three parietal subsystems is correct, it is an anatomical fact that those activations sites are strikingly reproducible. It is remarkable that the HIPS, AG, and PSPL are systematically activated in different subjects, often from different countries, with different educational strategies and achievements in mathematics (Stevenson & Stigler, 1992), and with a diversity of linguistic schemes for expressing number (Hurford, 1987). Even the fine dissociation between subtraction and multiplication is reproducible with French vs. Korean subjects (Cohen et al., 2000; Lee, 2000). Such systematicity in the anatomical organisation of parietal numerical processes must be reconciled with the obvious fact that arithmetic is, in part, a recent cultural invention.

Our hypothesis is that the cultural construction of arithmetic is made possible by pre-existing cerebral circuits that are biologically determined and are adequate to support specific subcomponents of number processing (Dehaene, 1997). This hypothesis supposes an initial prespecialisation of the brain circuits that will ultimately support high-level arithmetic in adults. It implies that it should be possible to identify precursors of those circuits in infancy and childhood. Indeed, quantity processing is present at a very young age. Infants in their first year of life can discriminate collections based on their numerosity (Dehaene et al., 1998a; Starkey & Cooper, 1980; Wynn, 1992), even when the numbers are as large as 8 vs. 16 (Xu & Spelke, 2000). Although no brain-imaging evidence is available in infants yet, we speculate that this early numerical ability may be supported by a quantity representation similar to adults' (Dehaene, 1997; Spelke & Dehaene, 1999). This representation would serve as a foundation for the construction of higher-order arithmetical and mathematical concepts.

The hypothesis of an early emergence of quantity, verbal, and attentional systems leads to several predictions concerning normal and impaired number development:

*Brain activation in infancy and childhood.* A precursor of the HIPS region should be active in infants and young children during numerosity manipulation tasks. At present, this prediction has only been tested with 5-year-old children in a number comparison task (E. Temple & Posner, 1998). Event-related potentials revealed the scalp signature of a numerical distance effect, with a topography similar to adults, common to numbers presented as Arabic numerals or as sets of dots. There is a clear need to extend those data to an earlier age and with a greater anatomical accuracy.

*Developmental dyscalculia and the parietal lobe.* Deficits of number processing should be observed in case of early left parietal injury or disorganisation. Developmental dyscalculia is relatively frequent, affecting 3–6% of children (Badian, 1983; Kosc, 1974; Lewis, Hitch, & Walker, 1994). We predict that a fraction of those children may suffer from a core conceptual deficit in the numerical domain. Indeed, a "developmental Gerstmann syndrome" has been reported (Benson & Geschwind, 1970; Kinsbourne & Warrington, 1963; Spellacy & Peter, 1978; C. M. Temple, 1989, 1991). In those children, dyscalculia is accompanied by most or all of the following symptoms: dysgraphia, left–right disorientation, and finger agnosia, which suggest a neurological involvement of the parietal lobe. Interestingly, even in a sample of 200 normal children, a test of finger knowledge appears to be a better predictor of later arithmetic abilities than is a test of general intelligence (Fayol, Barrouillet, & Marinthe, 1998).

Two recent reports directly relate developmental dyscalculia to an underlying left parietal disorganisation. Levy, Reis, and Grafman (1999) report the case of an adult with lifelong isolated dyscalculia together with superior intelligence and reading ability, in whom the standard anatomical MRI appeared normal, yet MR spectroscopy techniques revealed a metabolic abnormality in the left inferior parietal area. Similarly, Isaacs, Edmonds, Lucas, and Gadian (2001) used voxel-based morphometry to compare gray matter density in adolescents born at equally severe grades of prematurity, half of whom suffered from dyscalculia. They found a single region of reduced gray matter in the left intraparietal sulcus. The Talairach coordinates of this region (−39, −39, +45) are quite close to the coordinates of the HIPS.

*Subtypes of developmental dyscalculia.* As in adult acalculia, at least two subtypes of developmental dyscalculia should be observed, and those should be traceable to a differential impairment of quantity vs. language processing circuits. Although several distinctions between subtypes of developmental dyscalculia have been proposed (e.g., Ashcraft, Yamashita, & Aram, 1992; Geary, Hamson, & Hoard, 2000; Rourke & Conway, 1997; C. M. Temple, 1991), most are based on group studies and standardised batteries of tests, which are inappropriate for testing the predicted subtle distinctions between, e.g., subtraction and multiplication. One exception is the single-case study of patient HM (C. M. Temple, 1991), who suffered from developmental phonological dyslexia. His deficit in arithmetic was mostly limited to multiplication facts, while he experienced no difficulty in solving simple addition and subtraction problems with numbers of the same size. Our view predicts that the association of verbal and multiplication impairments observed in this study should be generalisable. Multiplication deficits should be present in cases of dyscalculia accompanied by dysphasia and/or dyslexia, while subtraction and quantity-manipulation deficits should be present in patients with dyscalculia but without any accompanying dyslexia or language retardation. Although this proposal remains largely untested, Geary et al. (2000) do report interesting differences between developmental dyscalculics with or without associated dyslexia. When faced with the same simple addition problems, nondyslexics tend to use fact retrieval much more often than do dyslexics, who rather use finger-counting strategies. This is consistent with the hypothesis that an impairment of rote verbal memory is partially responsible for dyscalculia in children with dyslexia.

*Genetics of developmental dyscalculia.* If the biological predisposition view is correct, specific combinations of genes should be involved in setting up the internal organisation of the parietal lobe and, in particular, the distinction between quantity and language circuits. Thus, it should be possible to identify dyscalculias of genetic origin. The available data, indeed, indicate that when a child is dyscalculic, other family members are also frequently affected, suggesting that genetic factors may contribute to the disorder (Shalev et al., 2001). Although the search for dyscalculias of genetic origin has only very recently begun, the possibility that Turner syndrome may conform to this typology has recently attracted attention. Turner syndrome is a genetic disorder characterised by partial or complete absence of one X chromosome in a female individual. The disorder occurs in approximately 1 girl in 2000 and is associated with well-documented physical disorders and abnormal oestrogen production and pubertal development. The cognitive profile includes deficits in visual memory, visual-spatial and attentional tasks, and social relations, in the context of a normal verbal IQ (Rovet, 1993). Most interestingly in the present context is the documentation of a mild to severe deficit in mathematics, particularly clear in arithmetic (Mazzocco, 1998; Rovet, Szekely, & Hockenberry, 1994; C. M. Temple & Marriott, 1998).

Anatomically, the data suggest possible bilateral parieto-occipital dysfunction in Turner syndrome. A positron emission tomography study of five adult women demonstrated a glucose hypometabolism in bilateral parietal and occipital regions (Clark, Klonoff, & Hadyen, 1990). Two anatomical MR studies, one with 18 and the other with 30 affected women, demonstrated bilateral reductions in parieto-occipital brain volume, together with other subcortical regions (Murphy et al., 1993; see also Reiss et al., 1993; Reiss, Mazzocco, Greenlaw, Freund, & Ross, 1995). Interestingly, the phenotype of Turner syndrome can differ depending on whether the remaining X chromosome is of paternal or maternal origin (Xm or Xp subtypes; Bishop, Canning, Elgar, Morris, Jacobs, & Skuse, 2000; Skuse, 2000; Skuse et al., 1997). Such a genomic imprinting effect was first demonstrated on tests of social competence (Skuse et al., 1997). It will be interesting to see if a similar effect exists in the arithmetic domain.

## CONCLUSION

We have reviewed the evidence for a subdivision of calculation-related processes in the parietal lobe. A broader discussion of the specificity of the number processing system should also consider the satellite systems that serve as input and outputs to calculation processes. At the visual identification level, pure alexic patients who fail to read words often show a largely preserved ability to read and process digits (Cohen & Dehaene, 1995; Déjerine, 1891, 1892). Conversely, a case of impaired number reading with preserved word reading is on record (Cipolotti, Warrington, & Butterworth, 1995). In the writing domain, severe agraphia and alexia may be accompanied by a fully preserved ability to write and read Arabic numbers (Anderson, Damasio, & Damasio, 1990). Even within the speech production system, patients who suffer from random phoneme substitutions, thus resulting in the production of an incomprehensible jargon, may produce jargon-free number words (Cohen, Verstichel, & Dehaene, 1997). These dissociations, however, need not imply a distinct semantic system for number. Rather, they can probably be explained by considering that the particular syntax of number words and the peculiarities of the positional notation for Arabic numeral place special demands on visual recognition, speech production, and writing systems.

Even within the parietal lobe, our review of number-related activations suggests that much of the human capacity for number processing relies on representations and processes that are not specific to the number domain. At least two of the parietal circuits that we have described, the posterior superior parietal attention system and the left angular verbal system, are thought to be associated with broader functions than mere calculation. The third circuit, in the bilateral horizontal intraparietal region (HIPS), is a more plausible candidate for domain specificity. As reviewed above, it is systematically activated during mental arithmetic; it is more activated by number words than by other words such as names of animals; and its activation increases with the amount or duration of quantity manipulation required, but is completely independent of the notation used for numbers. Still, we are reluctant to use the term "category-specific" for this brain region, and prefer the terms "core quantity system" or "number-essential" region instead. For a purely empirical point of view, deciding whether a given region is "specific" for numbers seems an extremely difficulty enterprise. Testing for specificity would seem to require a systematic comparison of the target category (e.g., number) against a potentially infinite list of alternatives. It is also complicated by the limited resolution of brain-imaging techniques, which cannot yet resolve the fine-grained neuronal and columnar organisation of human cortex. Comparison of group studies, as was done here, may overestimate the amount of overlap between tasks. Studies of multiple tasks within the same subjects will be required to examine whether (1) the very same voxels can be activated by multiple quantity-related paradigms, and (2) those voxels cannot be activated by any other non-numerical operation. Because such studies are lacking (although see Simon et al., 2002), it is still premature to conclude for or against category-specificity in number semantics.

## REFERENCES


Anderson, S. W., Damasio, A. R., & Damasio, H. (1990). Troubled letters but not numbers. Domain specific cognitive impairments following focal damage in frontal cortex. *Brain, 113*, 749–766.

Ashcraft, M. H., Yamashita, T. S., & Aram, D. M. (1992). Mathematics performance in left and right brain-lesioned children and adolescents. *Brain and Cognition, 19*, 208–252.

Badian, N. A. (1983). Dyscalculia and nonverbal disorders of learning. In H. R. Myklebust (Ed.), *Progress in learning disabilities* (Vol. 5, pp. 235–264). New York: Stratton.

Benson, D. F., & Geschwind, N. (1970). Developmental Gerstmann syndrome. *Neurology, 20*, 293–298.

Benton, A. L. (1961). The fiction of the Gerstmann syndrome. *Journal of Neurology, 24*, 176–181.

Benton, A. L. (1992). Gerstmann's syndrome. *Archives of Neurology, 49*, 445–447.

Bishop, D. V., Canning, E., Elgar, K., Morris, E., Jacobs, P. A., & Skuse, D. H. (2000). Distinctive patterns of memory function in subgroups of females with Turner syndrome: Evidence for imprinted loci on the X-chromosome affecting neurodevelopment. *Neuropsychologia, 38*, 712–721.

Burbaud, P., Camus, O., Guehl, D., Bioulac, B., Caille, J. M., & Allard, M. (1999). A functional magnetic resonance imaging study of mental subtraction in human subjects. *Neuroscience Letters, 273*, 195–199.

Butterworth, B. (1999). *The mathematical brain*. London: Macmillan.

Butterworth, B., Cappelletti, M., & Kopelman, M. (2001). Category specificity in reading and writing: The case of number words. *Nature Neuroscience, 4*, 784–786.

Cappelletti, M., Butterworth, B., & Kopelman, M. (2001). Spared numerical abilities in a case of semantic dementia. *Neuropsychologia, 39*, 1224–39.

Chochon, F., Cohen, L., van de Moortele, P. F., & Dehaene, S. (1999). Differential contributions of the left and right inferior parietal lobules to number processing. *Journal of Cognitive Neuroscience, 11*, 617–630.

Cipolotti, L., Butterworth, B., & Denes, G. (1991). A specific deficit for numbers in a case of dense acalculia. *Brain, 114*, 2619–2637.

Cipolotti, L., Warrington, E. K., & Butterworth, B. (1995). Selective impairment in manipulating arabic numerals. *Cortex, 31*, 73–86.

Clark, C., Klonoff, H., & Hadyen, M. (1990). Regional cerebral glucose metabolism in Turner syndrome. *Canadian Journal of Neurological Sciences, 17*, 140–144.

Cohen, L., & Dehaene, S. (1995). Number processing in pure alexia: The effect of hemispheric asymmetries and task demands. *NeuroCase, 1*, 121–137.

Cohen, L., & Dehaene, S. (1996). Cerebral networks for number processing: Evidence from a case of posterior callosal lesion. *NeuroCase, 2*, 155–174.

Cohen, L., & Dehaene, S. (2000). Calculating without reading: Unsuspected residual abilities in pure alexia. *Cognitive Neuropsychology, 17*, 563–583.

Cohen, L., Dehaene, S., Chochon, F., Lehéricy, S., & Naccache, L. (2000). Language and calculation within the parietal lobe: A combined cognitive, anatomical and fMRI study. *Neuropsychologia, 38*, 1426–1440.

Cohen, L., Verstichel, P., & Dehaene, S. (1997). Neologistic jargon sparing numbers: a category specific phonological impairment. *Cognitive Neuropsychology, 14*, 1029–1061.

Corbetta, M., Kincade, J. M., Ollinger, J. M., McAvoy, M. P., & Shulman, G. L. (2000). Voluntary orienting is dissociated from target detection in human posterior parietal cortex. *Nature Neuroscience, 3*, 292–297.

Coull, J. T., & Nobre, A. C. (1998). Where and when to pay attention: The neural systems for directing attention to spatial locations and to time intervals as revealed by both PET and fMRI. *Journal of Neuroscience, 18*, 7426–7435.

Culham, J. C., & Kanwisher, N. G. (2001). Neuroimaging of cognitive functions in human parietal cortex. *Current Opinions in Neurobiology, 11*, 157–63.

Dagenbach, D., & McCloskey, M. (1992). The organization of arithmetic facts in memory: Evidence from a brain-damaged patient. *Brain and Cognition, 20*, 345–366.

Dehaene, S. (1992). Varieties of numerical abilities. *Cognition, 44*, 1–42.

Dehaene, S. (1995). Electrophysiological evidence for category-specific word processing in the normal human brain. *NeuroReport, 6*, 2153–2157.

Dehaene, S. (1996). The organization of brain activations in number comparison: Event-related potentials and the additive-factors methods. *Journal of Cognitive Neuroscience, 8*, 47–68.

Dehaene, S. (1997). *The number sense.* New York: Oxford University Press.

Dehaene, S., Bossini, S., & Giraux, P. (1993). The mental representation of parity and numerical magnitude. *Journal of Experimental Psychology: General, 122*, 371–396.

Dehaene, S., & Cohen, L. (1995). Towards an anatomical and functional model of number processing. *Mathematical Cognition, 1*, 83–120.

Dehaene, S., & Cohen, L. (1997). Cerebral pathways for calculation: Double dissociation between rote verbal and quantitative knowledge of arithmetic. *Cortex, 33*, 219–250.

Dehaene, S., Dehaene-Lambertz, G., & Cohen, L. (1998a). Abstract representations of numbers in the animal and human brain. *Trends in Neuroscience, 21*, 355–361.

Dehaene, S., & Marques, F. (2002). Cognitive euroscience: Scalar variability in price estimation and the cognitive consequences of switching to the euro. *Quarterly Journal of Experimental Psychology, 55A*, 705–731.

Dehaene, S., Naccache, L., Le Clec'H, G., Koechlin, E., Mueller, M., Dehaene-Lambertz, G., Van de Moortele, P. F., & Le Bihan, D. (1998b). Imaging unconscious semantic priming. *Nature, 395*, 597–600.

Dehaene, S., Spelke, E., Stanescu, R., Pinel, P., & Tsivkin, S. (1999). Sources of mathematical thinking: Behavioral and brain-imaging evidence. *Science, 284*, 970–974.

Dehaene, S., Tzourio, N., Frak, V., Raynaud, L., Cohen, L., Mehler, J., & Mazoyer, B. (1996). Cerebral activations during number multiplication and comparison: A PET study. *Neuropsychologia, 34*, 1097–1106.

Déjerine, J. (1891). Sur un cas de cécité verbale avec agraphie suivi d'autopsie. *Mémoires de la Société de Biologie, 3*, 197–201.

Déjerine, J. (1892). Contribution à l'étude anatomo-pathologique et clinique des différentes variétés de cécité verbale. *Mémoires de la Société de Biologie, 4*, 61–90.

Delazer, M., & Benke, T. (1997). Arithmetic facts without meaning. *Cortex, 33*, 697–710.

Duffau, H., Denvil, D., Lopes, M., Gasparini, F., Cohen, L., Capelle, L., et al. (2002). Intraoperative mapping of the cortical areas involved in multiplication and subtraction: An electrostimulation study in a patient with a left parietal glioma. *Journal of Neurology, Neurosurgery, and Psychiatry, 73*, 733–738.

Fayol, M., Barrouillet, P., & Marinthe, X. (1998). Predicting arithmetical achievement from neuropsychological performance: A longitudinal study. *Cognition, 68*, B63–B70.

Fiez, J. A., & Petersen, S. E. (1998). Neuroimaging studies of word reading. *Proceedings of the National Academy of Sciences USA, 95*, 914–921.

Fulbright, R. K., Molfese, D. L., Stevens, A. A., Skudlarski, P., Lacadie, C. M., & Gore, J. C. (2000). Cerebral activation during multiplication: A functional MR imaging study of number processing. *American Journal of Neuroradiology, 21*, 1048–1054.

Geary, D. C., Hamson, C. O., & Hoard, M. K. (2000). Numerical and arithmetical cognition: A longitudinal study of process and concept deficits in children with learning disability. *Journal of Experimental Child Psychology, 77*, 236–263.

Gerstmann, J. (1940). Syndrome of finger agnosia, disorientation for right and left, agraphia, and acalculia. *Archives of Neurology and Psychiatry, 44*, 398–408.

Gobel, S., Walsh, V., & Rushworth, M. F. (2001). The mental number line and the human angular gyrus. *Neuroimage, 14*, 1278–1289.

Gruber, O., Indefrey, P., Steinmetz, H., & Kleinschmidt, A. (2001). Dissociating neural correlates of cognitive components in mental calculation. *Cerebral Cortex, 11*, 350–359.

Hauser, M. D., Carey, S., & Hauser, L. B. (2000). Spontaneous number representation in semi-free-ranging rhesus monkeys. *Proceedings of the Royal Society of London B, Biological Science, 267*, 829–833.

Hécaen, H., Angelergues, R., & Houillier, S. (1961). Les variétés cliniques des acalculies au cours des lésions rétro-rolandiques: Approche statistique du problème. *Revue Neurologique, 105*, 85–103.

Henschen, S. E. (1919). Über Sprach- Musik- und Rechenmechanismen und ihre Lokalisationen im Grosshirn. *Zeitschrift für die desamte Neurologie und Psychiatrie, 52*, 273–298.

Hittmair-Delazer, M., Sailer, U., & Benke, T. (1995). Impaired arithmetic facts but intact conceptual knowledge: A single case study of dyscalculia. *Cortex, 31*, 139–147.

Hurford, J. R. (1987). *Language and number.* Oxford: Basil Blackwell.

Isaacs, E. B., Edmonds, C. J., Lucas, A., & Gadian, D. G. (2001). Calculation difficulties in children of very low birthweight: A neural correlate. *Brain*, *124*, 1701–1707.

Kiefer, M., & Dehaene, S. (1997). The time course of parietal activation in single-digit multiplication: Evidence from event-related potentials. *Mathematical Cognition*, *3*, 1–30.

Kinsbourne, M., & Warrington, E. K. (1963). The developmental Gerstmann syndrome. *Archives of Neurology*, *8*, 490.

Kosc, L. (1974). Developmental dyscalculia. *Journal of Learning Disabilities*, *7*, 165–177.

Lampl, Y., Eshel, Y., Gilad, R., & Sarova-Pinhas, I. (1994). Selective acalculia with sparing of the subtraction process in a patient with left parietotemporal hemorrhage. *Neurology*, *44*, 1759–1761.

Langdon, D. W., & Warrington, E. K. (1997). The abstraction of numerical relations: A role for the right hemisphere in arithmetic? *Journal of International Neuropsychological Society*, *3*, 260–268.

Le Clec'H, G., Dehaene, S., Cohen, L., Mehler, J., Dupoux, E., Poline, J. B., Lehericy, S., Van de Moortele, P. F., & Le Bihan, D. (2000). Distinct cortical areas for names of numbers and body parts independent of language and input modality. *Neuroimage*, *12*, 381–391.

Lee, K. M. (2000). Cortical areas differentially involved in multiplication and subtraction: A functional magnetic resonance imaging study and correlation with a case of selective acalculia. *Annals of Neurology*, *48*, 657–661.

Lee, K. M., & Kang, S. Y. (2002). Arithmetic operation and working memory: Differential suppression in dual tasks. *Cognition*, *83*, B63–B68.

Lefevre, J.-A. (1996). Selection of procedures in mental addition: Reassessing the problem-size effect in adults. *Journal of Experimental Psychology: Learning, Memory, and Cognition*, *22*, 216–230.

Levy, L. M., Reis, I. L., & Grafman, J. (1999). Metabolic abnormalities detected by H-MRS in dyscalculia and dysgraphia. *Neurology*, *53*, 639–641.

Lewis, C., Hitch, G. J., & Walker, P. (1994). The prevalence of specific arithmetic difficulties and specific reading difficulties in 9- and 10-year-old boys and girls. *Journal of Child Psychology and Psychiatry*, *35*, 283–292.

Mayer, E., Martory, M. D., Pegna, A. J., Landis, T., Delavelle, J., & Annoni, J. M. (1999). A pure case of Gerstmann syndrome with a subangular lesion. *Brain*, *122*, 1107–1120.

Mazzocco, M. M. (1998). A process approach to describing mathematics difficulties in girls with Turner syndrome. *Pediatrics*, *102*, 492–496.

McNeil, J. E., & Warrington, E. K. (1994). A dissociation between addition and subtraction with written calculation. *Neuropsychologia*, *32*, 717–728.

Menon, V., Rivera, S. M., White, C. D., Glover, G. H., & Reiss, A. L. (2000). Dissociating prefrontal and parietal cortex activation during arithmetic processing. *NeuroImage*, *12*, 357–365.

Moyer, R. S., & Landauer, T. K. (1967). Time required for judgements of numerical inequality. *Nature*, *215*, 1519–1520.

Murphy, D. G., DeCarli, C., Daly, E., Haxby, J. V., Allen, G., White, B. J., McIntosh, A. R., Powell, C. M., Horwitz, B., Rapoport, S. I., et al. (1993). X-chromosome effects on female brain: A magnetic resonance imaging study of Turner's syndrome. *Lancet*, *342*, 1197–1200.

Naccache, L., & Dehaene, S. (2001). The priming method: Imaging unconscious repetition priming reveals an abstract representation of number in the parietal lobes. *Cerebral Cortex*, *11*, 966–974.

Paulesu, E., Frith, C. D., & Frackowiak, R. S. J. (1993). The neural correlates of the verbal component of working memory. *Nature*, *362*, 342–345.

Pesenti, M., Seron, X., & Van der Linden, M. (1994). Selective impairment as evidence for mental organisation of arithmetical facts: BB, a case of preserved subtraction? *Cortex*, *30*, 661–671.

Pesenti, M., Thioux, M., Seron, X., & De Volder, A. (2000). Neuroanatomical substrates of arabic number processing, numerical comparison, and simple addition: A PET study. *Journal of Cognitive Neuroscience*, *12*, 461–479.

Piazza, M., Mechelli, A., Butterworth, B., & Price, C. J. (2002a). Are subitizing and counting implemented as separate or functionally overlapping processes? *Neuroimage*, *15*, 435–446.

Piazza, M., Mechelli, A., Price, C., & Butterworth, B. (2002b). *The quantifying brain: Functional neuroanatomy of numerosity estimation and counting*. Manuscript submitted for publication.

Pinel, P., Dehaene, S., Riviere, D., & LeBihan, D. (2001). Modulation of parietal activation by semantic distance in a number comparison task. *Neuroimage*, *14*, 1013–1026.

Price, C. (1998). The functional anatomy of word comprehension and production. *Trends in Cognitive Science*, *2*, 281–288.

Reiss, A. L., Freund, L., Plotnick, L., Baumgardner, T., Green, K., Sozer, A. C., Reader, M., Boehm, C., & Denckla, M. B. (1993). The effects of X monosomy on brain development: Monozygotic twins discordant for Turner's syndrome. *Annals of Neurology, 34*, 95–107.

Reiss, A. L., Mazzocco, M. M., Greenlaw, R., Freund, L. S., & Ross, J. L. (1995). Neurodevelopmental effects of X monosomy: A volumetric imaging study. *Annals of Neurology, 38*, 731–738.

Roland, P. E., & Friberg, L. (1985). Localization of cortical areas activated by thinking. *Journal of Neurophysiology, 53*, 1219–1243.

Rosselli, M., & Ardila, A. (1989). Calculation deficits in patients with right and left hemisphere damage. *Neuropsychologia, 27*, 607–617.

Rourke, B. P., & Conway, J. A. (1997). Disabilities of arithmetic and mathematical reasoning. Perspectives from neurology and neuropsychology. *Journal of Learning Disabilities, 30*, 34–46.

Rovet, J. F. (1993). The psychoeducational characteristics of children with Turner syndrome. *Journal of Learning Disabilities, 26*, 333–341.

Rovet, J., Szekely, C., & Hockenberry, M. N. (1994). Specific arithmetic calculation deficits in children with Turner syndrome. *Journal of Clinical Experimental Neuropsychology, 16*, 820–839.

Rueckert, L., Lange, N., Partiot, A., Appollonio, I., Litvar, I., Le Bihan, D., & Grafman, J. (1996). Visualizing cortical activation during mental calculation with functional MRI. *NeuroImage, 3*, 97–103.

Seymour, S. E., Reuter-Lorenz, P. A., & Gazzaniga, M. S. (1994). The disconnection syndrome: Basic findings reaffirmed. *Brain, 117*, 105–115.

Shalev, R. S., Manor, O., Kerem, B., Ayali, M., Badichi, N., Friedlander, Y., & Gross-Tsur, V. (2001). Developmental dyscalculia is a familial learning disability. *Journal of Learning Disabilities, 34*, 59–65.

Simon, O., Cohen, L., Mangin, J. F., Bihan, D. L., & Dehaene, S. (2002). Topographical layout of hand, eye, calculation and language related areas in the human parietal lobe. *Neuron, 33*, 475–487.

Skuse, D. H. (2000). Imprinting, the X-chromosome, and the male brain: Explaining sex differences in the liability to autism. *Pediatric Research, 47*, 9–16.

Skuse, D. H., James, R. S., Bishop, D. V., Coppin, B., Dalton, P., Aamodt-Leeper, G., Bacarese-Hamilton, M., Creswell, C., McGurk, R., & Jacobs, P. A. (1997). Evidence from Turner's syndrome of an imprinted X-linked locus affecting cognitive function. *Nature, 387*, 705–708.

Spelke, E., & Dehaene, S. (1999). On the foundations of numerical thinking: Reply to Simon. *Trends in Cognitive Science, 3*, 365–366.

Spelke, E. S., & Tsivkin, S. (2001). Language and number: A bilingual training study. *Cognition, 78*, 45–88.

Spellacy, F., & Peter, B. (1978). Dyscalculia and elements of the developmental Gerstmann syndrome in school children. *Cortex, 14*, 197–206.

Stanescu-Cosson, R., Pinel, P., Van de Moortele, P.-F., Le Bihan, D., Cohen, L., & Dehaene, S. (2000). Cerebral bases of calculation processes: Impact of number size on the cerebral circuits for exact and approximate calculation. *Brain, 123*, 2240–2255.

Starkey, P., & Cooper, R. G. (1980). Perception of numbers by human infants. *Science, 210*, 1033–1035.

Stevenson, H. W., & Stigler, J. W. (1992). *The learning gap*. New York: Simon & Schuster.

Takayama, Y., Sugishita, M., Akiguchi, I., & Kimura, J. (1994). Isolated acalculia due to left parietal lesion. *Archives of Neurology, 51*, 286–291.

Temple, C. M. (1989). Digit dyslexia: A category-specific disorder in development dyscalculia. *Cognitive Neuropsychology, 6*, 93–116.

Temple, C. M. (1991). Procedural dyscalculia and number fact dyscalculia: Double dissociation in developmental dyscalculia. *Cognitive Neuropsychology, 8*, 155–176.

Temple, C. M., & Marriott, A. J. (1998). Arithmetic ability and disability in Turner's syndrome: A cognitive neuropsychological analysis. *Developmental Neuropsychology, 14*, 47–67.

Temple, E., & Posner, M. I. (1998). Brain mechanisms of quantity are similar in 5-year-olds and adults. *Proceedings of the National Academy of Science USA, 95*, 7836–7841.

Thioux, M., Pesenti, M., De Volder, A., & Seron, X. (2002). Category-specific representation and processing of numbers and animal names across semantic tasks: A PET study. *NeuroImage, 13*, (6 suppl. 2/2), S617.

Thioux, M., Pillon, A., Samson, D., De Partz, M.-P., Noel, M.-P., & Seron, X. (1998). The isolation of numerals at the semantic level. *NeuroCase, 4*, 371–389.

Van Harskamp, N. J., & Cipolotti, L. (2001). Selective impairments for addition, subtraction and multiplication. Implications for the organisation of arithmetical facts. *Cortex*, *37*, 363–88.

Vuilleumier, P., & Rafal, R. (1999). "Both" means more than "two": Localizing and counting in patients with visuospatial neglect. *Nature Neuroscience*, *2*, 783–784.

Whalen, J., McCloskey, M., Lesser, R. P., & Gordon, B. (1997). Localizing arithmetic processes in the brain: Evidence from transient deficit during cortical stimulation. *Journal of Cognitive Neuroscience*, *9*, 409–417.

Wojciulik, E., & Kanwisher, N. (1999). The generality of parietal involvement in visual attention. *Neuron*, *23*, 747–764.

Wynn, K. (1992). Addition and subtraction by human infants. *Nature*, *358*, 749–750.

Xu, F., & Spelke, E. S. (2000). Large number discrimination in 6-month-old infants. *Cognition*, *74*, B1–B11.

Zago, L., Pesenti, M., Mellet, E., Crivello, F., Mazoyer, B., & Tzourio-Mazoyer, N. (2001). Neural correlates of simple and complex mental calculation. *NeuroImage*, *13*, 314–327.

Zorzi, M., Priftis, K., & Umiltà, C. (2002). Brain damage: Neglect disrupts the mental number line. *Nature*, *417*(6885), 138–139.

COGNITIVE NEUROPSYCHOLOGY, 2003, 20 (3/4/5/6), 507–523

# THE INFLUENCE OF CONCEPTUAL KNOWLEDGE ON VISUAL DISCRIMINATION

Isabel Gauthier, Thomas W. James, and Kim M. Curby
*Vanderbilt University, Nashville, USA*

Michael J. Tarr
*Brown University, Providence, USA*

Does conceptual knowledge about objects influence their perceptual processing? There is some evidence for interactions between semantic and visual knowledge in tasks requiring both long-term memory and lexical access. Here we assessed whether similar perceptual/semantic interactions arise during sequential visual matching, a task that does not require access to semantic information. Matching of two-dimensional or three-dimensional novel objects was facilitated when the objects were associated with arbitrarily assigned distinctive artificial semantic concepts as compared to similar semantic concepts. In contrast to prior demonstrations, this effect was obtained in a task that did not require naming objects, and was not affected by participants rehearsing consonant strings, suggesting a direct influence from semantic associations on visual object recognition.

## INTRODUCTION

Successful object recognition requires that visual input interface with visual memory. There is considerable evidence that conceptual knowledge that is nonvisual interacts with visual input to facilitate or interfere with recognition. For instance, supplying participants with verbal information about faces improves subsequent face recognition (Kerr & Winograd, 1982; Klatzky, Martin, & Kane, 1982), while supplying them with verbal information unrelated to a scene can facilitate recognition of that scene for days (Wiseman, MacLeod, & Lootsteen, 1985). In addition, learning to categorise objects into arbitrarily assigned sets changes the perceived similarity of those objects. For example, Goldstone and his colleagues (Goldstone, Lippa, & Shiffrin, 2001) found that faces were perceived as less similar when participants first learned to group them into different categories.

Bub and colleagues (Arguin, Bub, Dixon, Caille, & Fontaine, 1996a; Arguin, Bub, & Dudek, 1996b; Dixon, Bub, & Arguin, 1997, 1998) have investigated the interaction between visual input and conceptual knowledge by associating arbitrary names with either novel or familiar objects. They report on a patient (ELM) who presents with severe prosopagnosia, as well as a category-specific agnosia for living things. Although ELM's perceptual abilities remain intact (for instance, he is able tell whether two faces presented simultaneously are the same or different), he is unable to identify or recognise faces or other living things such as animals, fruits, or vegetables. Interestingly, when

Requests for reprints should be addressed to Isabel Gauthier, Department of Psychology, Vanderbilt University, 502 Wilson Hall, Nashville, TN 37240, USA (Email: isabel.gauthier@vanderbilt.edu).

We thank R. Marois, G. Logan, and the members of the Perceptual Expertise Network for comments. This work was supported by the National Science Foundation (IG), the James S. McDonnell Foundation (IG), and the Canadian Institutes of Health Research (TWJ).





http://www.tandf.co.uk/journals/pp/02643294.html DOI:10.1080/02643290244000275

such objects are arbitrarily paired with names that are semantically distinct, ELM can learn to identify a limited number of stimuli (objects or faces that would normally be difficult for him to identify). Thus, when ELM was asked to learn name–face pairings between a set of three unfamiliar faces and three famous names that were semantically unrelated (e.g., a famous actor, a pop singer, and a politician), he committed a similar number of naming errors to normal controls. When the faces were paired with three famous names that were semantically related (e.g., three famous figure skaters), however, ELM was unable to learn the pairings and performed far worse than controls (Dixon et al., 1998).

ELM also participated in similar experiments using name–object pairings with familiar or novel nonface objects, and living and nonliving object names (Arguin et al., 1996a, 1996b; Dixon et al., 1997). Again, ELM's performance was more similar to that of normal controls when the object names were semantically unrelated than when the names were related. These results have been replicated with a second patient who has a similar agnosia to ELM's (Schweizer, Dixon, Westwood, & Piskopos, 2001) and with a group of patients with Alzheimer's dementia (Dixon, Bub, Chertkow, & Arguin, 1999). Such results suggest that associating dissimilar semantic concepts with objects makes said objects more perceptually discriminable and thus easier to name.

## Two types of conceptual influence on visual perception

Conceptual influences on perception may be classified into two different experimental methodologies (Figure 1). First, the *effects of category learning on perception* (category learning—CL) have been studied by manipulating the categorisation of visual stimuli. For example, participants learn to categorise four objects, two into Group A and two into Group B. In such experiments, similarity ratings or psychophysical discriminations differ before and after categorisation training and this difference depends on whether the judged objects were categorised into the same or different groups. After training, objects in the same group are discriminated more slowly and judged as more similar than are objects in the different group (Goldstone, 1994; Goldstone et al., 2001; Sigala, Gabbiani, & Logothetis, 2002). In these experiments, the

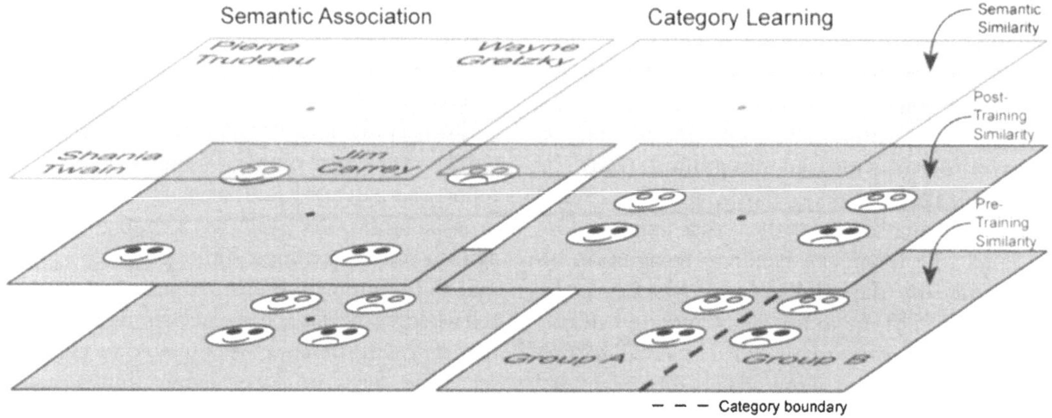


**Figure 1.** *Schematic representation of how perceived similarity of objects is affected by two different learning paradigms, semantic associations and category learning.* Semantic associations: *When names of famous people from dissimilar occupations are arbitrarily associated with face stimuli, those faces are perceived as more dissimilar after training. Post-training perceived similarity appears to depend on a combination of pre-training perceptual similarity and the similarity of the associated semantic information (Dixon et al., 1998).* Category learning: *When face stimuli are categorised into one of two groups, faces in different groups are perceived as more dissimilar after training. In this example, category membership was decided (arbitrarily) based on mouth expression, not on eye darkness. Post-training perceived similarity appears to depend mostly on the feature that was diagnostic for categorisation, in this case mouth expression (Goldstone et al., 2001).*

conceptual knowledge takes the form of the particular groups into which the objects were (arbitrarily) categorised. The speculation is that during category learning, perceptual dimensions that are diagnostic for a given category are given more weight than nondiagnostic dimensions, for instance, as described in the generalised context model (Nososfky, 1986).

Second, conceptual knowledge can influence perception *through the association of specific semantic features with objects* (semantic association—SA), as in the studies with patient ELM (Arguin et al., 1996a, 1996b; Dixon et al., 1997, 1998, 1999). In such experiments, the association of dissimilar semantic information with objects facilitates ELM's ability to name the objects.

Although both CL and SA are examples of a conceptual influence on perception, there are important differences between the two paradigms, in particular, how objects are categorised in the two cases as well as the relationship between perceptual and conceptual information. In SA experiments, objects are identified at the individual level during training (i.e., no two objects are given the same label), so that there is no between- versus within-category comparisons, the crucial manipulation in CL experiments. In contrast to CL experiments, where objects are explicitly put into categories, in SA manipulations any category would be implicitly formed (e.g., all faces given individual politicians' names can be grouped in a "politician" category). More importantly, however, in CL experiments the categories can be learned by attending selectively to one of the perceptual dimensions of the stimulus set (e.g., Goldstone et al., 2001), whereas in SA studies, there is typically no systematic relationship between perceptual features of the objects and the category (e.g., there is no perceptual dimension that separates faces of politicians from non-politicians). Thus, in an SA experiment, a novel stimulus (e.g., a new face) could not be categorised solely on the basis of perceptual information, whereas it could in a CL experiment.

One property common to both CL and SA experiments has been the use of tasks that involve recognition memory or naming. Because naming involves both semantic and lexical access, studies using naming tasks to investigate the interaction between visual processing and cognitive processes may not actually reflect an influence of semantic knowledge on early vision (Pylyshyn, 1999). Rather, such studies may be measuring a conceptual influence on the naming process. For instance, Humphreys, Lloyd-Jones, and Fias (1995) hypothesised that the influence of semantics on visual judgements occurs at the mapping between semantics and phonology. In other words, they claim that conceptual knowledge influences access to an object's name but not the perceptual processes that are performed as a precursor to naming.

Humphreys et al.'s argument was based on a "post-cue" procedure in which the presentation of a pair of coloured objects that are semantically related or unrelated is *followed by* a cue (the colour of one object) indicating which of the two objects is to be named. Semantic interference on naming is inferred when naming is slower for objects paired with semantically-related distractors. Using a modified version of the same post-cue procedure, Dean, Bub, and Masson (2001) obtained results suggesting that semantic interference affects more than object naming. As in the post-cue procedure, they presented a pair of objects that were either semantically related or unrelated followed by a cue. The cue, however, was an achromatic object (one of the pair) and the participants were to respond with the *colour* of the cued object. Crucially, in this case, retrieving the name of the object was not required to perform the task. Dean et al. still obtained evidence for semantic interference, suggesting that conceptual knowledge influences a visual task that does not require a naming response and, in fact, requires participants to remember only a single visual feature.

In summary, there appear to be at least two different ways in which conceptual knowledge can influence perceptual judgments. First, category learning affects perceptual judgments, presumably because perceptual information diagnostic for the learned categorisation is weighted more heavily in visual memory. Second, effects of semantic associations may reflect a more direct link between perceptual and conceptual representations. Such a link is at least hinted at in studies demonstrating that associating nonperceptual information with particular objects improves naming performance in patients with category-specific visual agnosia, especially when the associated concepts are relatively distinctive. In the present study, we consider whether such semantic associations affect perceptual judgements in normal individuals. Furthermore, we explore whether these effects necessarily require mediation through naming, that is, can they be obtained in the context of visual matching judgements that neither require nor encourage naming.

## Overview of experiments

In the following experiments, we examined the influence of semantic information on perceptual decisions in normal individuals. To circumvent the fact that semantics almost certainly influence visual processing through access to an object's name, we used novel objects (which have no names) and a visual sequential-matching task (in which naming is not required to generate a correct response). Critically, in the visual recognition literature sequential matching is often treated as cognitively impenetrable (e.g., Biederman & Gerhardstein, 1993). For instance, it is not necessary to endow an artificial system with semantic memories for it to be able to match two images of an object successfully (whether simultaneously or sequentially presented), even when those images present very different views of the object (Riesenhuber & Poggio, 1999).

This property of the sequential-matching task makes it an attractive tool for studying visual representation independently of other knowledge (Biederman & Gerhardstein, 1993; Ellis & Allport, 1986; Hayward & Williams, 2000; Lawson & Humphreys, 1996; Tarr, Williams, Hayward, & Gauthier, 1998) and to distinguish between perceptual and semantic impairments in neuropsychology. For instance, one of the factors used to distinguish patients with apperceptive and associative visual agnosia is their ability to perceptually match or copy objects (Farah, 1990; Humphreys & Riddoch, 1987; Kolb & Whishaw, 1996). It remains an open question, however, whether the information used to make a sequential-matching decision is exclusively visual. Here, rather than address the important but thorny question of whether there is any stage of visual processing that is cognitively impenetrable (Pylyshyn, 1999), we ask a more practical question: can participants' performance in matching judgements be assumed to reflect only perceptual knowledge?

One concern of particular importance in the study of conceptual influences on visual perception is the common confound between the semantic similarity and the structural similarity in visual stimuli. That is, objects that are semantically related (e.g., different vehicles) also tend to be visually similar. To address this issue, some studies have used novel stimuli and/or arbitrarily assigned semantic descriptions to the stimuli (for examples, see Dixon et al., 1997, 1998). In the experiments presented here, we addressed this problem in a similar way; by arbitrarily associating semantic information with novel shapes and objects. In Experiment 1, we used two-dimensional shapes rotated in the picture-plane and arbitrarily associated them with conceptual labels from a single basic-level category (to create similar concepts associated with each shape; Rosch, Mervis, Gray, Johnson, & Boyes-Braem, 1976) or from multiple basic-level categories (to create dissimilar concepts associated with each shape). In Experiments 2 and 3, we used three-dimensional objects rotated in depth and associated them with "artificial concepts" that were comprised of sets of three semantic features. The amount of overlap of these features between sets determined the semantic similarity. For both experiments, viewpoint manipulations were included to reduce idiosyncratic strategies based on salient local features (Boucart & Humphreys, 1997). Moreover, how observers generalise across changes in viewpoint is consider one of the most critical aspects of visual recognition (Biederman & Gerhardstein, 1993; Tarr et al., 1998). Thus, an effect of conceptual knowledge in this task would illustrate the importance of considering such information in any theory of object recognition.

Our overarching hypothesis was that conceptual information would facilitate the discrimination of visually similar objects when this information was semantically dissimilar. We expected a conceptual influence with only visually similar objects for one of the two following reasons: (1) visually similar objects are more confusable than visually dissimilar objects and thus would benefit from the addition of any type of information (including semantic) that would help distinguish them; and (2) visually similar objects take longer to differentiate than visually dissimilar objects, which in turn may allow more time for semantic associations to influence the discrimination process. Semantic knowledge, however, will only increase discriminability when the information associated with each object is relatively disparate, and therefore provides additional (useful) evidence for discriminating among them (Dixon et al., 1997, 1998). At the same time, it remains to be shown whether similar semantic associations actually interfere with object discriminations or not. The present study is not designed to address this question, in that we tested only the *relative* effect of similar and dissimilar semantic associations on visual recognition; whether any observed differences are due to facilitation or interference remains an open question.

## EXPERIMENT 1

Participants learned to associate four words with four shapes. The shapes were visually similar or dissimilar, and the words belonged either to different or to a common basic-level category (e.g., four species of fish). Following training, we tested whether, for only visually similar shapes (the more difficult discrimination), responses in a sequential-matching task were facilitated for shapes associated with words from *different* categories.

### Methods

*Participants*

Sixty-four participants who reported normal or corrected to normal vision participated in this experiment for payment or course credit (with informed written consent).

*Materials*

Sets of four 2-dimensional shape stimuli were selected from a larger set of 16 shapes (Figure 2) for the study and test phases of the experiment. Shapes were chosen to be either visually similar (V+) or visually dissimilar (V−). Shapes within a V+ set shared a common structure and could not be distinguished based on any one line-segment, whereas shapes within a V− set did not share a common structure. Thus, processing of the spatial relations of parts within a shape was necessary for V+ shape sets. In addition to the set of four shapes that was used during the study and test phases, two other shapes were also used for the test phase only (Figure 2), for a total of six test shapes for any given participant.

During the study phase, words were associated with the shape stimuli. Sets of 4 words were chosen from a larger set of 16 words that belonged to four categories: *birds* (crow, jay, pigeon, owl), *trees* (pine, palm, cedar, cypress), *flowers* (iris, violet, orchid, tulip), and *fish* (guppy, tuna, trout, carp). For the semantically similar condition (S+), words were chosen from within one category (e.g., crow, jay, pigeon, owl), whereas for the semantically dissimilar condition (S−), words were chosen across categories (e.g., crow, pine, iris, guppy).

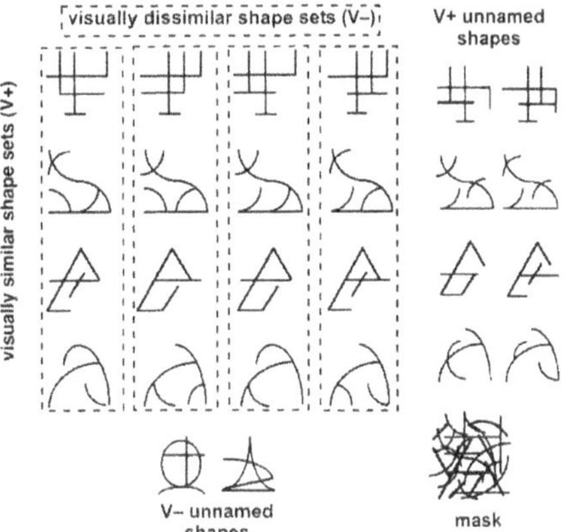


Figure 2. *Stimuli used in Experiment 1. Each participant learned four shapes, from either one of the four visually similar sets (V+, shaded areas) or from one of the four visually dissimilar sets (V−, dashed areas). The unnamed shapes used during sequential-matching test tasks in V+ and V− conditions are shown (two unnamed shapes per condition) as well as the pattern mask.*

All stimuli were presented to participants on a CRT monitor via an Apple Macintosh G3 computer running RSVP software (http://www.cog.brown.edu/~tarr/rsvp.html).

*Design and procedures*

Each participant was randomly assigned to one of four groups and learned four shapes and four words. The four groups were arrived at by crossing the V+ and V– conditions with the S+ and S– conditions, yielding four groups (V+S+, V+S–, V–S+, V–S–) with 16 participants each. Shape–word combinations were counterbalanced so that no two participants associated the same words with the same shapes. Participants were told that they were learning about four shapes on planet Zol, "where things look very different."

The experiment was divided into a study phase and a test phase. During the first part of the study phase, each shape was shown eight times, simultaneously with its word label, for 5 s. During the second part of the study phase, participants matched the shapes to these same-word labels. On each matching trial, a word was presented above the set of four shapes. Each shape was identified by a number that was presented below it on the screen. Participants responded by pressing the number key on the keyboard that corresponded to the shape that matched with the word. To prevent associations between the shapes and locations on the screen, and to encourage learning of shape–word pairings, the positions of the four shapes on the screen varied on each trial. Matching trials were presented in blocks of eight trials. Participants completed a minimum of three blocks and continued until they were able to complete two consecutive blocks with no errors.

After the shape–label pairings were learned to criterion, participants performed a speeded sequential-matching task. Six shapes were used in this test phase, the four shapes that were learned during the study phase, plus two more (Figure 2). Each trial consisted of the following events in order: a fixation cross for 200 ms, the first shape (S1) for 500 ms, a pattern mask for 1000 ms, and the second shape (S2). S2 was displayed until a "same" or "different" response was made (participants were asked to judge whether the two shapes were identical, although they could be rotated). S1 was always one of the four shapes from the study phase and was always shown at its studied orientation, denoted as zero degrees (0°). S2 was one of the four studied shapes or one of two unstudied shapes. S2 was rotated in the picture plane 0°, 55°, 110°, or 165° from the studied orientation. For each orientation, two shapes were rotated clockwise and the other two shapes were rotated counterclockwise. In total, there were 160 trials of the following types: 80 same trials, 48 different trials with a different studied shape, and 32 different trials with a different unstudied shape.

## Results and discussion

During the study phase, the number of blocks of matching trials that were required to learn the shape–word pairings was primarily determined by the visual similarity of the shapes. A 2 × 2 ANOVA with visual similarity and semantic similarity revealed a significant effect of visual similarity, $F(1, 60) = 7.9$, $MS_E = 5.957$, $p \leq .01$, but no effect of semantic similarity, $F < 1.0$, n.s., and no interaction between visual similarity and semantic similarity, $F < 1.0$, n.s. The visually similar shapes ($M_{(S-V+)} = 4.40$, $M_{(S+V+)} = 5.30$) required longer to learn than the visually dissimilar shapes ($M_{(S-V-)} = 3.06$, $M_{(S+V-)} = 3.13$). Importantly, there was no evidence that the level of semantic similarity influenced how quickly the participants learned the shape–word pairings.

For the post-training sequential-matching test task, both mean sensitivity (d′)[1] and mean response time for correct responses (RT)[2] were analysed. A 2 × 2 × 4 split-plot ANOVA with visual similarity and semantic similarity as between-subjects factors and orientation as a within-subjects factor was

[1] Mean hits and correct rejections were also analysed and showed the same pattern of results as d′.

[2] Mean RT was calculated as a geometric mean (Alf & Grossberg, 1979) for correct responses only. This estimate of central tendency is less susceptible to outliers than the arithmetic mean. See also Gauthier, Behrmann, and Tarr (1999) and Gauthier, Williams, Tarr, and Tanaka (1998).

performed on d′ and RT. As expected (Tarr & Pinker, 1989; Gauthier & Tarr, 1997), there was a significant main effect of orientation for both d′, $F(3, 180) = 4.14$, $MS_E = 1.30$, $p < .01$[3], and RT, $F(3, 180) = 40.2$, $MS_E = 3755.1$, $p < .001$. Also expected, due to the obvious difference in difficulty between the visually similar and visually dissimilar conditions, was a significant main effect of visual similarity for both d′, $F(1, 60) = 17.2$, $MS_E = 27.5$, $p < .001$, and RT, $F(1, 60) = 41.2$, $MS_E = 111861.6$, $p < .001$. There was also a significant interaction for RT between orientation and visual similarity, $F(3, 180) = 8.96$, $MS_E = 3755.1$, $p < .001$, due to a less pronounced effect of orientation in the V− condition compared to the V+ condition.

The interaction between visual similarity and semantic similarity that was predicted based on our hypothesis was not significant for either d′, $F(1, 60) = 2.63$, n.s., or RT, $F(1, 60) = 2.30$, n.s.; see Figure 3.[4]

To address our specific a priori hypothesis that performance for the V+S− condition would be better than for the V+S+ condition, we conducted a focused t-test. This comparison revealed no significant difference in d′ between these conditions, $t(30) = 1.61$, $p = .075$, with greater sensitivity for the V+S− condition. There was no significant difference in RT between the conditions, $t(30) = 1.11$, $p = .28$, however, the V+S− condition was faster than the V+S+ condition, ruling out a possible speed accuracy tradeoff. Thus, although our results were not conclusive, they do suggest that a more powerful experimental design might reveal effects consistent with our predictions.

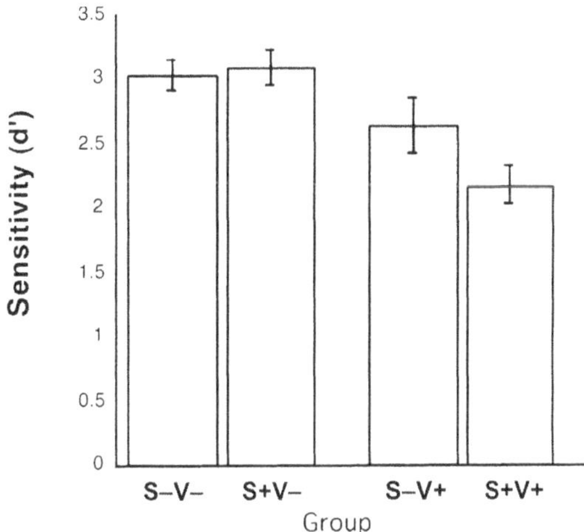


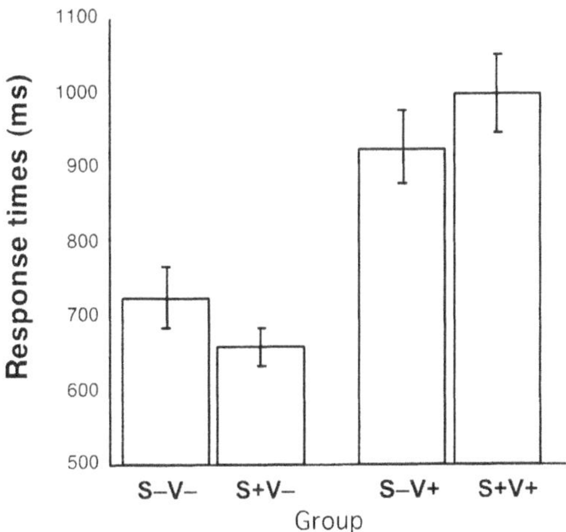


**Figure 3.** *Mean sensitivity and response times for correct responses in Experiment 1. Error bars show the standard error of the mean.*

## EXPERIMENT 2

In Experiment 2, we again tested whether arbitrary associations between semantic information and novel objects would affect subsequent performance in a perceptual task. To increase the influence of semantics on perceived similarity, we changed the way that semantic associations were generated. Participants learned to associate "artificial concepts" with three-dimensional novel objects (Figure 3). The objects were all visually similar and thus there was no visually dissimilar condition in Experiment 2. The artificial concepts were triads of nonvisual semantic features, which is an important difference between Experiment 1 and Experiment

[3] *F* statistics, $MS_E$, and *p* values have been corrected using Greenhouse-Geisser epsilon when necessary.

[4] Tests of significance for the visual similarity and semantic similarity factors were calculated in two ways, collapsing across orientation and by isolating only the 0 orientation. These analyses always produced the same effects.

2. With the shape–word pairings used in Experiment 1, activation of the word concept activated not only nonvisual semantic features, but also visual semantic features (e.g., a "crow" <is black>, <has wings>, etc.). The features that were used to create the artificial concepts were all nonvisual semantic features (Table 1). Also, sets of four artificial concepts were either made semantically similar (S+) or semantically dissimilar (S−) based on the overlap between features (Table 1), which was manipulated experimentally. Thus, the use of artificial concepts instead of single count noun labels may provide both a stronger and more direct test of semantic–perceptual interactions.

We again used a sequential-matching task to measure post-training performance with the objects. As mentioned earlier, it was unlikely that naming influences a sequential-matching task and participants did report that they were not naming the shapes in Experiment 1. Nevertheless, in an effort to further discourage participants from covertly naming the objects we introduced a subvocal verbal rehearsal task (Baddeley, 1986) for half of the sequential-matching trials. Furthermore, in Experiment 1, participants might have been encouraged to name the objects because their training task was to associate a single word with each shape and that word was always a concrete noun. In contrast, the objects in Experiment 2 were associated with triads of nonvisual semantic features.

## Methods

### *Participants*

Thirty-two participants who reported normal or corrected to normal vision participated for payment or course credit (with informed written consent).

### *Materials*

Four novel three-dimensional objects (YUFOs; Figure 4) were used. The four YUFOs were highly visually similar and could only be discriminated using subtle differences in shape. They were created using FormZ (Autodessys Inc., Columbus, OH) and rendered with a blue texture in Lightscape (Lightscape Technologies, Inc., San Jose, CA) to create highly realistic images. The four objects were rendered at an arbitrary canonical pose (referred to as 0°) as well as four other viewpoints generated by progressive 30° rotations in depth around the vertical axis. Artificial concepts were triads of features selected from a larger pool of 16 features. These features were "fast," "flexible," "friendly," "cold,"

**Table 1.** *Examples of similar and dissimilar nonvisual artificial concepts used in Experiment 2*

| | *Object 1* | *Object 2* | *Object 3* | *Object 4* |
|---|---|---|---|---|
| *Semantically dissimilar* | | | | |
| fast | ✓ | | | |
| flexible | ✓ | | | |
| friendly | ✓ | | | |
| cold | | ✓ | | |
| rare | | ✓ | | |
| sweet | | ✓ | | |
| fragile | | | ✓ | |
| hollow | | | ✓ | |
| nervous | | | ✓ | |
| sticky | | | | ✓ |
| soft | | | | ✓ |
| wet | | | | ✓ |
| *Semantically similar* | | | | |
| loud | ✓ | ✓ | ✓ | |
| heavy | | ✓ | ✓ | ✓ |
| nocturnal | ✓ | | ✓ | ✓ |
| strong | ✓ | ✓ | | ✓ |

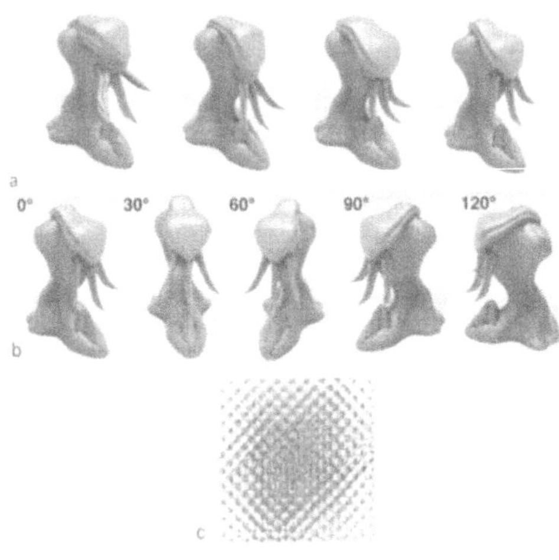


**Figure 4.** *Stimuli used in Experiment 2 (YUFOs). (a) The four YUFOs learned by each participant; (b) the five orientations in depth; and (c) the pattern mask used in the sequential-matching test task.*

"rare," "sweet," "fragile," "hollow," "nervous," "sticky," "soft," "wet," "loud," "heavy," "nocturnal," and "strong". In the semantically dissimilar (S−) condition, four artificial concepts were created by selecting three features per concept that did not overlap between concepts. Thus, for the S− condition, 12 features were used to create four concepts (Table 1). In the semantically similar (S+) condition, four concepts were created from just four features. Thus, each feature was used in three of the four concepts, leading to considerably feature overlap between the concepts (Table 1). The object–concept combinations were counterbalanced as in Experiment 1.

All stimuli were presented to participants on a CRT monitor via a MacIntosh G3 computer running RSVP software. Six sheets of paper with the pictures of the four YUFOs on them were also given to the participants.

*Design and procedures*

Participants were randomly assigned to either the S+ or S− conditions. The experiment was divided into a study phase and a test phase. For the study phase, a different training procedure was used for Experiment 2 than was used for Experiment 1, due to the assumption that learning to associate semantic feature triads with objects would be more difficult than associating single words.

During the first part of the study phase, each object was shown four times, simultaneously with two features from its three-feature concept, for 5 s. During the second part of the study phase, participants answered 16 questions about the association between pairs of features and the objects (e.g., "Is this one *cold* and *flexible*?"). During the third part of the study phase, two objects were shown six times, simultaneously with all three features from their associated concept, for 5 s. During the fourth part of the study phase, participants answered 24 questions about the association between single features and these two objects (e.g., "Is this one *sticky*?"). During the fifth part of the study phase, the remaining two objects were shown six times, simultaneously with all three features from the associated concept, for 5 s. During the sixth part of the study phase, participants then answered 50 questions about associations between single features and all four objects. These six parts of the study phase (110 trials) were then repeated, for a total of 220 study trials. To facilitate learning, at six points during the study phase, participants were asked to write down all of the adjectives (features) that they could remember about each object, on sheets of paper depicting pictures of the four YUFOs. This occurred after Part 2, Part 5, and Part 6 during each of the two repetitions.

In the final part of the study phase, matched triads of features with the correct object until they reached a criterion. On each matching trial, the three features of a single artificial concept were presented above three of the four YUFOs. Each YUFO was identified by a number that was presented below it on the screen. Participants responded by pressing the number key on the keyboard that corresponded to the YUFO that matched with the concept. To prevent associations between the YUFOs and locations on the screen, and to encourage learning of object–concept pairings, the positions of each YUFO on the screen varied on each trial. Matching trials were presented in blocks of 12 trials. Participants completed a minimum of two blocks and continued until they were able to complete a block with only two errors.

After the object–concept pairings were learned to criterion, participants performed a speeded sequential-matching task in the test phase of the experiment. Each trial consisted of the following events in order: a fixation cross for 1000 ms, the first YUFO (O1) for 1500 ms, a mask for 500 ms, and the second YUFO (O2). O2 was displayed until a "same" or "different" response was made. O1 was always shown at its studied orientation, denoted 0° here. O2 was about the vertical axis 0°, 30°, 60°, 90°, or 120° from the studied orientation. O1 and O2 were the same YUFO for half of the trials. It was made clear to the participants that they were to make this decision based on the images that were presented on the screen. No mention was made of the adjectives that had been associated with the objects. Debriefing revealed that a several participants believed that the matching part of the experiment was in fact a separate experiment that was not related to the association phase. Thus, it seemed unlikely that participants were explicitly recalling the associated information to aid them in matching task. To further study this possibility, though, participants performed two blocks of 120 trials and during one block of trials, they performed a subvocal verbal-rehearsal task. During the verbal rehearsal block (the order of which was counterbalanced), participants were presented with a string of seven consonants (e.g., H K T V X C F) and then rehearsed them while performing the sequential-matching trials. After each set of 20 trials, participants were prompted to recall the string, after which they were presented with a new string for the next 20 trials.

## Results and discussion

The number of blocks required to reach criterion during the final part of the study phase was small and not significantly different between the S− condition ($M$ = 3.06, SE = 0.25) and the S+ condition ($M$ = 4.31, SE = 3.11); $t(30) = 1.46$, n.s. The number of blocks required for the S+ condition was more variable due to two participants who took longer to reach criterion (10 and 13 blocks). Apart from these two participants, all others reached criterion in four blocks or less. The mean number of blocks without the largest two values in each condition was: S+, 3.21, SE = 0.11, and S−, 3.00, SE = 0.0; $t(26) = 1.88$, n.s. Thus, there was little evidence that the level of semantic similarity influenced how quickly the participants learned the object–concept pairings. Although it may seem paradoxical that similar concepts were learned as quickly as dissimilar concepts, it should be noted that highly similar objects had to be discriminated simultaneously with learning the semantic associations. Because of the high degree of visual similarity of the novel objects, it is likely that the factor that constrained the number of trials to reach criterion was the visual similarity (which was the same) as opposed to the semantic similarity (which was varied).

For the post-training sequential-matching test task, both mean sensitivity (d′) and mean response time for correct responses (RT) were analysed. A 2 × 2 × 4 split-plot ANOVA with semantic similarity as a between-subjects factor and verbal rehearsal and orientation as within-subjects factors was performed on d′ and RT. Again, there was a significant main effect of orientation for both d′, $F(4, 120) = 41.6$, $MS_E = 15.1$, $p < .001$, and RT, $F(4, 120) = 19.5$, $MS_E = 192683.3$, $p < .001$, but orientation did not interact with the other factors.

As illustrated in Figure 5, the effect of semantic similarity was obtained in RT, $F(1, 30) = 8.02$, $MS_E$

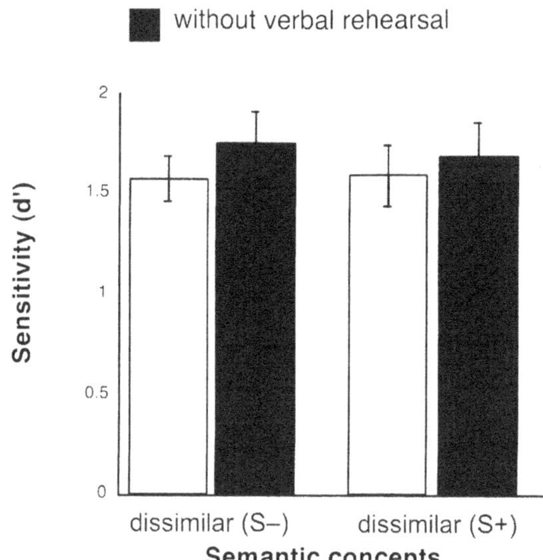


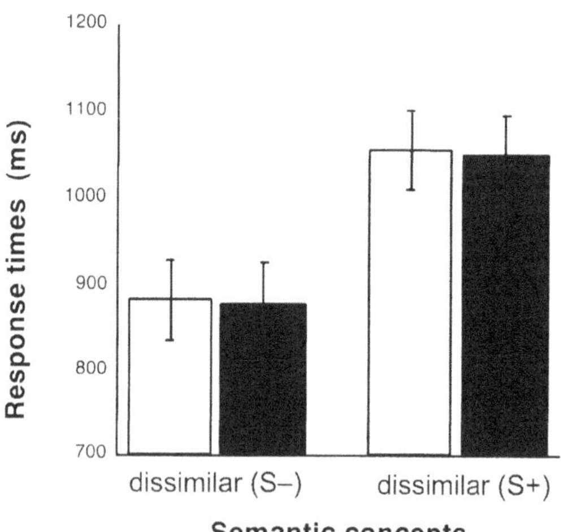


**Figure 5.** *Mean sensitivity and response times for correct responses in Experiment 2. Error bars show the standard error of the mean.*

= 2347032.7, $p < .01$, but not in d′, $F(1, 30) < 1.0$. There was no significant effect of verbal rehearsal on d′, $F(1, 30) = 3.92$, $MS_E = 0.382$, n.s., nor RT $F(1, 30) < 1.0$. Importantly, there was no interaction of verbal rehearsal with semantic similarity for either d′ or RT $F(1, 30) < 1.0$, suggesting that performing a sequential-matching task is more difficult during verbally rehearsal but that verbal rehearsal did not disrupt the effect of semantic similarity on the ability to perceptually match the objects.

Relatively dissimilar semantic associations facilitated the speed of matching over similar semantic associations three-dimensional objects. This result was in the same direction as the nonsignificant result described in Experiment 1. In addition, manipulating verbal rehearsal in Experiment 2 demonstrated that the effects of semantic similarity were not due to covert object naming.

By associating objects with artificial concepts comprised of triads of nonvisual semantic features instead of using single concrete nouns, we removed the possibility that the effects of semantic similarity were due to semantic information regarding visual properties. For instance, associating the label "crow" with an object would activate semantic information about visual properties (e.g., <has wings>, <is black>) in addition to activating semantic information about nonvisual properties (e.g., <eats carrion>, <is light>). Although dividing semantic information into only visual and nonvisual features may be overly simplistic in some contexts (McRae & Cree, 2002), because we are dealing with the visual perception of objects, this division suffices for the point we wish to make. Specifically, any influence obtained using the procedure in Experiment 1 could be interpreted as arising due to associations developed between *visual* semantic information and the stimulus shapes, with no contribution from the *nonvisual* semantic information. Because only nonvisual semantic features were used in Experiment 2, these results provide evidence that semantic information influences visual perception more generally. That is, although semantic information can be divided into different types, a correspondence between the perceptual sensory modality and the type of semantic information is not a necessary condition for perception and semantics to interact.

## EXPERIMENT 3

In Experiment 2, we obtained an effect of semantic associations on response times. To investigate whether this effect could also be observed in sensitivity, we made the sequential-matching task from Experiment 2 more difficult by restricting the presentation time of the second stimulus.

### Methods

#### *Participants*

Thirty-two participants who reported normal or corrected to normal vision participated for payment or course credit (with informed written consent).

#### *Materials*

The same stimuli as in Experiment 2 were used.

#### *Design and procedures*

Procedures were identical to those in Experiment 2, with the following differences in the sequential matching task that followed the study phase. Each trial consisted of the following events in order: a fixation cross for 1000 ms, the first YUFO presented centrally for 1500 ms, a 500 ms blank followed by the second YUFO for 175 ms, presented centred up to 70 pixels away from the centre of the screen (the position was randomly determined so that the YUFOs, each 283 pixels high × 203 pixels wide, would be randomly displayed within a window about 1.5 times their height and 1.7 times their width) and finally a square pattern mask (450 pixels wide) for 200 ms.[5] There was no verbal distractor task during the test phase.

[5] Details of the sequential matching task in Experiment 3 were set to provide a reasonable match to similar studies using lateralised presentation, albeit with central presentation (Curby, Hayward, & Gauthier, 2003). In particular, the second stimulus was masked (as it would be when presented to only one hemisphere) and it appeared with some position uncertainty.

## Results and discussion

The number of blocks required to reach criterion during the final part of the study phase was not significantly different between the S− ($M$ = 3.06, SE = 0.06) and S+ conditions ($M$ = 5.50, SE = 1.61); $t(30)$ = 1.51, n.s. The number of blocks to reach criterion was highly variable in the S+ condition due to two participants who took 20 blocks to reach criterion. Apart from these two participants, all others reached criterion in four blocks or less. Without these two participants, the mean number of blocks in the S+ condition was 3.14, SE = 0.10, and that in the S− condition was 3.00, SE = 0.0; $t(26)$ = 1.47, n.s.

Sensitivity and mean RT in the sequential matching judgements are shown in Figure 6. As expected, the effect of the semantic association on sequential matching was obtained in sensitivity, $F(1, 120)$ = 4.12, $MS_E$ = 3.170, $p$ = .05, which also showed an effect of orientation, $F(4, 120)$ = 24.62, $MS_E$ = 5.912, $p < .0001$, but no interaction of orientation with condition ($F < 1.0$). An ANOVA on mean response time for correct responses only revealed a significant effect of orientation, $F(4, 120)$ = 8.00, $MS_E$ = 36277.3, $p < .0001$. Response times in Experiment 3 were considerably faster than in Experiment 2, as can be appreciated by comparing Figures 5 and 6. This is undoubtedly due to the fast presentation of the second stimulus, preventing extended inspection times as permitted in Experiment 2.

Thus, depending on the allotted time course of visual processing, effects of nonvisual knowledge may manifest themselves in either the speed of processing or the accuracy of the discrimination. Here our results indicate that when the visual task is more difficult due to shortened processing time, relatively dissimilar semantic information associated with novel objects improves sensitivity on subsequent visual matching judgements.

## GENERAL DISCUSSION

We hypothesised that arbitrarily associating semantic information with objects would influence subsequent perceptual judgements of those objects. In addition, we argued that the influence should be independent of object naming. These hypotheses were derived from previous research on categorisation (Goldstone, 1994; Goldstone et al., 2001) and category-specific agnosia (Arguin et al., 1996a, 1996b; Dixon et al., 1997, 1998). Our results support these hypotheses and extend prior work in that we combined a manipulation consisting of the distinctiveness of nonperceptual information

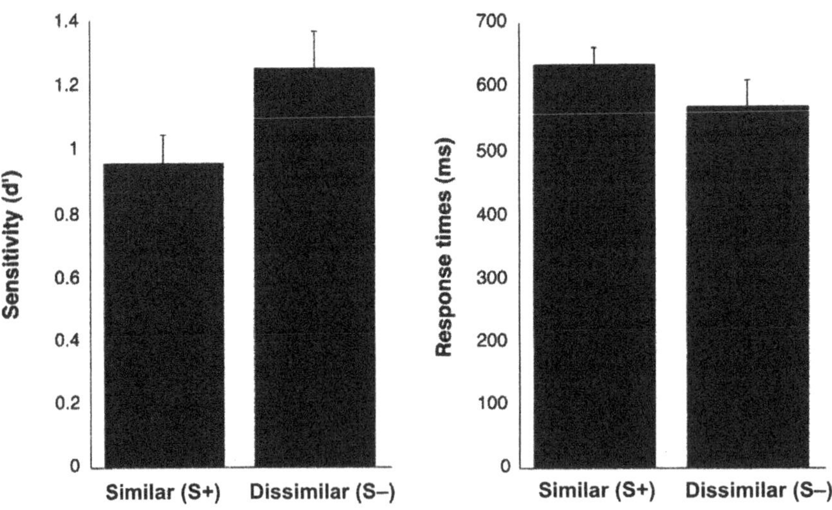


**Figure 6.** *Mean sensitivity and response times for correct responses in Experiment 3. Error bars show the standard error of the mean.*

associated with novel objects (as in studies with patients with category-specific agnosia) with a task that could be performed on the basis of perceptual information alone (as in studies of the effects of category learning), rather than using naming judgements. Associating novel objects with relatively semantically dissimilar concepts produced relatively better performance in sequential-matching judgements (as expressed either in response times or sensitivity, depending on task difficulty) than associating objects with semantically-similar concepts.

The influence of semantics on perception did not reach significance when the semantic information was a single concrete noun and when the objects were two-dimensional shapes rather than three-dimensional shapes. However, when two-dimensional shapes were visually similar the effect was in the same direction as for three-dimensional objects associated with "artificial concepts" (triads of semantic features), so it would seem that the same processing principles apply rather broadly across stimulus categories. We also found that the effect of semantic similarity can be obtained either in sensitivity or in response times depending on the specifics of the matching task: One possibility is that neither dependent variable reached significance in Experiment 1 because the effect was split between domains (visually similar shapes were matched both more accurately and faster when associated with semantically dissimilar concepts).

One somewhat surprising result is that we found no evidence that the associated conceptual information interacted with the viewpoint effects obtained when objects were matched across different orientations. One interpretation of this finding is that the "additive" nature of viewpoint and semantic similarity implies separate processing stages (Sternberg, 1966)—the former perceptual and the latter conceptual. However, given that we still do not have a clear model of how observers compensate for viewpoint (Tarr & Bülthoff, 1998), it is difficult to attribute viewpoint normalisation to a perceptual system and the effects of semantic similarity to a conceptual system. In particular, more recent models of viewpoint normalisation rely on an "accumulation of evidence" approach (see Perrett, Oram, & Ashbridge, 1998) that, plausibly, is occurring at an earlier point in object processing than once thought. Consistent with this hypothesis, a recent fMRI study comparing viewpoint effects for object recognition judgements to those obtained in mental rotation judgements found that activity related to viewpoint specifically during object recognition occurred at several points in the occipito-temporal pathway, including as early as BA 19 (Gauthier, Hayward, Tarr, Anderson, Skudlarski, & Gore, 2002). Thus, a great deal of *visual* processing may occur post-normalisation—for instance, visual processing to bind features together or to extract object structure. In short, there is a great deal of room for perceptually mediated semantic effects. Thus, the most that can be said is that the absence of an interaction between viewpoint and conceptual similarity suggests that these two factors recruit different stages of perceptual processing.

There is another interesting inference that may be based on the lack of an interaction between semantic similarity and viewpoint, namely that the effect of semantic similarity was not dependent on the time required to discriminate the objects. This supposition is further supported by the results of Experiment 3, in which participants responded almost twice as quickly as in Experiment 2, yet showed the same effect of semantic similarity. Taken together, these results suggest that semantic similarity interacted with visual similarity and not with the time taken to discriminate the objects; however, this issue deserves further investigation.

## Semantic, perceptual, and phonological interactions

We obtained an effect of semantic similarity on visual matching regardless of whether the matching task was performed while participants engaged in verbal rehearsal or not, that is, semantic similarity produced an effect under conditions that would generally not be expected to be affected by nonperceptual manipulations. Based on this result, we propose that semantic knowledge influences perceptual decisions without mediation by other nonvisual processes, such as phonological lookup or lexical access.

This claim stands in contrast to one by Humphreys and colleagues, who argued that semantic influences on perception are attributable to interference between semantic and phonological representations (Humphreys et al., 1995) or interference between two semantic representations (Boucart & Humphreys, 1992, 1994; Humphreys & Boucart, 1997). Beyond the post-cue procedure described earlier, Humphreys and colleagues also found that visual matching judgements that required attending to global shape were subject to interference from semantic information. As in the post-cue procedure, semantic interference was attributed to the semantic similarity between two matched images (e.g., more interference for matching the orientation of lines overlapping a helicopter and a truck than lines overlapping a helicopter and a rabbit). However, in this case the associations between semantic and visual features are not completely arbitrary, as they were in our design, and at least part of their effect may be attributed to greater visual similarity within than between classes (something that is accepted for visual categories). In contrast, our results indicate that matching two images of the *same object* can be influenced by an experimental manipulation of the semantic similarity of concepts associated with each of the objects in a stimulus set.

## Contextual effects of semantic associations

Having hypothesised that semantics does influence perception, that is, without mediation from other processes, we would caution that the posited interaction between perceptual and semantic representations need not have occurred during the test phase of our experiment, as we originally assumed. Our semantic manipulation may have exerted its influence during the study phase, during the test phase, or it may have influenced both phases. Our working assumption has been that associations are formed during the study phase between the perceptual representation of a given object and the semantic representation of the specified semantic information. During the test phase, these associations caused the automatic activation of associated semantic knowledge that then influences performance. An alternative explanation is that studying the novel objects in the presence of conceptual information changed the way that the perceptual representations were encoded. That is, the semantic information acted as a context within which the perceptual representations were learned. During the test phase, these different perceptual representations would produce differences in performance. Some categorisation research has favoured the latter account, in which categorisation influences the nature of the perceptual representation (Goldstone, 1994; Goldstone et al., 2001; Schyns & Rodet, 1997). A variant of this idea is that the learning phases of the two semantic conditions differed in difficulty and that this difference caused differences in the way that the perceptual representations of the objects were created. Specifically, if the S+ condition was more difficult, then the objects that were learned in the S+ condition would develop poorer representations, which might produce poorer performance during the test phase.

Our experiments were not designed to address this question directly; however, we did not find evidence of differential learning in the two semantic conditions in any of the experiments. This was perhaps because study phase duration was limited primarily by the difficulty of learning to discriminate the visually similar objects and not by learning of the artificial concepts. Interestingly, a small number of participants took a very long time to reach criterion in the study phase of Experiments 2 and 3—and these were all in the S+ condition. Although this suggests that the S+ condition may indeed have been slightly more difficult, it also suggests that participants in the S+ condition received more exposure to the objects than participants in the S− condition. Such additional experience should have, if anything, led to *better* performance during the test phase for the S+ condition, contrary to the results obtained. Thus, it is difficult to make any definitive claims about the precise locus of the effect of any semantic associations learned simultaneously with visual information. Whether different perceptual representations were built at study or associations automatically engaged at test is important to the question of the modularity of visual processes (Fodor, 1983; Pylyshyn, 1999), but in practice, both situations still suggest that it is difficult to study visual processes independently of semantic influences. As such, it may be unwarranted to assume that any visual task is protected from such influences or that novel visual stimuli would guard against this possibility.

## Implications of semantic–perceptual interactions

One implication of our findings concerns the interpretation of performance in tasks that can in principle be performed solely on the basis of perceptual information. We obtained an influence of semantic similarity in such a task and our effects arose from semantic–perceptual associations learned over a short period of time (much less than 1 hour). Furthermore, our criterion for having learned the associations successfully was not speeded and required only that participants remember them correctly. Given these parameters for learning arbitrary associations, our effects could be comparable to those of similar nonvisual associations spontaneously generated by participants as they become familiar with novel objects learned in many studies of visual cognition. Moreover, similar effects would be expected to be even more pronounced for familiar objects that have a rich pool of already-established semantic associations.

What is made clear by these results is that the field should be cautious in invoking the oft-made distinction between low-level perceptual and high-level visual recognition tasks. Such a distinction is typical in neuropsychology, where researchers often distinguish between brain-injured participants who can perform perceptual matching tasks and those who cannot (Farah, 1990; Humphreys & Riddoch, 1987; Kolb & Whishaw, 1996). Our present findings suggest that the low-level/high-level dichotomy may not be as strong as once supposed. For instance, brain-injured participants may perform more poorly than normal controls on perceptual tasks with novel objects because of perceptual impairments (the standard explanation) or, as implied by our results, due to an impaired ability to generate semantic associations with those objects. The extent to which participants automatically generate semantic attributes for novel objects they learn in the laboratory is often ignored and its impact may need to be reconsidered.

## Semantic–perceptual interactions investigated with neuroimaging

We close with the suggestion that one means for addressing some of the open questions in our work is through neuroimaging. Such methods might prove useful in differentiating between two possible mechanisms that may underlie our effect. Previous neuroimaging studies have determined that the posterior cortex is functionally heterogeneous. For example, regions have been found that respond preferentially to different perceptual attributes of objects, such as their colour, form, and movements (Corbetta, Miezin, Dobmeyer, Shulman, & Petersen, 1991). More recently, regions have been identified that respond selectively during semantic retrieval of object-related knowledge. Interestingly, these regions also appear to be somewhat heterogeneous. Martin and his colleagues (Martin, Ungerleider, & Haxby, 1999) have investigated the neural substrates that underlie the representation of both perceptual and semantic features or attributes. Their work suggests semantic and perceptual information related to a particular attribute (i.e., colour) is stored in neighbouring regions of cortex. For instance, perceptual access to an attribute activates an area of cortex that neighbours the area of cortex that is activated during semantic access to the same attribute. In particular, the regions that respond to semantic access appear to be just anterior to the related regions that respond to perceptual access. Thus, combining neuroimaging techniques with our training and testing procedure may allow us to identify some of the neural substrates through which an influence of semantics on perceptual judgements occurs.

## Conclusion

The association of nonvisual semantic features with novel objects can influence object discrimination judgements that may be made on the basis of visual information alone. Beyond complicating the task of studying perceptual processes in isolation from other higher-level processes (contrary to Fodor, 1983), it is our belief that future models of visual processing should more carefully consider the role of top-down knowledge (e.g., Mumford, 1992) and, in particular, whether or not perceptual systems can be engaged independently of non-perceptual systems.

## REFERENCES


Alf, E. F., & Grossberg, J. M. (1979). The geometric mean: Confidence limits and significance tests. *Perception and Psychophysics*, *26*, 419–421.

Arguin, M., Bub, D., Dixon, M., Caille, S., & Fontaine, S. (1996a). Shape integration and semantic proximity effects in visual agnosia for biological objects: A replication. *Brain and Cognition*, *32*, 259–261.

Arguin, M., Bub, D., & Dudek, G. (1996b). Shape integration for visual object recognition and its implication in category-specific visual agnosia. *Visual Cognition*, *3*, 221–275.

Baddeley, A. D. (1986). *Working memory*, London: Oxford University Press.

Biederman, I., & Gerhardstein, P. C. (1993). Recognizing depth-rotated objects: Evidence and conditions for three-dimensional viewpoint invariance. *Journal of Experimental Psychology: Human Perception and Performance*, *19*, 1162–1182.

Boucart, M., & Humphreys, G. W. (1992). Global shape cannot be attended without object identification. *Journal of Experimental Psychology: Human Perception and Performance*, *18*, 785–806.

Boucart, M., & Humphreys, G. W. (1994). Attention to orientation, size, luminance, and color: Attentional failure within the form domain. *Journal of Experimental Psychology: Human Perception and Performance*, *20*, 61–80.

Boucart, M., & Humphreys, G. W. (1997). Integration of physical and semantic information in object processing. *Perception*, *26*, 1197–1209.

Corbetta, M., Miezin, F. M., Dobmeyer, S., Shulman, G. L., & Petersen, S. E. (1991). Selective and divided attention during visual discriminations of shape, color, and speed: Functional anatomy by positron emission tomography. *The Journal of Neuroscience*, *11*, 2383–2402.

Curby, K. M., Hayward, W. G., & Gauthier, I. (2003). *Laterality effects in the recognition of depth rotated objects.* Manuscript submitted for publication.

Dean, M. P., Bub, D. N., & Masson, M. E. J. (2001). Interference from related items in object identification. *Journal of Experimental Psychology: Learning, Memory, and Cognition*, *27*, 733–743

Dixon, M. J., Bub, D. N., & Arguin, M. (1997). The interaction of object form and object meaning in the identification performance of a patient with category-specific visual agnosia. *Cognitive Neuropsychology*, *14*, 1085–1130.

Dixon, M. J., Bub, D. N., & Arguin, M. (1998). Semantic and visual determinants of face recognition in a prosopagnosic patient. *Journal of Cognitive Neuroscience*, *10*, 362–376.

Dixon, M. J., Bub, D. N., Chertkow, H., & Arguin, M. (1999). Object identification deficits in dementia of the Alzheimer type: Combined effects of semantic and visual proximity. *Journal of the International Neuropsychological Society*, *5*, 330–345.

Ellis, R., & Allport, D. A. (1986). Multiple levels of representation for visual objects: A behavioural study. In A. G. Cohn & J. R. Thomas (Eds.), *Artificial intelligence and its applications* (pp. 245–247). New York: Wiley.

Farah, M. J. (1990). *Visual agnosia: Disorders of object recognition and what they tell us about normal vision.* Cambridge, MA: MIT Press.

Fodor, J. A. (1983). *Modularity of mind.* Cambridge, MA: The MIT Press.

Gauthier, I., Behrmann, M., & Tarr, M. J. (1999). Can face recognition really be dissociated from object recognition? *Journal of Cognitive Neuroscience*, *11*, 349–370.

Gauthier, I., Hayward, W. G., Tarr, M. J., Anderson, A. W., Skudlarski, P., & Gore, J. C. (2002). Bold activity during mental rotation and viewpoint-dependent object recognition. *Neuron*, *34*, 161–171.

Gauthier, I., & Tarr, M. J. (1997). Orientation priming of novel shapes in the context of viewpoint-dependent recognition. *Perception*, *26*, 51–73.

Gauthier, I., Williams, P., Tarr, M. J., & Tanaka, J. W. (1998). Training "Greeble" experts: A framework for studying expert object recognition processes. *Vision Research*, *38*, 2401–2428.

Goldstone, R. (1994). Influences of categorization on perceptual discrimination. *Journal of Experimental Psychology: General, 123*, 178–200.

Goldstone, R., Lippa, Y., & Shiffrin, R. M. (2001). Altering object representations through category learning. *Cognition, 78*, 27–43.

Hayward, W. G., & Williams, P. (2000). Viewpoint dependence and object discriminability. *Psychological Science, 11*, 7–12.

Humphreys, G. W., & Boucart, M. (1997). Selection by color and form in vision. *Journal of Experimental Psychology: Human Perception and Performance, 23*, 136–153.

Humphreys, G. W., Lloyd-Jones, T. J., & Fias, W. (1995). Semantic interference effects on naming using a postcue procedure: Tapping the links between semantics and phonology with pictures and words. *Journal of Experimental Psychology: Learning, Memory, and Cognition, 21*, 961–980.

Humphreys, G. W., & Riddoch, M. J. (1987). The fractionation of visual agnosia. In G. W. Humphreys & M. J. Riddoch (Eds.), *Visual object processing: A cognitive neuropsychological approach*. Hove, UK: Lawrence Erlbaum Associates Ltd.

Kerr, N. H., & Winograd, E. (1982). Effects of contextual elaboration on face recognition. *Memory and Cognition, 10*, 603–609.

Klatzky, R. L., Martin, G. L., & Kane, R. A. (1982). Semantic interpretation effects on memory for faces, *Memory and Cognition, 10*, 195–206.

Kolb, B., & Whishaw, I. Q. (1996). *Fundamentals of human neuropsychology*. New York: W. H. Freeman.

Lawson, R., & Humphreys, G. W. (1996). View specificity in object processing: Evidence from picture matching. *Journal of Experimental Psychology: Human Perception and Performance, 22*, 395–416.

Martin, A., Ungerleider, L. G., & Haxby, J. V. (1999). Category specificity and the brain: The sensory/motor model of semantic representations of objects. In M. Gazzaniga (Ed.), *The new cognitive neuroscience* (2nd ed.). Cambridge, MA: MIT Press.

McRae, K., & Cree, G. (2002). Factors underlying category-specific semantics deficits. In E. M. E. Forde & G. Humphreys (Eds.), *Category-specificity in mind and brain*. Hove, UK: Psychology Press.

Mumford, D. (1992). On the computational architecture of the neo-cortex: II. The role of the cortico-cortical loop. *Biological Cybernetics, 66*, 241–251.

Nososfky, R. M. (1986). Attention, similarity, and the identification-categorization relationship. *Journal of Experimental Psychology: General, 115*, 39–61.

Perrett, D. I., Oram, M. W., & Ashbridge, E. (1998). Evidence accumulation in cell populations responsive to faces: An account of generalisation of recognition without mental transformations. *Cognition, 67*, 111–145.

Pylyshyn, Z. (1999). Is vision continuous with cognition? The case of impenetrability of visual perception. *Behavioral and Brain Sciences, 22*, 341–423.

Riesenhuber, M., & Poggio, T. (1999). Hierarchical models of object recognition in cortex. *Nature Neuroscience, 2*, 1019–1025.

Rosch, E., Mervis, C. B., Gray, W. D., Johnson, D. M., & Boyes-Braem, P. (1976). Basic objects in natural categories. *Cognitive Psychology, 8*, 382–439.

Schweizer, T. A., Dixon, M. J., Westwood, D., & Piskopos, M. (2001). Contribution of visual and semantic proximity to identification performance in a viral encephalitis patient. *Brain and Cognition, 46*, 260–264.

Schyns, P. G., & Rodet, L. (1997) Categorization creates functional features. *Journal of Experimental Psychology: Learning, Memory, and Cognition, 23*, 681–696.

Sigala, N., Gabbiani, F., & Logothetis, N. K. (2002). Visual categorization and object representation in monkeys and humans. *Journal of Cognitive Neuroscience, 14*, 187–198.

Sternberg, S. (1966). High-speed scanning in human memory. *Science, 153*, 652–654.

Tarr, M. J., & Bülthoff, H. H. (1998). Image-based object recognition in man, monkey, and machine. *Cognition, 67*, 1–20.

Tarr, M. J., & Pinker, S. (1989). Mental rotation and orientation-dependence in shape recognition. *Cognitive Psychology, 21*, 233–282.

Tarr, M. J., Williams, P., Hayward, W. G., & Gauthier, I. (1998). *Nature Neuroscience, 1*, 275–277.

Wiseman, S., MacLeod, C. M., & Lootsteen, P. J. (1985). Picture recognition improves with subsequent verbal information. *Journal of Experimental Psychology: Learning, Memory, and Cognition, 11*(3), 588–595.

Wiseman, S., & Neisser, U. (1974). Perceptual organization as a determinant of visual recognition memory. *American Journal of Psychology, 87*, 675–681.

COGNITIVE NEUROPSYCHOLOGY, 2003, 20 (3/4/5/6), 525–540

# ROLE OF MENTAL IMAGERY IN A PROPERTY VERIFICATION TASK: FMRI EVIDENCE FOR PERCEPTUAL REPRESENTATIONS OF CONCEPTUAL KNOWLEDGE

Irene P. Kan
*University of Pennsylvania, Philadelphia, USA*

Lawrence W. Barsalou
*Emory University, Atlanta, GA, USA*

Karen Olseth Solomon
*Willamette University, Salem, MA, USA*

Jeris K. Minor and Sharon L. Thompson-Schill
*University of Pennsylvania, Philadelphia, USA*

Is our knowledge about the appearance of objects more closely related to verbal thought or to perception? In a behavioural study using a property verification task, Kosslyn (1976) reported that there are both amodal and perceptual representations of concepts, but that amodal representations may be more easily accessed. However, Solomon (1997) argued that due to the nature of Kosslyn's stimuli, subjects may be able to bypass semantics entirely and perform this task using differences in the strength of association between words in true trials (e.g., cat–whiskers) and those in false trials (e.g., mouse–stinger). Solomon found no evidence for amodal representations when the task materials were altered to include *associated* false trials (e.g., cat–litter), which require semantic processing, as opposed to associative strategies. In the current study, we used fMRI to examine the response of regions of visual association cortex while subjects performed a property verification task with either associated or unassociated false trials. We found reliable activity across subjects within the left fusiform gyrus when true trials were intermixed with *associated* false trials but not when true trials were intermixed with *unassociated* false trials. Our data support the idea that conceptual knowledge is organised visually and that it is grounded in the perceptual system.

One of the leading theories of the organisation of semantic knowledge holds that conceptual information is distributed across distinct attribute domains, such as vision, touch, and action (Allport, 1985). Numerous investigators have drawn distinctions between visual knowledge and nonvisual (e.g., functional) knowledge, in areas ranging from language acquisition (e.g., Gentner, 1978; Nelson,

Requests for reprints should be addressed to Irene P. Kan, Department of Psychology, University of Pennsylvania, 3815 Walnut Street, Philadelphia, PA 19104-6196, USA (Email: ikan@psych.upenn.edu).

Supported by grants from National Institute of Health (NIH R01 MH60414) and Searle Scholars Program awarded to STS, and grant from National Science Foundation (SBR-9905024) awarded to LWB. We thank Jessica Pickard for assistance with data collection, Geoff Aguirre and Joseph Kable for assistance with data analysis, and two anonymous reviewers for helpful comments on an earlier version of this manuscript.





http://www.tandf.co.uk/journals/pp/02643294.html DOI:10.1080/02643290244000257

1974) to object categorisation (e.g., Rosch, Mervis, Gray, Johnson, & Boyes-Braem, 1976). Many neuroimaging studies have supported the distinction between visual and nonvisual knowledge (see Thompson-Schill, 2003, for a review). One interpretation of these studies is that our knowledge about the visual attributes of an object is represented differently from our knowledge of other, nonvisual attributes. This claim is related to a fundamental question that has been debated by philosophers (e.g., Locke, 1690/1959) and psychologists (e.g., Kosslyn, 1994; Pylyshyn, 1981) for centuries: To what extent does conceptual knowledge rely on perceptual representations, as opposed to propositional, amodal representation? That is, are the underlying representations descriptive (i.e., more akin to verbal thoughts and nonperceptual) or are they depictive (i.e., perceptual and possess visual-spatial qualities)? Until the mid-twentieth century, the view that conceptual knowledge is perceptually based was widely accepted (e.g., Locke, 1690/1959; Price, 1953). However, this assumption was called into question, and the nature of the internal representations of conceptual knowledge has undergone much scrutiny over the past few decades.

One approach that researchers have taken to address these questions is to examine the processes involved in mental imagery. It is assumed that in order to create a mental image of an object, access to conceptual knowledge is necessary. That is, in order to create a mental image of an apple, one must retrieve the stored knowledge about the concept "apple." Thus, it seems that understanding the nature of mental imagery may help us address more fundamental questions about the representation of long-term conceptual knowledge, especially knowledge about visual attributes. According to depictive theories of conceptual knowledge, mental imagery involves the same representations and mechanisms normally used during visual perception (e.g., Kosslyn, 1994; Shepard & Cooper, 1982; Zatorre, Halpern, Perry, Meyer, & Evans, 1996). That is, conceptual representations are grounded in the perceptual systems and that information is represented in a spatial and pictorial format. One line of evidence in support of this theory came from visual scanning experiments. In Kosslyn, Ball, and Reiser's (1978) classic study, subjects were instructed to focus their attention on one part of a mental image and "move" that part to the location of some other part of the image. They reported that the time taken to complete a mental scan was directly proportional to the physical distance between the two locations. Kosslyn and colleagues inferred from these findings that mental imagery and visual perception must share similar mechanisms.

However, the validity of these conclusions has been questioned. For example, Pylyshyn (1981) argued that subjects interpreted the task demands as simulating the use of visual-spatial knowledge. Similarly, Intons-Peterson (1983) suggested that subjects were responding to experimenters' expectations, and that their performance was biased by the experimenters' presumptions. These investigators have proposed that subjects' expectations resulted in performance that appeared to support a perceptual-based theory, even though the underlying representations were not perceptual. Instead, Pylyshyn and others have argued that there is a complete independence between the perceptual system and the conceptual system, such that when an object is perceived, its visual features will be represented in the perceptual system, and the conceptual system will reinterpret that information as a list of propositional features. For example, on perceiving an apple, the perceptual system represents it in a visual form, and the conceptual system reinterprets that information into an amodal feature list, with entries such as "shiny," "red," "round." Proponents of propositional theories argued that since much of cognition depends on a "language of thought," it is only natural that mental images are represented propositionally, and that this amodal list is retrieved when conceptual knowledge is accessed (Fodor & Pylyshyn, 1988; Pylyshyn, 1984). However, as Barsalou (1999) noted, nearly all evidence for amodal theories is indirect, relying either on theoretical arguments, or on the ability to implement amodal representations formally and computationally.

The only exception seems to be Kosslyn's (1975, 1976) property verification experiments, in which he investigated whether visual imagery and other forms of internal representations can be differentiated. In this task, subjects were asked to determine whether certain properties are true or false of certain concepts. For example, when presented with the concept word "cat," subjects were asked to verify whether the property "claws" is true of that concept. To determine whether individuals would consult amodal knowledge or perceptual knowledge when verifying properties, Kosslyn (1976) manipulated task instructions within the same group of subjects. For the first block of trials, subjects did not receive explicit instructions on how to perform the task. They were simply told to verify the properties as quickly as possible without sacrificing accuracy. For the second block of trials, subjects were given explicit imagery instructions. They were told to first form a vivid mental image and then to verify each property by consulting their mental picture. Furthermore, Kosslyn systematically varied two other factors: size of a property relative to its concept and the associative strength between a property and its concept.

Under neutral instructions, subjects were significantly faster at verifying properties than under the imagery condition. Furthermore, reaction times collected under the neutral instructions were correlated with associative strength between properties and their concepts, which support theories of amodal representations. On the other hand, reaction times collected under the imagery condition were not correlated with associative strength; instead, the reaction times were inversely correlated with property size. These results support theories of perceptual representations. In sum, Kosslyn concluded that there are both amodal and perceptual representations of concepts, but that amodal representations may be more easily accessed.

Although these findings have been cited extensively, recent work challenges the extent to which these findings can elucidate the representation of conceptual information. Solomon (1997) questioned the nature of the stimuli used in Kosslyn's (1976) original studies (see also Barsalou, Solomon, & Wu, 1999), noting that the true trials and the false trials actually differed on two dimensions: (1) whether the properties belong to the concepts, and (2) whether the properties are associated with the concepts. One way of assessing associative strength between two concepts is how frequently the two concepts co-occur in the same context. The more frequently they occur together, the more associated they are. Another way of thinking about associative strength is how readily a concept becomes available when another concept is accessed. For example, consider the two concept–property pairs "cat–head" and "mouse–stinger." The words in the first pair are associated because these words often appear together within the same context. On the other hand, the words "mouse" and "stinger" rarely occur within the same context, and it is unlikely that these two words are associated with each other. In other words, not only do these word pairs differ on whether the property belongs with the concept, they also differ on associative strength.

The inadvertent variation in association strength between false and true trials may have had consequences for the results reported by Kosslyn (1976). Solomon (1997) pointed out that while all of the true properties in Kosslyn's original study were associated to their concepts (e.g., cat–head), all of the false properties were unassociated to their concepts (e.g., mouse–stinger). It was possible for subjects in the neutral condition to perform the task based on a simple word association strategy. That is, subjects might have adopted a strategy of answering "yes" if the concept and property are at all associated and answering "no" if the concept and property are unassociated. Furthermore, it has been shown that when using a simple word association strategy, access to conceptual knowledge is not obligatory (Glaser, 1992). Glaser proposed a model that includes a direct connection between the printed words and the verbal lexicon, and this route is independent from the conceptual system. If subjects in Kosslyn's experiment were in fact not accessing conceptual knowledge to perform the task in the neutral condition, then the findings from that experiment do not bear on the question of the nature of conceptual knowledge representations.

Solomon (1997) replicated Kosslyn's property verification experiments (1975, 1976), with one important variation: To ensure that conceptual processing would be engaged in all property verification trials, Solomon replaced the unassociated false trials with *associated* false trials (e.g., steak–grill) in one condition of the experiment. Solomon reasoned that subjects would not be able to rely on a simple word-association strategy when the concepts and properties of both true and false trials were equivalently associated. Under these conditions, subjects' performance was predicted by perceptual factors (e.g., size) and not linguistic factors (e.g., associative strength). Contrary to Kosslyn's (1976) results, Solomon obtained this pattern of data even when subjects received neutral instructions (i.e., associated-neutral subjects). The author interpreted these data as support for the idea that conceptual knowledge is grounded in perceptual simulation. The present experiment follows from this study, but additionally addresses differences in neural activity between associated and unassociated conditions.

One approach to investigating the relation between conceptual knowledge and perception has been to compare neural mechanisms of each. This approach has been motivated, in part, by the unresolved questions from behavioural experiments. Neuropsychological studies of patients with perceptual and imagery deficits as a result of brain damage have been used to bolster the hypothesis that mental imagery and perception share common processes (e.g., Bisiach & Luzzatti, 1978; Farah, Soso, & Dasheiff, 1992; Servos & Goodale, 1995). Recently, functional neuroimaging has been used to investigate this question in normal subjects. Some studies have reported activation in visual cortex during mental imagery (e.g., Charlot, Tzourio, Zilbovicius, Mazoyer, & Denis, 1992; D'Esposito et al., 1997; Goldenberg, Podreka, Steiner, Franzen, & Deecke, 1991; Goldenberg, Podreka, Steiner, & Willmes, 1987; Roland & Friberg, 1985), in extrastriate and occasionally primary visual areas (see Kosslyn & Thompson, 2000, for a full review of this topic). As this approach will be used in the present investigation, we briefly review some relevant findings here.

Using functional magnetic resonance imaging (fMRI), D'Esposito and colleagues (1997) used a mental image generation task to examine the neural bases of mental imagery. Subjects listened to alternating blocks of concrete words (e.g., apple, horse) and abstract words (e.g., treaty, guilt) while in the scanner. Subjects were instructed to generate mental images of the concrete words' referents, and they were told to listen passively to the abstract words. D'Esposito and colleagues reported that in neurologically intact adults, visual association cortex was recruited during mental imagery. Specifically, when compared to passive listening of abstract words, generating images in response to concrete words resulted in significantly greater activity that was asymmetrically lateralised to the left fusiform gyrus, left premotor area, and the left anterior cingulate gyrus. These data were also consistent with other neuroimaging studies of mental imagery (e.g., Goldenberg et al., 1987, 1991).

Thompson-Schill, Aguirre, D'Esposito, and Farah (1999) reported similar findings in their investigation of the neural bases of semantic knowledge using fMRI. Subjects in their experiment were asked a series of yes/no questions about visual or nonvisual characteristics of living and nonliving objects. For example, the following questions were posed to the subjects: visual/living—"Does a parrot have a curved beak?"; nonvisual/living—"Are pandas found in China?"; visual/nonliving—"Are bows of violins longer than violins?"; and nonvisual/nonliving—"Does a toaster use more electricity than a radio?" Consistent with D'Esposito et al.'s (1997) results, Thompson-Schill and colleagues also found differential patterns of activations between visual knowledge retrieval and nonvisual knowledge retrieval. Specifically, greater left fusiform gyrus activity was found when subjects engaged in visual knowledge retrieval than when they executed nonvisual knowledge retrieval. Additionally, in one subject who participated in both experiments, when activation during visual knowledge retrieval was compared to the explicit imagery task used by D'Esposito et al., considerable overlap in the left fusiform gyrus was found between these two tasks. On the basis of these results, the left fusiform gyrus was a crucial region of interest in the present investigation.

The aim of the present study was to demonstrate the involvement of visual cortical regions during semantic processing—even with no explicit imagery instructions—and furthermore to show that such involvement depends on the extent to which semantic knowledge, as opposed to lexical association information, is required to perform the task. Specifically, we used fMRI to examine the involvement of the left fusiform gyrus in the property verification task. Activity in the visual association cortex during property verification would support the assertion that semantic knowledge is indeed grounded in the perceptual system. However, this prediction only applies to tasks that require the retrieval of semantic knowledge. Thus, we hypothesised that different patterns of activation would be observed depending on whether the false trials in the experiment were associated or unassociated pairs. To test this hypothesis, subjects were randomly assigned to the associated condition, in which both true and false trials were associated pairs (as in Solomon, 1997), or the unassociated condition, in which true trials were associated but false trials were unassociated pairs (as in Kosslyn, 1976). Following from Solomon, we predicted that left fusiform activity during property verification would only be observed in the associated condition because this condition forces subjects to retrieve semantic knowledge. In contrast, activation of the left fusiform gyrus during property verification would not be expected to reliably occur in the unassociated condition, in which subjects are able to adopt a word association strategy to perform the task. If semantic knowledge is represented amodally (Pylyshyn, 1981, 1984), then no activation in the visual association cortex is expected in either condition.

## METHODS

### Subjects

Fourteen subjects from the University of Pennsylvania participated in this experiment. Subjects were randomly assigned to either the associated or unassociated task condition. Subjects in the associated group were two males and five females, aged 19–21 years (mean age = 19.9 years). Subjects in the unassociated group were five males and two females, aged 18–22 years (mean age = 20.6 years). All subjects met the following inclusion criteria: They were (1) high-school educated, (2) native English speakers, and (3) right-handed. General exclusionary criteria were (1) history of neurological or psychiatric illness or (2) current use of medication affecting the central nervous system (e.g., psychotropic drugs). Informed consent was obtained from all subjects. Each subject was paid $20 for his or her participation.

### Materials

#### *Property verification task*

Each subject performed a property verification task, in which the task was to determine whether a property (e.g., frosting) was part of a concept (e.g., cake). Subjects were told that each stimulus pair was arranged in a top–bottom configuration and that all concept words were presented on the top and all property words were presented on the bottom. All of the concept–property pairs used in this experiment were originally developed by Solomon (1997). To construct the 100 true trials, 100 properties (e.g., hood, udder, drawer) were paired with 100 concepts (e.g., car, cow, dresser) from 18 different superordinate categories (e.g., vehicle, mammal, furniture), and all properties were limited to physical parts of concepts. For example, "hill" could be loosely considered a property of "ant," but here it was considered a false property because it was not a physical part of the concept. These pairings varied widely along both association strength and size of property, and no property or concept was ever repeated.

For the false trials, two sets of materials were constructed. The associated set was constructed by pairing 100 concepts with 100 associated false properties (i.e., canary–sing). The unassociated set was constructed by pairing the same 100 concepts with a random order of the same 100 false properties (i.e., canary–wine), thereby creating unassociated pairs, but also keeping the concepts and properties constant. No false property or concept was repeated or used as a true property or concept.

To assess the association strength of both the true and false pairs, an independent group of 20 subjects from University of Chicago rated the association strength of all possible pairs. For this task, subjects first read a concept word, then a property word, and then rated how much the property word had come to mind while reading the concept word. Subjects made their rating from a scale of 1 (*did not come to mind*) to 9 (*immediately came to mind*). The true pairs varied widely in association strength, with the 50 most-associated properties averaging 7.5 and the 50 least-associated properties averaging 4.6. The two kinds of false pairs differed markedly, with the associated false pairs averaging 5.0 and the unassociated false pairs averaging 1.2.

True pairs were also chosen to represent a wide variety of sizes of properties of the concepts. For example, a cat's head is larger than a cat's claw and therefore a head should be easier to resolve on an image of a cat than a claw. To assess the size of the property on the concept, 12 new subjects imagined each concept and estimated the percentage of the concept that the property occupied. For example, subjects were asked, "What percentage of the total volume of a fox is its nose?" Subjects gave a rating from 0 to 100 for each concept–property pair. The largest 50 properties averaged 29.7%, whereas the smallest 50 properties averaged 10.6%. Concept–property pairs were also chosen so that association strength and the size of the property was not correlated ($r = .13$, $p > .25$).

To summarise, there were three types of property verification trials—true, associated false, and unassociated false. The correct response for a true trial was "yes," and the correct answer for a false trial was "no." Subjects in both the associated and the unassociated groups encountered the same true trials (e.g., goat–ear). The critical trials that differed between the two groups were the false trials. Subjects in the associated condition received associated false trials (e.g., stapler–paper), and subjects in the unassociated condition received unassociated false trials (e.g., stapler–vegetable). Although both associated false trials and unassociated false trials required a "no" response, the relationships between the stimulus words differed in the two conditions. In the associated false trials, even though the two words were associated with each other, the property was not part of the object, but in the unassociated false trials, the property was neither part of the object nor an associate of the concept.

### *Baseline letter verification task*

In the letter verification task, subjects determined whether a single letter (e.g., "m") was part of a pronounceable nonword letter string (e.g., "smalum"). As in the property verification task, the stimulus pair was arranged in a top–bottom configuration, where the pronounceable nonword appeared on the top and the single letter appeared on the bottom. Average number of letters in the nonwords was matched to those of the experimental trials.

## Procedures

The procedure used in the associated and unassociated groups was identical, with the only difference being the stimuli in the critical false trials, as described above. Each trial began with a fixation point presented in the middle of the screen for 200 ms. The concept word (or nonword) followed the fixation and was presented for 2800 ms and remained on the screen for the duration of the trial. The stimulus onset asynchrony between the concept word (or nonword) and the property word (or letter) was 1300 ms. In other words, the total exposure time for the concept word (or nonword) was 2800 ms, and the total exposure time for the property word (or letter) was 1500 ms. The duration of each trial was 3000 ms. Subjects indicated their response with bilateral button presses on a four-button keypad, and their response times in milliseconds were recorded. If the answer was "yes," they pressed the two inner buttons, and if the answer was "no," they pressed the two outer buttons. They were told to respond as quickly as possible without sacrificing accuracy, and they were told that they must respond within the 1500 ms time window during which the property word remained on the screen. It is important to note that subjects were *not* given explicit instructions on *how* to make their decision (e.g., no imagery instructions were given); rather they were told to determine as accurately and as quickly as possible whether the property was part of the concept. Four sample items, using nontest pairs, were shown to the subjects to familiarise them with the task prior to the scanning session.

The timing and trial composition of the blocks were the same for both tasks. Each experimental run consisted of 20 blocks of trials, alternating between property verification blocks and letter verification blocks. True and false trials were intermixed within each property verification block (see Figure 1). There were 10 blocks (i.e., 100 trials) of trials in each run. There were 50 property verification trials and 50 letter verification trials. Among all of the trials within each run, half of them required a "yes" response, and half of them required a "no" response. A total of four runs (i.e., 400 trials) comprised the experiment.

Using PsyScope software (Cohen, MacWhinney, Flatt, & Provost, 1993), stimuli were presented by a Macintosh G3 Powerbook connected to an LCD projector. The image was projected to a screen that was placed at the subjects' feet. A mirror that was mounted to the head coil was placed right above the subjects' eyes, and it allowed them to see the projected image on the screen. However, a different stimulus presentation system was used for three of the subjects (one in the associated group and two in the unassociated group). For these three subjects, the Avotec Silent Vision Visual Presentation system was used (Avotec, 2002). A four-button fibre-optic response pad connected to the computer was used to record the subjects' button press responses.

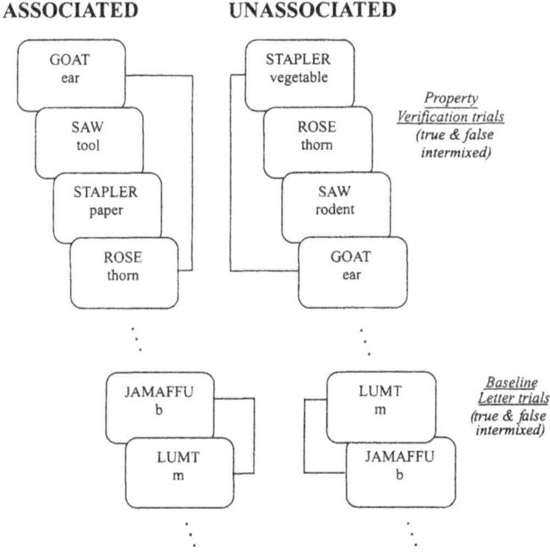


**Figure 1.** *Pictorial depiction of trial types.*

### *Image acquisition*

Following the acquisition of saggital and axial T1-weighted localiser images, gradient echo, echoplanar fMRI was performed in 21 contiguous 5 mm axial slices (TR = 2000, TE = 50, 64 × 64 pixels in a 24 cm field of view, voxel size = 3.75 mm × 3.75 mm × 5 mm) using a 1.5-T GE Signa system equipped with a fast gradient system and the standard quadrature head coil. To minimise head motion, foam padding was placed between the subject's head and the head coil. Twenty seconds of "dummy" gradient and rf pulse preceded the actual data acquisition to approach steady-state magnetisation.

### *Image processing*

Offline data processing was performed using VoxBo software (VoxBo, 2002). After image reconstruction, the data were sinc interpolated in time to correct for the fMRI acquisition sequence. A slicewise motion compensation method was utilised to remove spatially coherent signal changes by the application of a partial correlation method to each slice in time (Zarahn, Aguirre, & D'Esposito, 1997). Additional motion detection and correction was undertaken using a six-parameter, rigid-body transformation. None of the subjects had translational motion that exceeded 2 mm in any plane or angular motion that resulted in more than a 2 mm displacement. Additionally, spatial smoothing and normalisation were performed. Raw data for all runs from each subject were transformed to standardised MNI space (Evans, Collins, Mills, Brown, Kelly, & Peters, 1993) and spatially smoothed by convolution with a three-dimensional Gaussian kernel that has a FWHM of 1.5 × 1.5 × 2.0 (in voxels).

*Image analyses*

Voxelwise analysis was performed on each subject's data by using a general linear model for serially correlated error terms (Worsley & Friston, 1995), and an estimate of intrinsic temporal autocorrelation was included within the model (Aguirre, Zarahn, & D'Esposito, 1997). Furthermore, sine and cosine regressors for frequencies below that of the task (0.0148 Hz) were also included in the general linear model. Temporal data were smoothed with an empirically derived estimate of the haemodynamic response of the fMRI system; this analysis has been empirically demonstrated to hold the mapwise false positive rate at or below tabular values (Zarahn et al., 1997).

## RESULTS

### Behavioural results

The task employed in this experiment was a direct replication of Solomon's (1997) behavioural experiments. A summary of the relevant data from Solomon's study is reported in Table 1 (for a full report of the behavioural effects of these manipulations, please refer to Solomon's study). In this experiment, we collected and analysed behavioural data from nine of our subjects as a manipulation check. Overall, we replicated the basic findings reported by Solomon: Subjects were highly accurate at verifying properties for concepts and for verifying letters in nonwords. Specifically, individuals in the associated condition ($M$ = 98.0%) were equally accurate at letter verification as subjects in the unassociated condition ($M$ = 97.8%). However, subjects in the associated condition ($M$ = 93.7%) were less accurate at verifying properties than subjects in the unassociated condition ($M$ = 99.8%). In terms of reaction times, on correct true trials, subjects in the associated condition responded slightly slower on the true trials ($M$ = 829 ms) than subjects in the unassociated condition ($M$ = 809 ms). Furthermore, on correct false trials, subjects in the associated condition responded slower on the associated false trials ($M$ = 885 ms) than subjects in the unassociated condition on the unassociated false trials ($M$ = 833 ms).

### fMRI results

The same analysis was performed on data from both the associated and the unassociated groups: To identify a significant property verification main effect, all property verification trials were compared to all baseline letter verification trials. In both conditions, all subjects showed significant increases in fMRI activity during the property verification condition relative to the baseline condition, mapwise $\alpha$ = .05 (see Figure 2). Two analyses were performed to examine group differences in the pattern of activation between subjects in the associated and unassociated groups: First, we performed a focused region of interest analysis to test for group differences in the specific area of visual cortex hypothesised to be involved in imagery and visual semantics. Second, we conducted an exploratory analysis across the whole brain to identify other candidate regions displaying group differences, in either direction.

**Table 1.** *Summary of behavioural results (mean reaction times and mean error rates) from Solomon's (1997) study and the current study*

| | *Mean reaction times (SD)* | | | | *Mean error rate* | | | |
|---|---|---|---|---|---|---|---|---|
| | *Solomon (n = 96)* | | *Current study (n = 9)* | | *Solomon (n = 96)* | | *Current study (n = 9)* | |
| *Conditions* | *True* | *False* | *True* | *False* | *True* | *False* | *True* | *False* |
| Associated | 842 (182) | 979 (276) | 829 | 885 | 0.07 | 0.07 | 0.06 | 0.07 |
| Unassociated | 731 (169) | 748 (150) | 809 | 833 | 0.05 | 0.02 | 0.01 | 0.01 |

a

Subject RB, ASSOCIATED condition

L R

b

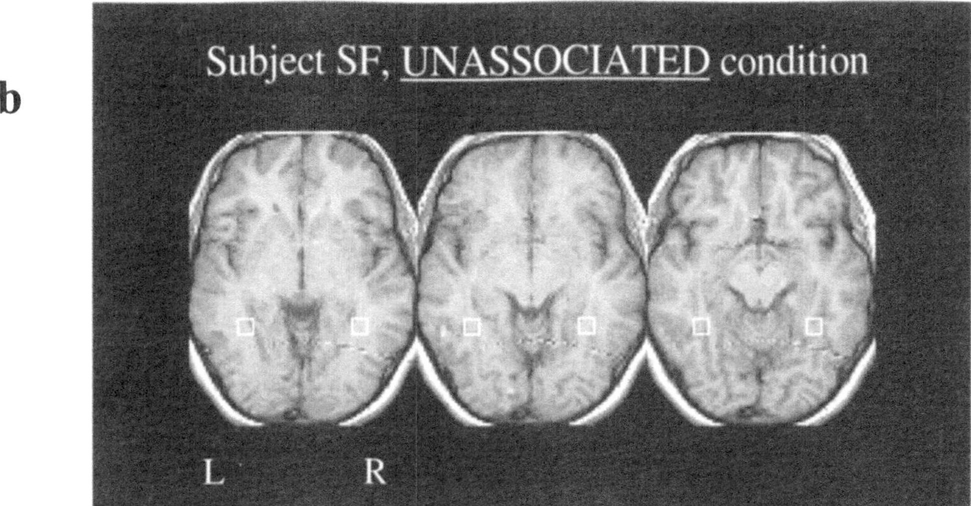


Figure 2. *Data from representative subjects in (a) the associated condition and (b) the unassociated condition. Both subjects showed significant increases in fMRI activity during property verification condition relative to baseline condition (mapwise $\alpha$ = .05). However, only the associated subject showed significant activation in the left fusiform gyrus. Furthermore, neither subject showed significant activation in the right fusiform gyrus. Anatomically defined regions of interest in the left and right fusiform gyri are indicated by the white outline boxes.*

*ROI analyses.* In each subject, an anatomically defined region of interest (ROI) in the left fusiform gyrus was created. Specifically, the local maxima coordinates for the left fusiform activity reported by D'Esposito et al. (1997) were used as a landmark (Talairach coordinates: −33, −48, −18). Subsequently, using those coordinates as the centre, a sphere that encompassed 30 voxels (~2.11 cm$^3$) was created. This ROI was then used to examine the effects of property verification. The time series from all 30 voxels were averaged, and the effect size for property verification relative to baseline trials

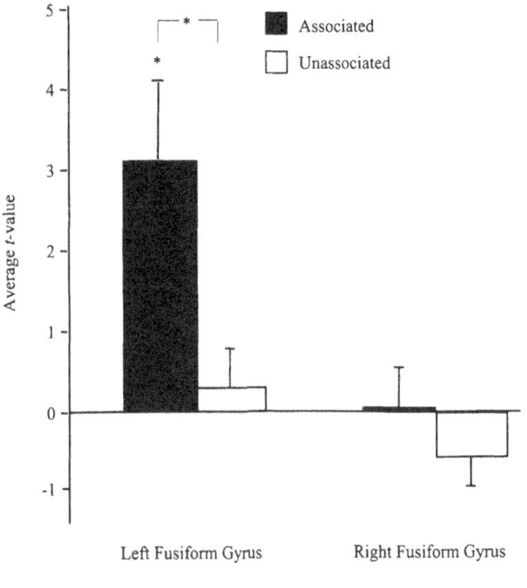


**Figure 3.** *Average* t*-value of property verification minus baseline letter verification comparison within the left fusiform gyrus and the right fusiform gyrus.*

was calculated for the averaged time series for each subject. An unpaired $t$-test of these effect sizes, with subjects as a random variable and condition as a between-subject variable, was used to test for group differences. Furthermore, to examine potential hemispheric differences, the same approach was used to analyse activity within the right fusiform gyrus (Figure 2).

As a group, subjects in the associated condition showed significant activation in the left fusiform gyrus, $M = 3.09$; $t(6) = 3.05, p < .05$ (Figure 3). On the other hand, subjects in the unassociated group did not show significant activity in the same anatomical region $M = 0.26$; $t(6) = 0.451, p = .67$ (Figure 3). An unpaired $t$-test revealed a significant difference between the two groups, $M = 2.83$; $t(12) = 2.44, p < .05$.

To investigate laterality differences, a 2 (condition) × 2 (hemispheres) mixed ANOVA was conducted. A significant interaction was found, $F(1, 12) = 4.80, p = .05$. Probing with simple effects revealed a significant hemispheric difference in the associated group, $F(1, 6) = 10.27, p < .05$, but not in the unassociated group, $F(1, 6) = 3.85, p = .10$.

*Whole-brain analyses.* We performed an exploratory whole-brain analysis that directly compared all voxels in the associated and the unassociated conditions, using a random effects group analysis of normalised data from all subjects. Due to the small number of subjects in each group, we did not have enough power to detect above-threshold differences using the conservative Bonferroni correction for ~18,000 voxels. We identified all voxels above a threshold of $t = 3.5$, based on an uncorrected alpha level of .005. To guard against Type I error, we initially included only activation with an extent of seven or more contiguous voxels. Using these criteria, the only area found to be different between the two conditions, with greater activation in the associated condition than the unassociated condition, was the left fusiform gyrus (see Figure 4). This region was slightly superior (~10 mm) to the hypothesised region in the ROI analysis. When the cluster size was lowered to two contiguous voxels, the left middle frontal gyrus also revealed greater activation for the associated condition. Furthermore, right middle temporal gyrus showed greater activation for the unassociated condition than the associated condition (see Table 2).

**Table 2.** *Local maxima for areas of activation in the random effects group analysis of the whole brain*

| *Region (Brodmann's area)* | | *Talairach coordinates (x, y, z)* | | | *Cluster size*[a] | *t* |
|---|---|---|---|---|---|---|
| *Associated > Unassociated* | | | | | | |
| Fusiform gyrus (37) | L | −45 | −53 | −6 | 9 | 4.33 |
| Middle frontal gyrus (10) | L | −33 | 55 | −6 | 2 | 4.05 |
| *Unassociated > Associated* | | | | | | |
| Middle temporal gyrus (21) | R | 48 | −24 | −6 | 2 | 3.81 |

[a]No. of voxels.

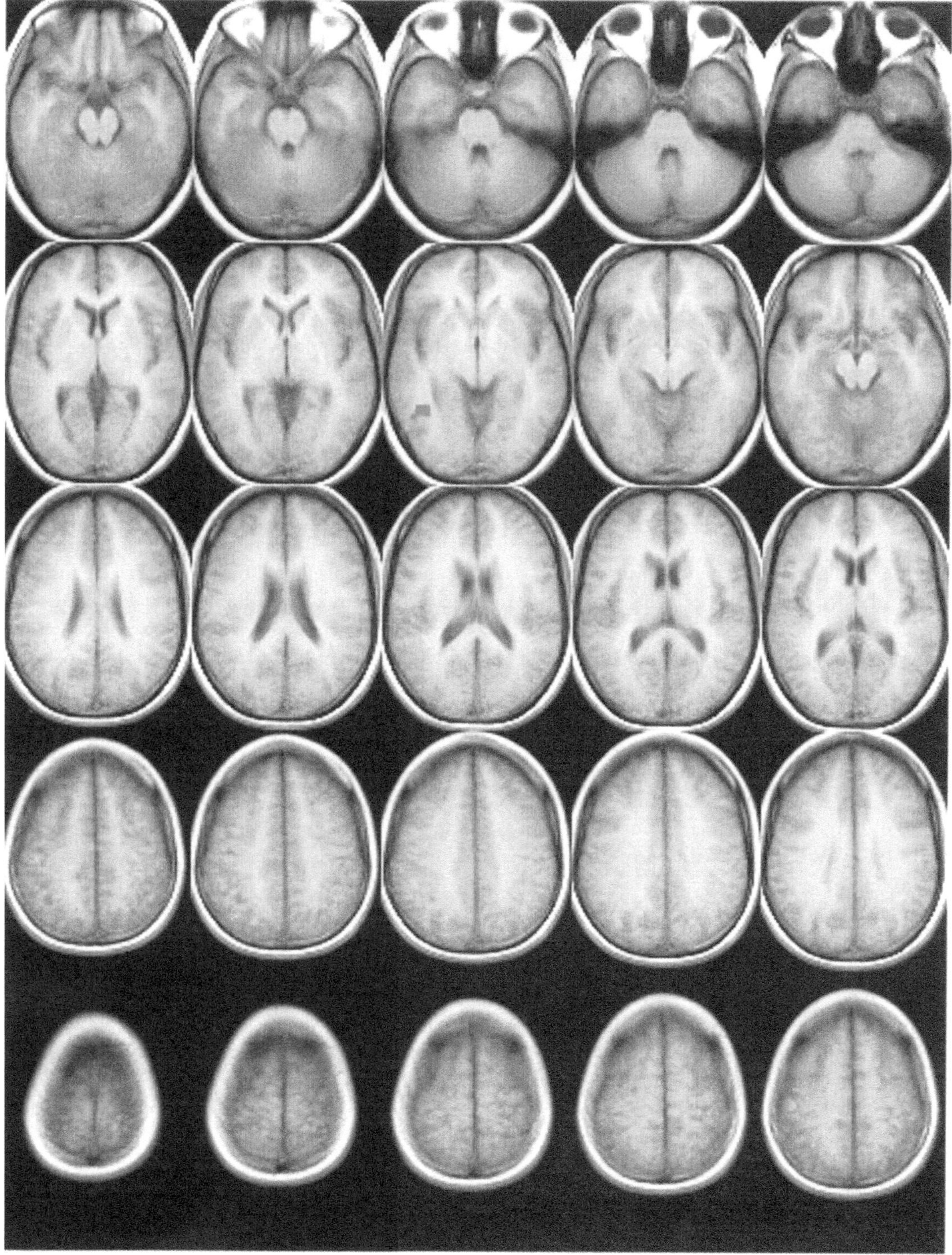

**Figure 4.** *Random effects group analysis of the whole brain. (Associated–Unassociated, cluster size = 7 contiguous voxels.)*

## DISCUSSION

In this study, we investigated the involvement of visual cortex during conceptual processing, in order to test claims about the representation of semantic knowledge. Specifically, we investigated the extent to which the left occipito-temporal region of the brain is involved in the property verification task. We examined a region of interest in the left fusiform gyrus, which has been associated with mental imagery in previous studies (D'Esposito et al., 1997; Thompson-Schill et al., 1999). We hypothesised that if semantic knowledge is indeed grounded in the perceptual system, we should find significant activity in the left fusiform gyrus during property verification, but only when conceptual information is required (i.e., when associated false trials were present). Two aspects of the results of this study are noteworthy: The location of activation associated with the property verification task and the conditions under which this activation was observed. Each of these points is elaborated below.

The first important finding of this study was that retrieval of semantic knowledge, in the absence of explicit mental imagery instructions, activated a region of visual association cortex that has been associated with visual object recognition (e.g., Ishai, Ungerleider, Martin, & Haxby, 2000; for a review, see Kanwisher, Downing, Epstein, & Kourtzi, 2001) and visual imagery (e.g., D'Esposito et al., 1997). Activation of visual association cortex during semantic processing supports the idea that conceptual knowledge is grounded in the perceptual system. Furthermore, we replicated the hemispheric asymmetry reported in other studies on mental imagery (e.g., D'Esposito et al., 1997; Farah, 1984; Riddoch, 1990). The absence of activation in the right fusiform gyrus serves as a control region to show that effects reported here are specific to areas involved in mental imagery rather than nonspecific increases in activation related to task difficulty or duration of processing. In addition, the hemispheric differences may have implications for understanding the processes involved in retrieval of semantic knowledge. Farah (1995) has claimed that the process of mental image formation is lateralised to the left hemisphere, despite the fact that visual perception occurs, at least in its initial stages, symmetrically in both hemispheres. Barsalou (1999) argued that retrieval of conceptual knowledge requires the simulation of perceptual information; our results suggest that the process of visual simulation during semantic retrieval is, like mental imagery, a left-hemisphere lateralised process. Differential involvement of the left and right fusiform gyri has also been reported in studies of object recognition. In an fMRI experiment using a repetition priming paradigm, Koutstaal, Wagner, Rotte, Maril, Buckner, and Schacter (2001) reported differential neural effects of priming in left and right fusiform gyri. Specifically, it was reported that visual form changes between first and second exposures were more "costly" in the right fusiform than in the left fusiform. That is, perceptual changes of stimuli led to a greater reduction of neural priming effects in the right fusiform than the left fusiform. Future studies may help elucidate the nature of hemispheric specialisation in the fusiform gyrus, as it relates to both image formation and object recognition.

The second important finding was that activation of this region only occurred under conditions hypothesised to require conceptual knowledge. Within the left fusiform gyrus, we found reliable activity across subjects when true trials were intermixed with associated false trials, but not when true trials were intermixed with unassociated false trials. This pattern of activation follows from the task analysis provided by Solomon (1997). Based on patterns of response times, she argued that two processes are available to perform the property verification task: First, one can consult information about lexical co-occurrence, or strength of association between two words; this process will only be effective when associative strength is a reliable indicator of the correct response (i.e., in the unassociated condition). Second, one can retrieve semantic information about the properties of an object by perceptually simulating the representation; this process is assumed to be less efficient than the former, and will thus be preferred only when the other process is ineffective (i.e., in the associated condition). According to this framework, differences in activation between the associated and unassociated condition will reflect the semantic retrieval and perceptual simulation demands that are unique to the associated condition. As predicted, these differences were observed in visual association cortex.

It is possible that activation in other regions of cortex would also differ between the two conditions, either as a result of an extended network of cortex that supports perceptual simulation or as a consequence of other cognitive differences between the two tasks (e.g., conflict monitoring in the more difficult, associated condition). In order to evaluate other, unanticipated differences, we conducted an exploratory analysis of effects across the entire brain. With a cluster size of seven contiguous voxels, the left fusiform gyrus was the only region that revealed greater activity in the associated than the unassociated condition. This result is consistent with the region of interest analysis reported above, although the location of the cluster is slightly superior to the a priori region of interest based on the results of D'Esposito et al. (1997). Although the results of the whole-brain analysis must be interpreted with caution because a conservative threshold was not applied, the trend in the data indicates that the left fusiform gyrus is selectively recruited by whatever processing differences exist between the two conditions. Based on previous research, differences in the left fusiform gyrus are likely to reflect perceptual simulation (or image formation) that accompanies semantic knowledge retrieval.

The task analysis described above would seem to support the prediction that regions associated with retrieval of lexical associations would be more active in the unassociated condition relative to the associated condition. In the unassociated minus associated contrast, the only area that showed a hint of activation was in the right middle temporal gyrus. However, note that this activation is present only when the cluster threshold is lowered to two contiguous voxels (see Table 2), so it would be premature to draw any strong inferences based on this result. One possible reason for the lack of greater activation in the unassociated condition may be due to automatic word association processing, which is common to both conditions. According to the priming literature, word association is assumed to be a relatively automatic process (e.g., Meyer & Schvaneveldt, 1971; Shelton & Martin, 1992). When subjects perform the task, word association processes may be triggered automatically. Thus, brain areas that are recruited for word associations would be activated for subjects in both associated and unassociated conditions, and a direct comparison would reveal no differences in relevant brain regions. Another possible explanation for the lack of increased activation in the unassociated condition is that perhaps there is more between-subject variability in the patterns of activation associated with retrieval of linguistic information. Since a group analysis was performed, only areas that are reliably activated for all subjects were identified. Therefore, increased between-subject variability associated with a given process would result in fewer common areas found to be active in the group analysis.

Thus far, we have illustrated how one manipulation (i.e., relationship between true and false trials in a property verification task) modulates activity in the visual association cortex. It is reasonable to further examine how other factors may affect activity in this part of the brain. Data from neuroimaging (e.g., Martin, Wiggs, Ungerleider, & Haxby, 1996; Mummery, Patterson, Hodges, & Wise, 1996; Thompson-Schill et al., 1999) and neuropsychological studies (e.g., Farah, McMullen, & Meyer, 1991; Warrington & McCarthy, 1987; Warrington & Shallice, 1984) have indicated that there may be category-specific effects in the retrieval of semantic knowledge. It is, then, reasonable to suppose that the effects that we have observed in the current study may differ across different types of stimuli. For example, perhaps the processes involved in verifying properties of living things may differ from verifying properties of nonliving things. Unfortunately, since a blocked design was used, we are unable to address that issue in this study. Thus, it will be informative to investigate these effects in an imaging study using an event-related design.

For the past few decades, Pylyshyn has maintained that subjects in mental imagery experiments are merely simulating the use of visual spatial representations, even though the internal representations are organised amodally (for a review, see Pylyshyn, 1981). He further argued that this is particularly true in experiments that explicitly ask subjects to imagine a certain object or scenario. He postulated that the subjective experience of "seeing with the mind's eye" is purely epiphenomenal. Researchers who support the idea that conceptual knowledge is grounded perceptually have tried to use neuroimaging data to counter Pylyshyn's argument. For example, in a review chapter, Kosslyn and Thompson (2000) concluded that visual perception and mental imagery share many common neural mechanisms on the basis of many neuroimaging studies. Although it is difficult to imagine a way in which subjects could "simulate" blood flow to certain regions of the brain, Pylyshyn (in press) has recently extended his criticisms to the functional neuroimaging literature as well.

We believe that our current study addresses part of Pylyshyn's concern. In the present experiment, although subjects were told to verify each property with the corresponding concept, they were *not* given explicit imagery (or nonimagery) instructions on how to perform the task. Thus, it seems improbable that subjects would interpret the task as requiring them to simulate the use of visual representations. Furthermore, it is even less plausible that all of the associated subjects would choose to simulate the use of visual spatial representations and that the unassociated subjects would choose not to simulate that experience. Our finding that manipulating the type of false trials modulates activation of the visual association areas presents a strong argument against Pylyshyn's (in press) claims. If neural activity is purely epiphenomenal, there is no reason to expect the group differences observed in this experiment. It is difficult to explain the group differences observed in this study with Pylyshyn's reasoning. In contrast, our results are easily explained by differences between the two conditions with regard to requirements for conceptual knowledge, which is grounded in the perceptual system.

## REFERENCES

Aguirre, G. K., Zarahn, E., & D'Esposito, M. (1997). Empirical analyses of BOLD fMRI statistics. II. Spatially smoothed data collected under null-hypothesis and experimental conditions. *NeuroImage, 5,* 199–212.

Allport, D. A. (1985). Distributed memory, modular subsystems and dysphasia. In S. K. Newman & R. Epstein (Eds.), *Current perspectives in dysphasia* (pp. 207–244). Edinburgh: Churchill Livingstone.

Avotec. (2002). Retrieved February 8, 2002, from http://www.avotec.org

Barsalou, L. W. (1999). Perceptual symbol systems. *Behavioral and Brain Sciences, 22,* 577–660.

Barsalou, L. W., Solomon, K. O., & Wu, L. L. (1999). *Perceptual simulation in conceptual tasks.* Paper presented at the Proceedings of the 4th conference of the International Cognitive Linguistics Association, Amsterdam, The Netherlands.

Bisiach, E., & Luzzatti, C. (1978). Unilateral neglect of representational space. *Cortex, 14,* 129–133.

Charlot, V., Tzourio, M., Zilbovicius, M., Mazoyer, B., & Denis, M. (1992). Different mental imagery abilities result in different regional cerebral blood flow activation patterns during cognitive tasks. *Neuropsychologia, 30,* 565–580.

Cohen, J. D., MacWhinney, B., Flatt, M., & Provost, J. (1993). PsyScope: A new graphic interactive environment for designing psychology experiments. *Behavioral Research Methods, Instruments, and Computers, 25,* 257–271.

D'Esposito, M., Detre, J. A., Aguirre, G. K., Stallcup, D., Alsop, D. C., Tippett, L. J., & Farah, M. J. (1997). A functional MRI study of mental image generation. *Neuropsychologia, 35,* 725–730.

Evans, A. C., Collins, D. L., Mills, S. R., Brown, E. D., Kelly, R. L., & Peters, T. M. (1993). *3D statistical neuroanatomical models from 305 MRI volumes.* Paper presented at the IEEE-Nuclear Science Symposium and Medical Imaging Conference.

Farah, M. J. (1984). The neurological basis of mental imagery: A componential analysis. *Cognition, 18,* 245–272.

Farah, M. J. (1995). Current issues in the neuropsychology of image generation. *Neuropsychologia, 33,* 1455–1471.

Farah, M. J., McMullen, P. A., & Meyer, M. M. (1991). Can recognition of living things be selectively impaired? *Neuropsychologia, 29,* 185–193.

Farah, M. J., Soso, M. J., & Dasheiff, R. M. (1992). Visual angle of the mind's eye before and after unilateral occipital lobectomy. *Journal of Experimental Psychology: Human Perception and Performance, 18*, 241–246.

Fodor, J. A., & Pylyshyn, Z. W. (1988). Connectionism and cognitive architecture: A critical analysis. *Cognition, 28*, 3–71.

Gentner, D. (1978). On relational meaning: The acquisition of verb meaning. *Child Development, 49*, 988-998.

Glaser, W. R. (1992). Picture naming. *Cognition, 42*, 61–106.

Goldenberg, G., Podreka, I., Steiner, M., Franzen, P., & Deecke, L. (1991). Contributions of occipital and temporal brain regions to visual and acoustic imagery—a SPECT study. *Neuropsychologia, 29*, 695–702.

Goldenberg, G., Podreka, I., Steiner, M., & Willmes, K. (1987). Patterns of regional cerebral blood flow related to memorizing of high and low imagery words: An emission computer tomography study. *Neuropsychologia, 25*, 473–485.

Intons-Peterson, M. J. (1983). Imagery paradigms: How vulnerable are they to experimenters' expectations? *Journal of Experimental Psychology: Human Perception and Performance, 9*, 394–412.

Ishai, A., Ungerleider, L. G., Martin, A., & Haxby, J. V. (2000). The representation of objects in the human occipital and temporal cortex. *Journal of Cognitive Neuroscience, 12*(suppl. 2), 35–51.

Kanwisher, N., Downing, P., Epstein, R., & Kourtzi, Z. (2001). Functional neuroimaging of human visual recognition. In R. Cabeza & A. Kingstone (Eds.), *The handbook of functional neuroimaging* (pp. 109–152). Cambridge, MA: MIT Press.

Kosslyn, S. M. (1975). Information representation in visual images. *Cognitive Psychology, 7*, 341–370.

Kosslyn, S. M. (1976). Can imagery be distinguished from other forms of internal representation? Evidence from studies of information retrieval time. *Memory and Cognition, 4*, 291–297.

Kosslyn, S. M. (1994). *Image and brain.* Cambridge, MA: MIT Press.

Kosslyn, S. M., Ball, T. M., & Reiser, B. J. (1978). Visual images preserve metric spatial information: Evidence from studies of image scanning. *Journal of Experimental Psychology: Human Perception and Performance, 4*, 47–60.

Kosslyn, S. M., & Thompson, W. L. (2000). Shared mechanisms in visual imagery and visual perception: Insights from cognitive neuroscience. In M. S. Gazzaniga (Ed.), *The new cognitive neurosciences.* Cambridge, MA: MIT Press.

Koutstaal, W., Wagner, A. D., Rotte, M., Maril, A., Buckner, R. L., & Schacter, D. L. (2001). Perceptual specificity in visual object priming: Functional magnetic resonance imaging evidence for a laterality difference in fusiform cortex. *Neuropsychologia, 39*, 184–199.

Locke, J. (1959). *An essay concerning human understanding, Vol. 1 & 2* (1st ed.) (original work published in 1960). New York: Dover.

Martin, A., Wiggs, C. L., Ungerleider, L. G., & Haxby, J. V. (1996). Neural correlates of category-specific knowledge. *Nature, 379*, 649–651.

Meyer, D. E., & Schvaneveldt, R. W. (1971). Facilitation in recognizing pairs of words: Evidence of a dependence between retrieval operations. *Journal of Experimental Psychology, 90*, 227–234.

Mummery, C. J., Patterson, K., Hodges, J. R., & Wise, R. J. (1996). Generating "tiger" as an animal name or a word beginning with T: Differences in brain activation [published erratum appears in Proc R Soc Lond B Biol Sci 1996 Dec 22;263(1377):1755–6]. *Proceedings of the Royal Society of London - Series B: Biological Sciences, 263*, 989–995.

Nelson, K. (1974). Concept, word, and sentence: Interrelations in acquisition and development. *Psychological Review, 81*, 267-285.

Price, H. H. (1953). *Thinking and experience.* London: Hutchinson's Universal Library.

Pylyshyn, Z. W. (1981). The imagery debate: Analogue media versus tacit knowledge. *Psychological Review, 88*, 16–45.

Pylyshyn, Z. W. (1984). *Computation and cognition: Toward a foundation for cognitive science.* Cambridge, MA: MIT Press.

Pylyshyn, Z. W. (in press). Mental imagery: In search of a theory. *Behavioral and Brain Sciences.*

Riddoch, M. J. (1990). Loss of visual imagery: A generation deficit. *Cognitive Neuropsychology, 7*, 249–273.

Roland, P. E., & Friberg, L. (1985). Localization of cortical areas activated by thinking. *Journal of Neurophysiology, 53*, 1219–1243.

Rosch, E., Mervis, C. B., Gray, W., Johnson, D., & Boyes-Braem, P. (1976). Basic objects in natural categories. *Cognitive Psychology, 8*, 382–439.

Servos, P., & Goodale, M. A. (1995). Preserved visual imagery in visual form agnosia. *Neuropsychologia, 33*, 1383–1394.

Shelton, J. R., & Martin, R. C. (1992). How semantic is automatic semantic priming? *Journal of Experimental Psychology: Learning, Memory, and Cognition*, *18*, 1191–1210.

Shepard, R. N., & Cooper, L. A. (1982). *Mental images and their transformations*. New York: Cambridge University Press.

Solomon, K. O. (1997). *The spontaneous use of perceptual representations during conceptual processing*. Chicago: University of Chicago.

Thompson-Schill, S. L. (2003). Neuroimaging studies of semantic memory: Inferring "how" from "where." *Neuropsychologia*, *43*, 280–292.

Thompson-Schill, S. L., Aguirre, G. K., D'Esposito, M., & Farah, M. J. (1999). A neural basis for category and modality specificity in semantic knowledge. *Neuropsychologia*, *37*, 671–676.

VoxBo. (2002). Retrieved February 8, 2002, from http://www.voxbo.org

Warrington, E. K., & McCarthy, R. (1987). Categories of knowledge: Further fractionations and an attempted integration. *Brain*, *110*, 1273–1296.

Warrington, E. K., & Shallice, T. (1984). Category specific semantic impairments. *Brain*, *107*, 829–854.

Worsley, K. J., & Friston, K. (1995). Analysis of fMRI time-series revisited—again. *NeuroImage*, *2*, 173–182.

Zarahn, E., Aguirre, G. K., & D'Esposito, M. (1997). Empirical analyses of BOLD fMRI statistics. I. Spatially unsmoothed data collected under null-hypothesis conditions. *NeuroImage*, *5*, 179–197.

Zatorre, R. J., Halpern, A. R., Perry, D. W., Meyer, E., & Evans, A. C. (1996). Hearing in the mind's ear: A PET investigation of musical imagery and perception. *Journal of Cognitive Neuroscience*, *8*, 29–46.

COGNITIVE NEUROPSYCHOLOGY, 2003, 20 (3/4/5/6), 541–559

# DO SEMANTIC CATEGORIES ACTIVATE DISTINCT CORTICAL REGIONS? EVIDENCE FOR A DISTRIBUTED NEURAL SEMANTIC SYSTEM

L. K. Tyler, P. Bright, E. Dick, P. Tavares, L. Pilgrim, P. Fletcher, M. Greer, and H. Moss

*University of Cambridge, UK*

A key issue in cognitive neuroscience concerns the neural representation of conceptual knowledge. Currently, debate focuses around the issue of whether there are neural regions specialised for the processing of specific semantic attributes or categories, or whether concepts are represented in an undifferentiated neural system. Neuropsychological studies of patients with selective semantic deficits and previous neuroimaging studies do not unequivocally support either account. We carried out a PET study to determine whether there is any regional specialisation for the processing of concepts from different semantic categories using picture stimuli and a semantic categorisation task. We found robust activation of a large semantic network extending from left inferior frontal cortex into the inferior temporal lobe and including occipital cortex and the fusiform gyrus. The only category effect that we found was additional activation for animals in the right occipital cortex, which we interpret as being due to the extra visual processing demands required in order to differentiate one animal from another. We also carried out analyses in specific cortical regions that have been claimed to be preferentially activated for various categories, but found no evidence of any differential activation as a function of category. We interpret these data within the framework of cognitive accounts in which conceptual knowledge is represented within a nondifferentiated distributed system.

## INTRODUCTION

Patients who show category-specific semantic impairments following brain damage raise important issues about the organisation of conceptual knowledge. Typically, such patients have disproportionate difficulty with living things (e.g., animals, fruits/vegetables) although deficits for artefact concepts (e.g., tools, vehicles) have also been reported, albeit less frequently (see Gainotti, Silveri, Daniele, & Giustolisi, 1995; Saffran & Schwartz, 1994, for reviews). Such deficits raise the issue of how conceptual knowledge is organised such that damage can lead to deficits for a specific category or domain of knowledge.

Various theoretical accounts have been proposed to explain such deficits. According to one influential account, the neural substrate for the representation of animate objects such as animals and plant life is evolutionarily adapted and independent of the areas involved in the processing of other categories of knowledge (Caramazza & Shelton, 1998), although the account makes no assumptions regarding which anatomical regions

Requests for reprints should be addressed to L. K. Tyler, Dept of Experimental Psychology, University of Cambridge, Cambridge, UK (Email: lktyler@csl.psychol.cam.ac.uk).

We thank Tim Donovan and Victoria Liversidge of the Wolfson Brain Imaging Centre for their invaluable assistance in running these studies. This research was funded by an MRC programme grant to LKT. PT was supported by the Foundation for Science and Technology, Lisbon, Portugal.





http://www.tandf.co.uk/journals/pp/02643294.html

DOI:10.1080/02643290244000211

subserve each domain. Thus, certain entities (such as animals and plant life) have played a special role in human evolution, and this has lead to their representation by distinct neural mechanisms. However, attempts to locate neural substrates that are specific to living things have proved difficult. For example, although lesion studies show some broad correlations between medial temporal and associated temporal neocortex damage and a living things deficit, there are patients who do not show this pattern (Caramazza & Shelton, 1998; Hillis & Caramazza, 1991; Perani et al., 1995). For example, Caramazza and Shelton' s patient, EW, has a selective deficit for animals as a result of damage in the left posterior frontal and parietal lobes. Living things deficits have also been reported in patients with Alzheimer's dementia, where cortical damage is arguably patchy and widespread (Garrard, Lambon Ralph, Watson, Powis, Patterson, & Hodges, 2001; Garrard, Patterson, Watson, & Hodges, 1998; Gonnerman, Andersen, Devlin, Kempler, & Seidenberg, 1997; Silveri, Daniele, Giustolisi, & Gainotti, 1991).

Category-specific deficits have also been explained as evidence for the existence of separate stores of knowledge for different types of semantic features—e.g., sensory and functional features (Warrington & McCarthy, 1983) and features corresponding to visual form and motion (Martin, 2001; Martin & Chao, 2001). On the sensory-functional account, damage to the store of sensory knowledge leads to a disproportionate deficit for living things since these concepts are more dependent upon sensory than functional features. In contrast, damage to the store of functional knowledge has a greater effect on artefact concepts since these are more dependent upon functional information (Warrington & McCarthy, 1983, 1987; Warrington & Shallice, 1984). The sensory-functional account has been questioned on a number of grounds. Patients have been reported with a living things deficit who show equal impairments for visual/perceptual and functional properties. It is possible that the greater deficits for sensory properties associated with living things impairments in some of the earlier studies was due to the greater difficulty of the sensory property questions for living things (Caramazza & Shelton, 1998). Similarly, in the few reported cases of patients with artefact deficits who have been tested on the relevant contrasts, there is either no difference between sensory and functional properties (Moss & Tyler, 2000), or an effect in the reverse direction (Lambon Ralph, Howard, Nightingale, & Ellis, 1998). Moreover, we have argued elsewhere that the contribution of functional information to the concepts of living things has been underestimated due to an overly narrow definition of what counts as a functional property. For example, animals have important *biological* functions, such as *running, breathing, eating*, and so on, that are central to our conceptual knowledge of this domain (see Tyler & Moss, 1997, for a discussion), but which tend to be overlooked in analyses of their properties. Finally, recent neuroimaging studies have shown no consistent differences in cortical activation as a function of sensory or functional properties (Devlin et al. 2002b; Kellenbach, Brett, & Patterson, 2001; Moore & Price, 1999; Perani, Schnur, Tettamanti, Gorno-Tempini, Cappa, & Fazio, 1999; Spitzer et al., 1998).

A modified version of the sensory-functional account has recently been proposed by Martin and colleagues (Chao, Haxby, & Martin, 1999; Martin, & Chao, 2001; Martin, Wiggs, Ungerleider, & Haxby, 1996). On the basis of neuroimaging data with healthy subjects, focusing on the object processing system, Martin, Haxby and colleagues have proposed that different object categories are represented in an extensive distributed and partially overlapping network involving the occipital, temporal, and parietal lobes and pre-motor cortex. Within this system there is some specialisation as a function of category. For example, in bilateral ventral regions of the posterior temporal lobe (fusiform gyrus), where attributes of visual form are stored, they claim that peak activation for animals is more lateral and tools more medial. On the lateral surface of the temporal lobe animals elicit more activation than tools in posterior superior temporal sulcus while posterior middle temporal activations are activated more for tools than animals. The authors stress the point that tools activate areas close to regions thought to mediate perception of artefact motion (left posterior middle temporal lobe, Martin, 2001) and animals activate regions associated with the perception of biological motion (superior temporal sulcus: Bonda, Petrides, Ostry, & Evans, 1996; Puce, Allison, Bentin, Gore, & McCarthy, 1998), although this latter effect was only observed in approximately half the subjects tested (Martin & Chao, 2001).

However, this account also has its problems. Even though increased activation for tools in the left posterior middle temporal lobe is the most robust finding (e.g., Chao et al., 1999; Martin et al., 1996; Moore & Price, 1999; Perani et al., 1999), not all studies show this effect (Devlin et al., 2002b; Grabowski, Damasio, & Damasio, 1998; Perani et al., 1995). A recent meta-analysis of seven PET studies also identified an effect in left posterior middle temporal lobe, which was stronger for tools than other man-made items such as vehicles (Devlin et al., 2002a). However, the region was not tool-specific but also responded during motion relative to perceptual decisions for fruits, and furthermore, naming body parts produced more activation here than naming tools, animals, or faces. Indeed, the most striking finding in the neuroimaging studies of category and domain specificity is that most categories activate the same neural regions with only weak and inconsistent category-specific effects.

In contrast to these accounts, which assume some degree of neural specialisation for semantic information, we have recently argued that category-specific deficits can emerge as a function of the content and structure of concepts within a nondifferentiated distributed neural system (Durrant-Peatfield, Tyler, Moss, & Levy, 1997; Tyler & Moss, 2001; Tyler, Moss, Durrant-Peatfield, & Levy, 2000). Our claim is that concepts vary in number and type of features, in the degree to which those features are shared or distinctive, and in the strength of the correlations between different features. Correlated features support each other with mutual activation and thus are more resistant to damage than features without this support. This distributed neural system involves a number of brain areas including frontal, temporal, parietal, and occipital regions. Temporal regions are clearly critically involved in the representation and processing of concepts, with other cortical regions more or less involved depending on a number of factors, such as the nature of the input (e.g., spoken, written, pictures), the nature of the task (e.g., naming, reading, matching) and the additional nonlinguistic cognitive demands required. Within this system, category-specific deficits will emerge because some concepts are more robust to damage than others due to their internal structure. Specifically, for living things, shared properties (e.g., eyes, legs) are numerous and densely intercorrelated, while distinctive properties (e.g., a zebra's stripes, a lion's mane) are fewer and weakly correlated with other properties of the concept. In contrast, the distinctive properties of artefacts are supported by form–function correlations (e.g., blade–cut, handle–turn), while the shared properties are fewer and less intercorrelated. It is through this disadvantage for distinctive relative to shared properties of living things over artefacts that the disproportionate living things deficit emerges. This account predicts no specialised activation for different categories in the normal brain, as long as the materials are carefully matched on variables such as familiarity and visual complexity.

In a recent series of PET and fMRI studies, using written words and matching items across categories (animals, fruits, tools, and vehicles) and domains on the crucial variables of frequency, letter length, and visual complexity, we found no neural specialisation for the processing of any category or domain. We used two tasks—lexical decision and semantic categorisation—and found that all categories of knowledge activated a common extensive neural system, primarily in the left hemisphere, involving the inferior frontal cortex, inferior and middle temporal gyri, and the temporal pole (Devlin et al., 2002b). We argued, on the basis of these results, that the conceptual system is represented in a distributed neural network with no differentiation as a function of category or domain. However, it could be argued that since our imaging studies used written words rather than pictures they did not tap directly into the object processing network, and that the strongest evidence for a differentiated semantic neural system comes from work on the object processing system in the ventral temporal lobes (Martin & Chao, 2001; Martin et al., 1996).

We thus carried out a study using the same paradigm (semantic categorisation) as in our earlier experiments (Devlin et al., 2002b) but used pictures instead of written words. Our secondary aim was to evaluate claims for category-specificity made by Martin and colleagues by including the same categories that feature in many of their studies (animals and tools). Since these categories vary on a number of dimensions, most notably in their visual complexity, we added two more categories (vehicles and fruits/vegetables), so that we could match living and nonliving things on visual complexity. Thus, within the living things domain we included a visually simple (fruits/vegetables) and visually complex (animals) category, and within the nonliving domain there was a visually complex (vehicles) and visually simple (tools) category.

Given the dangers of both statistical leniency and conservatism, we took a multi-analysis approach to analysing our imaging data by conducting our analyses at two levels of threshold. In the first analysis, we adopted a conservative threshold of $p$ = .05 after correcting for multiple comparisons (Worsley, Marrett, Neelin, Vandal, Friston, & Evans, 1996) in order to reduce the possibility of obtaining false positives. In a second set of analyses we took a more lenient approach and lowered our statistical threshold substantially (to an uncorrected level of $p$ = .05) in order to maximise our chances of detecting any small category effects.

# METHODS

## Subjects

We tested nine right-handed, male native English speakers whose mean age was 28 years (range: 21–43 years). Each gave informed consent and they were medically screened for PET prior to entering the scanning room.

## Stimuli and design

For this study, we modified the semantic categorisation task that we had previously used with written words (Devlin et al., 2002b; Tyler, Russell, Fadili, & Moss, 2001) so that it could be used with picture stimuli. In the picture version of the task, subjects saw three cue pictures presented sequentially in the centre of a computer screen and made a speeded same/different decision as to whether a fourth (target) picture belonged to the same subcategory. For example, subjects might see cue pictures of a sheep, a pig, and a horse followed by a target picture of a donkey, to which they would respond "same." On another trial, they might see the cue pictures of a butterfly, a caterpillar, and a beetle followed by the target picture of a cow, to which they would respond "different."

The pictures (which were all coloured photographs) came from one of four categories: two were from the domain of natural kinds (animals; vegetables & fruit) and two were from the domain of nonliving things (tools; vehicles). Stimuli within each of the four categories were sorted into subcategories. For example, items within the animal category were subcategorised into birds, mammals, and insects. We constructed triplets out of these subcategories, enabling us to construct "different" trials in which the target was from a different subcategory, but within the main category. Thus, the cue and target pictures (whether in "same" or "different" trials) were always from the same category. Within each category there were equal numbers of same and different trials. The triples and their targets were pre-tested to ensure that, across the categories, they were equally semantically related (see Semantic Relatedness Pre-test below).

The cue triples and targets in each category were matched as closely as possible on familiarity using the MRC Psycholinguistic databases (Coltheart, 1981) and our own norms (see Table 1). Since pictures vary in their visual complexity, and this in turn can affect naming and decision latencies (Gaffan & Haywood, 1993; Stewart, Parkin, & Hunkin, 1992), we attempted to match the pictures within the two domains on this variable. Items within the categories of tools and fruits/vegetables

Table 1. *Statistics of the stimuli: Mean (and SD)*

| | *Animals* | *Fruits/veg* | *Vehicles* | *Tools* |
|---|---|---|---|---|
| Target familiarity | 3.1 (0.5) | 4.1 (0.6) | 3.1 (0.9) | 3.6 (0.8) |
| Target visual complexity | 3.3 (0.2) | 2.1 (0.5) | 3.1 (0.6) | 1.6 (0.4) |
| Triple familiarity | 2.5 (0.3) | 3.7 (0.4) | 3.0 (0.8) | 3.6 (0.5) |
| Triple visual complexity | 3.3 (0.2) | 2.3 (0.6) | 3.1 (0.2) | 1.8 (0.3) |

were more visually simple than pictures of animals and vehicles, as determined by our rating pre-tests carried out on 17 subjects. Thus, the tools and fruits/vegetables were matched on rated visual complexity, as were the vehicles and animals (see Table 1).

We also constructed a baseline consisting of sets of quadruples of meaningless, simple shapes made up of combinations of small squares, varying the colour and number of squares in each object. A set of three simple shapes were presented sequentially and followed by a target shape that was either from the same "family" of shapes or from a different family (see Figure 1 for examples). All items (both test and baseline) were scaled to the same size and pre-tested for relatedness in the same way as the test items (see above). There were 96 picture trials and 48 baseline trials.

## Semantic relatedness pre-test

Semantic relatedness was determined by means of a pre-test in which we presented each cue triplet followed by its target to 11 subjects and asked them to decide the relatedness of each triplet to its target, using a scale of 1–7, where 1 was very unrelated and 7 was very related. For the same sets we rejected any quadruple with a mean relatedness score of less than 5.5. The mean relatedness score for the final same

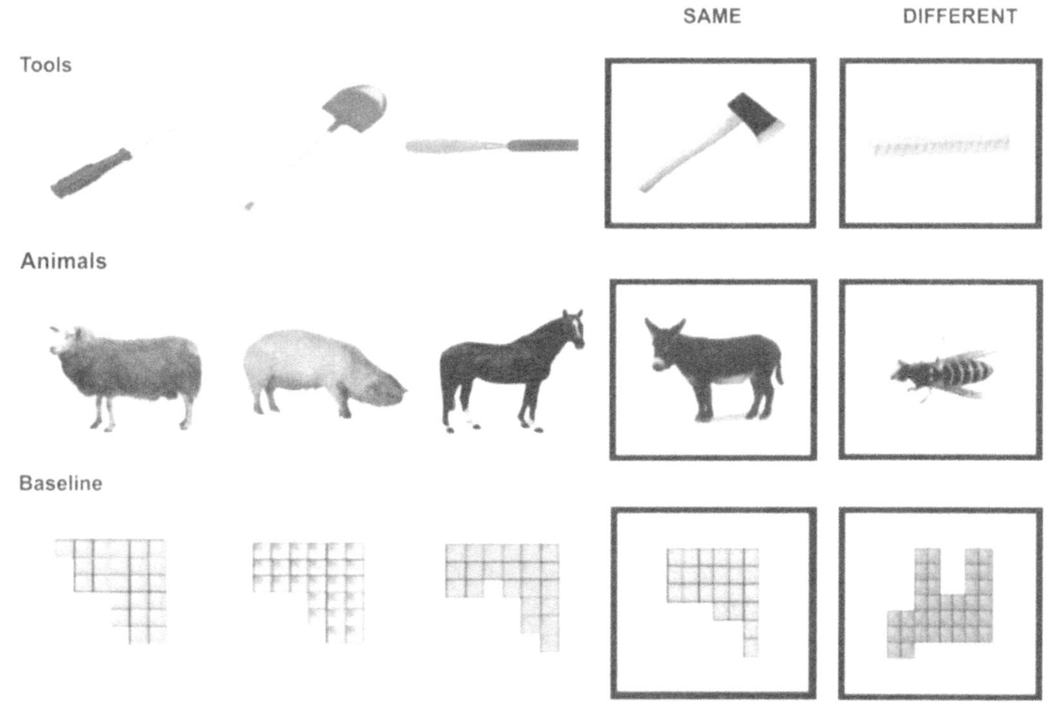


Figure 1. *Examples of the experimental stimuli. Please note that the stimuli were presented to participants in colour. To view the colour version of this figure, please go to the online version of this journal issue.*

set of items in each of the categories was: animals = 6.3; vehicles = 6.11; tools = 6.31; fruits = 6.39; baseline = 6.11; $F(1, 10) = 1.539, p = .209$.

## Procedure

The three cue stimuli were displayed against a white background. The fourth stimulus was framed by a thin black line to indicate that it was the target and that subjects were required to make a response. Each trial lasted 4416 ms, with each stimulus presented for 400 ms, separated by a 200 ms interval. There was then a 2217 ms interval between the presentation of the target and the first cue of the following trial. Subjects made a same response by pressing the left mouse button and a different response by pressing the right mouse button. We delivered the stimuli and recorded latencies and error rates using the DMDX software (Forster & Forster, 1991).

Stimuli were presented within the first 53 s of each 90 s scan to coincide with the critical period of tracer uptake and thus optimise the sensitivity of the design (Silbersweig et al., 1993). Within each 53 s period we presented a block of 12 trials. In total, each subject received 12 scans of 90 s, 2 from each of the 4 categories (vehicles, tools, animals, fruits & vegetables) and 4 from the baseline condition. The scan order was varied across sessions and subjects.

Scans were performed at the Wolfson Brain Imaging Centre in Cambridge, England on a GE Advance PET Scanner (General Electric Medical Systems, Milwaukee, Wisconsin). It comprises 18 rings of crystals, which results in 35 image planes, each 4.25 mm thick. The axial field-of-view is 15.3 cm, thus allowing for whole brain acquisition. Each subject received a bolus of 300 MBq of $H_2O^{15}$ before each scan for a total radiation exposure of 4.2 mSv. The emission data was acquired with the septa retracted (3D mode) and reconstructed using the PROMIS algorithm (Kinahan & Rogers, 1989) with an unapodised Colsher filter. Corrections were applied for randoms, scatter, attenuation and dead time. The voxel sizes were 2.34, 2.34, and 4.25 mm.

# RESULTS

## Behavioural data

The subjects' raw RT data was inverse transformed prior to statistical analysis in order to reduce the effects of outliers (Ulrich & Miller, 1994). There were no significant differences in the mean RTs in the four semantic conditions: animals = 805 ms, fruits/vegetables = 811 ms, tools = 822 ms, vehicles = 811 ms, $F_2(3, 95) < 1, p = .907$ . However, these RTs were slower than the mean RT for the baseline of 775 ms, $F_2(4, 143) = 2.971, p = .022$. An analysis of the errors showed that there were no significant differences in error rates between any of the five conditions, $F_2(4, 134) = 1.2, p = .301$. RTs were also not affected by the visual complexity of the pictures, $F_2(1, 95) = 1.180, p = .280$.

## Imaging data

The functional images were realigned using SPM (Friston et al., 1995; SPM99, Wellcome Institute of Cognitive Neurology, www.fil.ion.ucl.ac.uk). Translation and rotation corrections did not exceed 4 mm and 3°, respectively, for any of the participants. The mean image created by the realignment procedure was used to determine the parameters for transforming the images onto the Montreal Neurological Institute (MNI) mean brain. These parameters were then applied to the functional images (Ashburner & Friston, 1997; Ashburner, Neelin, Collins, Evans, & Friston, 1997) and the image was resampled into isotropic 2 $mm^3$ voxels. Finally, each image was smoothed with a 16 mm at full-width half-maximum (FWHM) Gaussian filter. The SPM software was used to compute a within-subjects analysis (fixed-effects) using the general linear model (Friston, Holmes, Worsley, Poline, Frith, & Frackowiak, 1995b). Results are reported at a $p < .05$ level after correcting for multiple comparisons (Worsley et al., 1996).

### *Semantic activations*

To determine the semantic network activated by the combined set of categories, we contrasted all semantic categories against baseline (animals, vehicles, fruits/vegetables, tools minus baseline). There were two very large clusters of activation (one of over 13,000 voxels) that were significant at a threshold of $p < .05$. To identify individual peaks within these large clusters the contrast was run at a raised uncorrected threshold of $p = .0001$. This broke the cluster into several separate regions, which are shown in Table 2 and Figure 2.

We found large clusters of activation in the LH stretching from the inferior/middle occipital gyrus through the anterior part of the fusiform (BA37), and extending laterally into the middle and superior temporal cortex. There was also significant activation in the inferior and medial frontal cortex, including Broca' s area and anterior portions of the cingulate gyrus. Similar regions of occipital cortex and fusiform gyrus were activated in the RH, although activation did not extend as far forward into anterior regions as in the LH, and there was significant cerebellar activation. In addition, we found significant bilateral medial frontal activation.

A subsequent analysis was carried out to determine the semantic network that was *commonly* activated for all four categories. For this, we computed a main effect of semantic categories relative to baseline, as before, but inclusively masked it with each of the individual contrasts (animals minus baseline, fruits/vegetables minus baseline, tools minus baseline, vehicles minus baseline at an uncorrected $p <$ .05 threshold. This ensures that the main effect for semantic categories relative to baseline will represent only those regions active for all four categories (i.e., the common semantic system). In other words, if activations were present for some but not all categories these would be excluded from the results. Once again, we found large clusters of activation and therefore we computed the same contrast at an uncorrected threshold of .0001. This broke the cluster into smaller regions, which are shown in Table 3 and Figure 3.

One cluster of activation was located in the left fusiform extending posteriorly into the cingulate and lingual gyrus and anteriorly into the parahippocampal gyrus and middle temporal gyrus. A second large LH cluster was in the medial frontal lobe, and a third in inferior frontal gyrus, including Broca' s area. There was also significant activation in the middle frontal gyrus. In the RH, we found significant activations in the cerebellum extending into the fusiform, and also in the medial frontal lobe. There were also significant bilateral activations in the cingulate gyrus.

There was considerable overlap between the semantic network activated in the masked and unmasked analyses, suggesting that each of the four

**Table 2.** *Semantic activations (animals + fruits + tools + vehicles minus baseline)*

| *Region* | *BA* | *x* | *y* | *z* | *SPM{t}* | *Extent* |
|---|---|---|---|---|---|---|
| *Right hemisphere* | | | | | | |
| Cerebellum | | 46 | −73 | −30 | 6.81 | 1796 |
| Fusiform gyrus | 37 | 40 | −49 | −16 | 5.95 | |
| Fusiform gyrus | 18 | 42 | −74 | −10 | 5.56 | |
| Cuneus | 18 | 6 | −71 | 20 | 6.40 | 1275 |
| Cerebellum | | 18 | −85 | −28 | 5.75 | 524 |
| *Left hemisphere* | | | | | | |
| Medial frontal lobe | 9 | −4 | 48 | 27 | 6.55 | 1171 |
| Fusiform gyrus | 37 | −38 | −45 | −13 | 6.41 | 1503 |
| | 36 | −34 | −32 | −19 | 5.62 | |
| *Bilateral* | | | | | | |
| Cingulate gyrus | 23/31 | 0 | −57 | 16 | 5.16 | |

Peaks shown for all clusters significant at $p < .05$ using Talairach coordinates. Cluster extents are presented at a threshold of .0001.

**Table 3.** *Semantic activations (animals + fruits/vegetables + vehicles + tools minus baseline) inclusively masked with each of the individual contrasts (animals minus baseline, fruits/vegetables minus baseline, tools minus baseline, vehicles minus baseline) at a $p < .05$ corrected threshold*

| *Region* | *BA* | *x* | *y* | *z* | *SPM{t}* | *Extent* |
|---|---|---|---|---|---|---|
| *Right hemisphere* | | | | | | |
| Cerebellum | | 46 | −73 | −30 | 6.81 | 1617 |
| Fusiform gyrus | 37 | 40 | −49 | −16 | 5.95 | |
| Fusiform gyrus | 8/19 | 42 | −74 | −10 | 5.56 | |
| Cuneus | 17 | 6 | −71 | 20 | 6.40 | 1174 |
| Cerebellum | | 18 | −85 | −28 | 5.75 | 329 |
| *Left hemisphere* | | | | | | |
| Medial frontal lobe | 9 | −4 | 48 | 27 | 6.55 | 1101 |
| Fusiform gyrus | 36 | −38 | −45 | −13 | 6.41 | 1457 |
| | 36 | −34 | −32 | −19 | 5.62 | |
| *Bilateral* | | | | | | |
| Cingulate gyrus | 23 | 0 | −57 | 16 | 5.16 | |

Peaks shown for all clusters significant at $p < .05$ using Talairach coordinates. Cluster extents are presented at an uncorrected threshold of .0001.

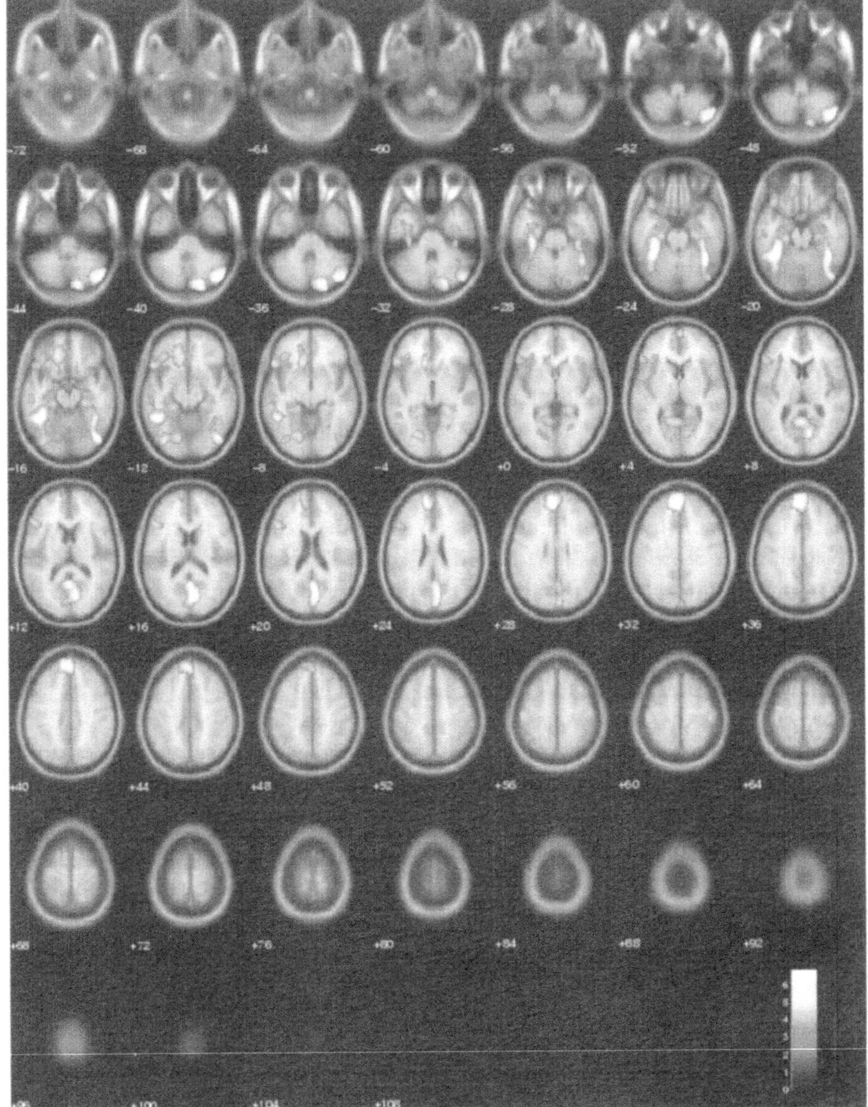

**Figure 2.** *The areas activated in the semantic minus baseline (unmasked) contrasts in the semantic categorisation task. Activations are shown superimposed on a structural image. The image is in neurological convention (L = L). Red and yellow areas were reliably (p < .05) active at the cluster level after statistical correction. The height threshold was set at 3.89.*

semantic categories activates essentially the same set of neural regions.

Additional analyses were carried out to ensure that the experiment was sufficiently sensitive to detect small differences in activation, if they were present in the data. Rather than using an introspective approach that uses the voxel scores as typical observations to calculate the power of the analysis (Van Horn, Ellmore, Esposito, & Berman, 1998), we used a more stringent retrospective approach that utilises the whole data set to estimate the effect size and the proportion of active voxels. We then fit a Receiver Operating Characteristic curve (ROC), using a finite mixture-based model, to the observed

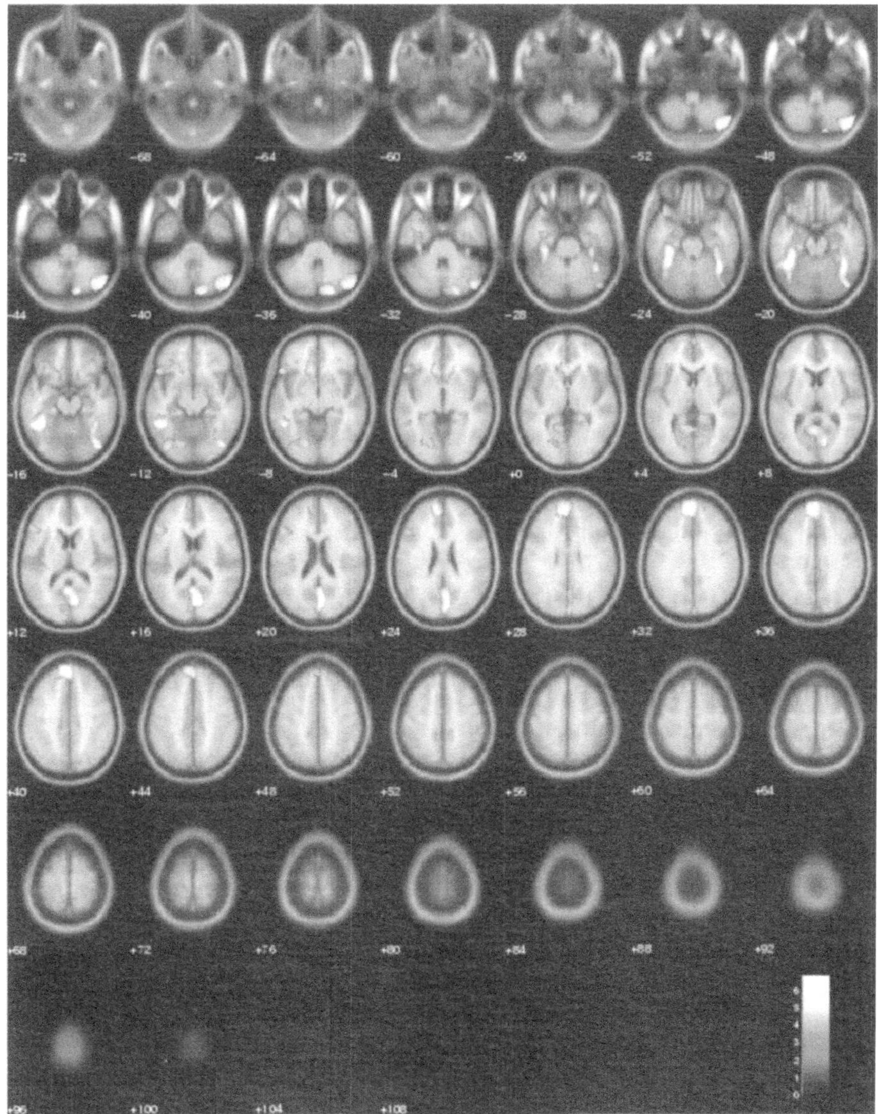

Figure 3. *The areas activated in the semantic minus baseline (masked) contrasts. Activations are shown superimposed on a structural image. The image is in neurological convention (L = L). Red and yellow areas were reliably ($p < .05$) active at the cluster level after statistical correction. The height threshold was set at 3.89.*

data (Gustard et al., 2001). This model overcomes the binormal assumption of the classical parametric methods and can be generalised to any statistical score (Genovese, Noll, & Eddy, 1997); it is directly applicable in our context using either the $t$ or the $F$ SPMs. The data provided by the $t$ maps given in SPM were fitted with a mixture of two $t$-distributions representing the $t$ values of individual voxels under the null hypothesis ($H_0$) and under an active hypothesis ($H_1$). The algorithm provides us with the mixing proportion (the estimated proportion of activated voxels) and effect size which best fit the data. These were estimated using a maximum likelihood procedure (Gustard et al., 2001).

Comparing semantic conditions to the baseline we found $\lambda = .209$ and $\delta = 2.76$. That is, the mean effect size elicited an approximately 2.8% change in regional cerebral blood flow (rCBF) and 21% of voxels were activated in this condition. The detection power was of 81% at false positives fraction (FPF) of .03.

*Effects of domains*

We examined domain effects by directly comparing living things with artefacts. At an uncorrected threshold of .001, one RH cluster (330 voxels) was just significant at $p < .05$ (see Table 4) for living things compared to artefacts. This was situated in the sylvian fissure between superior temporal gyrus (BA 22) and inferior parietal gyrus (BA 40), a region anterior and superior to that reported as specific to animals by Chao et al. (1999). No further clusters were significant at this threshold for living things or for artefacts.

*Effects of categories*

To determine whether there were regions of the semantic network that were more activated for one category than another, we directly contrasted each semantic category against the three other semantic categories. There were no clusters significant at $p < .05$ for vehicles, fruits/vegetables, or tools. However, we found a region in the right inferior occipital gyrus extending into the right cerebellum that was significantly more active for animals than other categories (see Table 5 and Figure 4). A subsequent analysis, in which we inclusively masked this contrast with the three other simple contrasts (animals minus fruits/vegetables, animals minus tools, animals minus vehicles) as well as the baseline (animals minus baseline), showed significant activation for animals in the same right inferior occipital region (see Table 6), suggesting that this activation was specific to animals only.

**Table 4.** *Domain-specific activations: Living things compared to artefacts [(animals + fruits/vegetables) minus (vehicles + tools)]*

| *Region* | *BA* | *x* | *y* | *z* | *SPM{t}* | *Extent* |
|---|---|---|---|---|---|---|
| *Right hemisphere* | | | | | | |
| Superior temporal gyrus/ inferior parietal gyrus | 22/40 | 57 | −34 | 22 | 5.02 | 330 |

Peaks shown for all clusters significant at $p < .05$ using Talairach coordinates. Cluster extents are presented at an uncorrected threshold of .001. There were no significant effects found for artifacts over living things [(vehicles + tools) − (animals + fruits/vegetables)].

**Table 5.** *Animal-specific activations: [animals minus (fruits/vegetables + vehicles + tools)]*

| *Region* | *BA* | *x* | *y* | *z* | *SPM{t}* | *Extent* |
|---|---|---|---|---|---|---|
| *Right hemisphere* | | | | | | |
| Inferior occipital gyrus | 19 | 50 | −76 | −1 | 4.75 | 740 |
| Cerebellum | | 40 | −55 | −19 | 4.10 | |

Peaks shown for all clusters significant at $p < .05$ using Talairach coordinates. Cluster extents are presented at an uncorrected threshold of .001.

**Table 6.** *Animal-specific activations: Animals minus (fruits + vehicles + tools) inclusively masked with each of the individual contrasts (animals - tools, animals - fruits, tools - vehicles, animals - baseline) at a p < .05 corrected threshold*

| *Region* | *BA* | *x* | *y* | *z* | *SPM{t}* | *Extent* |
|---|---|---|---|---|---|---|
| *Occipital/Cerebellar activations* | | | | | | |
| Right hemisphere | | | | | | |
| Inferior occipital gyrus | 19 | 50 | −76 | −1 | 4.75 | 707 |
| Cerebellum | | 40 | −55 | −19 | 4.10 | |

Peaks shown for all clusters significant at $p < .05$ using Talairach coordinates. Cluster extents are presented at an uncorrected threshold of .001.

*Effects of visual complexity*

To determine whether activations varied as a function of the visual complexity of the stimuli, we compared the two visually complex object categories (animals, vehicles) against the two visually simple object categories (fruits/vegetables, tools). This produced a cluster of activation in right inferior occipital gyrus extending into the right inferior temporal gyrus (see Table 7).

**Table 7.** *Effects of visual complexity*

| *Region* | *x* | *y* | *z* | *SPM{t}* | *Extent* |
|---|---|---|---|---|---|
| *Visually complex (animals + tools) relative to visually simple (tools + fruits)* | | | | | |
| R inferior occipital gyrus (BA 19) | 46 | −80 | −4 | 4.26 | 398 |

Peaks shown for all clusters significant at $p < .05$ using Talairach coordinates. Cluster extents are presented at an uncorrected threshold of .001.

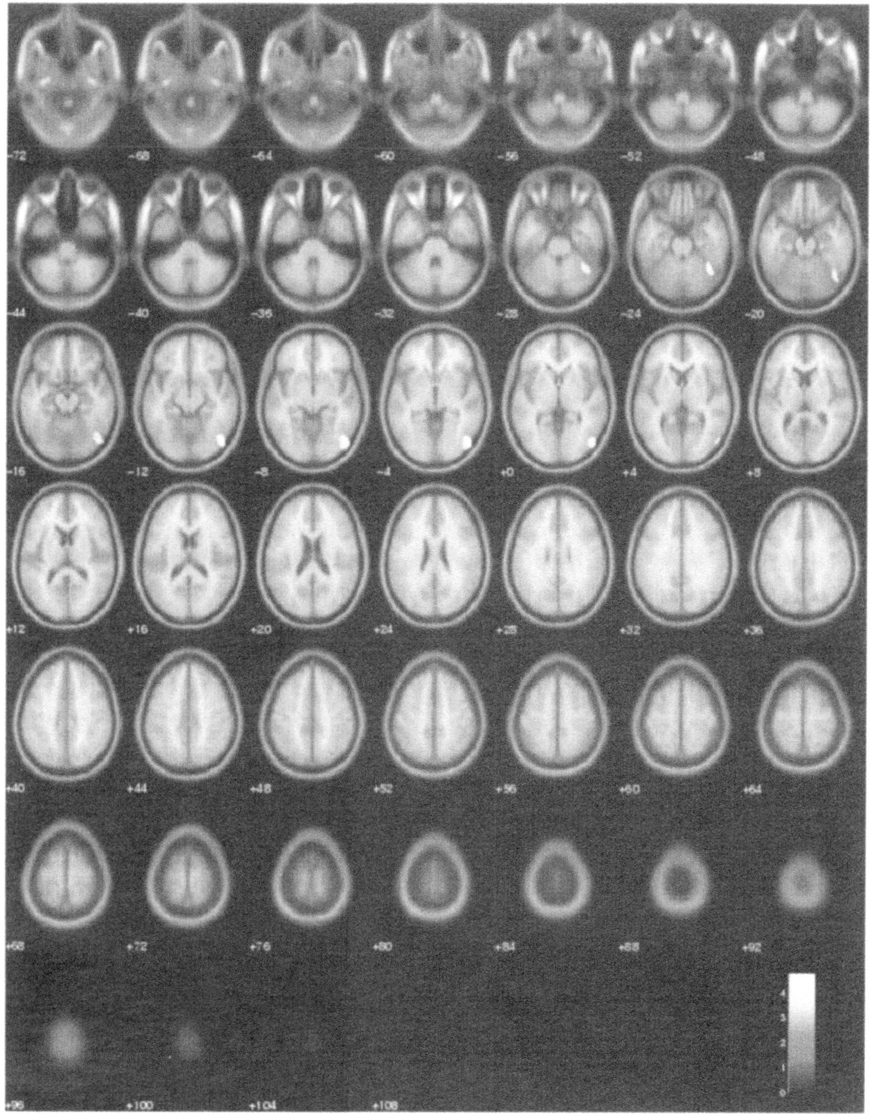


**Figure 4.** *The areas activated in the animals minus (tools + fruit/vegetables + vehicles) contrast. Activations are shown superimposed on a structural image. The image is in neurological convention (L = L). Red and yellow areas were reliably ($p < .05$) active after statistical correction.*

However, this activation was not produced by both visually complex categories (animals, vehicles) since, when we carried out a masked analysis, there were no significant activations. For the masked analysis we contrasted the two visually complex object categories with the two visually simple object categories and masked this with the four simple contrasts (animals minus fruits, animals minus tools, vehicles minus fruits, vehicles minus tools). There were no clusters significant at $p < .05$, suggesting that the effect of visual complexity seen in the unmasked analysis was due to only one of the categories. Comparing the activation for the unmasked visually complex categories with the activation for each of the categories individually, we see that the additional activation for visually complex categories overlaps with that found for the animals.

## Summary

The results show that our task successfully activated a large network in occipital, fusiform, and frontal regions, which largely overlaps with the object processing system identified by Martin and others (Chao et al., 1999; Chao & Martin, 2000; Martin et al., 1996). However, unlike Martin et al., we did not find evidence for category effects in temporal cortex. Martin et al. claim that animals activate regions of lateral temporal cortex, whereas tools activate more medial regions of the temporal lobe. We found no cortical regions that were more active for tools. The only increased activation that we found for animals was in right occipital cortex, which overlapped with the additional activation we observed for visually complex stimuli. We consider the implications of these results in the Discussion.

One possible reason for this difference in results is that we were too conservative in analysing the data and thus reduced the possibility of detecting small differences in activation as a function of category. In order to test this hypothesis, we carried out additional analyses in which we lowered the threshold of our statistical maps and then plotted the activations for each category in those regions which have been claimed by Martin and colleagues to be preferentially involved in the processing of objects in different semantic categories.

## Additional analyses

*Sensorimotor network for tools*

In a series of papers, Martin and colleagues (Chao et al., 1999; Chao & Martin, 2000; Martin & Chao, 2001) have reported that in addition to activating medial fusiform regions, tools preferentially activate several cortical areas, including middle temporal gyrus (motion attributes), left ventral premotor cortex and left posterior parietal cortex, which are associated with retrieval of information about the hand movements involved in using manipulable objects. In order to determine whether the same regions were involved in processing pictures of tools in the present experiment, we carried out analyses analogous to those used by Martin et al. (Chao et al., 1999; Chao & Martin, 2000). For these analyses we obtained an SPM map for the semantics (animals, tools, vehicles, fruits) minus baseline contrast, using a very low uncorrected threshold of .05. We used this low threshold in order to detect the maximum set of voxels activated by the semantic conditions. Our next step was to locate the coordinates of the activations in left ventral pre-motor and posterior parietal regions reported in Chao and Martin (2000), and in the left middle temporal gyrus and the bilateral medial fusiform reported in Chao et al. (1999). We then plotted the parameter estimates of the effects of interest for each of the four categories (animals, tools, vehicles, fruits/vegetables) at each of those coordinates. These parameter estimates provide an estimate of the activation generated by each of the four categories, enabling us to determine whether tools generated the largest effects in these specific regions, as predicted by Chao, Martin, and colleagues.

In order to maximise our chances of obtaining differential activation in the regions specified by Martin and colleagues, we carried out further analyses in which we looked for differential activation in specific cortical regions rather than only focusing on individual voxels. In order to define a volume, we calculated an average coordinate based on the coordinates published in Chao and Martin (2000) and Chao et al. (1999) for a specific region. From this point of origin we selected a volume of interest (VOI) as a sphere large enough to encompass all of the coordinates for that region. We used a VOI radius of 5 mm for left ventral pre-motor and left middle temporal gyrus regions, and a radius of 4 mm for the left posterior parietal region. To increase our chances of detecting any differential effects, we again set the threshold to a very low level ($p$ = .6). Within each volume we estimated effect sizes by comparing activations averaged across all of the voxels for each of the four categories against the baseline and applied a small volume correction (Worsley, 1996).

*Left ventral premotor.* Within the low thresholded SPM map of semantics minus baseline we located the coordinates given in Chao and Martin (2000) and plotted parameter estimates, which are shown in Figure 5a. There was no evidence of any preferential activation for tools at any of these coordinates. Rather, at each coordinate a different subset of categories produced the largest effect (as can be seen in Figure 5a). When we tested the active voxels within the VOI in this region to determine whether tools generated more activation than the other categories, we obtained the same lack of any differential effects.

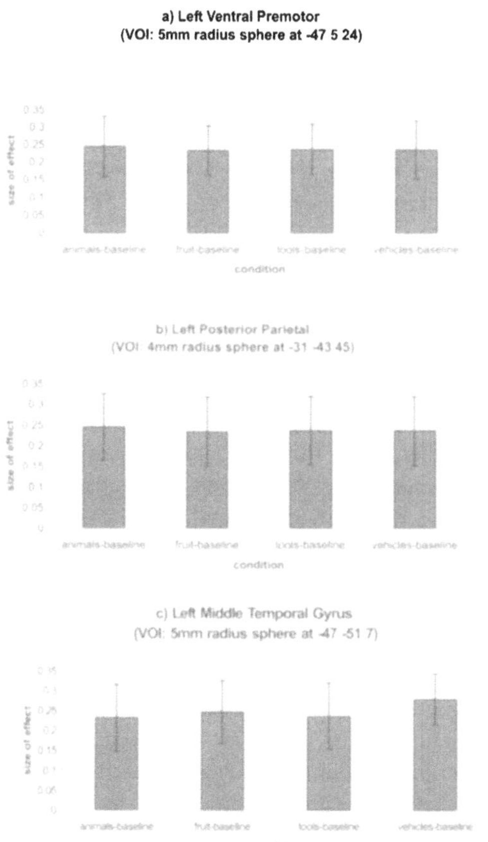


Figure 5. *The figure shows size of effect (in arbitrary units) for each of the four conditions in relation to the baseline for three volumes of interest derived from Chao, Martin, and colleagues' proposed network for the conceptual processing of tools. Volumes of interest specified as spheres with radius of 5mm (a and c) or 4mm (b). Points of origin shown in Talairach coordinates.*

*Left posterior parietal.* Following the procedure described above, we also plotted effects sizes at the two peak coordinates for tools in left parietal cortex (Chao & Martin, 2000). At one (−30,−39,47) there was no activation at all in our maps, while at the other, the categories of fruits and tools generated more activation than animals or vehicles (see Figure 5b). The VOI analysis of activated voxels in this region showed no differential effects as a function of category.

*Middle temporal gyrus.* We also plotted effects size for several coordinates in left middle temporal gyrus reported in Chao et al. (1999). Once again, we found wide variation in the effects produced by various categories at these coordinates, with a considerable degree of overlap across the categories. In the LH there tended to be a slightly larger effect for fruits at some coordinates (but not in all), whereas in comparable locations in the RH the category of vehicles tended to have a larger effect on activation. However, the most notable feature of these analyses was the absence of selective activation, the fact that most categories showed some degree of activation at almost all locations, and the variation in effect sizes for a specific category at locations differing by just a few millimeters (see Figure 5c). Once again, the VOI analysis also showed no additional activation for tools in this region.

*Animals vs. tools in the fusiform gyrus.* Martin and colleagues (Chao et al., 1999) claim that animals activate the more lateral regions of the fusiform whereas tool activation is found in more medial fusiform regions. We plotted effects sizes for all four categories using the coordinates in lateral and medial fusiform reported in Chao et al., and within the VOI for these regions (calculated as spheres large enough to encompass all the coordinates for that region, using small volume correction as described in Worsley et al., 1966). We used a VOI radius of 7 mm for left lateral and medial regions of the fusiform gyrus, 6 mm for right lateral fusiform gyrus, and 9 mm for right medial fusiform gyrus. Once again, we found no differences in the extent to which each category activated voxels in these two

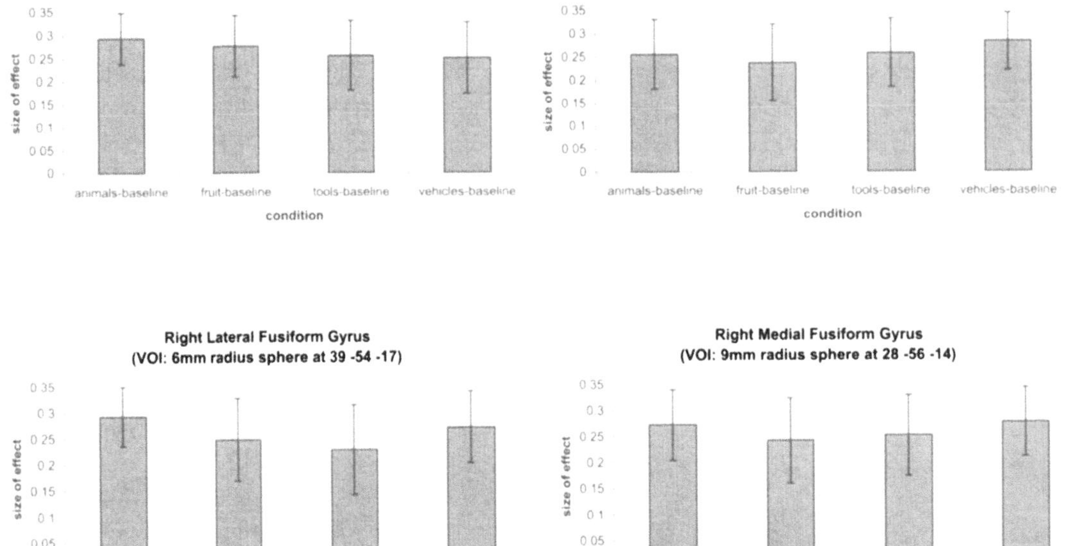


Figure 6. *The figure shows size of effect (in arbitrary units) for each of the four conditions in relation to the baseline for four volumes of interest derived from the cortical regions that Chao, Martin, and colleagues have claimed generate more activation for animals compared to tools. Volumes of interest specified as spheres with radius of 7 mm for left lateral and medial regions of the fusiform gyrus, 6 mm for right lateral fusiform gyrus, and 9 mm for right medial fusiform gyrus. Points of origin for volumes of interest shown in Talairach coordinates.*

regions (see Figure 6). Direct contrasts of animals against tools within the VOI in lateral fusiform gyrus, and tools against animals within the VOI in medial fusiform gyrus, also failed to produce significant activations.

## DISCUSSION

In this experiment, we found that pictures of common objects and entities activated an extensive conceptual system primarily in left occipital, temporal, and frontal regions but also including the right occipital and fusiform gyrus. Many of these areas have been reported in other studies using a variety of tasks such as silent naming, viewing, and matching to sample (e.g., Mummery, Shallice, & Price, 1999; Thompson-Schill, Aguirre, D'Esposito, & Farah, 1999; Tyler et al., 2001; Vandenberghe, Price, Wise, Josephs, & Frackowiak, 1996). We also found a large swathe of activation in left middle frontal gyrus extending to the anterior cingulate. Previous studies have reported increased anterior cingulate activity during conditions of high relative to low response competition (e.g., Botvinick, Nystrom, Fissell, Carter, & Cohen, 1999; Carter, Braver, Barch, Botvinick, Noll, & Cohen, 1998; Menon, Adleman, White, Glover, & Reiss, 2001), suggesting that anterior cingulate activity most likely reflects cognitive processes that subjects invoke to minimise errors rather than as a direct response to errors. In the present study, although error in the semantic conditions was equivalent to that in the baseline condition, reaction time was significantly longer, suggesting a higher level of overall demand. Although the maximal medial prefrontal activation in the present study lay rostrally to anterior cingulate, the limited spatial resolution of PET, the imprecision of the Talairach–Tournoux coordinate system, and the fact that the observed activations extend to the anterior cingulate, suggest that our findings might also be interpreted in terms of differences in response competition across conditions.

The activations in this study largely overlap with those found in our previous study using the same task with written words (Devlin et al., 2002b). Here we found a similar semantic network involving temporal and frontal activations, although the frontal activation was more posterior than in the present study. The major difference between the two studies was that the present study, perhaps not surprisingly given that we used pictures as stimuli, elicited more occipital activation. Thus, the semantic categorisation task, whether using words or pictures as stimuli, is sufficiently sensitive to robustly activate the neural system involved in conceptual processing. This point was reinforced by the power analyses, which showed that the experiment was highly sensitive to neural activity.

Even though the paradigm was very sensitive to neural activation, we found very little evidence for any category-specific differences. For example, a comparison of each category against the baseline condition activated essentially the same semantic network. The only category-specific activation was for animals in right inferior occipital cortex, which was slightly more lateralised and anterior than the right occipital activation for animals reported by Perani et al. (1999), and Chao et al. (1999). However, this region cannot be considered to be specific only for the processing of pictures of animals, since Ishai, Ungerleider, Martin, and Haxby (2000) have reported stronger activation in this region for faces compared to chairs and houses. These findings are consistent with a nonspecialised role of inferior occipital regions in the processing of different categories of objects.

We found considerable overlap between this region and that activated for visually complex compared to visually simple pictures. By comparing the masked and unmasked visual complexity analyses we were able to establish that the visual complexity activation came from the animal category and not from the vehicles. Given that we carefully matched the animals and vehicles on visual complexity, this result suggests that visual complexity per se cannot account fully for the differences in processing different semantic categories. Indeed, other variables—such as structural similarity—have also been claimed to account for differences between categories. For example, Humphreys, Riddoch, and Quinlan (1988) have argued that it is especially difficult to discriminate between different animals because of structural similarity within the category—that is, because most animals share many of the same visual features. Thus, the increased activation that we observe for animals in right occipital cortex may well be due to the extra visual processing required to be able to discriminate one animal from another. This does not imply any regional specialisation for object-specific attributes since this region was not selectively activated for animals in our previous study using the same semantic categorisation task with written words instead of pictures (Devlin et al., 2002b). Instead, it suggests that this region was activated because of the nonspecific visual processing demands involved in processing pictures of animals. This claim is supported by data from Moore and Price (1999) showing that both animals and complex objects elicited additional activation in right medial extrastriate.

Martin and Chao (2001) have raised the possibility that the stronger occipital activation for animals might reflect top-down modulation from more anterior temporal sites, implying that the meaning of the picture/object affects perceptual processing, and this interacts with category. Some recent studies of category-specific effects using ERPs render this hypothesis unlikely. Kiefer (2001) has reported that objects from natural kinds categories elicit early processing in occipital cortex. He found a larger N1 ERP component over inferior occipital sites compared to objects from artefact categories. This early N1 (obtained between 160–200 ms after target onset) is associated with perceptual processing (Mangun & Hillyard, 1991). Since enhanced perceptual processing only occurred for pictures and not for written words, this suggests that it is associated specifically with processing the pictures and does not reflect perceptual processing of properties intrinsic to the concept.

The detailed analysis of our activations, with reference to the claims made by Chao, Martin, and colleagues, concerning the distribution and processing of objects within different semantic categories, failed to find reliable differential activation for either animals or tools. This was the case in spite of the fact that we substantially lowered the threshold of our SPM maps and focused specifically on the neural regions they claim to be involved in category-specific processing. When we plotted the parameter estimates within the regions claimed by Chao et al. (1999) and Chao and Martin (2000) to constitute the neural pathway involved in the processing of animals and tools, in the majority of cases we found no differential effects whatsoever. On the rare occasion when we did see larger activation for one category compared to another this was only at a very low threshold and did not approach significance at a corrected level.

How do we account for the apparent discrepancy between the findings of the current experiment and those of Martin and colleagues (Martin & Chao, 1999), who showed category-specific activations in a number of brain regions? While it is possible that there are systematic differences in the functional organisation of the different groups of subjects, we believe this to be highly unlikely. We must therefore confront two possible explanations. One is that our analysis has produced Type II error (i.e., false negatives). While our initial use of a stringent threshold does indeed carry with it the risk of failing to find activations, we feel that the second stage of our analysis, in which the threshold was lowered and the task-specific activity across separate regions was plotted, rules this out since not even a trend towards systematic category differences was observed. A further possibility is that our use of the PET technique is inherently less sensitive than fMRI, used by Martin et al. However, we think this an unlikely explanation since fMRI studies that we have carried out using the same tasks and materials as used in our PET studies show the lack of domain or category differences (Devlin et al., 2002b; Pilgrim, Fadili, Fletcher, & Tyler, 2002). Moreover, a number of PET studies have reported category effects (Cappa, Perani, Schnur, Tettamanti, & Fazio, 1998; Damasio, Grabowski, Tranel, Hichwa, & Damasio, 1996; Moore & Price, 1999; Perani et al., 1999). The alternative explanation is that the reported category specificity arises from a Type I error (false positive). While Martin et al.' s analysis uses a similar implementation of the general linear model and parametric statistics to our own, one important issue concerns the extent to which individual variability has an influence on the group statistic. This is a major problem with fMRI and has led to the development of mixed effect modeling to validate group findings. Martin et al. conscientiously report the numbers of individual subjects who show category-specific effects. However, without further discussion and clarification of the group level analyses (including random effects), the possibility of Type I error arising from individual idiosyncrasies remains a possibility which must be excluded.

In conclusion, we found no evidence in this study for the claim that objects and entities are associated with differential activation in different neural regions. The only "category-specific" activation we found was in right occipital cortex, which was associated with the perceptual processing of the visual properties of pictures of animals. Our results are most consistent with the claim that conceptual knowledge is represented in a single distributed system which is not partitioned according to category or type of semantic knowledge (Tyler & Moss, 2001). This account predicts that the same semantic system will be activated whenever a word or object is processed, with some variation as a function of the nature of the input and the task that the subject is performing on that input. Thus, if the stimuli consist of pictures or objects, there may well be some category-specific regional specialisation in brain regions that process visual stimuli as a function of the differences in visual processing required for different objects, as we see in the present study. Similarly, if the task requires access to different levels of the conceptual representation (e.g., naming versus categorisation of an object), this may also generate apparent category-specific activations.

## REFERENCES


Ashburner, J., & Friston, K. (1997). Multimodal image coregistration and partitioning—a unified framework. *NeuroImage*, *6*, 209–217.

Ashburner, J., Neelin, P., Collins, D. L., Evans, A., & Friston, K. (1997). Incorporating prior knowledge into image registration. *NeuroImage*, *6*, 344–352.

Bonda, E., Petrides, M., Ostry, D., & Evans, A. (1996). Specific involvement of human parietal systems and the amygdala in the perception of biological motion. *Journal of Neuroscience*, *16*, 3737–3744

Botvinick, M., Nystrom, L. E., Fissell, K., Carter, C. S., & Cohen, J. D. (1999). Conflict monitoring versus selection-for-action in anterior cingulate cortex. *Nature*, *402*, 179–181.

Cappa, S. F., Perani, D., Schnur, T., Tettamanti, M., & Fazio, F. (1998). The effects of semantic category and knowledge type on lexical-semantic access: A PET study. *NeuroImage*, *8*, 350–359.

Caramazza, A., & Shelton, J. R. (1998). Domain-specific knowledge systems in the brain: The animate–inanimate distinction. *Journal of Cognitive Neuroscience*, *10*, 1–34.

Carter, C. S., Braver, T. S., Barch, D. M., Botvinick, M. M., Noll, D., & Cohen, J. D. (1998). Anterior cingulate cortex, error detection, and the online monitoring of performance. *Science*, *280*, 747–749.

Chao, L. L., Haxby, J. V., & Martin, A. (1999). Attribute-based neural substrates in temporal cortex for perceiving and knowing about objects. *Nature Neuroscience*, *2*, 913–919.

Chao, L. L., & Martin, A. (2000). Representation of manipulable man-made objects in the dorsal stream. *NeuroImage*, *12*, 478–84.

Coltheart, M. (1981). The MRC Psycholinguistic Database. *Quarterly Journal of Experimental Psychology*, *33*, 497–505.

Damasio, H., Grabowski, T., Tranel, D., Hitchwa, R., & Damasio, A. (1996). A neural basis for lexical retrieval. *Nature*, *380*, 499–505.

Devlin, J. T., Moore, C. J., Mummery, C. J., Gorno-Tempini, M. L., Phillips, J. A., Noppeney, U., Frackowiak, R. S. J., Friston, K. J., & Price, C. J. (2002a). Anatomic constraints on cognitive theories of category specificity. *NeuroImage*, *15*, 675–685.

Devlin, J. T., Russell, R. P., Davis, M. H., Price, C. J., Moss, H. E., Fadili, M. J., & Tyler, L. K. (2002b). Is there an anatomical basis for category-specificity? Semantic memory studies in PET and fMRI. *Neuropsychologia*, *40*, 54–75.

Durrant-Peatfield, M., Tyler, L. K., Moss, H. E., & Levy, J. (1997). The distinctiveness of form and function in category structure: A connectionist model. In *Proceedings of the Nineteenth Annual Conference of the Cognitive Science Society* (pp. 193–198). Stanford University, Mahwah, NJ: Lawrence Erlbaum Associates Inc.

Forster, K. I., & Forster, J. C. (1990). *The DMASTR display system for mental chronometry*. Tucson, AZ: University of Arizona.

Friston, K. J., Ashburner, J., Frith, C. D., Poline, J.-B., Heather, J., & Frackowiack, R. S. J. (1995a). Spatial registration and normalisation of images. *Human Brain Mapping*, *2*, 165–189.

Friston, K. J., Holmes, A. P., Worsley, K. J., Poline, J.-B., Frith, C. D., & Frackowiak, R. S. J. (1995b). Statistical parametric maps in functional imaging: A general linear approach. *Human Brain Mapping*, *2*, 189–210.

Gaffan, D., & Heywood, C. A. (1993). A spurious category-specific visual agnosia for living things in normal human and non-human primates. *Journal of Cognitive Neuroscience*, *5*, 118–128.

Gainotti, G., Silveri, M. C., Daniele, A., & Giustolisi, L. (1995). Neuroanatomical correlates of category-specific semantic disorders: A critical survey. *Memory*, *3*, 247–264.

Garrard, P., Lambon Ralph, M. A., Watson, P. C., Powis, J., Patterson, K., & Hodges, J. R. (2001). Longitudinal profiles of semantic impairment for living and nonliving concepts in dementia of Alzheimer's type. *Journal of Cognitive Neuroscience*, *13*, 892–909.

Garrard, P., Patterson, K., Watson, P. C., & Hodges, J. R. (1998). Category specific semantic loss in dementia of Alzheimer's type: Functional-anatomical correlations from cross-sectional analyses. *Brain*, *121*, 633–646.

Genovese, C. R., Noll, D. C., & Eddy, W. F. (1997). Estimating test–retest reliability in functional MR imaging. I: Statistical methodology. *Magnetic Resonanance in Medicine*, *38*, 497–507.

Gonnerman, L. M., Andersen, E. S., Devlin, J. T., Kempler, D., & Seidenberg, M. S. (1997). Double dissociation of semantic categories in Alzheimer's disease. *Brain and Language*, *57*, 254–79.

Grabowski, T. J., Damasio, H., & Damasio, A. R. (1998). Premotor and prefrontal correlates of category-related lexical retrieval. *NeuroImage*, *7*, 232–243.

Gustard S., Fadili M. J., Williams, E., Hall, L. D., Carpenter, A. T., Bretty, M., & Bullmore, E. T. (2001). Effect of slice orientation on reproducibility of fMRI motor activation at 3T. *Magnetic Resonance Imaging, 19*, 1323–1331.

Hillis, A. E., & Caramazza, A. (1991). Mechanisms for accessing lexical representations for output: Evidence from a category-specific semantic deficit. *Brain and Language, 40*, 106–144.

Hodges, J. R., Garrard, P., & Patterson, K. (1998). Semantic dementia. In A. Kertesz & D. G. Munoz (Eds.), *Pick' s disease and Pick complex* (pp. 83–104). New York: Wiley-Liss.

Humphreys, G. W., Riddoch, M. J., & Quinlan, P. (1998). Cascade processes in picture identification. *Cognitive Neuropsychology, 5*, 67–103.

Ishai, A., Ungerleider, L. G., Martin, A., & Haxby, J. V. (2000). The representation of objects in the human occipital and temporal cortex. *Journal of Cognitive Neuroscience, 2000, 12(Suppl 2)*, 35–51.

Kellenbach, M. L., Brett, M., & Patterson, K. (2001). Large, colourful or noisy? Attribute and modality-specific activations during retrieval of perceptual attribute knowledge. *Cognitive, Affective and Behavioral Neuroscience, 1*, 207–221.

Kiefer, M. (2001). Perceptual and semantic sources of category-specific effects: Event-related potentials using picture and word categorisation. *Memory and Cognition, 29*, 100–116.

Kinahan, P. E., & Rogers, J. G. (1989). Analytic 3D image reconstruction using all detected events. *IEEE Transactions of Nuclear Science, 35*, 680–684.

Lambon Ralph, M. A., Graham, K. S., Ellis, A. W., & Hodges, J. R. (1998). Naming in semantic dementia-what matters? *Neuropsychologia, 36*, 775–84.

Lambon Ralph, M. A., Howard, D., Nightingale, G., & Ellis, A. W. (1998). Are living and nonliving category-specific deficits causally linked to impaired perceptual or associative knowledge? Evidence from a category-specific double dissociation, *Neurocase, 4*, 311–338.

Mangun, G. R., & Hillyard, S. A. (1991). Modulations of sensory-evoked brain potentials indicate changes in perceptual processing during visual-spatial priming. *Journal of Experimental Psychology: Human Perception and Performance, 17*, 1057–74.

Martin, A. (2001). Functional neuroimaging of semantic memory. In R. Cabaza & A. Kingstone (Eds.), *Functional neuroimaging of semantic memory* (pp. 153–186). Cambridge, MA: MIT Press.

Martin, A., & Chao, L. L. (2001). Semantic memory and the brain: structure and processes. *Current Opinion in Neurobiology, 11*, 194–201.

Martin, A., Wiggs, C. L., Ungerleider, L. G., & Haxby, J. V. (1996). Neural correlates of category-specific knowledge. *Nature, 379*, 649–652.

Menon, V., Adleman, N. E., White, C. D., Glover, G. H., & Reiss, A. L. (2001). Error-related brain activation during a Go/NoGo response inhibition task. *Human Brain Mapping, 12*, 131–143.

Moore, C. J., & Price, C. J. (1999). A functional neuroimaging study of the variables that generate category-specific object processing differences. *Brain, 122*, 943–962.

Moss, H. E., & Tyler, L. K. (2000). A progressive category-specific semantic deficit for non-living things. *Neuropsychologia, 38*, 60–82.

Mummery, C. J., Patterson, K., Price, C. J., Ashburner, J., Frackowiak, R. S., & Hodges, J. R. (2000). A voxel-based morphometry study of semantic dementia: Relationship between temporal lobe atrophy and semantic memory. *Annals of Neurology, 47*, 36–45.

Mummery, C. J., Shallice, T., & Price, C. J. (1999). Dual-process model in semantic priming: A functional imaging perspective. *NeuroImage, 9*, 516–525.

Perani, D., Cappa, S. F., Bettinardi, V., Bressi, S., Gorno-Tempini, M., Matarrese, M., & Fazio, F. (1995). Different neural systems for the recognition of animals and man-made tools. *Neuroreport, 6*, 1637–41.

Perani, D., Schnur, T., Tettamanti, M., Gorno-Tempini, M., Cappa, S. F., & Fazio, F. (1999). Word and picture matching: a PET study of semantic category effects. *Neuropsychologia, 37*, 293–306.

Pilgrim, L. K., Fadili, J., Fletcher, P., & Tyler, L. K. (2002). Overcoming confounds of stimulus blocking: An event-related fMRI design of semantic processing. *NeuroImage, 16*, 713–723.

Puce, A., Allison, T., Bentin, S., Gore, J. C., & McCarthy, G. (1998). Temporal cortex activation in humans viewing eye and mouth movements. *Journal of Neuroscience, 18*, 2188–2199.

Saffran, E. M., & Schwartz, M. F. (1994). Of cabbages and things: Semantic memory from a neuropsychological perspective—a tutorial review. *Attention and Performance, XV*, 507–536.

Silbersweig, D. A., Stern, E., Frith, C. D., Cahill, C., Schnorr, L., Grootoonk, S., Spinks, T., Clark, J., Frackowiak, R., & Jones, T. (1993). Detection of thirty-second cognitive activations in single subjects with positron emission tomography: A new low-dose

H2(15)O regional cerebral blood flow three-dimensional imaging technique. *Journal of Cerebral Blood Flow and Metabolism*, *13*, 617–629.

Silveri, M. C., Daniele, A., Giustolisi, L., & Gainotti, G. (1991). Dissociation between knowledge of living and nonliving things in dementia of the Alzheimer type. *Neurology*, *41*, 545–546.

Spitzer, M., Kischka, U., Guckel, F., Bellemann, M., Kammer, T., Seyyedi, S., Weisbod, M., Schwartz, A., & Brix, G. (1998). Functional magnetic resonance imaging of category-specific cortical activation: Evidence for semantic maps. *Cognitive Brain Research*, *6*, 309–319.

Stewart, F., Parkin, A. J., & Hunkin, N. M. (1992). Naming impairments following recovery from herpes simplex encephalitis: Category-specific? *Quarterly Journal of Experimental Psychology*, *44A*, 261–284.

Thompson-Schill, S. L., Aguirre, G. K., D'Esposito, M., & Farah, M. J. (1999). A neural basis for category and modality specificity of semantic knowledge. *Neuropsychologia*, *37*, 671–676.

Tyler, L. K., & Moss, H. E. (1997). Functional properties of concepts: Studies of normal and brain-damaged patients. *Cognitive Neuropsychology*, *14*, 511–545.

Tyler, L. K., & Moss, H. E. (2001). Towards a distributed account of conceptual knowledge. *Trends in Cognitive Sciences*, *5*, 244–252.

Tyler, L. K., Moss, H. E., Durrant-Peatfield, M. R., & Levy, J. P. (2000). Conceptual structure and the structure of concepts: a distributed account of category-specific deficits. *Brain and Language*, *75*, 195–231.

Tyler, L. K., Russell, R., Fadili, J., & Moss, H. E. (2001). The neural representation of nouns and verbs: PET studies. *Brain*, *124*, 1619–1634.

Ulrich, R., & Miller, J. (1994). Effects of truncation on reaction time analysis. *Journal of Experimental Psychology: General*, *123*, 34–80.

Vandenberghe, R., Price, C., Wise, R., Josephs, O., & Frackowiak, R. S. (1996). Functional anatomy of a common semantic system for words and pictures. *Nature*, *383*, 254–256.

Van Horn, J. D., Ellmore, T. M., Esposito, G., & Berman, K. F. (1998). Mapping voxel-based statistical power on parametric images. *NeuroImage*, *7*, 97–107.

Warrington, E. K., & McCarthy, R. (1983). Category specific access dysphasia. *Brain*, *106*, 859–878.

Warrington, E. K., & McCarthy, R. A. (1987). Categories of knowledge: Further fractionations and an attempted intergration. *Brain*, *110*, 1273–1296.

Warrington, E. K., & Shallice, T. (1984). Category specific semantic impairments. *Brain*, *107*, 829–854.

Worsley, K. J., Marrett, S., Neelin, P., Vandal, A. C., Friston, K. J., & Evans, A. C. (1996). A unified statistical approach for determining significant signals in images of cerebral activation. *Human Brain Mapping*, *4*, 58–73.

COGNITIVE NEUROPSYCHOLOGY, 2003, 20 (3/4/5/6), 561–574

# HOW IS THE FUSIFORM GYRUS RELATED TO CATEGORY-SPECIFICITY?

C. J. Price, U. Noppeney, and J. Phillips
*University College, London, UK*

J. T. Devlin
*University of Oxford, UK*

There is growing evidence from functional imaging studies that distinct regions in the fusiform gyri are differentially sensitive to object category. In this paper, we investigate how the areas that are more sensitive to animals than tools respond to other visual and semantic variables. We illustrate that (1) category effects in the fusiform areas are stronger for pictures of objects than their written names; (2) retrieving information on the colour or size of objects activates a left lateralised fusiform area that lies anterior to the category-sensitive areas; and (3) both left and right category-sensitive areas respond strongly to visual feature detection on false fonts—meaningless visual stimuli with no semantic associations. These results dissociate the responses in two fusiform areas: The posterior category-sensitive areas are primarily modulated by visual input, whereas a more anterior polymodal region is involved in the retrieval of visual information. In addition, we demonstrate that the posterior areas which are more active for animals than tools are also more active for fruits than tools. Our data are therefore consistent with the proposal that activation in the lateral posterior fusiform gyri reflects the demands on structural differentiation. Since animals and fruits tend to have more structurally similar neighbours than man-made kinds of objects, category effects are likely to be observed during most picture identification tasks. In contrast, when the stimuli are written or auditory names, category effects may only be observed when the task requires access to fine spatial details in the objects' structures.

## INTRODUCTION

Several functional neuroimaging studies have shown that, within the large expanse of occipito-temporal cortex that responds to pictures of all objects, individual categories evoke different *patterns* of activation (Chao, Haxby, & Martin, 1999; Chao, Weisberg, & Martin, 2002; Gorno-Tempini & Price, 2001; Ishai, Ungerleider, Martin, Schouten, & Haxby, 1999; Martin & Chao, 2001; Thompson-Schill, Aguirre, D'Esposito, & Farah, 1999; Whatmough, Chertkow, Murtha, & Hanratty, 2002). For example, pictures of animals tend to increase activation in lateral posterior fusiform areas relative to tools, and the reverse contrast results in medial fusiform activations (Chao et al., 1999, 2002). Similar effects of category have been observed for written names when subjects make category decisions about animals and tools (Chao et al., 1999) and in the absence of picture or word input, when subjects generate mental images of different

Requests for reprints should be addressed to Cathy J. Price, PhD, Wellcome Department of Imaging Neuroscience, University College London, 12 Queen Square, London WC1N 3BG, UK (Email: cprice@fil.ion.ucl.ac.uk).

This work was supported by the Wellcome Trust. We thank the radiographers at the Functional Imaging Laboratory for their assistance in collecting these data, the volunteers who participated in these studies, and Karl Friston for his helpful comments.





http://www.tandf.co.uk/journals/pp/02643294.html DOI:10.1080/02643290244000284

categories of object (Ishai et al., 1999). Martin and Chao (2001) have therefore suggested that category effects in the fusiform areas "are driven by stored object information" with objects from the same category tending to share similar forms or structures.

There is, however, a debate as to whether the category effects in the fusiform gyri reflect differences at the perceptual (Gerlach, Aaside, Humphreys, Grade, Paulson, & Law, 2002; Whatmough et al., 2002) or the semantic (Martin & Chao, 2001) level, which in turn depends on one's definition of semantics. For example, if our conceptual representations of objects are distributed in the sensory and motor cortices that perceive and respond to the presence of objects (Damasio, 1989), semantic areas become synonymous with sensory and motor areas. The distinction between perception and semantics then rests on whether activation in an area is driven by the sensory input or the mechanisms that enable the retrieval of learnt information in the absence of the stimulus. Nevertheless, it is clear that conceptual representations of objects involve more than distributed patterns of activity in unimodal sensory and motor cortices. Polymodal association areas in parietal, anterior, and posterior middle temporal areas also respond to familiar relative to unfamiliar stimuli (Gorno-Tempini & Price, 2001; Gorno-Tempini et al., 1998) and when subjects make semantic association judgements (Vandenberghe, Price, Wise, Josephs, & Frackowiak, 1996). These areas might represent the convergence of information from multiple modalities and correspond to high-level object representations—our amodal semantic system. According to Damasio (1989), the higher-order convergence zones are not accumulators of all information described in earlier regions; rather they serve to reactivate sensory and motor cortices during recall. Thus, the retrieval of sensory or motor information can only be achieved by recourse to unimodal cortices. Although it is well established that early sensory cortices can be activated during imagery (see Kosslyn, Ganis, & Thompson, 2001, for review), there are many reports of patients who have preserved object knowledge even when perception is impaired following bilateral occipital lesions (Bartolomeo et al., 1998; Servos & Goodale, 1995; Shuren, Brott, Scheff, & Houston, 1996). This dissociation suggests that at least some visual information can be retrieved from high level representations without recourse to perceptual areas.

With respect to the category-sensitive areas in the posterior fusiform gyri, we need to establish the level of object representation that is being processed. Is activity in these areas primarily driven by visual input, or is it also required when visual form information is being retrieved from spoken and written words? Previous studies have highlighted a left mid-fusiform area, anterior to the category-sensitive areas, during colour retrieval (Martin, Haxby, Lalonde, Wiggs, & Ungerleider, 1995), imagining concrete objects (D'Esposito et al., 1997) and when the imageability of heard and seen words increased (Wise et al., 2000). Despite consistent reports of left mid-fusiform activation, none of these studies reported activation in the posterior category-sensitive areas. The association of the left mid-fusiform with semantic retrieval is consistent with the anterior shift in fusiform activity that is observed as objects become more recognisable (Bar et al., 2001). The posterior (category-sensitive) areas are activated by both meaningful and meaningless objects relative to visual noise (Van Turennout, Ellmore, & Martin, 2000), whereas the left mid-fusiform is more responsive to meaningful than meaningless objects even when the task and attentional demands are held constant (Gerlach et al., 2002; Moore & Price, 1999b); see Table 1 for anatomical details.

In this paper, we reconsider whether the category effects in the fusiform areas are primarily driven by visual or semantic input. In the first study, we compare the effect of category when the stimuli are pictures and written words. If the category effects are only present for pictures, they are more likely to arise from bottom-up processing of the stimuli. On the other hand, if they are present for both pictures and words, they are more likely to reflect access to stored object representations. Each of these hypotheses is then explored further. The second study investigates the retrieval of visual

Table 1. *Previous studies*

| *First author* | *Year* | *Stimuli* | *Activation* | *Baseline* | *L post fus* | *R post fus* | *L mid fus* |
|---|---|---|---|---|---|---|---|
| Chao | 1999 | Pictures | Animals | Tools | −37 −55 −20 | 37 −52 −20 | |
| Chao | 2002 | Pictures | Animals | Tools | −38 −58 −10 | 36 −57 −10 | |
| Van Turennout | 2000 | Pictures | Nonobjects | Noise | −38 −56 −20 | 36 −52 −20 | |
| Moore | 1999b | Pictures | Objects | Nonobjects | ---- | ---- | −32 −40 −20 |
| Gerlach | 2002 | Pictures | Objects | Nonobjects | ---- | ---- | −34 −40 −18 |
| Martin | 1995 | Pictures | Colour | Action | ---- | ---- | −42 −46 −12 |
| D'Esposito | 1997 | Aud words | High img | Low img | ---- | ---- | −33 −48 −18 |
| Wise | 2000 | Aud/Vis words | High img | Low img | ---- | ---- | −31 −40 −18 |
| | | | | | | | −35 −50 −14 |

L post fus = left posterior fusiform (y = −54 to −66); R post fus = right posterior fusiform (y = −52 to −63); L mid fus = left mid fusiform (y = −40 to −50); aud = auditory; vis = visual; img = imageability.
Note that Martin et al. (1995) also report right mid-fusiform activation at 42, −42, −20.

information when the stimuli are auditory and visual words using paradigms that depend on access to object representations. The third study identifies regions driven by meaningless visual rather than semantic input. In summary, if the category effects are driven by stored object form, we would expect a correspondence in the activation observed in Studies 1 and 2. In contrast, if category effects are primarily driven by visual input, we would expect a correspondence between activations in Studies 1 and 3.

## METHODS

Three studies are reported in order to investigate (1) category effects; (2) retrieval of visual information from object names; and (3) visual processing of meaningless items. We focused on characterising the functional responses in two adjacent regions of the fusiform: (1) the category-sensitive fusiform areas identified by Chao and colleagues (2002), and (2) the more anterior mid-fusiform area identified by D'Esposito et al. (1997), Wise et al. (2000), and Martin et al. (1995); see Table 1 for coordinates.

### Study 1: Category effects

This study consisted of seven different experiments, which each manipulated object category with separate conditions for natural kind and man-made objects. The stimulus modality and task varied between experiments. In two experiments stimuli were black-and-white line drawings (Gorno-Tempini, Cipolotti, & Price, 2000; Moore & Price, 1999b); in two the stimuli were written or auditory words (Mummery, Patterson, Hodges, & Wise, 1996; Mummery, Patterson, Hodges, & Price, 1998); and in three the stimuli were both drawings and written words (Moore & Price, 1999a, Exp. 1 and 2; Phillips, Humphreys, Noppeney, & Price, 2002). The effect of category (natural vs. man-made) was computed for each experiment separately by including only the conditions where subjects named the stimuli (Gorno-Tempini et al., 2000; Moore & Price, 1999b, 1999a, Exp. 1); performed semantic decisions (Moore & Price, 1999a, Exp. 2; Mummery et al., 1998; Phillips et al., 2002); or retrieved exemplars of a particular category (Mummery et al., 1996). In other words, conditions without a strong semantic component were not included in the category comparisons. The common effects of category were computed for pictures and words separately over experiments. Then we tested for the category by stimulus type interaction in the two studies that manipulated these variables independently and looked at the simple main effects of category in each experiment. A total of 60 subjects participated (6–12 in each experiment). Further details can be found in Table 2 and Devlin et al. (2002).

**Table 2.** *Summary of the stimuli and tasks used in the experiments included in Study 1*

| *Study* | *Task* | *Categories*[a] | *Subjects* |
|---|---|---|---|
| 1. Gorno-Tempini et al. (2000) | Naming outline drawings | A, T | 8 |
| 2. Moore and Price (1999a) | Naming outline drawings | A, F, MC, MS | 8 |
| 3. Moore and Price (1999b) | Naming outline drawings<br>Reading object names | N, M | 10 |
| 4. Mummery et al. (1998) | Semantic decisions on written names | F, T | 12 |
| 5. Moore and Price (1999a) | Matching drawings to written names | A, F, V, T | 6 |
| 6. Phillips et al. (2002) | Semantic decisions outline drawings<br>Semantic decisions written names | N, M | 10 |
| 7. Mummery et al. (1996) | Category fluency, auditory names | N, M | 6 |

Categories included animals (A), fruit (F), natural kinds (N, i.e., animals and fruit in same block), vehicles (V), tools (T), man-made objects with complex structures such as vehicles and furniture (MC), man-made objects with simple shapes, mainly tools (MS), and mixed categories of man-made items (M).

## Study 2: Retrieval of visual information from object names

This study consisted of two experiments. The first had two conditions. In the activation condition, subjects listened to words (one per 4 s) depicting food items (mainly fruit and vegetables) and made a key press response to indicate if the physical form of the object was associated with the colour red. In the baseline condition, the same words were digitally reversed (to control for acoustic processing) and subjects were instructed to make a gender decision ("Is the voice female?") to control for decision processes and the manual key press response. There were nine subjects who were scanned three times in each condition. See Appendix A for full list of stimuli. Effects outside the fusiform gyri are being reported in Noppeney and Price (2003).

In the second experiment, stimuli were the written names of fruits (presented one per 4.5 s; see Appendix A) and there were three tasks, two semantic and one baseline. In the semantic tasks, subjects were engaged in either retrieval of action ("do you peel it with your hands?") or visual ("is it bigger than a kiwi?") information. The baseline task involved screen size judgements ("Is the physical size of the word on the screen, large or small?"). Twelve subjects participated in two scans per condition; see Phillips et al. (2002) for additional details.

In both experiments, activation differences were expected to include visual imagery of object form as subjects imagined the item in order to retrieve its semantic attributes (i.e. colour, actions, or real-life size).

## Study 3: Visual processing of meaningless features

This was a single experiment with two conditions. In the activation condition, subjects were presented with strings of meaningless false fonts at a rate of one string per 1.5 s. The task was to press a key if a predetermined visual feature was present. The baseline condition was resting with eyes closed. In this fashion, subjects were forced to focus on the visual form of the stimuli. The experiment is reported in order to compare early visual processing areas to category (Study 1) and semantic retrieval (Study 2 ) effects. Four subjects participated in four scans per condition. See Price, Wise, and Frackowiak (1996) for additional details.

*Imaging.* All studies were conducted on Siemens/CTI PET scanners (Knoxville, TN, USA) with septa retracted (model 962 for Studies 1 and 2 and model 953B for Study 3). Subjects gave written informed consent prior to receiving 12 PET scans each involving a bolus of $H_2O^{15}$ with a total radiation exposure of <5.0m Sv in accordance with the Administration of Radioactive Substances Advisory Committee of the Department of Health, UK. Correction for attenuation was made by a transmission scan with an exposed $^{68}Ge/^{68}Ga$ external source. All 12 scans were included in data preprocessing to maximise sensitivity, although the statistical contrasts included only the conditions of interest (see above).

*Data analysis.* Functional images were realigned to correct for head motion as implemented in Statistical Parametric Mapping (SPM99, Wellcome Department of Cognitive Neurology) (Friston, Ashburner, Frith, Poline, Heather, & Frackowiak, 1995a). The mean image created by the realignment procedure was used to determine the parameters for transforming the images onto the Montreal Neurological Institute (MNI) mean brain. These parameters were then applied to the functional images (Ashburner & Friston, 1997; Ashburner, Neelin, Collins, Evans, & Friston, 1997) and the image was re-sampled into isotropic 2 $mm^3$ voxels. Finally, each image was smoothed with a 16mm at full-width half-maximum Gaussian filter. The SPM software was used to compute multiple-linear regression analyses and global CBF counts were included as covariates of no interest (Friston, Holmes, Worsley, Poline, Frith, & Frackowiak, 1995b). In this paper we focus only on responses in the fusiform areas that have previously been associated with category-specific effects and semantic retrieval.

## RESULTS

### Study 1: Category effects for pictures and words

Pictures of natural relative to man-made objects activated the posterior category-sensitive fusiform areas that have previously been identified by Chao and colleagues (1999, 2002) and Whatmough et al. (2002). The advantage for pictures of natural objects survived correction for multiple comparisons in our regions of interest (10 mm spheres centred on the coordinates from Chao et al., 2002) with peaks at −42, −62, −20 ($z$ = 4.0, $p < .001$ corrected) in the left and 40, −54, −14 ($Z = 3.8, p <$ .005 corrected) in the right (see Table 2).[1] Figure 1 illustrates the spatial extent of these effects and shows the effect sizes for naming pictures of animals, fruits, and man-made items relative to viewing nonobjects. As can be seen, both animals and fruit increased activation more than man-made items. The Z scores for the comparison of fruits > tools (data from Phillips et al., 2002; Moore & Price, 1999a) were 2.7 in the left posterior fusiform (−38, −58, −18) and 1.9 in the right posterior fusiform (36, −58, −8).

In contrast to the strong category effects for pictures, there was no effect of natural relative to man-made objects when the stimuli were presented as written or auditory words, even when the search volume was restricted to 10 mm spheres as above ($Z < 1.6, p > .1$). The difference between the effects for pictures and words was investigated by computing the interaction of category and stimulus modality in the two experiments that manipulated both variables independently (Moore & Price, 1999b; Phillips et al., 2002). This revealed a highly significant interaction in the left fusiform ($Z = 3.2$ at −42, −58, −10, $p < .02$ after small volume correction) whereas in the right, the size of the interaction was smaller ($Z = 1.7$ at 40, −54, −18, $p = .34$ after small volume correction). Figure 2 illustrates the effect sizes for natural > man-made objects for pictures (black bars) and words (grey bars) in the left and right posterior fusiform. The data are plotted for two locations in each hemisphere—at the peak coordinates of the left and right posterior fusiform areas identified in the current study (top row) and in Chao et al. (2002, bottom row). Together these coordinates span the extent of the activation and indicate that the effects are not specific to indi-

[1] It is worth noting that this result was not reported by Devlin et al. (2002) because it did not reach significance when corrected for multiple comparisons across the entire brain. Likewise, the areas reported by Devlin et al. that were outside the fusiform gyrus are not reported here.

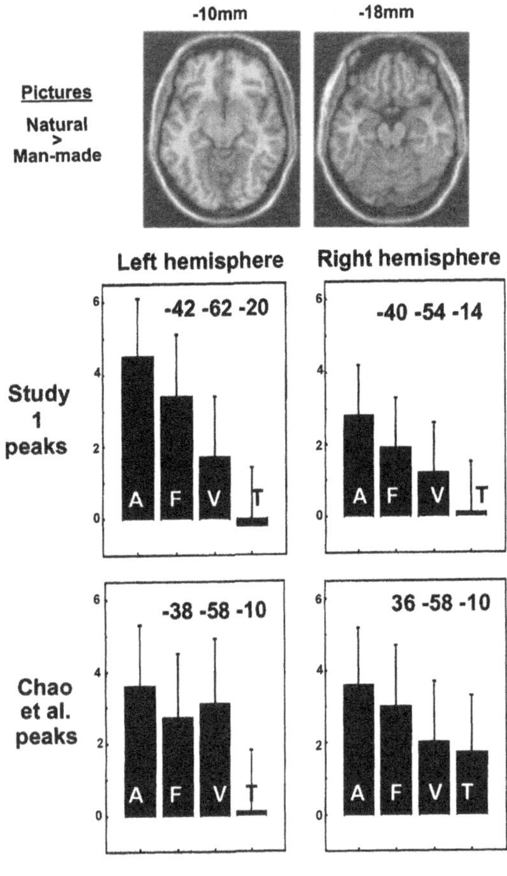


**Figure 1.** *Activation for pictures of natural relative to man-made items. Upper: Activation (threshold, Z > 2.8) for pictures of natural relative to man-made items is shown in red on two axial slices of the MNI T1 template image, 10 mm and 18 mm below the ac–pc line. Data from Study 1, Devlin et al. (2002). Lower: Effect sizes in the left and right category-sensitive fusiform areas (see Table 2) for naming animals (A), fruit and vegetables (F), man-made objects with complex shapes (mainly vehicles and furniture—V), and man-made objects with simple shapes (mainly tools-T) relative to saying "OK" to unfamiliar nonsense objects. Data from Moore and Price (1999a). Two points should be noted. First, as indicated in Table 1, nonobjects also activate these fusiform areas relative to visual noise (Van Turennout et al., 2000). We would therefore expect stronger effects for all conditions including tools if the baseline was fixation or visual noise (see Chao et al., 2002). Second, when subjects perform the same task (e.g., say "OK") on objects and nonobjects, activation is only higher for objects in the left anterior fusiform area (see Table 1). In contrast, Figure 1 (lower part) shows that naming objects is also increased activation in the category-sensitive fusiform areas relative to saying "OK" to nonobjects. In this case, activation for objects may reflect enhanced attention to the physical properties of the picture when a naming response was required.*

vidual locations but are generally true of the region. As can be seen, there was no advantage for natural kinds of objects when the stimuli were written words.

Finally, when man-made items were contrasted to natural stimuli, there were no significant effects in the fusiform gyri. The absence of medial fusiform activation for tools > animals (cf. Chao et al., 1999, 2002; Whatmough et al., 2002) may relate to (1) reduced sensitivity as a consequence of inhomogeneity in the man-made items included in different studies (see Table 2) and/or (2) the low spatial resolution of PET—although a strong lateral-medial fusiform division has been observed with the identical image acquisition and data processing when pictures of faces and buildings were compared (Gorno-Tempini & Price, 2001) and in another PET study comparing animals and tools (Whatmough et al., 2002).

## Study 2: Retrieval of visual information from object names

When subjects listened to object names and decided if the object was red (Experiment 1), peak activation was located in the left mid-fusiform area (anterior to the category-sensitive areas) and the left posterior inferior temporal cortex (lateral to the category-sensitive areas), see Table 3. There were no detectable effects in any right fusiform voxels (Z < 1.6). Figure 3 illustrates these activations in relation to the category-effects reported in Study 1. Although activation in the left hemisphere bordered the category-sensitive fusiform area, it is clear that the category-sensitive areas are distinct from the areas involved in retrieving visual information.

We considered the possibility that responses in the category-sensitive fusiform areas were small (Ishai, Ungerleider, & Haxby, 2000) and may have been lost due to our high spatial smoothing (16 mm FWHM). We therefore re-analysed the data using a 5 mm smoothing kernel. The same left mid-fusiform and left posterior inferior temporal activations were observed with slightly lower Z scores ($Z = 3.3$ and 4.4 respectively). Nonetheless, a two-voxel cluster in the left (−36, −56, −8; Z =

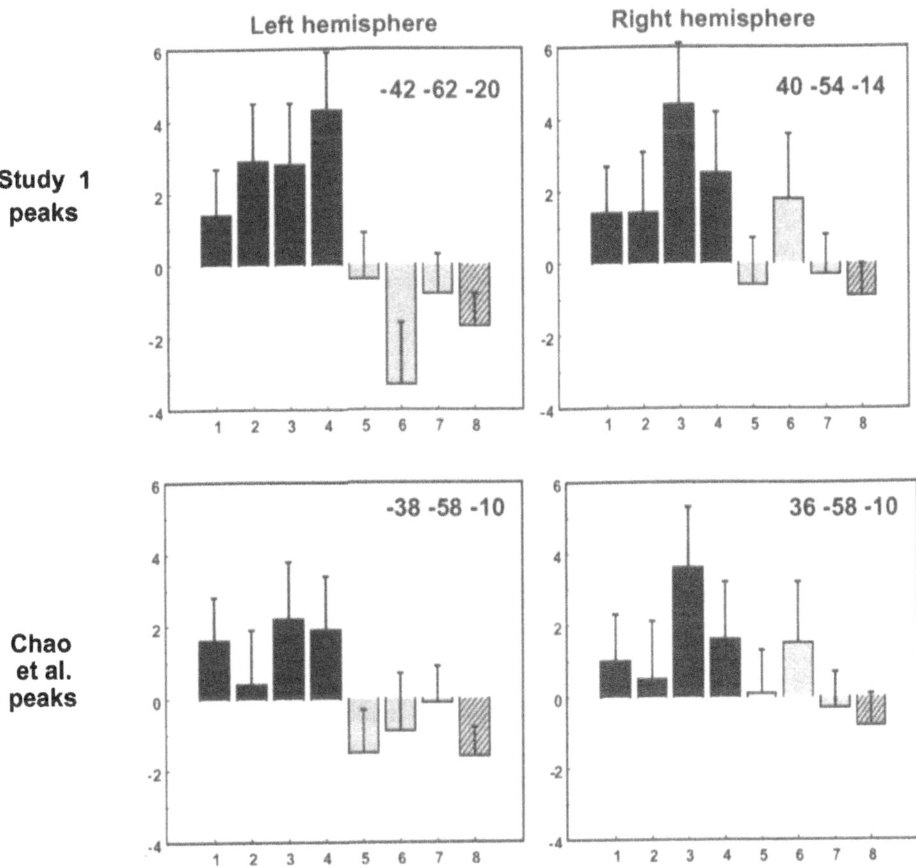


Figure 2. *Category effects for pictures and words. Effect sizes in the left and right category-sensitive fusiform areas for natural relative to man-made objects, see Tables 1 and 3. Black bars indicate picture stimuli, grey bars indicate the written names of objects; hashed grey bars indicate the auditory names of objects. Data are taken from the multi-study analysis reported in Study 1: Column 1, Phillips et al. (2002); Column 2, Moore and Price (1999a); Column 3, Gorno-Tempini et al. (2000); Column 4, Moore and Price (1999b); Column 5, Phillips et al. (2002); Column 6, Moore and Price (1999b); Column 7, Mummery et al. (1998); Column 8, Mummery et al. (1996).*

2.1) and a two voxel cluster in the right (40, −64, −12; $Z$ = 1.9) posterior fusiform areas were revealed when the threshold was reduced to $Z >$ 1.6. Although these voxels were in regions of interest, it should be noted that (1) 275 other areas were also identified across the cortex with two or more voxels at this threshold; and (2) even when the search volume was reduced to 10 mm, see above, activations did not reach significance ($p$ = .79 on the left and .86 in the right). We can only conclude that, as noted by Ishai, Ungerleider, and Haxby (2000), activation in the category-sensitive fusiform areas during mental imagery may be exceedingly small (or negligible), and this contrasts to the highly significant effects we observed in the more anterior left mid-fusiform.

The second experiment (action or size decisions on the written names of fruits) produced a virtually identical pattern of activation in the left mid-fusiform and left posterior inferior temporal area (see Table 3) with no detectable effects in either the left or right category-sensitive areas ($Z < 1.6$), see Figure 3. There was no significant difference in fusiform activation for action relative to size decisions, nor was there a significant RT difference (937 ms for action, 922 ms for size).

**Table 3.** *Results of Studies 1–3*

| | *L post fusiform* | *R post fusiform* | *L mid-fusiform* | *L post inf temporal* |
|---|---|---|---|---|
| Study 1 | −42, −62, −20 (4.2) | 40, −54, −14 (3.9) | | |
| | *−38, −58, −10 (2.6)* | *36, −57, −10 (3.2)* | | |
| Study 2, Exp 1 | | | −28, −40, −22 (4.5) | −54, −50, −18 (5.2) |
| Study 2, Exp 2 | | | −32, −40, −22 (3.0) | −60, −58, −16 (2.1) |
| Study 3 | −42, −68, −12 (6.1) | 46, −56, −16 (5.7) | | |
| | *−38, −58, −10 (5.6)* | *36, −57, −10 (4.9)* | | |

Italics indicate effect sizes at the coordinates identified as category sensitive by Chao et al. (2000), see Table 1. All other effects were identified by SPM as separable peaks. L = left, R = right, post = posterior, inf. = inferior.

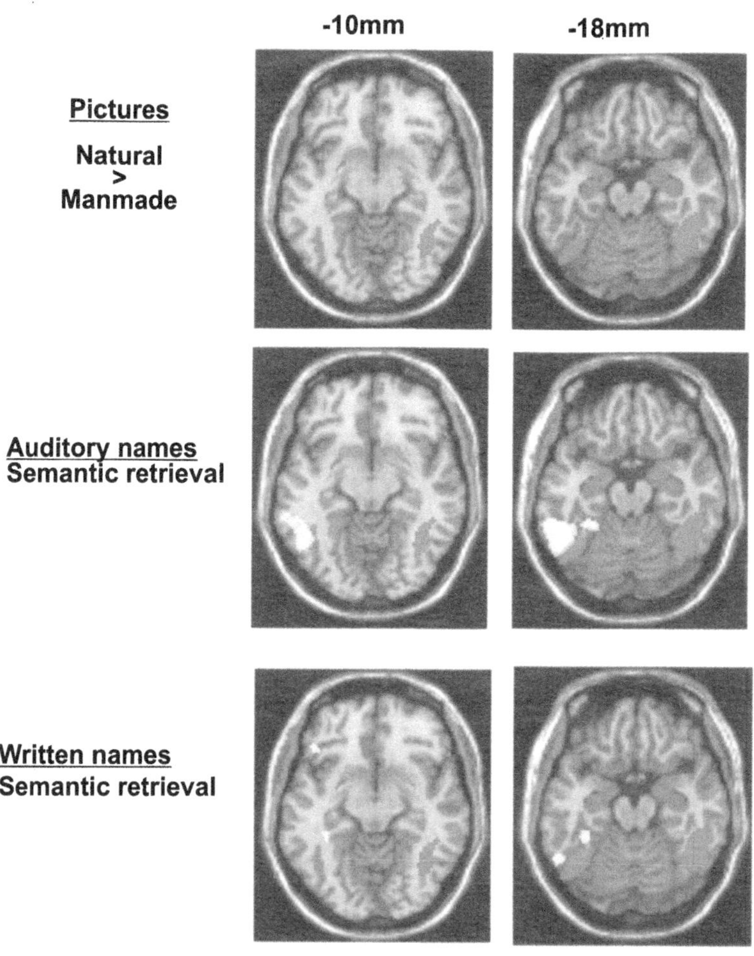


**Figure 3.** *Category and semantic effects in the fusiform gyri. Activation (threshold, Z > 2.8) for pictures of natural relative to man-made items (red) and retrieval of visual information (yellow) on two axial slices of the MNI T1 template image, 10 mm and 18 mm below the ac–pc line. Top row: category effects only, data from Study 1, Devlin et al. (2002). Second row: yellow = retrieval of object colour from auditory names (Study 2, Experiment 1). Third row: yellow = retrieval of object size from written names of fruit (Study 2, Experiment 2).*

### Study 3: Visual processing of meaningless features

The third study was included to determine whether the posterior category-sensitive fusiform areas were sensitive to visual form processing in general, even without any semantic content. Visual feature detection (mean RT 462 ms) resulted in highly significant posterior fusiform activation that encompassed the entire category-sensitive areas (Study 1) but did not extend into the semantic retrieval areas identified in Study 2 (see Table 3 and Figure 4).

## DISCUSSION

Previous imaging studies have reported category-sensitive patterns of activation in the fusiform gyri during picture processing (Chao et al., 1999, 2002; Gorno-Tempini & Price, 2001; Ishai et al., 2000, 1999; Whatmough et al., 2002). Our studies replicate the enhancement of lateral fusiform activation for pictures of animals relative to tools, and extend these results in three ways. First, we show the distinction between the bilateral posterior fusiform areas that are primarily driven by bottom-up visual processing and the left mid-fusiform area that is engaged during the retrieval of visual information. Second, posterior fusiform activation was more strongly modulated by category when the stimuli were pictures of objects relative to their written names; and third, we demonstrate that the area that responds more to pictures of animals than tools is also more active for pictures of fruit relative to tools. As we discuss below, these findings constrain the interpretation of category effects in the fusiform gyrus.

### The posterior and mid-fusiform areas

By comparing activation evoked by category changes (Study 1), retrieval of visual information (Study 2), and visual processing of meaningless input (Study 3), we demonstrate that category effects in the fusiform overlap with visual rather than semantic processing. The overlap between category effects and visual input suggests that the category-sensitive fusiform areas are part of the unimodal visual association cortex while the more anterior left mid-fusiform activation for semantic retrieval suggests that the left mid-fusiform region is a polymodal association area. Furthermore, the absence of posterior fusiform activation during semantic retrieval suggests that visual information can be retrieved from polymodal association cortex without recourse to the category-sensitive fusiform areas. Other functional imaging studies have also demonstrated mid- rather than posterior fusiform activation when visual information is retrieved (D'Esposito et al., 1997; Martin et al., 1995; O'Craven & Kanwisher, 2000; Wise et al., 2000). Nevertheless, posterior fusiform activation has been reported when subjects vividly imagine previously viewed objects (Ishai et al., 2000). Visual imagery tasks of this kind, that require retrieval of fine resolution detail, may be more likely to evoke activation in visual cortices (see Kosslyn et al., 2001). Future studies are therefore required to directly compare tasks that require retrieval of fine spatial details (Ishai et al., 2000) with those that require retrieval of colour and size information (Study 2). We would predict that the former would activate unimodal visual cortex whereas the latter can be accomplished by polymodal association cortex.

The same rostro-caudal shift from unimodal to polymodal cortex within the fusiform gyrus is also seen in anatomical studies in macaques. Using cytoarchetectonic data, von Bonin and Bailey (1947) identified two distinct regions of the macaque fusiform gyrus, TF and TH, which corresponded to equivalent regions in humans (cf. Von Economo, 1929). TF included most of the gyrus medial to the occipito-temporal sulcus[2] and is part of the ventral visual path based on its extensive and reciprocal connections with occipital areas V2, V3, and V4 and the inferior temporal regions TEO

[2] Although Von Bonin and Bailey (1974) call this fusiform gyrus, others have also referred to it as parahippocampal gyrus (e.g., Van Hoesen, 1982).

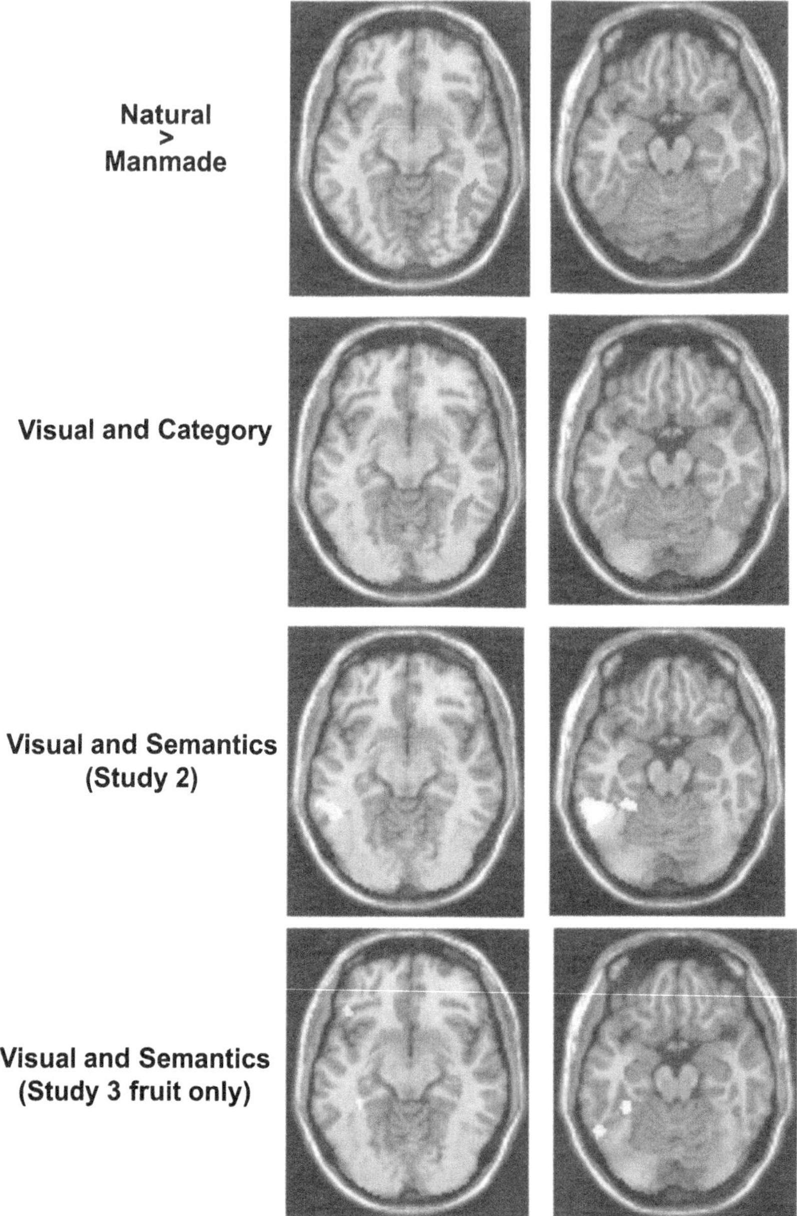


Figure 4. *Category, visual, and semantic effects in the fusiform gyri. Activation for pictures of natural relative to man-made items (red), retrieval of visual information (yellow), and visual feature processing (green) on two axial slices of the MNI T1 template image, 10 mm and 18 mm below the ac–pc line. Top row: category effects from Study 1, Devlin et al. (2002). Second row: category effects (Study 1) and visual effects (Study 3). Third row: visual effects (Study 3) and semantic effects (Study 2, Experiment 1). Bottom row: visual effects (Study 3) and semantic effects (Study 2, Experiment 2).*

and TE (Distler, Boussaoud, Desimone, & Ungerleider, 1993). TH, on the other hand, is more anterior, lying between TF and the hippocampal formation and receiving inputs from a number of different sensory systems (Van Hoesen, 1982). While there is no simple correspondence between TF in macaques and the posterior fusiform in humans, the rostro-causal shift from unimodal to polymodal cortex within the fusiform does appear to be maintained.

## Category effects in the fusiform

In contrast to the study reported by Chao et al. (1999), we did not find category effects when the stimuli were either written or auditory object names. One possible explanation is simply that the current study lacked sufficient sensitivity to detect these category effects. By focusing our search exclusively on the specific region of the fusiform gyrus identified by Chao et al. (2002), the statistical sensitivity within this region was greatly enhanced. Indeed, within this ROI, category effects were easily detected for pictures but not for words, even when the same subjects performed the same tasks. On average the effects for words were not simply small (and therefore obscured by the variance in the data), they were in the wrong direction (see Fig 2a). We therefore consider an explanation in terms of insufficient sensitivity unlikely. Below, we consider the possibility that differences in the visual input of picture stimuli contribute to category effects in the fusiform irrespective of the task, whereas category effects during written word processing are specific to particular task contexts.

Pictures of animals and tools differ in many ways. The most obvious relates to their visual complexity. Animals tend to have multi-component shapes whereas tools tend to have simple structures with few components. Our data, however, revealed that activation in the fusiform was almost as high for pictures of fruits with simple structures as it was for pictures of animals with complex structures. Indeed, the Z scores for the comparison of fruits > tools (data from Moore & Price, 1999a; Phillips et al., 2002) were 2.7 in the left posterior fusiform (−38, −58, −18) and 1.9 in the right posterior fusiform (36, −58, −8) replicating the animal > tool advantage. Thus visual complexity is not likely to be the cause of the advantage for natural kinds.

An alternative possibility is that category-specific effects in the lateral fusiform gyri for pictures reflect the increased structural differentiation required to identify natural kinds, which tend to have more structurally similar neighbours than man-made objects. Category-specific differences in the demands on structural differentiation have previously been emphasised by Humphreys et al. (Humphreys, Riddoch, & Price, 1997; Humphreys, Riddoch, & Quinlan, 1988). More recently, Joseph and Piper (2001) have shown that differentiating structurally similar objects and nonsense shapes enhances activation in the fusiform areas that are particularly sensitive to animals (see also Gerlach et al., 2002; Gerlach, Law, Gade, & Paulson, 1999). According to this account, category effects would be observed for pictures whenever an identification response is required. In contrast, when the stimuli are written and auditory words, category effects in the fusiform will not be driven by the visual input and may only be observed during specific tasks. For instance, differentiation of object structure is not required to match words on the basis of their colour and typical location (Mummery et al., 1998), to make action or size retrieval judgements (Phillips et al., 2002), or to read aloud (Moore & Price, 1999b), and therefore these studies do not show category effects in the fusiform. Differentiation of object structure may, however, be engaged for written words when subjects have to make decisions on structural details of the objects. This would explain the category effects that were observed in the posterior fusiform when subjects had to decide if written words refer to animals that live in the forest or tools that could be used as kitchen utensils (Chao et al., 1999). In summary, we are suggesting that category effects in the posterior fusiform gyri may be driven bottom-up from visual input when pictures of objects are identified; but may only be observed for written and auditory words when the task involves visual imagery and access to the structural details of objects.

### Lesion data

Most patients with category-specific deficits for natural kinds relative to man-made items have extensive damage to anterior temporal lobe structures, often subsequent to herpes simplex encephalitis, while very few have lesions to ventral temporal areas (Gainotti, 2000; Gainotti, Silveri, Daniele, & Giustolisi, 1995). Arguin, Bub, and Dudek (1996) and Humphreys et al. (1997) have reported patients with (1) large left occipito-temporal lesions; (2) category-specific deficits for pictures of natural relative to man-made items; and (3) deficits retrieving perceptual relative to functional associations of objects. These patients may have a single functional impairment that accounts for their deficits retrieving visual information and recognising natural kinds of object, as suggested by Arguin et al. (1996) and Humphreys et al. (1997). Alternatively, they may have two separate deficits as a consequence of damage to both the posterior and middle left fusiform regions. We do not know of any patients where posterior fusiform lesions have led to category-specific deficits in the absence of perceptual knowledge deficits or the reverse dissociation. Thus, at present, the lesion data are not particularly informative.

## CONCLUSION

Martin and colleagues (Chao et al., 1999, 2002; Martin & Chao, 2001) have noted category effects in occipital and posterior fusiform regions and argued that because occipital cortex is so early in the visual processing stream, these effects may be due to top-down modulation from more anterior areas. We argue that the same may apply to the posterior fusiform regions, which are still within the visual processing stream. Although category-sensitive activations are driven directly (bottom-up) by pictorial stimuli, other stimuli are unlikely to produce category effects in these areas from bottom-up processes. Nonetheless, in some cases, the names of objects do lead to category effects in the posterior fusiform (Chao et al., 1999), and this may reflect top-down modulation from more anterior polymodal regions. Future studies are required to investigate the tasks that elicit category effects with written and auditory words and the visual retrieval paradigms that evoke activation in the posterior category-sensitive fusiform areas.

## REFERENCES

Arguin, M., Bub, D., & Dudek, G. (1996). Shape integration for visual object recognition and its implication in category-specific visual agnosia. *Visual Cognition*, *3*, 221–275.

Ashburner, J., & Friston, K. (1997). Multimodal image coregistration and partitioning: A unified framework. *NeuroImage*, *6*, 209–217.

Ashburner, J., Neelin, P., Collins, D. L., Evans, A. C., & Friston, K. J. (1997). Incorporating prior knowledge into image registration. *NeuroImage*, *6*, 344–352.

Bar, M., Tootell, R. B., Schacter, D. L., Greve, D. N., Fischl, B., Mendola, J. D., Rosen, B. R., & Dale, A. M. (2001). Cortical mechanisms specific to explicit visual object recognition. *Neuron*, *29*, 529–535.

Bartolomeo, P., Bachoud-Levi, A.-C., De Gelder, B., Denes, G., Dalla Barba, G., Brugieres, P., & Degos, J.-D. (1998). Multiple-domain dissociation between impaired visual perception and preserved mental imagery in a patient with bilateral extrastriate lesions. *Neuropsychologia*, *36*, 239–249.

Chao, L., Haxby, J. V., & Martin, A. (1999). Attribute-based neural substrates in temporal cortex for perceiving and knowing about objects. *Nature Neuroscience*, *2*, 913–919.

Chao, L., Weisberg, J., & Martin, A. (2002). Experience dependent modulation of category-related cortical activity. *Cerebral Cortex*, *12*, 545–551.

Damasio, A. R. (1989). Time locked multiregional retroactivation: A systems level proposal for the neural substrates of recall and recognition. *Cognition*, *33*, 25–62.

D'Esposito, M., Detre, J. A., Aguirre, G. K., Stallcup, M., Alsop, D. C., Tippett, L. J., & Farah, M. J. (1997). A functional MRI study of mental image generation. *Neuropsychologia*, *35*, 725–730.

Devlin, J. T., Moore, C. J., Mummery, C. J., Gorno-Tempini, M., Phillips, J., Noppeney, U., Friston, K.

J., Frackowiak, R. S. J., & Price, C. J. (2002). Anatomic constraints on cognitive theories of category-specificity. *NeuroImage, 15*, 675–685.

Distler, C., Boussaoud, D., Desimone, R., & Ungerleider, L. (1993). Cortical connections of inferior temporal area TEO in macaque monkeys. *Journal of Comparative Neurology, 334*, 125–150.

Friston, K. J., Ashburner, J., Frith, C. D., Poline, J.-B., Heather, J. D., & Frackowiak, R. S. J. (1995a). Spatial registration and normalization of images. *Human Brain Mapping, 2*, 165–189.

Friston, K. J., Holmes, A. P., Worsley, K. J., Poline, J.-B., Frith, C. D., & Frackowiak, R. S. J. (1995b). Statistical parametric maps in functional imaging: A general linear approach. *Human Brain Mapping, 2*, 189–210.

Gainotti, G. (2000). What the locus of brain lesion tells us about the nature of the cognitive deficit underlying category-specific disorders: A review. *Cortex, 36*, 539–559.

Gainotti, G., Silveri, M. S., Daniele, A., & Giustolisi, L. (1995). Neuroanatomic correlates of category-specific semantic disorders: A critical survey. *Memory, 3*, 247–264.

Gerlach, C., Aaside, C. T., Humphreys, G. W., Gade, A., Paulson, O. B., & Law, I. (2002). Brain activity related to integrative processes in visual object recognition: Bottom-up integration and the modulatory influence of stored knowledge. *Neuropsychologia, 40*, 1254–1267.

Gerlach, C., Law, I., Gade, A., & Paulson, O. B. (1999). Perceptual differentiation and category effects in normal object recognition: A PET study. *Brain, 122*, 2159–2170.

Gorno-Tempini, M. L., Cipolotti, L., & Price, C. J. (2000). Which level of object processing generates category-specific differences in brain activation? *Proceedings of the Royal Society of London B*, 1253–1258.

Gorno-Tempini, M. L., & Price, C. J. (2001). Identification of famous faces and buildings: A functional neuroimaging study of semantically unique items. *Brain, 124*, 2087–2097.

Gorno-Tempini, M. L., Price, C. J., Josephs, O., Vandenberghe, R., Cappa, S. F., Kapur, N., & Frackowiak, R. S. J. (1998). The neural systems sustaining face and proper-name processing. *Brain, 121*, 2103–2118.

Humphreys, G. W., Riddoch, M. J., & Price, C. J. (1997). Top-down processes in object identification: Evidence from experimental psychology, neuropsychology and functional anatomy. *Philosophical Transactions of the Royal Society of London Series B: Biological Sciences, 352*, 1275–1282.

Humphreys, G. W., Riddoch, M. J., & Quinlan, P. T. (1988). Cascade processes in picture identification. *Cognitive Neuropsychology, 5*, 67–103.

Ishai, A., Ungerleider, L. G., & Haxby, J. V. (2000). Distributed neural systems for the generation of visual images. *Neuron, 26*, 979–990.

Ishai, A., Ungerleider, L. G., Martin, A., Schouten, J. L., & Haxby, J. V. (1999). Distributed representation of objects in the human ventral visual pathway. *Proceedings of the National Academy of Science, USA, 96*, 9379–9384.

Joseph, J. E., & Piper, G. A. (2001). Parametric variation of structural similarity in object recognition. *Journal of Cognitive Neuroscience (Suppl)*, 134.

Kosslyn, S. M., Ganis, G., & Thompson, W. L. (2001). Neural foundations of imagery. *Nature Reviews Neuroscience, 2*, 635–642.

Martin, A., & Chao, L. L. (2001). Semantic memory and the brain: Structure and processes. *Current Opinions in Neurobiology, 11*, 194–201.

Martin, A., Haxby, J., Lalonde, F., Wiggs, C., & Ungerleider, L. (1995). Discrete cortical regions associated with knowledge of color and knowledge of action. *Science, 270*, 102–105.

Moore, C. J., & Price, C. J. (1999a). A functional neuroimaging study of the variables that generate category-specific object processing differences. *Brain, 122*, 943-962.

Moore, C. J., & Price, C. J. (1999b). Three distinct ventral occipitotemporal regions for reading and object naming. *NeuroImage, 10*, 181–192.

Mummery, C. J., Patterson, K., Hodges, J., & Wise, R. J. (1996). Generating "tiger" as an animal name or a word beginning with T: Differences in brain activation. *Proceedings of the Royal Society of London B: Biological Sciences, 263*, 989–995.

Mummery, C. J., Patterson, K., Hodges, J. R., & Price, C. J. (1998). Functional neuroanatomy of the semantic system: Divisible by what? *Journal of Cognitive Neuroscience, 10*, 766–777.

Noppeney, U., & Price, C. J. (2003). Functional imaging of the semantic system: Retrieval of sensory experienced and verbally-learnt knowledge. *Brain and Language, 84*, 120–133.

O'Craven, K. M., & Kanwisher, N. (2000). Mental imagery of faces and places activates corresponding stimulus-specific brain regions. *Journal of Cognitive Neuroscience, 12*, 1013–1023.

Phillips, J., Noppeney, U., Humphreys, G. W., & Price, C. J. (2002). Can segregation within the semantic system account for category-specific deficits? *Brain, 125*, 2067–2080.

Price, C. J., Wise, R. J. S., & Frackowiak, R. S. J. (1996). Demonstrating the implicit processing of visually presented words and pseudowords. *Cerebral Cortex, 6*, 62–72.

Servos, P., & Goodale, M. A. (1995). Preserved visual imagery in visual form agnosia. *Neuropsychologia, 33*, 1383–1394.

Shuren, J. E., Brott, T. G., Scheff, B. K., & Houston, W. (1996). Preserved color imagery in an achromatopsic. *Neuropsychologia, 34*, 485–489.

Thompson-Schill, S. L., Aguirre, G. K., D'Esposito, M., & Farah, M. J. (1999). A neural basis for category and modality specificity of semantic knowledge. *Neuropsychologia, 37*, 671–676.

Vandenberghe, R., Price, C. J., Wise, R., Josephs, O., & Frackowiak, R. S. J. (1996). Functional anatomy of a common semantic system for words and pictures. *Nature, 383*, 254–256.

Van Hoesen, G. (1982). The parahippocampal gyrus. *Trends in Neuroscience, 5*, 345–350.

Van Turennout, M., Ellmore, T., & Martin, A. (2000). Long lasting cortical plasticity in the object naming system. *Nature Neuroscience, 3*, 1329–1334.

Von Bonin, G., & Bailey, P. (1947). *The neocortex of Macaca Mulatta.* Urbana, IL: University of Illinois Press.

Von Economo, C. (1929). *The cytoarchitectonics of human cerebral cortex.* London: Oxford University Press.

Whatmough, C., Chertkow, H., Murtha, S., & Hanratty, K. (2002). Dissociable brain regions process object meaning and object structure during picture naming. *Neuropsychologia, 40*, 174–186.

Wise, R. J., Howard, D., Mummery, C. J., Fletcher, P., Leff, A., Buchel, C., & Scott, S. K. (2000). Noun imageability and the temporal lobes. *Neuropsychologia, 38*, 985–994.

# APPENDIX A

## Auditory stimuli presented in Study 2, Experiment 1

| Scan 1 | Scan 2 | Scan 3 |
|---|---|---|
| milk | kiwi | date |
| apricot | lime | peanuts |
| garlic | curd | grapes |
| butter | magarine | pineapple |
| tangerine | cottage cheese | onion |
| cabbage | cress | ketchup |
| cucumber | cauliflower | brussels sprout |
| carrot | coffeebeans | raspberry |
| leek | peppers | radish |
| salt | lemon | spinach |
| mango | sugar | beetroot |
| flower | tomato | lettuce |
| water | strawberry | potatoes |
| grapefruit | cherry | broccoli |
| basil | parsley | banana |
| bread | mushrooms | chips |
| toast | turnip | squash |
| egg | baguette | asparagus |
| celery | crisps | bagels |

## Visual stimuli presented in Study 2, Experiment 2

| Fruit 1 | Fruit 2 |
|---|---|
| Onion | Banana |
| Cauliflower | Mushroom |
| Orange | Artichoke |
| Grapes | Cherry |
| Apple | Pear |
| Tomato | Carrot |
| Lemon | Cucumber |
| Lettuce | Celery |
| Potato | Pineapple |
| Pepper | Strawberry |
| Pumpkin | Asparagus |
| Grapefruit | Corn |

COGNITIVE NEUROPSYCHOLOGY, 2003, 20 (3/4/5/6), 575–587

# NEURAL FOUNDATIONS FOR UNDERSTANDING SOCIAL AND MECHANICAL CONCEPTS

**Alex Martin and Jill Weisberg**
*National Institute of Mental Health, Bethesda, USA*

Motivated by neuropsychological investigations of category-specific impairments, many functional brain imaging studies have found distinct patterns of neural activity associated with different object categories. However, the extent to which these category-related activation patterns reflect differences in conceptual representation remains controversial. To investigate this issue, functional magnetic resonance imaging (fMRI) was used to record changes in neural activity while subjects interpreted animated vignettes composed of simple geometric shapes in motion. Vignettes interpreted as conveying social interactions elicited a distinct and distributed pattern of neural activity, relative to vignettes interpreted as mechanical actions. This neural system included regions in posterior temporal cortex associated with identifying human faces and other biological objects. In contrast, vignettes interpreted as conveying mechanical actions resulted in activity in posterior temporal lobe sites associated with identifying manipulable objects such as tools. Moreover, social, but not mechanical, interpretations elicited activity in regions implicated in the perception and modulation of emotion (right amygdala and ventromedial prefrontal cortex). Perceiving and understanding social and mechanical concepts depends, in part, on activity in distinct neural networks. Within the social domain, the network includes regions involved in processing and storing information about the form and motion of biological objects, and in perceiving, expressing, and regulating affective responses.

## INTRODUCTION

Reports of category-specific impairments following brain injury or disease have motivated an ever-increasing number of functional imaging studies on category representation in the normal human brain. Many of these investigations have shown that object categories are represented by neural activity distributed across wide spread regions of cortex. It has also been established that many of these activations are found in processing streams associated with perception of specific object features such as form and colour (ventral occipitotemporal cortex), motion (posterior lateral temporal cortex; specifically, the middle temporal gyrus and superior temporal sulcus [STS], and with grasping and manipulating objects (left intraparietal sulcus and ventral premotor cortices). Moreover, different object categories evoke distinct patterns of activity in these regions (for recent reviews, see Josephs, 2001; Martin 2001; Martin & Chao, 2001; Thompson-Schill, 2002). For example, animate objects, as represented by pictures of human faces (e.g., Haxby, Ungerleider, Clark, Shouten, Hoffman, & Martin, 1999; Ishai, Ungerleider, Martin, Shouten, & Haxby, 1999; Kanwisher

Requests for reprints should be addressed to Alex Martin, PhD, Laboratory of Brain and Cognition, National Institute of Mental Health, Building 10, Room 4C-104, 10 Center Drive MSC 1366, Bethesda, Maryland 20892-1366, USA (Email: alex@codon.nih.gov).

We thank Susan Johnson of the Dartmouth College, Media Laboratory for creating the animations, and Jay Schulkin and Cheri Wiggs for valuable discussions.



http://www.tandf.co.uk/journals/pp/02643294.html
DOI:10.1080/02643290342000005

McDermott, & Chun, 1997), human figures (Beauchamp, Lee, Haxby, & Martin, 2002), and animals (e.g., Chao, Haxby, & Martin, 1999), show heightened activity in the lateral region of the fusiform gyrus and in STS, relative to a number of other object categories (houses, tools, chairs). In contrast, manipulable objects such as tools and utensils show heightened activity relative to animate objects in the medial portion of the fusiform gyrus (e.g., Chao et al., 1999), posterior region of the left middle temporal gyrus (e.g., Chao et al., 1999; Moore & Price, 1999), and in left intraparietal and ventral premotor cortices (e.g., Chao & Martin, 2000).

Although these object category-related patterns of activity have most often been found with tasks using object pictures, they have also been found when objects are represented by their written names (see above-cited reviews). These and related findings have led us to suggest that information about different object attributes and features are stored in these regions of cortex. Moreover, we have suggested that these regions are involved in both *perceiving* and *knowing* about features and properties critical for object identification (e.g., Martin, 1998).

For example, activity in posteriolateral left temporal cortex, just anterior to primary motion processing area MT, has been reported in multiple studies of object semantics. Naming pictures of tools, answering questions about tools, and generating action words in response to object pictures or their written names show enhanced activity in the left middle temporal gyrus. In contrast, naming pictures of animals and viewing human faces show enhanced activity in a more dorsal location centred on the STS, usually stronger in the right than the left hemisphere (see above-cited reviews). This region (STS) is of particular interest because it is involved in perceiving biological motion in both humans (e.g., Puce, Allison, Bentin, Gore, & McCarthy, 1998) and monkeys (e.g., Oram & Perrett, 1994). Moreover, we have recently shown that these regions are preferentially responsive to different types of object motion. Activity in the middle temporal gyrus was strongly and selectively enhanced by video clips of moving tools, while STS was selectively responsive to human movement (Beauchamp et al., 2002).

To explain these patterns of results, we suggested that, as a result of repeated experience with objects, regions in lateral temporal cortex become tuned to different properties of object-associated motion. For example, middle temporal gyrus may be tuned to unarticulated patterns of motion commonly associated with tools, whereas STS may be tuned to articulated patterns of motion commonly associated with biological objects (see Beauchamp et al., 2002, for details). In a similar fashion, ventral occipitotemporal cortex may become tuned to different properties of object form. Importantly, it is also proposed that, once these object-feature networks are established, they are active whenever an object *concept* is retrieved, regardless of the physical format of the stimuli used to elicit the concept (picture, word, moving shapes, mental imagery, etc.). Thus, activity in these regions can be driven bottom-up by features and properties, and top-down, as part of the representation of the concept.

The goal of the present experiment was to evaluate this idea by using the same stimuli to evoke different categories of conceptual representation. Specifically, we used functional magnetic resonance imaging to record changes in brain activity while subjects interpreted the motion of simple geometric forms (circles, rectangles, triangles) designed to elicit either social or mechanical concepts.

Behavioural studies, beginning with the seminal work of Heider and Simmel (1944), have documented that higher-order cognitive concepts such as causality and agency can be elicited from observing the motion of simple geometric stimuli (for review, see Scholl & Tremoulet, 2000). An interesting and important aspect of these demonstrations is that the moving shapes can elicit the concept of living beings (agents performing actions) who, in turn, are perceived as having goals and possessing intentional states such as beliefs and desires. If this is so, then it would be expected that the neural substrate associated with understanding the social world would include the same substrate that becomes active when perceiving animate objects, in tandem with other regions. Indeed, using positron emission tomography (PET), Castelli and colleagues (Castelli, Happé, Frith, & Frith, 2000) reported evidence consistent with this hypothesis. Specifically, viewing vignettes modelled after Heider and Simmel's original investigation, and designed to evoke theory of mind states (ToM; intention to deceive, surprise, etc.), elicited activity in several regions, including the fusiform gyrus and STS, relative to a random motion condition. The same findings held, although to a weaker extent, when the ToM vignettes were contrasted to animations depicting only simple, goal-directed activity (dancing, chasing, etc.; see also, Castelli, Frith, Happé, & Frith, 2002). One limitation of this study was that both of the meaningful conditions (ToM and simple, goal-directed animations) concerned the same conceptual domain (human interaction). Greater activity was elicited for the more complex or higher-level concepts, relative to the simpler ones. Thus, it is possible that the activations reported by Castelli and colleagues reflected only general, problem-solving processes involved in interpreting moving visual forms, rather than being specific to ToM or social interaction.

In the current study we designed vignettes to elicit two different types of conceptual representations: social interaction and mechanical action. Further, both vignette types were preceded by the same, ambiguous cue ("What is it?" cf. Castelli et al., 2000). Based on the above discussion, we predicted that animations interpreted as social would engage regions previously found to be associated with animate objects (humans and animals), whereas mechanical interpretations would be associated with sites previously linked to perceiving and knowing about tools. Specifically, within posterior regions, vignettes interpreted as social would be associated with bilateral activity in the lateral fusiform gyrus and STS, relative to vignettes interpreted as mechanical. In contrast, vignettes interpreted as mechanical would show enhanced bilateral activity in the medial fusiform, and the left middle temporal gyri. In addition, based on investigations of social cognition (see Adolphs, 2001, for review), we also expected to find activity in the amygdala, medial prefrontal cortex, and related areas for the social vignettes.

# METHODS

## Subjects

Twelve strongly right-handed individuals participated in the fMRI study (six female, mean age = 27.5 years, range 23–34, mean verbal intelligence quotient (VIQ) as estimated by the National Adult Reading Test = 121, range 112–128). Informed consent was obtained in writing under an approved NIMH protocol. Prior to the imaging study, responses to the vignettes were collected from a different group of subjects ($N$ = 12, seven female). These subjects were instructed to generate a label describing the action depicted in each vignette. These labels and their associated response times, measured from the onset of the animation, were collected.

## Stimuli and design

The stimuli consisted of animations created using ElectricImage software and converted to Quicktime for subject presentation. An initial set of 24 vignettes each lasting 21 s were constructed using simple geometric shapes (circles, squares, triangles, etc.) to depict either social or mechanical action (12 social, 12 mechanical). Based on pilot testing to determine consistency of interpretation, this set of meaningful animations was reduced to 16 vignettes used in the fMRI experiment (8 of each type). Human activities depicted in the social vignettes included interactions set in the context of a baseball game, dancing, fishing, sharing, scaring, playing on a seesaw, playing on a slide, and swimming. Mechanical depictions included actions designed to represent the movement of inanimate objects in the context of billiards, bowling, pinball, a cannon, a crane, a steam shovel, a conveyor belt, and a paper shredder. In addition, two control conditions were created in which the same stimuli used in the meaningful vignettes were presented either in random motion (four blocks; two each using objects from the social or the mechanical vignettes), or as static images. For the still condition, a different static configuration of the geometric forms was presented every 4.2 s to maintain subjects' attention.

During each of eight fMRI runs, subjects viewed 10 stimulus blocks of 30 s. Each block began with a cue screen (3 s), followed by either a motion or still condition (21 s), and ended with a response screen (6 s). Subjects were cued with the written question "What is it?" prior to each of the meaningful vignettes, and with "Stare" prior to the random motion and still conditions. The use of the "Stare" cue was necessary because behavioural pilot testing indicated that when the random motion animations were preceded by "What is it?," subjects commonly applied meaningful interpretations to them, and often chose a meaningful verbal label to describe the action even when the response choices included "nonsense." Thus subjects were cued as to which animations were meaningless so as to prevent them from engaging in the interpretive stance that was the focus of this study.

The response screens for the meaningful vignettes contained four written choices arranged in the same spatial configuration as the buttons on the response key held in the subject's left hand. Subjects were instructed to determine what action was being depicted and indicate their choice when the response screen appeared. The four choices included one likely and two less likely interpretations, along with the correct answer. For example, for the vignette illustrated in Figure 1, the choices were "playing tag," "playing volley ball," "picking apples," and "sharing ice cream." For the random motion and still conditions subjects were instructed to press a single button as indicated by the spatial location of the word "press" on the response screen. The location was randomly varied for each presentation of this condition. Prior to scanning, subjects performed a practice run with sample animations that were not included in the experiment.

Four of the 10 blocks consisted of meaningful vignettes (two social, two mechanical). The remaining blocks consisted of the random motion and still control conditions. Each of the eight runs began and ended with a still condition. Motion conditions were presented in pseudorandom order, with alternating blocks of the meaningful and random motion control conditions. All vignettes were presented during the first 4 runs and repeated during runs 5–8 in order to ensure adequate statistical power.

## Imaging parameters

High-resolution spoiled gradient recall (SPGR) anatomical images (124 sagittal slices 1.2 mm thick,

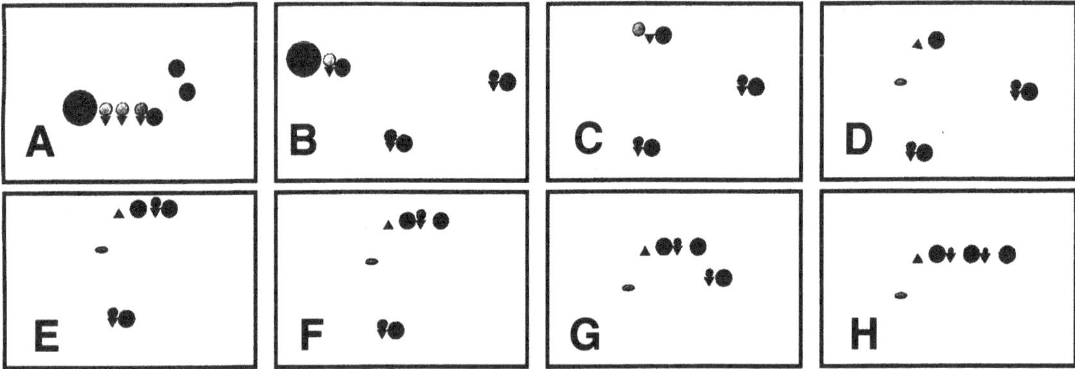


**Figure 1.** *Social vignette. Sample frames from a social vignette that elicited the concept of sharing. When viewing this animation, subjects interpreted the small purple circles as children receiving ice cream cones from a parent or adult figure (large blue circle) (panels A and B). In C and D, the first child drops her ice cream. In E and F, another child shares her ice cream with the first child. In G and H, the third child joins the other two and shares her ice cream, as well.*

field of view [FOV] = 24 cm, acquisition matrix = 256 × 256) and functional data (gradient-echo echo-planar imaging sequence, repetition time [TR] = 3 s, echo time [TE] = 40 ms, flip angle = 90°, 22 contiguous 5-mm axial slices, FOV = 24 cm, acquisition matrix = 64 × 64) were acquired on a 1.5 Tesla GE scanner.

### Image analysis

Functional images were motion corrected and a 1.2-voxel smoothing filter was applied to each scan. Regressors of interest for each of five stimulus types were convolved with a Gaussian estimate of the haemodynamic response and multiple regression was performed on each voxel's time series using AFNI v.2.40e (Cox, 1996). Individual subject Z-maps were normalised to the standardised space of Talairach and Tournoux (1988). Functional regions of interest (ROI) were determined in an unbiased manner by the group activation maps thresholded at $Z > 4.90$ ($p < 10^{-6}$) for the contrast of meaningful versus random motion conditions, and $Z > 3.09$ ($p < .001$) for the contrast of social versus mechanical vignettes. Regions discussed in this report include all those identified by this analysis except for regions in lateral prefrontal and medial parietal cortices, for which we had no a priori hypotheses. These ROIs served as a guide to extract MR time series and local maxima from each region in each subject. Time series data were obtained from voxels that exceeded a threshold of $Z > 3.09$ ($p < .001$) for meaningful versus random motion conditions, and $Z > 1.96$ ($p < .05$) for the contrast of social versus mechanical vignettes. The first three and last two time-points from each block (which represent the cue plus two TRs, and the response screen, respectively) were dropped from the time-series analysis. Beta weights resulting from a multiple regression analysis derived from the individual subject time series were submitted to a mixed effects analysis of variance, treating subjects as a random factor, to test for differences between conditions (social, mechanical, social control, mechanical control, stills).

## RESULTS

### Behavioural data

Subjects who viewed the vignettes outside the magnet were slower to spontaneously generate correct verbal labels for the social compared to the mechanical vignettes (means = 9.6 s and 6.6 s, respectively, $p < .001$). They were also slightly less accurate. Statistical comparison of the accuracy data was not valid because of ceiling effects. (The majority of the animations—four social, six mechanical—were correctly labeled spontaneously by all 12 subjects. During scanning, subjects' response choices were highly accurate: (> 97 % for both social and mechanical vignettes.)

### Imaging data

Direct comparison of the social and mechanical vignettes revealed different and highly selective patterns of activity in a number of regions (Table 1). These differences were confirmed by the mixed-effects ANOVA of the time-series data, which also revealed differences between other conditions. In ventral temporal cortex, vignettes interpreted as social elicited greater bilateral activity in the lateral portion of the fusiform gyrus, relative to mechanical vignettes, $F = 6.37$, $p < .05$ (Figure 2A). Moreover, in this region, activity associated with interpreting the mechanical animations was no greater than when subjects viewed these same objects, but were aware that their motion was random and meaningless, $F = 1.79$, $p > .10$ (Figure 2B). In contrast, vignettes interpreted as mechanical showed greater bilateral activity in the medial portion of the fusiform gyrus, relative to social animations, $F = 19.58$; $p < .001$ (Figure 2A). Here, activity associated with interpreting social animations was no greater than when viewing the random motion control condition composed of the same elements, $F < 1.0$ (Figure 2C). Both lateral and medial fusiform activations were bilateral, and, for the lateral fusiform, larger in the right than in the left hemisphere, $t(11) = 3.23$, $p < .01$.

**Table 1.** *Local maxima and Z values for each region based on the group data*

| *Region* | *Z value* | *X* | *Y* | *Z* |
|---|---|---|---|---|
| *Social > Mechanical* | | | | |
| L fusiform gyrus (lateral) | 3.95 | −44 | −57 | −23 |
| | 3.57 | −40 | −38 | −20 |
| R fusiform gyrus (lateral) | 4.49 | 41 | −52 | −15 |
| | 3.37 | 40 | −33 | −21 |
| R superior temporal sulcus | >7.0 | 56 | −58 | 19 |
| L superior temporal sulcus | >7.0 | −49 | −57 | 17 |
| R anterior STS | >7.0 | 53 | −20 | −4 |
| L anterior STS | 5.14 | −56 | −21 | 0 |
| R amygdala | 5.14 | 19 | −2 | −10 |
| R ventromedial prefrontal cortex | 3.76 | 3 | 52 | −11 |
| | 5.12 | 1 | 43 | −13 |
| *Mechanical > Social* | | | | |
| L fusiform gyrus (medial) | 4.22 | −25 | −44 | −18 |
| R fusiform gyrus (medial) | 6.95 | 27 | −57 | −16 |
| L middle temporal gyrus | 3.05 | −49 | −56 | −9 |
| | 3.16 | −34 | −58 | −7 |
| *Social = Mechanical* | | | | |
| *Meaningful > Random* | | | | |
| L polar frontal cortex | >7.0 | −28 | 40 | 37 |
| R polar frontal cortex | >7.0 | 35 | 50 | 27 |
| R anterior temporal cortex | >7.0 | 42 | −10 | 26 |

Vignettes interpreted as social or mechanical also produced differential activity along the lateral surface of posterior temporal cortex (Table 1). Relative to the mechanical vignettes, activity associated with interpreting the social vignettes was centred on the posterior region of STS, bilaterally: $F = 113.49$; $p < .0001$, and $F = 64.35$, $p < .001$ in the left and right STS, respectively (Figure 2D). The activity was bilateral but larger in the right than in the left hemisphere, $t(11) = 7.24$, $p < .0001$. Activity was particularly selective in right STS, where the haemodynamic response associated with the mechanical animations and its random motion control condition did not differ, $F = 1.52$, $p > 0.1$ (Figure 2E). In contrast, relative to the social animations, mechanical animations elicited greater activity in the left middle temporal gyrus, extending into the inferior temporal sulcus, $F = 24.89$, $p < .0001$. In this region, interpreting the social animations produced no more activity than its random motion control, $F < 1.0$ (Figure 2F).

Viewing and interpreting the social vignettes were also associated with activity in several other regions. These included a more anterior region of STS (bilaterally), the right amygdala, and right ventromedial prefrontal cortex (Table 1). Each of these areas showed an enhanced response when interpreting social relative to mechanical animations: left anterior STS, $F = 15.16$, $p < .001$; right anterior STS, $F = 48.85$, $p < .0001$; right amygdala, $F = 14.83$, $p < .001$; right ventromedial prefrontal cortex, $F = 8.71$, $p < .01$. In all regions, activity for mechanical vignettes did not exceed its control condition (Figure 3).

Finally, two other regions were identified where activity was strongly enhanced when subjects interpreted the meaningful vignettes, but failed to show differential activity for one type of meaningful vignette versus the other. These activations were located bilaterally in polar prefrontal cortex and in the anterior region of the right temporal lobe (Table 1).

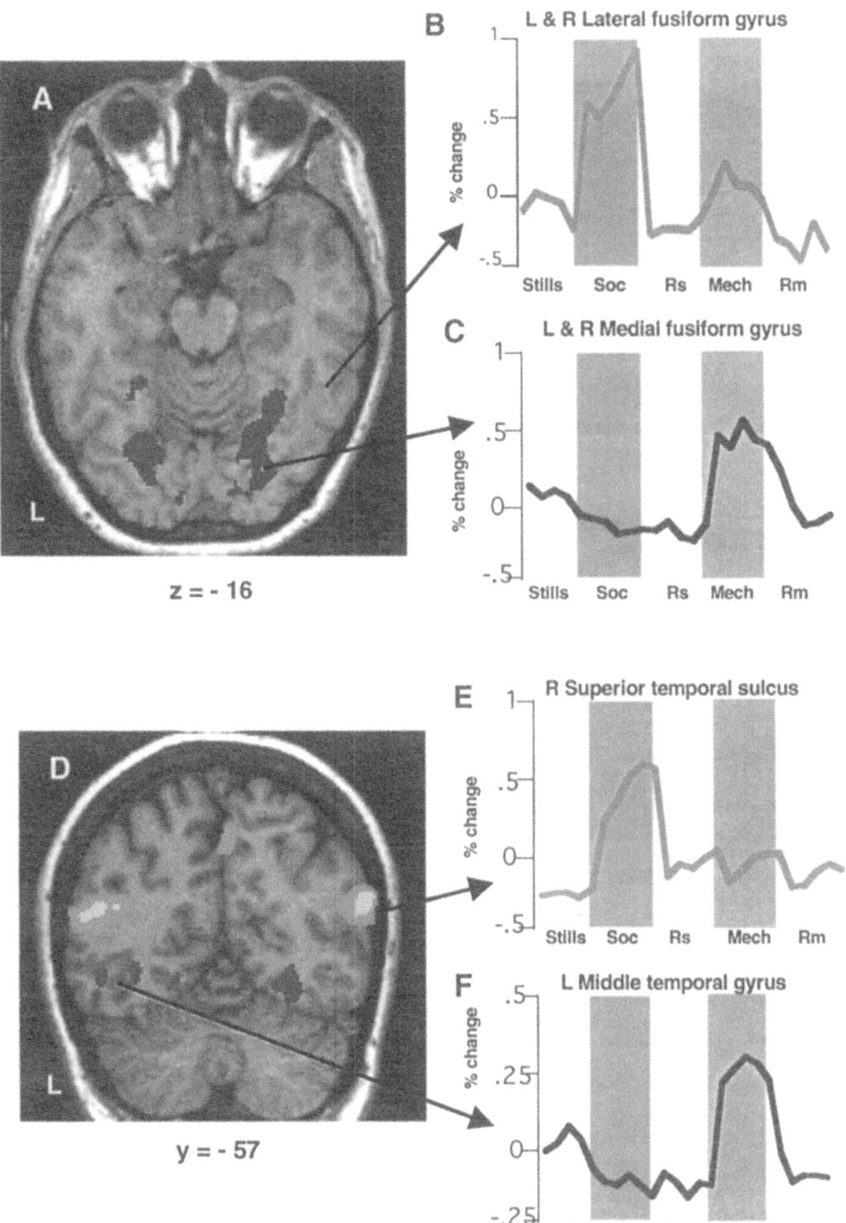


Figure 2. *Activations in posterior occipitotemporal cortex. Group averaged activity superimposed on a brain slice from an individual subject. Shown in colour are regions that responded more to meaningful than to random motion conditions. Regions in red were more active for social than mechanical vignettes, regions in blue were more active for mechanical than social vignettes. (A) Axial view at the Talairach and Tournoux coordinate of z = −16 showing differential activity in ventral occipitotemporal regions. Haemodynamic responses of voxels within lateral (B) and medial (C) fusiform gyrus that also showed enhanced activity to moving versus still geometric forms. These time series, as well as all others included in the figures, were averaged across subjects. (D) Coronal section at y = −57 showing activated regions in lateral temporal cortex. Haemodynamic response from voxels in the right STS (E) and left middle temporal gyrus/inferior temporal sulcus (F). Soc = social vignettes, Mech = mechanical vignettes, Rs and Rm = random control conditions for social and mechanical vignettes, respectively.*

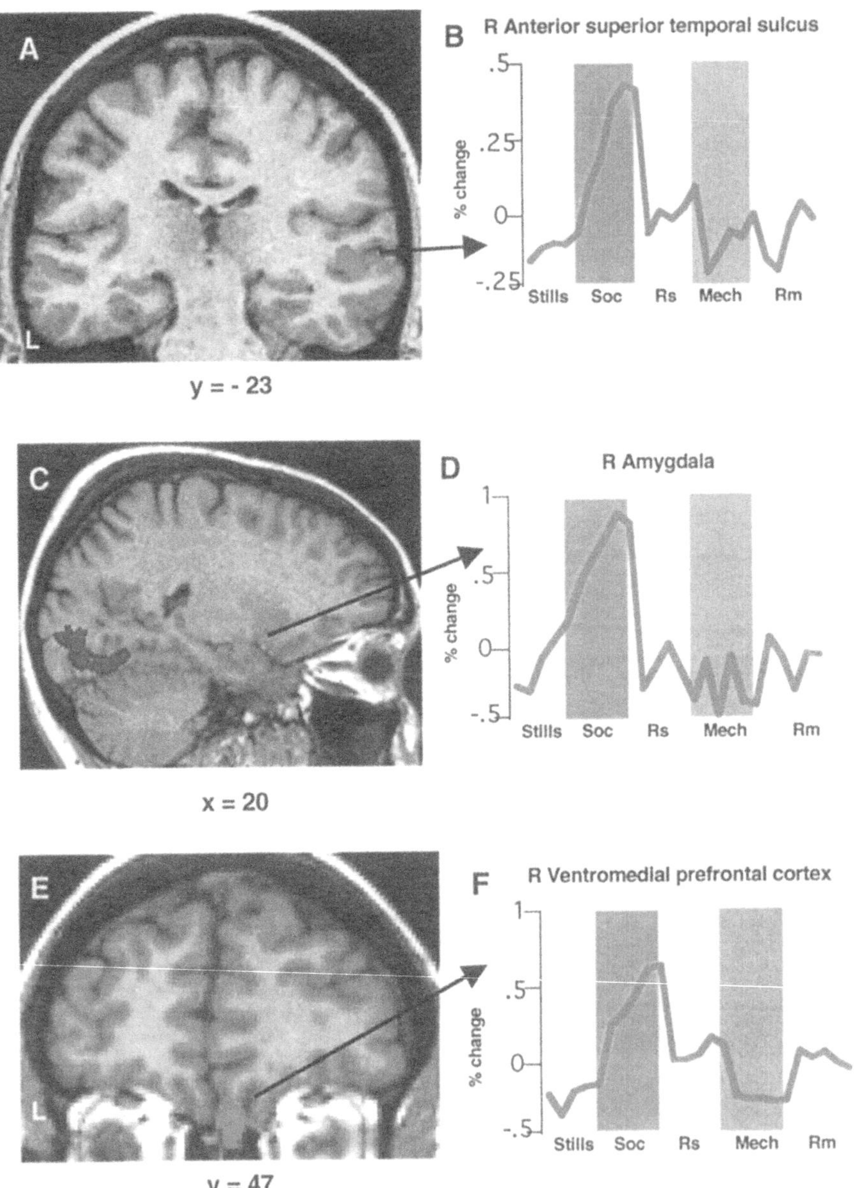


Figure 3. *Activations in right anterior STS, amygdala, and ventral prefrontal cortices. As in Figure 2: Coronal section (A) at y = −23 and haemodynamic response in region of anterior STS (B) responding more to social than mechanical vignettes. Sagittal section (C) at x = 20 and haemodynamic response (D) of right amygdala region responding more to social than mechanical vignettes. Coronal section (E) at y = 47 and haemodynamic response (F) in right ventromedial prefrontal region responding more to social than mechanical vignettes.*

## DISCUSSION

As predicted, social and mechanical vignettes showed differential activity in both the ventral and lateral regions of posterior temporal cortex. In addition, these regions showed highly specific patterns of response. In regions showing enhanced activity to social versus mechanical vignettes, the activity associated with interpreting the mechanical vignettes did not differ from the activity associated with viewing objects in random motion. Similarly, in mechanical-responsive regions, activity associated with interpreting the social vignettes did not differ from its random motion control condition.

Moreover, the regions showing differential activity were highly similar to those previously linked to viewing faces, human figures, and naming animals (lateral region of the fusiform gyrus, STS) and those linked to naming tools (medial fusiform gyrus, middle temporal gyrus). There is considerable evidence from studies of human and nonhuman primates that ventral and lateral occipitotemporal regions subserve different functions in object identification. Whereas lateral temporal cortex is primarily involved in processing object motion, ventral temporal cortex is primarily concerned with form-related features like shape and colour (for review, see Desimone & Ungerleider, 1989). However, in the present study the objects used for both the social and mechanical vignettes differed in neither shape nor colour. Thus, the central determinant of the location of these activations must have been the semantic interpretation given to these moving objects, not their physical characteristics (shape and colour).

The social, compared to the mechanical, vignettes also elicited activity in a more anterior region of STS, the amygdala, and ventromedial prefrontal cortex. As with regions identified in ventral and lateral aspects of posterior cortex, the responses were highly selective. Converging evidence from animal, human neuropsychological, and functional imaging studies of normal individuals has established that these regions form a network involved in perceiving and regulating emotion, social communication, and social decision making. Anterior STS has been implicated in the perception of complex mouth and hand movements and gestures (for review, see Allison, Puce, & McCarthy, 2000). Amygdala activity has been repeatedly shown to be modulated by attributes of human faces related to expression, especially emotions such as fear (for review, see Adolphs, 2002), but also by other emotional expressions and attributions (e.g., happiness, Breiter et al., 1996; trustworthiness, Winston, Strange, O'Doherty, & Dolan, 2002). It has also been shown that damage to the amygdala can impair identification of facial affect (e.g., Adolphs, Tranel, Damasio, & Damasio, 1994), and that the amygdala may be especially important for recognising "social" emotions such as guilt and arrogance relative to more basic emotions such as happiness and sadness (Adolphs, Baron-Cohen, & Tranel, 2002; see also Adolphs, Tranel, & Damasio, 1998). Affectively loaded verbal material can also activate the amygdala, highlighting that the response of this region is not limited to faces or other nonverbal, pictorial stimuli (Isenberg et al., 1999). In the current study, the activity was located in the dorsal portion of the amygdala, consistent with previous studies using positively valenced stimuli (for review, see Davis & Whalen, 2001). Activation of the dorsal portion of the amygdala in response to the social vignettes is also consistent with the proposal that this region plays a role in resolving ambiguity for biological relevant stimuli (Whalen, 1998). Ventromedial prefrontal cortex, a region strongly connected with the amygdala (e.g., Stefanacci & Amaral, 2002), was also selectively active during interpretation of social, relative to mechanical, vignettes. Damage to ventromedial prefrontal cortex has been associated with impaired social functioning and deficits in properly interpreting stimulus reward value as a guide to behavioural control (Bechara, Damasio, Tranel, & Damasio, 1997).

The present findings extend these previous reports by showing that the amygdala, ventromedial prefrontal cortex, as well as the anterior region of STS can be activated by stimuli that, in and of themselves, have neither affective valence nor social significance.[1] They are also highly consistent with the previous study by Castelli and colleagues (2000). In their study, the ToM animations elicited bilateral activity in the posterior fusiform gyrus, STS, and the amygdala region, stronger in the right than in the left hemisphere. Medial prefrontal activity was also observed, although in a more dorsal region compared to the present investigation. The close correspondence between our findings and those of Castelli and colleagues, using a different set of animations, instils confidence that these regions are part of a network associated with, if not directly mediating, social knowledge. Further, these studies suggest that activity in this network is associated with conceptual representations, not simply the physical characteristics of the stimuli evoking the concept.

The fact that the moving stimuli used in the social and mechanical vignettes did not differ in either their physical form or affective valence suggests that the activations discussed here are likely to result from top-down activity originating elsewhere. Candidate regions identified in this study that were equally active for both social and mechanical animations included the anterior region of the right temporal lobe and bilateral regions of polar prefrontal cortex. Previous studies of brain-injured patients and fMRI studies of normal individuals have implicated these regions in the representation and retrieval of nonverbal information (Simons, Graham, Galton, Patterson, & Hodges, 2001) as well as in reasoning and problem solving (Koechlin, Basso, Pietrini, Panzer, & Grafman, 1999).

These findings provide compelling evidence that reasoning about social events requires activation of a distributed system that includes regions involved in perceiving and knowing about specific objects (animate beings) and emotional states. Importantly, this system is separate and distinct from at least one other cognitive domain—mechanical knowledge. Our findings suggest that the major components of this social processing system are the ventral (lateral fusiform) and lateral (STS) regions of posterior temporal cortex, the amygdala, and the ventromedial region of prefrontal cortex. These findings are broadly consistent with the regions identified by studies of nonhuman primates as candidate areas for a network mediating social understanding (Brothers, 1990). They are also highly consistent with a growing body of evidence on the neural substrate of social cognition in humans (e.g., Adolphs, 2001).

In one view, this network may, in total or in part, form a "core system" for understanding social interaction (Brothers, 1990; Frith & Frith, 1999, 2001) and animate concepts (Caramazza & Shelton, 1998). This core system may have evolved as a direct result of evolutionary pressure for a system specialised for perceiving and knowing about animacy, causality, deception, and the like. Alternatively, this system may have developed from a more general learning capacity interacting with predetermined mechanisms for perceiving and learning about object features (how they look, how they move), and their affective valence (Martin, 1998).

Thus, within this view, higher-order concepts emerge from the interaction of more elemental processing capacities (U. Frith & Frith, 2001; Martin, 1998), rather than as a manifestation of innately determined conceptual domains (Caramazza & Shelton, 1998). For example, in the context of the current study the concept "animate" may be represented by information about human form (stored in the lateral portion of the fusiform gyrus), biological motion (stored in STS), and affect (mediated by the amygdala and ventromedial

[1] Although the stimuli were neutral, several of the social vignettes were perceived as having an affective component; and in particular, as being humorous. Thus the extent to which right amygdala and ventromedial prefrontal activity were related to this affective response was unclear. To examine this issue we compared activity for the four social vignettes judged to be most affectively loaded relative to the remaining four social animations (as determined by five independent raters). This analysis revealed that activity in ventromedial prefrontal cortex, but not in the amygdala, was influenced by perceived affect. Interestingly, the region identified by this analysis (1, 53, −12) was nearly identical to the region previously shown to be correlated with humour ratings of aurally presented jokes (3, 48, −12; Goel & Dolan, 2001). Whether ventromedial prefrontal cortex is activated by any humorous or rewarding stimulus, or only those of a social nature, remains to be determined.

prefrontal cortex). Combined activity in these regions (and perhaps others) is the neural correlate of the concept "animate". Similarly, the concept "mechanical" may be represented, at least in part, by information about the form of machine-like objects (stored in the medial fusiform gyrus), and information about their characteristic motion (stored in the left middle temporal gyrus).[2]

It is possible, however, that these activations are simply epiphenomenal, rather than causal. For example, they may have occurred as a by-product of visual imagery processes associated with interpreting the moving geometric forms. In fact, the lateral fusiform gyrus can be activated by asking subjects to imagine human faces (Ishai, Ungerleider, & Haxby, 2000; O'Craven & Kanwisher, 2000). However, studies of patients suggest that normal function of at least some of these regions may be necessary for understanding of social events. For example, impaired performance on ToM tasks has been demonstrated in patients with damage to the amygdala (Fine, Lumsden, & Blair, 2001; Stone, Baron-Cohen, Calder, Keane, & Young, 2003), and to right ventromedial prefrontal cortex (Stuss, Gallup, & Alexander, 2001). As with the neuroimaging data, the patient data suggest a stronger role for the right than the left hemisphere in mediating understanding of social concepts (Happé, Brownell, & Winner, 1999). It has also been shown that recognition and retrieval of information about tools can be disrupted by a lesion of the posterior middle temporal gyrus (Tranel, Damasio, & Damasio, 1997). Whether these patients also have a more general impairment in understanding mechanical concepts requires further investigation.

Finally, it must be noted that the true nature of the processing characteristics and type of information stored in the different brain regions discussed in this report remain to be determined. For example, the existing evidence strongly indicate that ventral and lateral regions of posterior cortex subserve processing and storage of object form and motion information, respectively. The data also strongly suggest that neither of these regions are homogeneous, but rather have an intrinsic organisation. Moreover, it *appears* that each region may be organised by conceptual category. It remains to be determined whether this category-like organisation can be further reduced to an organisation by properties of form (for ventral cortex) and motion (for lateral cortex) shared by category members, or whether this organisation is dictated by innately determined conceptual domains (Caramazza & Shelton, 1998). A model incorporating both types of organizational schemes (by properties and domains) would be an attractive alternative.

## CONCLUSION

Interpreting the movement of simple geometric shapes was associated with distinct neural systems depending on whether they were interpreted as depicting social or mechanical events. The active regions included those previously associated with animate objects (for the social vignettes) and tools (for the mechanical vignettes). Understanding social interactions was also associated with activity in regions linked to the perception and regulation of affect. It was suggested that these findings reveal putative "core systems" for social and mechanical understanding that are divisible into constituent parts or elements with distinct processing and storage capabilities. These elements may be viewed as semantic primitives that, in turn, form the foundation or scaffolding for realising a variety of complex mental constructs.

[2] Naming tools also activates the left intraparietal sulcus and ventral premotor cortex (e.g., Chao & Martin, 2000). These regions are associated with grasping, and object manipulation, suggesting that information about motor movements associated with the use of objects is stored here (Martin, 2001). In the current study, these areas were not differentially activated by the mechanical animations, nor were they expected to be. The mechanical vignettes did not depict small manipulable tool-like objects. Rather they evoked more machine-like actions (e.g., conveyor belt, paper shredder, cannon).

## REFERENCES


Adolphs, R. (2001). The neurobiology of social cognition. *Current Opinion in Neurobiology, 11*, 231–239.

Adolphs, R. (2002). Recognizing emotion from facial expressions: Psychological and neurological mechanisms. *Behavioral and Cognitive Neuroscience Reviews, 1*, 21–62.

Adolphs, R., Baron-Cohen, S., & Tranel, D. (2002). Impaired recognition of social emotions following amygdala damage. *Journal of Cognitive Neuroscience, 14*, 1264–1274.

Adolphs, R., Tranel, D., & Damasio, A. R. (1998). The human amygdala in social judgment. *Nature, 393*, 470–474.

Adolphs, R., Tranel, D., Damasio, H., & Damasio, A. R. (1994). Impaired recognition of emotion in facial expressions following damage to the human amygdala. *Nature, 372*, 669–672.

Allison, T., Puce, A., & McCarthy, G. (2000). Social perception from visual cues: Role of the STS region. *Trends in Cognitive Science, 4*, 267–278.

Beauchamp, M. S., Lee, K. E., Haxby, J. V., & Martin, A. (2002). Parallel visual motion processing streams for manipulable objects and human movements. *Neuron, 34*, 149–159.

Bechara, A., Damasio, H., Tranel, D., & Damasio, A. R. (1997). Deciding advantageously before knowing the advantageous strategy. *Science, 275*, 1293–1295.

Breiter, H. C., Etcoff, N. L., Whalen, P. J., Kennedy, W. A., Rauch, S. L., Buckner, R. L., Strauss, M. M., Hyman, S. E., & Rosen, B. R. (1996). Response and habituation of the human amygdala during visual processing of facial expression. *Neuron, 17*, 875–887.

Brothers, L. (1990). The social brain: A project for integrating primate behavior and neurophysiology in a new domain. *Concepts in Neuroscience, 1*, 27–51.

Caramazza, A., & Shelton, J. R. (1998). Domain-specific knowledge systems in the brain: The animate-inanimate distinction. *Journal of Cognitive Neuroscience, 10*, 1–34.

Castelli, F., Frith, C., Happé, F., & Frith, U. (2002). Autism, Asperger syndrome and brain mechanisms for the attribution of mental states to animated shapes. *Brain, 125*, 1839–1849.

Castelli, F., Happé, F., Frith, U., & Frith, C. (2000). Movement and mind: A functional imaging study of perception and interpretation of complex intentional movement patterns. *NeuroImage, 12*, 314–325.

Chao, L. L., & Martin, A. (2000). Representation of manipulable man-made objects in the dorsal stream. *NeuroImage, 12*, 478–484.

Chao, L. L., Haxby, J. V., & Martin, A. (1999). Attribute-based neural substrates in temporal cortex for perceiving and knowing about objects. *Nature Neuroscience, 2*, 913–919.

Cox, R. W. (1996). AFNI: Software for analysis and visualization of functional magnetic resonance neuroimages. *Computers and Biomedical Research, 29*, 162–173.

Davis, M., & Whalen, P. J. (2001). The amygdala: Vigilance and emotion. *Molecular Psychiatry, 6*, 13–34.

Desimone, R., & Ungerleider, L G. (1989). Neural mechanisms of visual processing in monkeys. In F. Boller & J. Grafman (Eds.), *Handbook of neuropsychology, Vol. 2* (pp. 267–299). Amsterdam: Elsevier.

Fine, C., Lumsden, J., & Blair, R. J. R. (2001). Dissociation between "theory of mind" and executive functions in a patient with early left amygdala damage. *Brain, 124*, 287–298.

Frith, C. D., & Frith, U. (1999). Interacting minds: A biological basis. *Science, 286*, 1692–1695.

Frith, U., & Frith, C. (2001). The biological basis of social interaction. *Current Directions in Psychological Science, 10*, 151–155.

Goel, V., & Dolan, R. J. (2001). The functional neuroanatomy of humor: Segregating cognitive and affective components. *Nature Neuroscience, 4*, 237–238.

Happé, F., Brownell, H., & Winner, E. (1999). Acquired "theory of mind" impairments following stroke. *Cognition, 70*, 211–240.

Haxby, J. V., Ungerleider, L. G., Clark, V. P., Shouten, J. L., Hoffman, E. A., & Martin, A. (1999). The effect of face inversion on activity in human neural systems for face and object perception. *Neuron, 22*, 189–199.

Heider, F., & Simmel, M. (1944). An experimental study of apparent behavior. *American Journal of Psychology, 57*, 243–249.

Isenberg, N., Silbersweig, D., Engelien, A., Emmerich, S., Malavade, K., Beattie, B., & Leon, A. C. (1999). Linguistic threat activates human amygdala. *Proceedings of the National Academy of Science, 96*, 10456–10459.

Ishai, A., Ungerleider, L. G., & Haxby, J. V. (2000). Distributed neural systems for the generation of visual images. *Neuron, 28*, 979–990.

Ishai, A., Ungerleider, L. G., Martin, A., Shouten, J. L., & Haxby, J. V. (1999). Distributed representation of objects in the ventral visual pathway. *Proceedings of the National Academy of Sciences, USA, 96*, 9379–9384.

Josephs, J. E. (2001). Functional neuroimaging studies of category specificity in object recognition: A critical review and meta-analysis. *Cognitive, Affective, and Behavioral Neuroscience, 1*, 119–136.

Kanwisher, N., McDermott, J., & Chun, M. M. (1997). The fusiform face area: A module in human extrastriate cortex specialized for the perception of faces. *Journal of Neuroscience, 17*, 4302–4311.

Koechlin, E., Basso, G., Pietrini, P., Panzer, S., & Grafman, J. (1999). The role of the anterior prefrontal cortex in human cognition. *Nature, 399*, 148–151.

Martin, A. (1998). The organization of semantic knowledge and the origin of words in the brain. In N. G. Jablonski & L. C. Aiello (Eds.), *The origins and diversification of language* (pp. 69–88). San Francisco, CA: California Academy of Sciences.

Martin, A. (2001). Functional neuroimaging of semantic memory. In R. Cabeza & A. Kingstone (Eds.), *Handbook of functional neuroimaging of cognition* (pp. 153–186). Cambridge, MA: MIT Press.

Martin, A., & Chao, L. L. (2001). Semantic memory and the brain: Structure and processes. *Current Opinion in Neurobiology, 11*, 194–201.

Moore, C. J., & Price, C. J. (1999). A functional neuroimaging study of the variables that generate category-specific object processing differences. *Brain, 112*, 943–962.

O'Craven, K. M., & Kanwisher, N. (2000). Mental imagery of faces and places activates corresponding stimulus-specific brain regions. *Journal of Cognitive Neuroscience, 12*, 1013–1023.

Oram, M. W., & Perrett, D. I. (1994). Responses of anterior superior temporal polysensory (STPa) neurons to "biological motion" stimuli. *Journal of Cognitive Neuroscience, 6*, 99–116.

Puce, A., Allison, T., Bentin, S., Gore, J. C., & McCarthy, G. (1998). Temporal cortex activation in humans viewing eye and mouth movements. *Journal of Neuroscience, 18*, 2188–2199.

Scholl, B. J., & Tremoulet, P. D. (2000). Perceptual causality and animacy. *Trends in Cognitive Science, 8*, 299–309.

Simons, J. S., Graham, K. S., Galton, C. J., Patterson, K., & Hodges, J. R. (2001). Semantic knowledge and episodic memory for faces in semantic dementia. *Neuropsychology, 15*, 101–114.

Stefanacci, L., & Amaral, D. G. (2002). Some observations on cortical inputs to the macaque monkey amygdala: An anterograde tracing study. *Journal of Comparative Neurology, 451*, 301–323.

Stone, V. E., Baron-Cohen, S., Calder, A., Keane, J., & Young, A. (2003). Acquired theory of mind impairments in individuals with bilateral amygdala lesions. *Neuropsychologia, 41*, 209–220.

Stuss, D. T., Gallup, G. G., & Alexander, M. P. (2001). The frontal lobes are necessary for "theory of mind". *Brain, 124*, 279–286.

Talairach, J., & Tournoux, P. (1988). *Co-planar stereotatic atlas of the human brain.* New York: Thieme.

Thompson-Schill, S. L. (2002). Neuroimaging studies of semantic memory: Inferring "how" from "where". *Neuropsychologia, 41*, 280–292.

Tranel, D., Damasio, H., & Damasio, A. R. (1997). A neural basis for the retrieval of conceptual knowledge. *Neuropsychologia, 35*, 1319–1328.

Whalen, P. J. (1998). Fear, vigilance, and ambiguity: Initial neuroimaging of the human amygdala. *Current Directions in Psychological Science, 7*, 177–188.

Winston, J. S., Strange, B. A., O'Doherty, J., & Dolan, R. J. (2002). Automatic and intentional brain responses during evaluation of trustworthiness of faces. *Nature Neuroscience, 5*, 277–283.

COGNITIVE NEUROPSYCHOLOGY, 2003, 20 (3/4/5/6), 588–592

# SUBJECT INDEX






http://www.tandf.co.uk/journals/pp/02643294.html